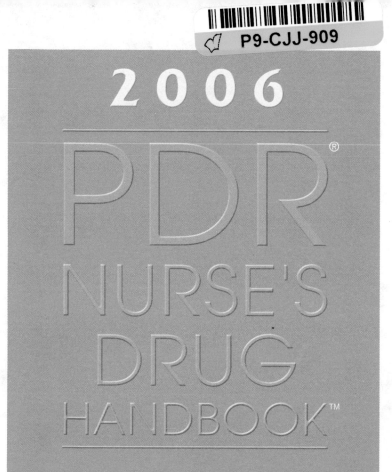

2006

PDR®
NURSE'S
DRUG
HANDBOOK™

CARDIOVASCULAR
EDITION

George R. Spratto • Adrienne L. Woods

2006

PDR®
NURSE'S
DRUG
HANDBOOK™

CARDIOVASCULAR EDITION

George R. Spratto, PhD
Dean and Professor of Pharmacology,
School of Pharmacy
West Virginia University
Morgantown, West Virginia

Adrienne L. Woods, MSN, ARNP, NP-C
Nurse Practioner
Primary Care at the
Department of Veterans Affairs Medical
and Regional Office Center,
Wilmington, Delaware

THOMSON

DELMAR LEARNING

2006 Edition PDR® Nurse's Drug Handbook™
Cardiovascular Edition
by
George R. Spratto, PhD and Adrienne L. Woods, MSN, ARNP, NP-C

Vice President,
Health Care Business Unit:
William Brottmiller

Editorial Director:
Cathy L. Esperti

Executive Editor:
Matthew Kane

Developmental Editor:
Maria D'Angelico

Editorial Assistant:
Michelle Leavitt

Marketing Director:
Jennifer McAvey

Marketing Channel Manager:
Heather Sisley

Marketing Coordinator:
Michele Gleason

Database Program Manager:
Linda Helfrich

Technology Director:
Laurie Davis

Technology Project Manager:
Mary Colleen Liburdi

Production Director:
Carolyn Miller

Production Editor:
Jack Pendleton

THOMSON

PDR

Executive Vice President:
Kevin Sanborn

Vice President, Product
Management:
William T. Hicks

Senior Director, Brand and Product
Management:
Valerie E. Berger

Director, Product Management:
Swan Oey

Director, Product Management/
Clinical Liaison:
Thomas Fleming, PharmD

Vice President, PDR Services:
Brian Holland

Director of Operations:
Robert Klein

Director, Editorial Services:
Bette LaGow

Manager, Professional Services:
Michael DeLuca, PharmD

Drug Information Specialists:
Majid Kerolous, PharmD;
Nermin Shenouda, PharmD;
Greg Tallis, RPh

Production Design Supervisor:
Adeline Rich

Production Specialist:
Christina Klinger

Project Manager:
Donald Pond

Table of Contents

Notice to the Reader

The monographs in this edition of the PDR™ Nurse's Drug Handbook™ Cardiovascular Edition are the work of two distinguished authors: George R. Spratto, PhD, Dean and Professor of Pharmacology of the School of Pharmacy at West Virginia University, Morgantown, West Virginia, and Adrienne L. Woods, MSN, ARNP, NP-C, Nurse Practitioner, Primary Care, at the Department of Veterans Affairs Medical and Regional Office Center, Wilmington, Delaware.

The publisher and the authors do not warrant or guarantee any of the products described herein or perform any independent analysis in connection with any of the product information contained herein. The publisher and the authors do not assume and expressly disclaim any obligation to obtain and include information other than that provided by the manufacturer.

The reader is expressly warned to consider and adopt all safety precautions that might be indicated by the activities described herein and to avoid all potential hazards. By following the instructions contained herein, the reader willingly assumes all risks in connection with such instructions.

The publisher and the authors make no representations or warranties of any kind, including but not limited to the warranties of fitness for a particular purpose or merchantability nor are any such representations implied with respect to the material set forth herein, and the publisher and the authors take no responsibility with respect to such material. The publisher and the authors shall not be liable for any special, consequential, or exemplary damages resulting, in whole or in part, from the reader's use of, or reliance upon, this material.

The authors and publisher have made a conscientious effort to ensure that the drug information and recommended dosages in this book and companion website are accurate and in accord with accepted standards at the time of publication. However, pharmacology and therapeutics are rapidly changing sciences, so readers are advised, before administering any drug, to check the package insert provided by the manufacturer for the recommended dose, for any contraindications for administration, and for any added warnings and precautions. This recommendation is especially important for new, infrequently used, or highly toxic drugs.

Preface

The PDR® Nurse's Drug Handbook™ is a trusted resource used by nursing students, practicing nurses, and other health care professionals. This special Cardiovascular Edition focuses specifically on drugs used to treat cardiovascular conditions. Drug information changes rapidly, including the development of new drugs, new uses for established drugs, revised and new administration routes (dosage forms), newly identified side effects and drug interactions, and changes in dosing and use recommendations based on feedback from health care professionals, researchers, and consumers. Nurses and other health care professionals depend on the PDR Nurse's Drug Handbook to provide the latest information on drug therapy, guidelines for monitoring efficacy of the therapy, and recommendations for teaching the client and family about important aspects of the drug therapy.

ORGANIZATION OF CONTENT

This guide contains individual drug monographs in alphabetical order by generic name. The purpose and meaning of each of the components of a monograph are described under "Using the Drug Monographs". See also the "Quick Reference Guide to a Drug Monograph". Following this list of drugs is general information on important therapeutic or chemical classes of drugs. The classes are listed alphabetically. Consult the Table of Contents for a listing of the therapeutic/chemical classes included in this section. Each class begins with a list of drugs for which a monograph appears in Chapter 1. The information provided in the class applies to all drugs listed for the class. Information that is specific to one of the drugs listed is included in the drug monograph. For complete knowledge of a specific drug, consult the class information as well as the appropriate monograph.

The FDA has added a boxed warning to prescribing information for numerous drugs whose side effects can be life-threatening and in some cases have resulted in death. In this handbook, these "Black Box Warnings" are indicated by an icon ■ following the drug name and by the icon and highlighted content in the "Special Concerns" portion of the monograph. A key to all of the icons in the book is included later in this preface.

The **general index** found at the back of this book is extensively cross-referenced: each generic drug name entry includes the major trade name(s) entry in parentheses and each trade name entry is followed by the generic drug name in parentheses. Each page of the general index contains a key identifying boldface as the generic drug name, italics as the therapeutic drug class, regular type as the trade name, and capitals as the combination drug name.

USING THE DRUG MONOGRAPHS

The following components are described in the order in which they appear in the monographs. All components may not appear in each monograph but are represented where appropriate and when information is available. Refer also to the sample monograph with explanatory notes for the purpose and use of each component.

Drug Name: The generic drug name is the first item in the name block (in color at the beginning of each monograph). One or more icons may follow the drug name:

■   Black box to indicate that the FDA has issued a boxed warning about potentially life-threatening side effects

© Ear to indicate that sound-alike drug names are linked to medication errors

Phonetic Pronunciation: Pronunciation guide for generic name to assist in mastering often complex names.

Classification: Defines the type of drug or the class under which the drug is listed. A classification or descriptor is provided for each drug name. If the drug class is new and only a few drugs are available in the class at the time of printing the handbook, the classification will not appear in the class monographs at the end of the book. It will be added at a later date as more drugs in the class reach the market.

Pregnancy Category: Lists the FDA pregnancy category (A, B, C, D, or X) assigned to the drug.

Trade Name: Trade names are identified as Rx (prescription) or OTC (over the counter, no prescription required). If numerous forms of the drug are available, the trade names are identified by form. Trade names available only in Canada are identified by a maple leaf icon ✦.

Controlled Substance: If the drug is controlled under the U. S. Federal Controlled Substances Act, the schedule in which the drug is placed follows the trade name listing (C-I, C-II, C-III, C-IV, C-V).

Combination Drug: This heading at the top of the name block indicates that the drug is a combination of two or more drugs in the same product.

The following components may appear in the body of a drug monograph.

Cross Reference: "See also . . ." directs the reader to the classification entry that matches the classification of the drug being reviewed or to another drug. General information about the drugs in the class is provided in the class monographs at the end of the book.

General Statement: This appears in a few drug monographs but is more common in the class entries. Information about the drug class and/or anything specific or unusual about a group of drugs is presented. Information may also be presented about the disease(s) or condition(s) for which the drugs are indicated.

Content: For combination drugs, provides the generic name and amount of each drug in the combination product.

Action/Kinetics: The action portion describes the proposed mechanism(s) by which a drug achieves its therapeutic effect. Not all mechanisms of action are known, and some are self-evident, as when a hormone is administered as a replacement. The kinetics portion lists critical information, if known, about the rate of drug absorption, distribution, time for peak plasma levels or peak effect, minimum effective serum or plasma level, biological half-life, duration of action, metabolism, and excretion route(s). Metabolism and excretion routes may be important for clients with systemic liver disease, kidney disease, or both.

Many drugs, when metabolized, bind to plasma proteins. If a client is prescribed several drugs that bind to plasma proteins, there is the potential for increased, reduced or altered drug effects because of competition for binding sites. It may be necessary to change one or more of the drugs to improve the therapeutic action.

The half-life ($t\frac{1}{2}$) is the time required for half the drug to be removed from the blood, serum, or plasma. Half-life is important in determining how often a drug is to be administered and how long the client is to be assessed for side effects. Therapeutic levels indicate the desired concentration, in serum or plasma, for the drug to exert its beneficial effect and are helpful in predicting the onset of side effects or the lack of effect. Drug therapy is often monitored in this manner (e.g., antibiotics, theophylline, phenytoin, amiodarone).

Uses: Approved therapeutic uses for the drug are listed. Some investigational uses are also listed for selected drugs.

Contraindications: Disease states or conditions in which the drug should not be used are noted. The safe use of many of the newer pharmacologic agents during pregnancy, lactation, or childhood has not been established. As a general rule, the use of drugs during pregnancy is contraindicated unless the benefits of drug therapy are determined to far outweigh the potential risks.

Special Concerns: Covers considerations for use with pediatric, geriatric, pregnant, or lactating clients. Situations and disease states when the drug should be used with caution are also listed. Numerous drugs have life-threatening side effects that may lead to irreversible organ/system damage and possibly death. The FDA provides boxed warnings with the prescribing information for these drugs to alert health care professionals to the potential for serious side effects. A black box icon ■ and highlighted content in this section of the monograph draw attention to the warning information.

Side Effects: Undesired or bothersome effects the client may experience while taking a particular agent are described. Side effects are listed by the body organ or system affected, and are presented when possible with the most common side effects in descending order of incidence. Nearly all potential side effects are listed. In any given clinical situation, however, a client may experience no side effects, one or two side effects, or several side effects. If potentially life-threatening, the side effect is displayed in ***bold italic*** type.

OD **Overdose Management**: When appropriate, this section provides a list of the symptoms observed following an overdose or toxic reaction (Symptoms) as well as treatment approaches and/or antidotes for the overdose (Treatment).

Drug Interactions: Alphabetical listing of drugs and herbals that may interact with the drug under discussion. The study of drug interactions is an important area of pharmacology that changes constantly. Because of the significant increase in the use of herbal products, interactions of medications with herbals are included in this section if known or suspected. These interactions are designated by the icon H. The listing of drug/drug and drug/herbal interactions is far from complete; therefore, listings in this handbook are to be considered only as general cautionary guidelines.

Drug interactions may result from a number of different mechanisms: (1) additive or inhibitory effects; (2) increased or decreased metabolism of the drug; (3) increased or decreased rate of elimination; (4) decreased absorption from the GI tract; (5) competition for or displacement from receptor sites or plasma protein binding sites. Such interactions may manifest themselves in a variety of ways; however, an attempt has been made throughout the handbook to describe these interactions whenever possible as an increase ($\uparrow$) or a decrease ($\downarrow$) in the effect of the drug, and a reason for the change. It is important to realize that any side effects that accompany the administration of a particular agent may be increased as a result of a drug or herbal interaction. Drug/herbal interactions are often listed for classes of drugs.

Laboratory Test Considerations: The manner in which a drug may affect laboratory test values is presented. Some of the effects are caused by the therapeutic or toxic effects of the drugs; others result from interference with the testing method itself. The laboratory considerations are described as increased ($\uparrow$) or false positive (+) values and as decreased ($\downarrow$) or false negative (-) values. Also included, when available, are drug-induced changes in blood or urine levels of endogenous substances (e.g., glucose, electrolytes, and so on).

How Supplied: The various dosage forms available for the drug and amounts of the drug in each of the dosage forms is presented. Such information is important as one dosage form may be more appropriate for a client than another. This information also allows the user to ensure the appropriate dosage form and strength is being administered.

Dosage: The dosage form and route of administration is followed by the disease state or condition (in italics) for which the dosage is recommended. This is followed by the adult and pediatric doses, when available. The listed dosage is to be considered as a general guideline; the exact amount of the drug to be given is determined by the provider. However, one should question orders when dosages differ markedly from the accepted norm.

Nursing Considerations: The guidelines provided in this section are designed to help the practitioner in applying the nursing process to pharmacotherapeutics to ensure safe practice. When applicable this section begins with sound alike drug warnings denoted by an ear icon 👂. In each monograph the following sections are provided when applicable.

- *Administration/Storage*: Guidelines for preparing medications for administration, administering the medication, and storage and disposal of the medication. Guidelines for administration by IV are indicated by an icon IV.
- *Assessment*: Guidelines for monitoring/assessing client before, during, and after prescribed drug therapy.
- *Interventions*: Guidelines for specific nursing actions related to the drug being administered.
- *Client/Family Teaching*: Guidelines to promote education, active participation, understanding, and adherence to drug therapy by the client and/or care givers. Precautions about the drug therapy are also noted for communication to the client/care giver.
- *Outcomes/Evaluate*: Desired outcomes of the drug therapy and client response. These will help determine the effectiveness and positive therapeutic outcome of the prescribed drug therapy.

Notes on Assessment and Interventions. The following tasks are critical in assessing the client for drug therapy and for planning the interventions needed to undertake the therapy.

- Gather physical data and client history
- Assess specific physiologic functions likely to be affected by the drug therapy
- Determine specific laboratory tests needed to monitor the course of the drug therapy
- Identify sensitivities/interactions and conditions that may preclude a particular drug therapy
- Document specific indications for therapy and describe symptom characteristics related to this condition
- Know the physiologic, pharmacologic, and psychologic effects of the drug and how these may affect the client and impact the nursing process
- Know side effects that can arise as a result of drug therapy and be prepared with appropriate nursing interventions
- Monitor the client for side effects and document/report them to the provider. Severe side effects generally require dosage modification or discontinuation of the drug.
- Ensure client safety when receiving drug therapy

When taking the nursing history, place emphasis on the client's ability to read and to follow directions. Language barriers must be identified and appropriate written translations should be provided to promote adherence to the drug therapy. In addition, client lifestyle, culture, income, availability of health insurance, and access to transportation are important factors that may affect adherence with therapy and follow-up care.

The assessment should include the potential for the client being/becoming pregnant, and if a mother is breastfeeding her infant.

The age and orientation level of the client, whether learned from personal observation or from discussion with close friends or family members, can be critical in determining potential relationships between drug therapy and/or drug interactions.

Including these factors in the nursing assessment will assist all members of the health care team to determine the type of pharmacotherapy, drug delivery system, and monitoring and follow-up plan best suited to a particular client to promote the highest level of adherence.

Notes on Client/Family Teaching. Specific understandable information for the client is provided for each drug. Client/family teaching assists the client/family to recognize side effects and avoid potentially dangerous situations, and alleviates anxiety associated with starting and maintaining drug therapy.

Details on administration are included to enhance client understanding and adherence. Side effects that require medical intervention are included, as are recommendations for minimizing the side effects for certain medications (e.g., take medication with food to decrease GI upset, or take at bedtime to minimize daytime sedative effects).

The proper education of clients is one of the most challenging aspects of nursing. The instructions must be tailored to the needs, awareness, and sophistication of each client. For example, clients who take medication to lower blood pressure should assume responsibility for taking their own blood pressure or having it taken and recorded.

Clients should carry identification listing the drugs currently prescribed. They should know what they are taking and why, and develop a mechanism to remind themselves to take their medication as prescribed. Clients should always carry this drug list with them whenever they go for a checkup or seek medical care, and it should be updated by providers at each visit. The drug list may also be shared with the pharmacist if there is a question concerning drugs prescribed, if the client is considering taking an over-the-counter medication, or if the client has to change pharmacies.

The records, especially blood pressure readings, should be shared with the health care provider to ensure accurate evaluation of the response to the prescribed drug therapy. This may also alert the provider to any drug/food/herbal consumption by the client that they did not prescribe, were not aware of, or that may interfere with (i.e., potentiate or antagonize) the current pharmacologic regimen. The provider may also encourage the client to call with any questions or concerns about the drug therapy.

Remember: The components described previously are covered for all drugs or drug classes. When drugs are presented as a group the information for each component is given only once for the group. Check each component for information relevant to all drugs covered in the class. Note that many of the drug monographs are cross-referenced to the general class information in the back of the book. Critical information or information relevant to a specific drug is provided in the individual drug monograph under appropriate headings, such as Additional Contraindications or Additional Side Effects. These are **in addition to** and **not instead of** the class entry which is referenced and must be consulted.

Acknowledgments

We would like to extend our thanks and appreciation to the Thomson Delmar Learning team who works so diligently to ensure that the manuscript process flows smoothly and to keep us on the appropriate time schedule. Team members include Matthew Kane, Executive Editor; Maria D'Angelico, Developmental Editor; Linda Helfrich, Database Program Manager; Marjorie Bruce, Market Research Specialist; Jack Pendleton, Production Editor; and Michelle Leavitt, Editorial Assistant. A special note of thanks is extended to Marge Bruce who, over the years, has provided countless hours of service to the project and is always willing to assist, regardless of the issue or questions. She is an inspiration for us to keep going.

George Spratto extends appreciation to his colleagues at West Virginia University. Special thanks are extended to Dr. Matthew Blommel of the West Virginia Center for Drug and Health Information, West Virginia University and his students, who assisted in researching information on new and existing drugs. Greatest appreciation and love go to his wife, Lynne, sons, Chris and Gregg, daughters-in-law, Kim and Mary Alice, granddaughters, Alexandra and Victoria, and grandsons, Dominic and Patrick, all of whom make the work of this project worthwhile by their unfailing support and encouragement.

Adrienne Woods would like to extend her appreciation to her colleagues at the VA and to her husband, Howard. He is the best father, and friend, she has ever known, and she thanks him for all his patience, caring, love, and understanding. To her children, Katy and Nate, she extends thanks for enduring hectic schedules, dirty/lost uniforms, and a few missed soccer, baseball, hockey, wrestling and lacrosse games. Finally, thanks to Fudge, her German short hair pointer, and Oreo, their kitty, for their patience and undying affection.

QUICK REFERENCE GUIDE TO A DRUG MONOGRAPH

Here is a quick guide to reading and understanding the drug monographs found in Chapter 1.

❶ GENERIC NAME OF DRUG:
One or more icons may be found here: black box (side effects warning), camera (photo), ear (sound-alike drug)

Cyclosporine ■
(sye-kloh-**SPOR**-een)

❷ PHONETIC PRONUNCIATION of generic name

CLASSIFICATION(S):
Immunosuppressant

❸ CLASSIFICATION: Defines the type of drug or the class under which the drug is listed.

PREGNANCY CATEGORY: C

❹ PREGNANCY CATEGORY assigned by the FDA. Defined in Appendix 6.

Rx: Cyclosporine Softgel Capsules, Gengraf, Neoral , Sandimmune
✦Rx: Sandimmune I.V.

❺ TRADE NAMES: names by which a drug is marketed. If numerous forms of the drug are available, the trade names are identified by form. **Rx** denotes prescription drugs. **OTC** denotes over-the-counter, nonprescription drugs **CANADIAN** trade names are indicated by a maple leaf. (✦)

ACTION/KINETICS
Thought to act by inhibiting the immunocompetent lymphocytes in the G_0 or G_1 phase of the cell cycle. T-lymphocytes are specifically inhibited; both the T-helper cell and the T-suppressor cell may be affected. Also in-

❻ CONTROLLED SUBSTANCES: If the drug is controlled by the U. S. Federal Controlled Substances Act, the schedule in which the drug is placed follows the trade name listing. Controlled substance schedules are placed after Rx drugs. (ex: **C-II**) (See Appendix 5.)

❼ ACTION/KINETICS: Critical information about the rate of drug absorption, distribution, time for peak plasma levels or peak effect, minimum effective serum or plasma level, duration of action, metabolism, and excretion route(s). Metabolism and excretion routes may be important for clients with systemic liver disease, kidney disease, or both.

CROSS REFERENCE (for selected drugs):"See also ..." directs the reader to the classification entry in Chapter 2 or to other parts of Chapter 1 that give a complete profile of the drug.

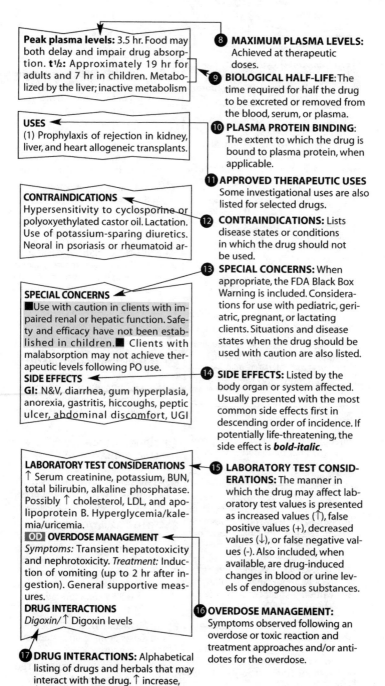

Peak plasma levels: 3.5 hr. Food may both delay and impair drug absorption. **t½:** Approximately 19 hr for adults and 7 hr in children. Metabolized by the liver; inactive metabolism

USES
(1) Prophylaxis of rejection in kidney, liver, and heart allogeneic transplants.

CONTRAINDICATIONS
Hypersensitivity to cyclosporine or polyoxyethylated castor oil. Lactation. Use of potassium-sparing diuretics. Neoral in psoriasis or rheumatoid ar-

SPECIAL CONCERNS
■Use with caution in clients with impaired renal or hepatic function. Safety and efficacy have not been established in children.■ Clients with malabsorption may not achieve therapeutic levels following PO use.

SIDE EFFECTS
GI: N&V, diarrhea, gum hyperplasia, anorexia, gastritis, hiccoughs, peptic ulcer, abdominal discomfort, UGI

LABORATORY TEST CONSIDERATIONS
↑ Serum creatinine, potassium, BUN, total bilirubin, alkaline phosphatase. Possibly ↑ cholesterol, LDL, and apolipoprotein B. Hyperglycemia/kalemia/uricemia.

OD OVERDOSE MANAGEMENT
Symptoms: Transient hepatotoxicity and nephrotoxicity. *Treatment:* Induction of vomiting (up to 2 hr after ingestion). General supportive measures.

DRUG INTERACTIONS
Digoxin/ ↑ Digoxin levels

8 MAXIMUM PLASMA LEVELS: Achieved at therapeutic doses.

9 BIOLOGICAL HALF-LIFE: The time required for half the drug to be excreted or removed from the blood, serum, or plasma.

10 PLASMA PROTEIN BINDING: The extent to which the drug is bound to plasma protein, when applicable.

11 APPROVED THERAPEUTIC USES Some investigational uses are also listed for selected drugs.

12 CONTRAINDICATIONS: Lists disease states or conditions in which the drug should not be used.

13 SPECIAL CONCERNS: When appropriate, the FDA Black Box Warning is included. Considerations for use with pediatric, geriatric, pregnant, or lactating clients. Situations and disease states when the drug should be used with caution are also listed.

14 SIDE EFFECTS: Listed by the body organ or system affected. Usually presented with the most common side effects first in descending order of incidence. If potentially life-threatening, the side effect is ***bold-italic***.

15 LABORATORY TEST CONSIDERATIONS: The manner in which the drug may affect laboratory test values is presented as increased values (↑), false positive values (+), decreased values (↓), or false negative values (-). Also included, when available, are drug-induced changes in blood or urine levels of endogenous substances.

16 OVERDOSE MANAGEMENT: Symptoms observed following an overdose or toxic reaction and treatment approaches and/or antidotes for the overdose.

17 DRUG INTERACTIONS: Alphabetical listing of drugs and herbals that may interact with the drug. ↑ increase, ↓ decrease, → leading to.

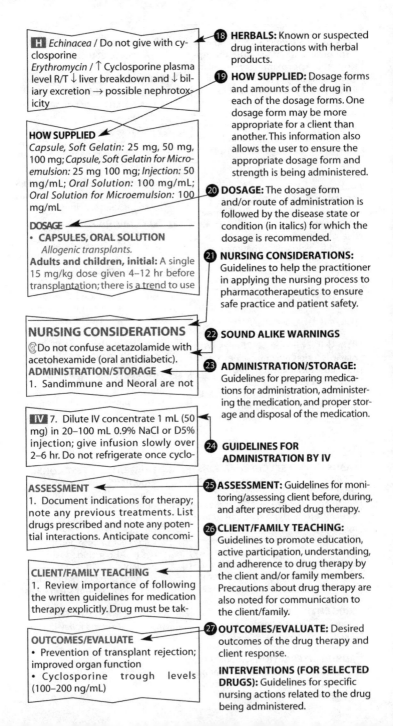

H *Echinacea* / Do not give with cyclosporine
Erythromycin / ↑ Cyclosporine plasma level R/T ↓ liver breakdown and ↓ biliary excretion → possible nephrotoxicity

18 HERBALS: Known or suspected drug interactions with herbal products.

HOW SUPPLIED
Capsule, Soft Gelatin: 25 mg, 50 mg, 100 mg; *Capsule, Soft Gelatin for Microemulsion:* 25 mg 100 mg; *Injection:* 50 mg/mL; *Oral Solution:* 100 mg/mL; *Oral Solution for Microemulsion:* 100 mg/mL

19 HOW SUPPLIED: Dosage forms and amounts of the drug in each of the dosage forms. One dosage form may be more appropriate for a client than another. This information also allows the user to ensure the appropriate dosage form and strength is being administered.

DOSAGE
• **CAPSULES, ORAL SOLUTION**
Allogenic transplants.
Adults and children, initial: A single 15 mg/kg dose given 4–12 hr before transplantation; there is a trend to use

20 DOSAGE: The dosage form and/or route of administration is followed by the disease state or condition (in italics) for which the dosage is recommended.

21 NURSING CONSIDERATIONS: Guidelines to help the practitioner in applying the nursing process to pharmacotherapeutics to ensure safe practice and patient safety.

NURSING CONSIDERATIONS
©Do not confuse acetazolamide with acetohexamide (oral antidiabetic).
ADMINISTRATION/STORAGE
1. Sandimmune and Neoral are not

22 SOUND ALIKE WARNINGS

23 ADMINISTRATION/STORAGE: Guidelines for preparing medications for administration, administering the medication, and proper storage and disposal of the medication.

IV 7. Dilute IV concentrate 1 mL (50 mg) in 20–100 mL 0.9% NaCl or D5% injection; give infusion slowly over 2–6 hr. Do not refrigerate once cyclo-

24 GUIDELINES FOR ADMINISTRATION BY IV

ASSESSMENT
1. Document indications for therapy; note any previous treatments. List drugs prescribed and note any potential interactions. Anticipate concomi-

25 ASSESSMENT: Guidelines for monitoring/assessing client before, during, and after prescribed drug therapy.

26 CLIENT/FAMILY TEACHING: Guidelines to promote education, active participation, understanding, and adherence to drug therapy by the client and/or family members. Precautions about drug therapy are also noted for communication to the client/family.

CLIENT/FAMILY TEACHING
1. Review importance of following the written guidelines for medication therapy explicitly. Drug must be tak-

OUTCOMES/EVALUATE
• Prevention of transplant rejection; improved organ function
• Cyclosporine trough levels (100–200 ng/mL)

27 OUTCOMES/EVALUATE: Desired outcomes of the drug therapy and client response.

INTERVENTIONS (FOR SELECTED DRUGS): Guidelines for specific nursing actions related to the drug being administered.

Abciximab

(ab-**SIX**-ih-mab)

CLASSIFICATION(S):
Antiplatelet drug
PREGNANCY CATEGORY: C
Rx: ReoPro

ACTION/KINETICS
Abciximab is the Fab fragment of the chimeric human-murine monoclonal antibody 7E3. It binds to a glycoprotein receptor on human platelets, thus inhibiting platelet aggregation by preventing the binding of fibrinogen, von Willebrand factor, and other adhesive molecules to receptor sites on activated platelets. **t ½, after IV bolus:** 30 min. Recovery of platelet function: About 48 hr, although the drug remains in the circulation bound to platelets for up to 10 days. Following IV infusion, free drug levels in the plasma decrease rapidly for about 6 hr and then decline at a slower rate.

USES
Inhibition of platelet aggregation. Adjunct to percutaneous coronary intervention (PCI) to prevent acute cardiac ischemic complications in clients at high risk for abrupt closure of the treated coronary vessel. Used with aspirin and heparin. *Investigational:* Early treatment of acute MI.

CONTRAINDICATIONS
Due to a potential for drug-induced bleeding, abciximab is contraindicated as follows: history of CVA (within 2 years) or CVA with a significant residual neurologic deficit; active internal bleeding; within 6 weeks of GI or GU bleed-ing of clinical significance; bleeding diathesis; within 7 days of administration of oral anticoagulants unless the PT is less than 1.2 times control; thrombocytopenia (less than 100,000 cells/μL); within 6 weeks of major surgery or trauma; intracranial neoplasm; arteriovenous malformation or aneurysm; severe uncontrolled hypertension; presumed or documented history of vasculitis; use of IV dextran before PCI or intent to use it during PCI; hypersensitivity to murine proteins.

SPECIAL CONCERNS
Assess benefits versus the risk of increased bleeding in clients who weigh less than 75 kg, are 65 years of age or older, have a history of GI disease, and are receiving thrombolytics and heparin. Conditions also associated with an increased risk of bleeding in the angioplasty setting and which may be additive to that of abciximab: PCI within 12 hr of onset of symptoms for acute MI, PCI lasting more than 70 min, and failed PCI. Use with caution during lactation and when abciximab is used with other drugs that affect hemostasis, including thrombolytics, oral anticoagulants, NSAIDs, dipyridamole, and ticlopidine. Safety and efficacy have not been determined in children.

SIDE EFFECTS
Bleeding tendencies: *Major bleeds, including intracranial hemorrhage*. Minor bleeding, including spontaneous gross hematuria/hematemesis. Loss of hemoglobin. **CV:** Hypotension, bradycardia, atrial fibrillation/flutter, vascular disorder, pulmonary edema, incomplete or *complete AV block,* VT, weak pulse, palpitations, nodal arrhythmia, limb embolism, thrombophlebitis, inter-

mittent claudication, pericardial effusion, pseudoaneurysm, AV fistula, ventricular arrhythmia. **GI:** N&V, abdominal pain, diarrhea, dry mouth, dyspepsia, ileus, gastroesophageal reflux. **Hematologic:** Thrombocytopenia, anemia/hemolytic anemia, leukocytosis, petechiae. **CNS:** Hypesthesia, confusion, abnormal thinking, agitation, anxiety, dizziness, *coma, brain ischemia,* insomnia. **Respiratory:** Pleural effusion, pleurisy, pneumonia, rales, bronchitis, bronchospasm, *PE,* rhonchi. **Musculoskeletal:** Myopathy, cellulitis, muscle contraction/pain. **GU:** UTI, urinary retention, abnormal renal function, dysuria, frequent micturition, cystalgia, incontinence, prostatitis. **Ophthalmic:** Diplopia, abnormal vision. **Miscellaneous:** Pain, peripheral edema, development of human antichimeric antibody, dysphonia, pruritus, increased sweating, asthenia, incisional pain, wound abscess, cellulitis, peripheral coldness, injection site pain, pallor, diabetes mellitus, hypertonia, enlarged abdomen, bullous eruption, inflammation.

DRUG INTERACTIONS

H *Bromelain* / Possible ↑ bleeding risk

H *Evening primrose oil* / Possible ↑ antiplatelet effect

H *Feverfew* / Possible ↑ antiplatelet effect

H *Garlic* / Possible ↑ antiplatelet effect

H *Ginger* / Possible ↑ antiplatelet effect

H *Ginkgo biloba* / Possible ↑ antiplatelet effect

H *Ginseng* / Possible ↑ antiplatelet effect

H *Grapeseed extract* / Possible ↑ antiplatelet effect

HOW SUPPLIED

Injection: 2 mg/mL

DOSAGE

• **IV BOLUS FOLLOWED BY IV INFUSION**

Clients undergoing percutaneous coronary intervention (PCI) with concomitant use of heparin and aspirin.

IV bolus: 0.25 mg/kg given 10–60 min before the start of the intervention. Followed by **continuous IV infusion:** 0.125 mcg/kg/min (maximum of 10 mcg/min) for 12 hr. Those with unstable angina not responding to usual therapy and who require PCI within 24 hr may be given abciximab, 0.25 mg/kg IV bolus, followed by an 18–24 hr IV infusion of 10 mcg/min, ending 1 hr after the PCI.

NURSING CONSIDERATIONS

ADMINISTRATION/STORAGE

IV 1. Stop infusion after 12 hr to avoid prolonged platelet receptor blockade effects.

2. Stop continuous infusion with failed PCIs; no evidence effective in such situations.

3. Discontinue abciximab and heparin if serious bleeding occurs not controlled by compression.

4. Do not use if preparations contain visibly opaque particles.

5. If symptoms of an allergic reaction or anaphylaxis occur, stop infusion immediately and institute appropriate treatment. Have available epinephrine, dopamine, theophylline, antihistamines, and corticosteroids for immediate use.

6. Withdraw drug (2 mg/mL) through a sterile, nonpyrogenic, low-protein-binding 0.2- or 0.22-μm filter into a syringe; give bolus 10–60 min before procedure.

7. For continuous infusion, withdraw 4.5 mL of abciximab as #6 directs into a syringe. Inject into 250 mL of 0.9% NSS or D5W and infuse at a rate of 17 mL/hr (10 mcg/min) for 12 hr by infusion pump with an in-line sterile, nonpyrogenic, low-protein-binding 0.2- or 0.22-μm filter. Discard any unused drug after 12 hr.

8. Give drug through a separate IV line with no other medications added to infusion solution. No incompatibilities have been noted with glass bottles or PVC bags or IV sets.

9. Store vials at 2–8°C (36–46°F); do not freeze or shake vials.

ASSESSMENT

1. Obtain a thorough nursing history; note indications/goals of therapy.

2. Note any history of CVA, bleeding disorders, recent episodes of bleeding, trauma, or surgery.

Bold Italic = life threatening side effect   ■ = black box warning   ✦ = Available in Canada

3. List other agents prescribed/OTC and when last consumed to prevent any bleeding potential.

4. Monitor PT, INR, PTT, CBC, VS, and EKG. Check platelet count 2–4 hr after initial bolus and again in 24 hr.

INTERVENTIONS

1. Anticipate client undergoing PCI will receive a bolus of abciximab (0.25 mg/kg) 10–60 min before procedure followed by a continuous IV infusion (10 mcg/min) for 12 hr.

2. Insert separate IV lines with saline locks for blood draws.

3. Observe carefully during infusion; anaphylaxis may occur at any time.

4. Administer 325 mg aspirin orally 2 hr before procedure and prepare heparin bolus and infusion for administration as prescribed.

5. Observe for any potential bleeding sites: catheter insertion sites, needle punctures, GI, GU, and retroperitoneal sites. Remove tape/dressings gently.

6. If serious bleeding develops (not controlled with pressure), stop infusions of abciximab and heparin.

7. Keep on complete bedrest while vascular access sheath in place. Restrain limb straight and raise HOB no more than 30 degrees. Stop heparin infusion at least 4 hr before sheath removal. Palpate/monitor distal pulses of involved extremity.

8. Apply pressure for 30 min over femoral artery once sheath is removed. When hemostasis evident, apply a pressure dressing with sandbag and check frequently for evidence of bleeding. Monitor hematoma for enlargement. Enforce bedrest for 6–8 hr after infusion completed and sheath removed.

CLIENT/FAMILY TEACHING

1. Review indications for therapy, what to expect, clinical management, and anticipated results.

2. Review risks associated with this therapy, e.g., bleeding from intracranial hemorrhage, which may be lethal, or bloody urine/vomit; may require blood/platelet transfusions.

3. Report any fever, chills, rash, or other adverse effects. Be aware it may take longer to stop bleeding and pressure will be applied to bleeding sites to help stop the flow.

4. Drug may cause formation of human antichimeric antibody, which may cause hypersensitivity reactions, low platelets, or diminished response on re-administration.

OUTCOMES/EVALUATE

Prevention of abrupt coronary vessel closure with associated ischemic complications

---

Acetazolamide ©

(ah-set-ah-**ZOE**-la-myd)

CLASSIFICATION(S):
Anticonvulsant, carbonic anhydrase inhibitor

PREGNANCY CATEGORY: C

Rx: Dazamide, Diamox, Diamox Sequels

✦Rx: Apo-Acetazolamide

Acetazolamide sodium

Rx: Diamox

SEE ALSO *ANTICONVULSANTS* AND *DIURETICS*.

ACTION/KINETICS

Sulfonamide derivative possessing carbonic anhydrase inhibitor activity. As an anticonvulsant, beneficial effects may be due to inhibition of carbonic anhydrase in the CNS, which increases carbon dioxide tension resulting in a decrease in neuronal conduction. Systemic acidosis may also be involved. As a diuretic, the drug inhibits carbonic anhydrase in the kidney, which decreases formation of bicarbonate and hydrogen ions from carbon dioxide, thus reducing the availability of these ions for active transport. Use as a diuretic is limited because the drug promotes metabolic acidosis, which inhibits diuretic activity. This may be partially circumvented by giving acetazolamide on alternate days. Also reduces intraocular pressure.

Absorbed from the GI tract and widely distributed throughout the body, including the CNS. Excreted unchanged in the urine. **Tablets: Onset,** 60–90 min; **peak:** 1–4 hr; **duration:** 8–12 hr. **Sustained-release capsules: Onset,** 2 hr; **peak:** 3–6 hr; **duration:** 18–24 hr. **Injection (IV): Onset,** 2 min; **peak:** 15 min; **duration:** 4–5 hr. Eliminated mainly unchanged through the kidneys.

USES
(1) Adjunct in the treatment of edema due to CHF or drug-induced edema. (2) Absence (petit mal) and unlocalized seizures. (3) Open-angle, secondary, or acute-angle closure glaucoma when delay of surgery is desired to lower IOP. (4) Prophylaxis or treatment of acute mountain sickness in climbers attempting a rapid ascent or in those susceptible to mountain sickness even with gradual ascent.

CONTRAINDICATIONS
Low serum sodium and potassium levels. Renal and hepatic dysfunction. Hyperchloremic acidosis, adrenal insufficiency, suprarenal gland failure, hypersensitivity to thiazide diuretics, cirrhosis. Chronic use in noncongestive angle-closure glaucoma.

SPECIAL CONCERNS
Use with caution in the presence of mild acidosis, advanced pulmonary disease, and during lactation. Increasing the dose does not increase effectiveness but may increase the risk of drowsiness or paresthesia. Safety and efficacy have not been established in children.

SIDE EFFECTS
GI: Anorexia, N&V, melena, constipation, alteration in taste, diarrhea. **GU:** Hematuria, glycosuria, urinary frequency, renal colic/calculi, crystalluria, polyuria, phosphaturia, decreased/absent libido, impotence. **CNS:** *Seizures,* weakness, malaise, fatigue, nervousness, drowsiness, depression, dizziness, disorientation, confusion, ataxia, tremor, headache, tinnitus, flaccid paralysis, lassitude, paresthesia of the extremities. **Hematologic:** *Bone marrow depression,* thrombocytopenic purpura, thrombocytopenia, *hemolytic anemia,* leukopenia, pancytopenia, agranulocytosis. **Dermatologic:** Pruritus, urticaria, skin rashes, erythema multiforme, *Ste-*

vens-Johnson syndrome, toxic epidermal necrolysis, photosensitivity. **Other:** Weight loss, fever, acidosis, electrolyte imbalance, transient myopia, hepatic insufficiency. *NOTE:* Side effects similar to those produced by sulfonamides may also occur.

OD OVERDOSE MANAGEMENT
Symptoms: Drowsiness, anorexia, N&V, dizziness, ataxia, tremor, paresthesias, tinnitus. *Treatment:* Emesis or gastric lavage. Hyperchloremic acidosis may respond to bicarbonate. Administration of potassium may also be necessary. Observe carefully and give supportive treatment.

DRUG INTERACTIONS
ALSO SEE *DIURETICS.*
Amphetamine / ↑ Amphetamine effect by ↑ renal tubular reabsorption
Cyclosporine / ↑ Cyclosporine levels → possible nephrotoxicity and neurotoxicity
Diflunisal / Significant ↓ in IOP with ↑ side effects
Ephedrine / ↑ Ephedrine effect R/T ↑ renal tubular reabsorption
Lithium carbonate / ↓ Lithium effect R/T ↑ renal excretion
Methotrexate / ↓ Methotrexate effect R/T ↑ renal excretion
Primidone / ↓ Primidone effect R/T ↓ GI absorption
Pseudoephedrine / ↑ Pseudoephedrine effect by ↑ renal tubular reabsorption
Quinidine / ↑ Quinidine effect by ↑ renal tubular reabsorption
Salicylates / Accumulation and toxicity of acetazolamide (including CNS depression and metabolic acidosis). Also, acidosis due to ↑ CNS penetration of salicylates

HOW SUPPLIED
Acetazolamide: *Capsule, Extended Release:* 500 mg; *Tablet:* 250 mg.
Acetazolamide sodium: *Powder for injection:* 500 mg

DOSAGE————————
• **EXTENDED-RELEASE CAPSULES, TABLETS, IV**
  Epilepsy.
Adults/children: 8–30 mg/kg/day in divided doses. Optimum daily dosage:

Bold Italic = life threatening side effect   ■ = black box warning   ✦ = Available in Canada

375–1,000 mg (doses higher than 1,000 mg do not increase therapeutic effect).
Adjunct to other anticonvulsants.
Initial: 250 mg/day; dose can be increased up to 1,000 mg/day in divided doses if necessary.
Glaucoma, simple open-angle.
Adults: 250–1,000 mg/day in divided doses. Doses greater than 1 g/day do not increase the effect.
Glaucoma, secondary or acute congestive (closed-angle).
Adults, short-term therapy: 250 mg q 4 hr or 250 mg twice a day **Adults, acute therapy:** 500 mg followed by 125–250 mg q 4 hr using tablets. For extended-release capsules, give 500 mg twice a day in the morning and evening. IV therapy may be used for rapid decrease in intraocular pressure. **Pediatric:** 5–10 mg/kg/dose IM or IV q 6 hr or 10–15 mg/kg/day in divided doses q 6–8 hr using tablets.
Acute mountain sickness.
Adults: 250 mg twice a day–q6h. (500 mg 1–2 times per day of extended-release capsules). During rapid ascent, 1 g/day is recommended.
Diuresis in CHF.
Adults, initial: 250–375 mg (5 mg/kg) once daily in the morning. If the client stops losing edema fluid after an initial response, do not increase doses; rather, skip medication for a day to allow the kidney to recover. The best diuretic effect occurs when the drug is given on alternate days or for 2 days alternating with a day of rest.
Drug-induced edema.
Adults: 250–375 mg once daily for 1 or 2 days. Most effective if given every other day or for 2 days followed by a day of rest. **Children:** 5 mg/kg/dose PO or IV once daily in the morning.

NURSING CONSIDERATIONS

℞ Do not confuse acetazolamide with acetohexamide (oral antidiabetic).

ADMINISTRATION/STORAGE

1. Change over from other anticonvulsant therapy should be gradual.
2. Acetazolamide tablets may be crushed and suspended in a cherry, chocolate, raspberry, or other sweet syrup. Do not use vehicles containing glycerin or alcohol. As an alternative, 1 tablet may be submerged in 10 mL of hot water and added to 10 mL of honey or syrup.
3. Tolerance after prolonged use may necessitate dosage increase.
4. Do not administer the sustained-release dosage form as an anticonvulsant; it should be used only for glaucoma and acute mountain sickness.
5. With prophylaxis of mountain sickness, initiate dosage 1–2 days before ascent and continue for at least 2 days while at high altitudes.
6. Due to possible differences in bioavailability, do not interchange brands.
IV 7. IV administration is preferred; IM administration is painful due to alkalinity of solution.
8. For direct IV use, administer over at least 1 min. For intermittent IV use, further dilute in dextrose or saline solution and infuse over 4-8 hr. Reconstitute each 500-mg vial with at least 5 mL of sterile water for injection.
9. Use within 24 hr after reconstitution, although reconstituted solutions retain potency for 1 week if refrigerated.

ASSESSMENT

1. Note indications for therapy, onset and characteristics of symptoms.
2. Review I&O, CBC, electrolytes, uric acid, and glucose. Assess for any liver/renal dysfunction.
3. List drugs prescribed to ensure no interactions.
4. With glaucoma, note baseline ophthalmic exam and intraocular pressures; assess for visual effects.
5. Perform CV/pulmonary assessment with CHF history. Obtain VS and weight.

CLIENT/FAMILY TEACHING

1. Taking drug with food may decrease GI upset/irritation.
2. Assess drug effects before undertaking tasks that require mental alertness.
3. Increases voiding frequency; take early to avoid interrupting sleep.
4. Take only as directed. If prescribed every other day, record to enhance adherence.
5. Increase fluids (2–3 L/day) to prevent urine crystals/stone formation.

6. Drug may increase blood glucose levels. Monitor FS and report increases; hypoglycemic agent may need adjustment. Avoid high sodium foods.

7. Report if nausea, dizziness, rapid weight gain, muscle weakness, cramps, or any changes in the color/consistency of stools occur.

8. Report for F/U visits and labs; may need potassium replacement.

OUTCOMES/EVALUATE
• ↓ Seizure activity
• ↓ Intraocular pressure
• ↓ CHF-associated edema
• Prevention of mountain sickness

Adenosine

(ah-**DEN**-oh-seen)

CLASSIFICATION(S):
Antiarrhythmic
PREGNANCY CATEGORY: C
Rx: Adenocard, Adenoscan

SEE ALSO *ANTIARRHYTHMIC DRUGS.*

ACTION/KINETICS
Found naturally in all cells of the body. It slows conduction time through the AV node, interrupts the reentry pathways through the AV node, and restores normal sinus rhythm in paroxysmal supraventricular tachycardia (PSVT). May cause a transient slowing of ventricular response immediately after use. Competitively antagonized by caffeine and theophylline; potentiated by dipyridamole. **Onset, after IV:** 34 sec. **t ½:** Less than 10 sec (taken up by erythrocytes and vascular endothelial cells). **Duration:** 1–2 min. Exogenous adenosine becomes part of the body pool and is metabolized mainly to inosine and AMP.

USES
(1) Conversion to sinus rhythm of PSVT (including that associated with accessory bypass tracts). (2) The phosphate salt is used for symptomatic relief of complications with stasis dermatitis in varicose veins. *Investigational:* With thallium-201 tomography in noninvasive assessment of clients with suspected CAD who cannot exercise adequately prior to being stress-tested. Adenosine is not effective in converting rhythms other than PSVT. The phosphate salt has been used to treat herpes infections and to increase blood flow to brain tumors and in porphyria cutanea tarda.

CONTRAINDICATIONS
Second- or third-degree AV block or sick sinus syndrome (except in clients with a functioning artificial pacemaker), atrial flutter, atrial fibrillation, ventricular tachycardia. History of MI or cerebral hemorrhage.

SPECIAL CONCERNS
At time of conversion to normal sinus rhythm, new rhythms (PVC, PACs, sinus bradycardia, skipped beats, varying degrees of AV block, sinus tachycardia) lasting a few seconds may occur. Use with caution in the elderly as severe bradycardia and AV block may occur and in clients with asthma due to possibility of bronchoconstriction. Safety and efficacy as a diagnostic agent have not been determined in clients less than 18 years of age.

SIDE EFFECTS
CV: Short lasting first-, second-, or ***third-degree heart block; cardiac arrest,*** sustained ventricular tachycardia, sinus bradycardia, ST-segment depression, sinus exit block, sinus pause, arrhythmias, T-wave changes, hypertension. prolonged asystole, Nonfatal MI, transient increase in BP, ***ventricular fibrillation***. Facial flushing (common), chest pain, sweating, palpitations, hypotension (may be significant). **CNS:** Lightheadedness, dizziness, numbness, headache, blurred vision, apprehension, paresthesia, drowsiness, emotional instability, tremors, nervousness. **GI:** Nausea, metallic taste, tightness in throat. **Respiratory:** SOB or dyspnea (common), urge to breathe deeply, chest pressure or discomfort, cough, hyperventilation, nasal congestion. **GU:** Urinary urgency, vaginal pressure. **Miscellaneous:** Pressure in head, burning sensation, neck and back pain, weakness, blurred vision, dry mouth, ear discomfort, pressure in groin, scotomas,

---

tongue discomfort, discomfort (tingling, heaviness) in upper extremities, discomfort in throat, neck, or jaw.

DRUG INTERACTIONS

H *Aloe; Buckthorn bark/berry; Cascara sagrada bark; Rhubarb root; Senna pod and leaf* / Possible ↑ adenosine effect
Caffeine / Competitively antagonizes adenosine effect
Carbamazepine / ↑ AV block
Digoxin / Possibility of ventricular fibrillation (rare)
Dipyridamole / ↑ Adenosine effect
Theophylline / Competitively antagonizes adenosine effect
Verapamil / Possibility of ventricular fibrillation (rare)

HOW SUPPLIED

Injection: 3 mg/mL

DOSAGE————————————————

- **RAPID IV BOLUS ONLY**
  Antiarrhythmic.

Adults, initial: 6 mg over 1–2 sec. If the first dose does not reverse the PSVT within 1–2 min, 12 mg should be given as a rapid IV bolus. The 12-mg dose may be repeated a second time, if necessary. Doses greater than 12 mg are not recommended. **Children, less than 50 kg, initial:** 0.05–0.1 mg/kg as a rapid IV bolus given either centrally or peripherally; follow by a saline flush. If conversion of PSVT does not occur within 1–2 min, additional bolus injections can be given at increasing doses of 0.05–0.1 mg/kg. Continue this until sinus rhythm is established or a maximum single dose of 0.3 mg/kg is given. Doses greater than 12 mg are not recommended. **Children, 50 kg or over:** Give the adult dose.

- **IV INFUSION ONLY**
  Diagnostic aid.

Adults: 140 mcg/kg/min infused over 6 min (total dose of 0.84 mg/kg).

- **IM ONLY**
  Varicose veins.

Initial: 25–50 mg 1–2 times daily until symptoms subside. **Maintenance:** 25 mg 2 or 3 times weekly.

NURSING CONSIDERATIONS

ADMINISTRATION/STORAGE

IV 1. Drug can be stored at room temperature; crystallization may result if the drug is refrigerated. If crystals form, dissolve by warming to room temperature. The solution must be clear when administered.

2. Discard any unused portion; contains no preservatives.

3. Administer directly into a vein over 1-2 sec. If given into an IV line, introduce in the most proximal line and follow with a rapid saline flush.

4. When used as a diagnostic aid, the dose of thallium-201 should be given at the midpoint of the adenosine infusion (i.e., after 3 min).

ASSESSMENT

1. Document indications for therapy, onset of symptoms, and ECG confirmation of arrhythmia.

2. Monitor rhythm strips closely for evidence of varying degrees of AV block and increased arrhythmias during conversion to sinus rhythm. These are usually only transient due to short half life of adenosine.

3. Monitor BP and pulse. Report complaints of numbness, tingling in the arms, blurred vision, or apprehensiveness, as this may be an indication to discontinue drug therapy.

4. Document chest pressure, SOB, heaviness of the arms, palpitations, or dyspnea. Note any history of MI or CVA as drug is contraindicated; with asthma may cause bronchoconstriction.

5. In stasis dermatitis carefully assess extremities and note findings.

CLIENT/FAMILY TEACHING

1. Drug helps restore heart to a normal, slower rhythm.

2. Avoid caffeine and report if concurrently prescribed theophylline, digoxin, or dipyridamole.

3. Facial flushing is a common temporary side effect of therapy. Report chest pain, numbness/tingling or increased SOB.

OUTCOMES/EVALUATE

- Conversion of PSVT to NSR
- Symptomatic relief with stasis dermatitis

A

Alteplase, recombinant

(**AL**-teh-playz)

CLASSIFICATION(S):
Thrombolytic, tissue plasminogen activator
PREGNANCY CATEGORY: C
Rx: Activase, Cathflo Activase
✤**Rx:** Activase rt-PA

ACTION/KINETICS
Alteplase, a tissue plasminogen activator, is synthesized by a human melanoma cell line using recombinant DNA technology. This enzyme binds to fibrin in a thrombus, causing a conversion of plasminogen to plasmin. This conversion results in local fibrinolysis and a decrease in circulating fibrinogen. Within 10 min following termination of an infusion, 80% of the alteplase has been cleared from the plasma by the liver. The enzyme activity of alteplase is 580,000 international units/mg. **t ½, initial:** 4 min; **final:** 35 min (elimination phase).

USES
Activase. (1) Improvement of ventricular function following AMI, including reducing the incidence of CHF and decreasing mortality. (2) Acute ischemic stroke, after intracranial hemorrhage has been excluded by CT scan or other diagnostic imaging. (3) Acute pulmonary embolism (confirm diagnosis by pulmonary angiography or noninvasive procedures as lung scanning). **Cathflo Activase.** Restoration of function to central venous access devices that have become occluded by a blood clot or thrombus. *Investigational:* Unstable angina pectoris.

CONTRAINDICATIONS
AMI or pulmonary embolism: Active internal bleeding, history of CVA, within 2 months of intracranial or intraspinal surgery or trauma, intracranial neoplasm, AV malformation or aneurysm, bleeding diathesis, severe uncontrolled hypertension.

Acute ischemic stroke: Symptoms of intracranial hemorrhage on pretreatment evaluation, suspected subarachnoid hemorrhage, recent intracranial surgery or serious head trauma, recent previous stroke, history of intracranial hemorrhage, uncontrolled hypertension (above 185 mm Hg systolic or above 110 Hg diastolic) at time of treatment, active internal bleeding, seizure at onset of stroke, intracranial neoplasm, AV malformation or aneurysm, bleeding diathesis.

SPECIAL CONCERNS
Use with caution in the presence of recent GI or GU bleeding (within 10 days), subacute bacterial endocarditis, acute pericarditis, significant liver dysfunction, concomitant use of oral anticoagulants, diabetic hemorrhagic retinopathy, septic thrombophlebitis or occluded arteriovenous cannula (at infected site), lactation, mitral stenosis with atrial fibrillation. Since fibrin will be lysed during therapy, careful attention should be given to potential bleeding sites such as sites of catheter insertion and needle puncture sites. Use with caution within 10 days of major surgery (e.g., obstetrics, coronary artery bypass) and in clients over 75 years of age. Safety and efficacy have not been established in children. *NOTE:* Doses greater than 150 mg have been associated with an increase in intracranial bleeding.
Use Cathflo Activase with caution in presence of suspected infection in a catheter.

SIDE EFFECTS
Bleeding tendencies: *Internal bleeding* (including the GI and GU tracts and intracranial or retroperitoneal site). Superficial bleeding (e.g., gums, sites of recent surgery, venous cutdowns, arterial punctures). Ecchymosis, epistaxis. **CV:** Bradycardia, hypotension, cardiogenic shock, arrhythmias, *heart failure, cardiac arrest, cardiac tamponade, myocardial rupture,* recurrent ischemia, reinfarction, mitral regurgitation, pericardial effusion, pericarditis, venous thrombosis and embolism, electromechanical dissociation, cholesterol embolism. **Allergic:** Rash, *laryngeal edema,*

---

orolingual angioedema, anaphylaxis.
GI: N&V. **Miscellaneous:** Fever, urticaria, pulmonary edema, cerebral edema.
Due to accelerated infusion: *Strokes, hemorrhagic stroke,* nonfatal stroke. Incidence increases with age.

OD OVERDOSE MANAGEMENT
Symptoms: Bleeding disorders. *Treatment:* Discontinue therapy immediately as well as any concomitant heparin therapy.

DRUG INTERACTIONS
Abciximab / ↑ Risk of bleeding
Aspirin / ↑ Risk of bleeding
Dipyridamole / ↑ Risk of bleeding
Heparin / ↑ Risk of bleeding, especially at arterial puncture sites
Nitroglycerin / ↓ Alteplase concentrations → ↓ thrombolytic effect
Vitamin K antagonists / ↑ Risk of bleeding

HOW SUPPLIED
Powder for injection: 50 mg, 100 mg; *Single-patient vial (Cathflo Activase):* 2 mg

DOSAGE————————————
• **IV INFUSION ONLY**
    AMI, accelerated infusion.
Weight > 67 kg: 100 mg as a 15-mg IV bolus, followed by 50 mg infused over the next 30 min and then 35 mg infused over the next 60 min. **Weight < 67 kg:** 15 mg IV bolus, followed by 0.75 mg/kg infused over the next 30 min (not to exceed 50 mg) and then 0.50 mg/kg infused over the next 60 min (not to exceed 35 mg). The safety and efficacy of this regimen have only been evaluated using heparin and aspirin concomitantly.
    AMI, 3-hr infusion.
100 mg total dose subdivided as follows: 60 mg (34.8 million international units) the first hour with 6–10 mg given in a bolus over the first 1–2 min and the remaining 50–54 mg given over the hour; 20 mg (11.6 million international units) over the second hour and 20 mg (11.6 million international units) given over the third hour. **Clients less than 65 kg:** 1.25 mg/kg given over 3 hr, with 60% given the first hour with 6–10% given by direct IV injection within the first 1–2 min; 20% is given the second

hour and 20% during the third hour. Doses of 150 mg have caused an increase in intracranial bleeding.
    Pulmonary embolism.
100 mg over 2 hr; heparin therapy should be instituted near the end of or right after the alteplase infusion when the partial thromboplastin or thrombin time returns to twice that of normal or less.
    Acute ischemic stroke.
0.9 mg/kg (maximum of 90 mg) infused over 60 min with 10% of the total dose given as an initial IV bolus over 1 min. Doses greater than 0.9 mg/kg may cause an increased incidence of intracranial hemorrhage. Use with aspirin and heparin during the first 24 hr after onset of symptoms has not been investigated.
    Restoration of function to central venous access device.
2 mg in 2 mL of solution for clients weighing 30 kg or more; for those weighing between 10 and 30 kg, use a dose of 1 mg/mL solution equivalent to 110% of the volume of the catheter's internal lumen but not more than 2 mg. A second dose may be instilled if the catheter is not functioning 120 min after the first dose.

NURSING CONSIDERATIONS
ADMINISTRATION/STORAGE
IV 1. Initiate alteplase therapy as soon as possible after onset of symptoms of acute MI and within 3 hr after the onset of stroke symptoms.
2. For acute MI, nearly 90% of clients also receive heparin concomitantly with alteplase and either aspirin or dipyridamole during or after heparin therapy.
3. Reconstitute with only sterile water for injection without preservatives immediately prior to use. The reconstituted preparation contains 1 mg/mL and is a colorless to pale yellow transparent solution. Do not add other medications to infusion solutions.
4. Using an 18-gauge needle, direct the stream of sterile water into the lyophilized cake. Leave product undisturbed for several minutes to allow dissipation of any large bubbles.

A

5. If necessary, the reconstituted solution may be further diluted immediately prior to use in an equal volume of 0.9% NaCl injection or D5W injection to yield a concentration of 0.5 mg/mL. Dilute by gentle swirling or slow inversion.

6. Either glass bottles or PVC bags may be used for administration.

7. Alteplase is stable for up to 8 hr following reconstitution or dilution. Stability will not be affected by light.

8. Do not use 50-mg vials if vacuum is not present (100-mg vials do not contain a vacuum). Reconstitute 50-mg vials with a large-bore needle (e.g., 18 gauge) directing stream of sterile water into lyophilized cake. For the 100-mg vial, use transfer device provided for reconstitution.

9. Use infusion device for administration. Do not add any other medications to the line. Anticipate 3 lines for access (1–alteplase; 1–heparin and other drugs such as lidocaine; 1–blood drawing and transfusions).

10. Store lyophilized alteplase at room temperatures not to exceed 30°C(86°F) or under refrigeration between 2–8°C (36–46°F).

11. Have available emergency drugs (especially aminocaproic acid) and resuscitative equipment.

ASSESSMENT

1. Note any history of hypertension, internal bleeding, PUD, or recent surgery.

2. Document onset and characteristics of chest pain and/or stroke symptoms; note deficits and monitor.

3. Assess and document overall physical condition; note CV and neurologic findings, weight, and ECG.

4. Obtain drug history. List those currently taking; note any anticoagulants/antiplatelets.

5. Obtain baseline hematologic parameters, type and cross, coagulation times, cardiac marker panel, and renal function studies.

INTERVENTIONS

1. Carefully review and follow instructions for drug reconstitution. Review contraindications before initiating therapy and document if accelerated or 3 hr infusion is prescribed.

2. Observe in a closely monitored environment; obtain VS and review and document monitor strips.

3. Anticipate and assess for reperfusion reactions such as:
- Reperfusion arrhythmias usually of short duration. These may include accelerated idioventricular rhythm and sinus bradycardia.
- Reduction of chest pain
- Return of the elevated ST segment to near baseline levels
- Smaller Q waves

4. Check all access sites for any evidence of bleeding. During IV therapy, arterial sticks require 30 min of manual pressure followed by application of a pressure dressing. In the event of any uncontrolled bleeding, terminate alteplase and heparin infusions and report.

5. Monitor neuro status; document every 15–30 min during infusion.

6. During treatment of stroke, note CT or MRI results.

7. During treatment for pulmonary embolism, ensure that the PTT or PT is no more than twice that of normal before heparin therapy is added.

8. Keep on bed rest and observe for S&S of abnormal bleeding (hematuria, hematemesis, melena, CVA, cardiac tamponade, ↑ HR, ↓ BP).

9. Obtain appropriate postinfusion labs (cardiac marker, platelets, H&H, PTT, ECG) as directed.

CLIENT/FAMILY TEACHING

1. Review the goals of therapy and inherent risks during acute coronary artery occlusion and/or stroke.

2. To be effective, the therapy should be instituted within 3 hr of stroke and 4–6 hr of MI symptoms.

3. Report any chest pain, SOB, N&V, heart palpitations or other adverse effects.

4. Encourage family members to learn CPR.

OUTCOMES/EVALUATE

- Lysis of thrombi with reperfusion of ischemic cardiac and/or cerebral tissue
- ↓ Infarct size with restoration of coronary perfusion and improved ventricu-

---

lar function (↑ CO, ↓ incidence of CHF, ↓ mortality)

Amiodarone hydrochloride ■

(am-ee-**OH**-dah-rohn)

CLASSIFICATION(S):
Antiarrhythmic, class III
PREGNANCY CATEGORY: D
Rx: Cordarone, Pacerone
✤**Rx:** Cordarone I.V., Gen-Amiodarone, Novo-Amiodarone, ratio-Amiodarone, Rhoxal-amiodarone

SEE ALSO *ANTIARRHYTHMIC DRUGS.*

ACTION/KINETICS
Blocks sodium channels at rapid pacing frequencies, causing an increase in the duration of the myocardial cell action potential and refractory period, as well as alpha- and beta-adrenergic blockade. The drug decreases sinus rate, increases PR and QT intervals, results in development of U waves, and changes T-wave contour. After IV use, amiodarone relaxes vascular smooth muscle, reduces peripheral vascular resistance (afterload), and increases cardiac index slightly. No significant changes are seen in left ventricular ejection fraction after PO use. Absorption is slow and variable but food increases the rate and extent of absorption. **Maximum plasma levels:** 3–7 hr after a single dose. **Onset:** Several days up to 1–3 weeks. Drug may accumulate in the liver, lung, spleen, and adipose tissue. **Therapeutic serum levels:** 0.5–2.5 mcg/mL. **t ½:** Biphasic: **initial t ½:** 2.5–10 days; **final t ½:** 26–107 days. Effects may persist for several weeks or months after therapy is terminated. Effective plasma concentrations are difficult to predict although concentrations below 1 mg/L are usually ineffective, whereas those above 2.5 mg/L are not necessary. Neither amiodarone nor its metabolite, desethylamiodarone, is dialyzable.

USES
Oral: Use should be reserved for life-threatening ventricular arrhythmias unresponsive to other therapy, such as recurrent ventricular fibrillation and recurrent, hemodynamically unstable ventricular tachycardia.
IV: Initial treatment and prophylaxis of frequently recurring ventricular fibrillation and hemodynamically unstable ventricular tachycardia in clients refractory to other therapy. Ventricular tachycardia/ventricular fibrillation clients unable to take PO medication. *Investigational:* Conversion of atrial fibrillation and maintenance of sinus rhythm, supraventricular tachycardia. IV to treat AV nodal reentry tachycardia.

CONTRAINDICATIONS
Parenteral use: Marked sinus bradycardia due to severe sinus node dysfunction, second- or third-degree AV block unless a functioning pacemaker is available, cardiogenic shock. **PO use:** Severe sinus-node dysfunction causing marked sinus bradycardia, second- and third-degree AV block, when bradycardia has caused syncope except when used with a pacemaker. **Parenteral and PO use:** Lactation.

SPECIAL CONCERNS
■(1) Due to significant possible toxicity, use only in certain life-threatening arrhythmias. (2) Possible fatal toxicities, including pulmonary toxicity (hypersensitivity pneumonitis or interstitial/alveolar pneumonitis). Overt liver disease can occur (may be fatal). (3) Amiodarone can exacerbate the arrhythmia by making it less well tolerated or more difficult to reverse. Significant heart block or sinus bradycardia are possible.■ Safety and effectiveness in children have not been determined. Although not recommended for use in children, minimize the potential for the drug to leach out di-(2-ethylhexyl)phthalate (DEHP) from IV tubing during administration to children (DEHP may alter development of the male reproductive tract when given in high amounts). The drug may be more sensitive in geriatric clients, especially in thyroid dysfunction. Carefully monitor the IV product in

geriatric clients and in those with severe left ventricular dysfunction.

SIDE EFFECTS

Adverse reactions, some potentially fatal, are common with doses greater than 400 mg/day. **Pulmonary:** Pulmonary infiltrates or fibrosis, interstitial/alveolar pneumonitis, hypersensitivity pneumonitis, alveolitis, pulmonary inflammation or fibrosis, *ARDS (after parenteral use)*, lung edema, cough and progressive dyspnea. Oral use may cause a clinical syndrome of cough and progressive dyspnea accompanied by functional, radiographic, gallium scan, and pathologic data indicating pulmonary toxicity. **CV:** *Worsening of arrhythmias, paroxysmal ventricular tachycardia,* proarrhythmias, symptomatic bradycardia, sinus arrest, SA node dysfunction, *CHF,* edema, hypotension (especially with IV use), *cardiac conduction abnormalities, coagulation abnormalities, cardiac arrest (after IV use).* IV use may result in atrial fibrillation, nodal arrhythmia, prolonged QT interval, and sinus bradycardia. **Hepatic:** Abnormal LFTs, overt liver disease, nonspecific hepatic disorders, cholestatic hepatitis, cirrhosis, hepatitis, steatohepatitis (with cumulative doses). **CNS:** Malaise, tremor, lack of coordination, fatigue, ataxia, paresthesias, peripheral neuropathy, abnormal involuntary movements, sleep disturbances, dizziness, insomnia, headache, decreased libido, abnormal gait. **Hematologic:** *Hemolytic anemia, aplastic anemia,* thrombocytopenia. **GI:** N&V, constipation, anorexia, abdominal pain, abnormal taste and smell, abnormal salivation. **Ophthalmologic:** Ophthalmic abnormalities, including optic neuropathy and/or optic neuritis (may progress to permanent blindness). Papilledema, corneal degeneration, photosensitivity, eye discomfort, scotoma, lens opacities, macular degeneration. Corneal microdeposits (asymptomatic) in clients on therapy for 6 months or more, photophobia, dry eyes, visual disturbances, blurred vision, halos. **Dermatologic:** Photosensitivity, solar dermatitis, blue discoloration of skin, rash, alopecia, spontaneous ecchymosis, flushing. **Miscellaneous:** Hypothyroidism or hyperthyroidism, myopathy, vasculitis, flushing, pseudotumor cerebri, epididymitis, angioedema. IV use may cause abnormal kidney function, *Stevens-Johnson syndrome,* respiratory syndrome, *fatal 'gasping syndrome' in neonates following IV use of benzyl alcohol-containing solutions,* and *shock.*

LABORATORY TEST CONSIDERATIONS

↑ AST, ALT, GGT. Alteration of thyroid function tests (↑ serum T_4, ↓ serum T_3).

OD OVERDOSE MANAGEMENT

Symptoms: Bradycardia, hypotension, *disorders of cardiac rhythm, cardiogenic shock,* AV block, hepatoxicity. *Treatment:* Use supportive treatment. Monitor cardiac rhythm and BP. Use a beta-adrenergic agonist or pacemaker to treat bradycardia; treat hypotension due to insufficient tissue perfusion with a vasopressor or positive inotropic agents. Cholestyramine may hasten the reversal of side effects by increasing elimination. Drug is not dialyzable.

DRUG INTERACTIONS

Anticoagulants / ↑ PT → bleeding disorders

Azithromycin / Potential for prolonged QTc interval and QT dispersion and dizziness

Beta-adrenergic blocking agents / ↑ Bradycardia and hypotension

Calcium channel blockers / ↑ Risk of AV block with verapamil or diltiazem or hypotension with all calcium channel blockers

Cholestyramine / ↑ Elimination of amiodarone → ↓ serum levels and half-life

Cimetidine / ↑ Serum levels of amiodarone

Cyclosporine / ↑ Plasma drug levels → elevated creatinine levels (even with ↓ cyclosporine doses)

Dextromethorphan / Chronic use of PO amiodarone (> 2 weeks) impairs dextromethorphan metabolism

Digoxin / ↑ Serum digoxin levels → toxicity

Disopyramide / ↑ QT prolongation → possible arrhythmias

Fentanyl / Possibility of hypotension, bradycardia, ↓ CO

Flecainide / ↑ Plasma flecainide levels

Fluoroquinolones / ↑ Risk of life-threatening cardiac arrhythmias, including torsades de pointes

Grapefruit juice / ↑ AUC and peak plasma amiodarone levels R/T inhibition of cytochrome P450 3A4 metabolism of amiodarone

Indinavir / ↑ Plasma levels of amiodarone due to ↓ breakdown by liver

Methotrexate / Chronic use of PO amiodarone (> 2 weeks) ↓ methotrexate metabolism → toxicity

Phenytoin / ↑ Serum phenytoin levels → toxicity; also, ↓ amiodarone levels

Procainamide / ↑ Serum procainamide levels→ toxicity

Pyridoxine / ↑ Amiodarone-induced photosensitivity

Quinidine / ↑ Quinidine toxicity, including fatal cardiac arrhythmias

Rifampin / ↓ Serum levels of amiodarone due to ↑ liver breakdown

Ritonavir / ↑ Levels of amiodarone → ↑ risk of amiodarone toxicity

Simvastatin / Possible severe myopathy with elevated creatine kinase

Theophylline / ↑ Serum theophylline levels → toxicity (effects may not be seen for 1 week and may last for a prolonged period after drug is discontinued)

HOW SUPPLIED

Injection: 50 mg/mL; *Tablet:* 100 mg, 200 mg, 400 mg

DOSAGE

Due to the drug's side effects, unusual pharmacokinetic properties, and difficult dosing schedule, administer amiodarone in a hospital only by physicians trained in treating life-threatening arrhythmias. Loading doses are required to ensure a reasonable onset of action.

• **IV INFUSION**

Life-threatening ventricular arrhythmias.

Loading dose, rapid: 150 mg over the first 10 minutes (15 mg/min). **Then, slow loading dose:** 360 mg over the next 6 hr (1 mg/min). **Maintenance dose:** 540 mg over the remaining 18 hr (0.5 mg/min). After the first 24 hr, continue maintenance infusion rate of 0.5 mg/min (720 mg/24 hr). This may be continued with monitoring for 2 to 3 weeks.

Once arrhythmias have been suppressed, the client may be switched to PO amiodarone. The following is intended only as a guideline for PO amiodarone dosage after IV infusion. **IV infusion less than 1 week:** Initial daily dose of PO amiodarone, 800–1,600 mg. **IV infusion from 1 to 3 weeks:** Initial daily dose of PO amiodarone, 600–800 mg. **IV infusion longer than 3 weeks:** Initial daily dose of PO amiodarone, 400 mg.

• **TABLETS**

Life-threatening ventricular arrhythmias.

Loading dose: 800–1,600 mg/day for 1–3 weeks (or until initial response occurs); **then,** reduce dose to 600–800 mg/day for 1 month. **Maintenance dose:** 400 mg/day (as low as 200 mg/day or as high as 600 mg/day may be needed in some clients). Give in divided doses with meals for total daily doses of 1,000 mg or higher or when GI intolerance occurs.

NURSING CONSIDERATIONS

ADMINISTRATION/STORAGE

1. Correct potassium or Mg deficiencies before initiation of therapy since antiarrhythmics may be ineffective or arrhythmogenic in clients with hypokalemia.

2. When initiating amiodarone therapy, gradually discontinue other antiarrhythmic drugs.

3. To minimize side effects, determine the lowest effective dose. If side effects occur, reduce the dose.

4. If dosage adjustments are required, monitor the client for an extended period of time due to the long and variable half-life of the drug and the difficulty in predicting the time needed to achieve a new steady-state plasma drug level.

5. Administer daily PO doses of 1000 mg or more in divided doses with meals.

6. If additional antiarrhythmic therapy is required, the initial dose of such

drugs should be about one-half the usual recommended dose.

IV 7. For the first rapid loading dose, add 3 mL amiodarone IV (150 mg) to 100 mL D5W for a concentration of 1.5 mg/mL; infuse at a rate of 100 mL/10 min. For the slower loading dose, add 18 mL amiodarone IV (900 mg) to 500 mL of D5W for a concentration of 1.8 mg/mL.

8. IV concentrations of amiodarone greater than 3 mg/mL in D5W cause a high incidence of peripheral vein phlebitis; concentrations of 2.5 mg/mL or less are not as irritating. Thus, for infusions greater than 1 hr, the IV concentration should not exceed 2 mg/mL unless a central venous catheter is used.

9. Because amiodarone adsorbs to PVC, IV infusions exceeding 2 hr must be given in glass or polyolefin bottles containing D5W.

10. Cordarone I.V. has been found to leach out plasticizers, such as DEHP, which can adversely affect male reproductive tract development in fetuses, infants, and toddlers. Cordarone I.V. is not indicated to treat arrhythmias in pediatric clients.

11. Amiodarone IV in D5W is incompatible with aminophylline, cefamandole nafate, cefazolin sodium, mezlocillin sodium, heparin sodium, and sodium bicarbonate.

12. Store the injection at room temperature protected from light.

ASSESSMENT

1. Note indications for therapy. Determine if taking any other antiarrhythmic medications.

2. Assess quality of respirations and breath sounds; note cardiac status, EKG, and CV findings.

3. Note baseline VS and perfusion (skin temperature, color). Document ABGs and assess for circulatory impairment and hypotension.

4. Assess vision before therapy.

5. Monitor thyroid studies because drug inhibits conversion of T_4 to T_3. May require replacement therapy with prolonged use.

6. Obtain baseline CBC, electrolytes, CXR, renal and LFTs.

7. During administration, observe for increased PR and QRS intervals, increased arrhythmias, and HR < 60 bpm. Obtain ECG and document rhythm strips; note EPS findings.

8. Anticipate reduced dosages of digoxin, warfarin, quinidine, procainamide, and phenytoin if administered concomitantly with amiodarone.

CLIENT/FAMILY TEACHING

1. Drug is used to control heart beat irregularities, so take as directed.

2. Report if crystals develop on the skin, producing a bluish color, so dosage can be adjusted.

3. Avoid direct exposure to sunlight. Wear protective clothing, sunglasses, and a sunscreen when exposed.

4. Report all side effects, especially any abnormal swelling, bleeding, or bruising.

5. Complaints of painful breathing, wheezing, fever, coughing, or SOB are S&S of pulmonary problems and require prompt attention.

6. Report CNS symptoms such as tremor, lack of coordination, numbness, and dizziness.

7. Complaints of headaches, depression, or insomnia as well as any change in behavior such as decreased interest in personal appearance or apparent hallucinations may require a change in therapy.

8. Schedule periodic eye exams because small yellow-brown granular corneal deposits may develop during prolonged therapy. Visual changes require prompt ophthalmic evaluation.

9. Therapy with this drug requires periodic lab studies and close medical evaluation.

OUTCOMES/EVALUATE

- Termination/control of arrhythmias
- Serum drug levels within therapeutic range (0.5–2.5 mcg/mL)

Amlodipine Ⓒ

(am-**LOH**-dih-peen)

CLASSIFICATION(S):
Calcium channel blocker

PREGNANCY CATEGORY: C
Rx: Amvaz, Norvasc

SEE ALSO *CALCIUM CHANNEL BLOCKING AGENTS.*

ACTION/KINETICS
Possible slight decrease in myocardial contractility. CO is increased; moderate decrease in peripheral vascular resistance. **Peak plasma levels:** 6–12 hr. **t ½, elimination:** 30–50 hr. About 93% plasma protein bound. 90% metabolized in the liver to inactive metabolites; 10% excreted unchanged in the urine.

USES
(1) Hypertension alone or in combination with other antihypertensives. (2) Chronic stable angina alone or in combination with other antianginal drugs. (3) Vasospastic (Prinzmetal's variant) angina alone or in combination with other antianginal drugs.

CONTRAINDICATIONS
Use with grapefruit juice.

SPECIAL CONCERNS
Use with caution in clients with CHF and in those with impaired hepatic function or reduced hepatic blood flow. Safety and efficacy have not been determined in children.

SIDE EFFECTS
CNS: Headache, fatigue, lethargy, somnolence, dizziness, lightheadedness, sleep disturbances, depression, amnesia, psychosis, hallucinations, paresthesia, asthenia, insomnia, abnormal dreams, malaise, anxiety, tremor, hand tremor, hypoesthesia, vertigo, depersonalization, migraine, apathy, agitation, amnesia. **GI:** Nausea, abdominal discomfort, cramps, dyspepsia, diarrhea, constipation, vomiting, dry mouth, thirst, flatulence, dysphagia, loose stools. **CV:** Peripheral edema, palpitations, hypotension, syncope, bradycardia, unspecified arrhythmias, tachycardia, ventricular extrasystoles, peripheral ischemia, *cardiac failure,* pulse irregularity, increased risk of MI. **Dermatologic:** Dermatitis, rash, pruritus, urticaria, photosensitivity, petechiae, ecchymosis, purpura, bruising, hematoma, cold/clammy skin, skin discoloration, dry skin. **Musculoskeletal:** Muscle cramps, pain, or inflammation; joint stiffness or pain, arthritis, twitching, ataxia, hypertonia. **GU:** Polyuria, dysuria, urinary frequency, nocturia, sexual difficulties. **Respiratory:** Nasal or chest congestion, sinusitis, rhinitis, SOB, dyspnea, wheezing, cough, chest pain. **Ophthalmologic:** Diplopia, abnormal vision, conjunctivitis, eye pain, abnormal visual accommodation, xerophthalmia. **Miscellaneous:** Tinnitus, flushing, sweating, weight gain, epistaxis, anorexia, increased appetite, taste perversion, parosmia.

ADDITIONAL DRUG INTERACTIONS
Diltiazem ↑ Plasma levels of amlodipine → further ↓ BP
Grapefruit juice / ↑ Plasma amlodipine levels

HOW SUPPLIED
Tablet: 2.5 mg, 5 mg, 10 mg

DOSAGE
• **TABLETS**
Hypertension.
Adults, usual, individualized: 5 mg/day, up to a maximum of 10 mg/day. Titrate the dose over 7–14 days.
Chronic stable or vasospastic angina.
Adults: 5–10 mg, using the lower dose for elderly clients and those with hepatic insufficiency. Most clients require 10 mg.

NURSING CONSIDERATIONS
ⓒ Do not confuse amlodipine with amiloride (a diuretic).

ADMINISTRATION/STORAGE
1. Food does not affect the bioavailability of amlodipine.
2. Elderly clients, small/fragile clients, or those with hepatic insufficiency may be started on 2.5 mg/day. This dose may also be used when adding amlodipine to other antihypertensive therapy.
3. Can be given safely with ACE inhibitors, beta-blockers, nitrates (long-acting), nitroglycerin (sublingual), or thiazides.

ASSESSMENT
1. Note indications for therapy and any history of CAD or CHF.
2. Review list of drugs currently prescribed to prevent interactions.

3. Monitor VS, ECG, CBC, renal and LFTs. Reduce dose in the elderly and clients with liver dysfunction.

CLIENT/FAMILY TEACHING
1. Take only as directed, once daily. May take with or without meals; food helps decrease stomach upset.
2. Report any symptoms of chest pain, SOB, dizziness, swelling of extremities, irregular pulse, or altered vision immediately. Record BP and pulse.
3. Use caution, may experience lightheadedness or dizziness.

OUTCOMES/EVALUATE
• Desired BP control
• ↓ Frequency/intensity of angina

Anagrelide hydrochloride

(an-**AG**-greh-lyd)

CLASSIFICATION(S):
Antiplatelet drug
PREGNANCY CATEGORY: C
Rx: Agrylin

ACTION/KINETICS
May act to reduce platelets by decreasing megakaryocyte hypermaturation; possible disruption in the postmitotic phase of megakaryocyte development and a reduction in megakaryocyte size and ploidy. Does not cause significant changes in white cell counts or coagulation parameters. Inhibits platelet aggregation at higher doses than needed to reduce platelet count. **Peak plasma levels:** 5 ng/mL at 1 hr. **t½:** 1.3 hr; **terminal t½:** About 3 days. Food modestly reduces bioavailability. Extensively metabolized in liver and excreted in urine and feces.

USES
Reduce elevated platelet count and the risk of thrombosis in thrombocythemia, secondary to myeloproliferative disorders; also to reduce associated symptoms, including thrombo-hemorrhagic events.

CONTRAINDICATIONS
Lactation.

SPECIAL CONCERNS
Use with caution in known or suspected heart disease and in impaired renal or hepatic function. Safety and efficacy have not been determined in those less than 16 years of age.

SIDE EFFECTS
CV: CHF, palpitations, chest pain, tachycardia, arrhythmias, angina pectoris, postural hypotension, hypertension, CVD, vasodilation, migraine, syncope, *MI, cardiomyopathy, CHB, fibrillation, CVA, pericarditis, hemorrhage, heart failure, pericardial effusion, thrombosis,* cardiomegaly, AF. **GI:** Diarrhea, abdominal pain, pancreatitis, gastric/duodenal ulcers, N&V, flatulence, anorexia, dyspepsia, constipation, GI distress, *GI hemorrhage,* gastritis, melena, aphthous stomatitis, eructations. **Respiratory:** Rhinitis, pharyngitis, cough, epistaxis, respiratory disease, sinusitis, pneumonia, bronchitis, asthma, pulmonary infiltrate, *pulmonary fibrosis, pulmonary hypertension, plerual effusion,* pulmonary infiltrates, dyspnea. **CNS:** Headache, *seizures,* dizziness, paresthesia, depression, somnolence, confusion, insomnia, nervousness, amnesia, asthenia. **Musculoskeletal:** Arthralgia, myalgia, leg cramps. **Dermatologic:** Pruritus, skin disease, alopecia, rash, urticaria. **Hematologic:** Anemia, thrombocytopenia, ecchymosis, lymphadenoma. **GU:** Dysuria, hematuria. **Body as a whole:** Fever, flu symptoms, chills, photosensitivity, dehydration, malaise, asthenia, edema, peripheral edema, pain. **Ophthalmic:** Amblyopia, abnormal vision, visual field abnormality, diplopia. **Miscellaneous:** Back pain, tinnitus.

LABORATORY TEST CONSIDERATIONS
↑ Liver enzymes.

OD **OVERDOSE MANAGEMENT**
Symptoms: Thrombocytopenia. *Treatment:* Close clinical monitoring. Decrease or stop dose until platelet count returns to the normal range.

DRUG INTERACTIONS
H *Evening primrose oil* / Potential for ↑ antiplatelet effect
H *Feverfew* / Potential for ↑ antiplatelet effect

Bold Italic = life threatening side effect   ▓ = black box warning   ♣ = Available in Canada

H *Garlic* / Potential for ↑ antiplatelet effect

H *Ginger* / Potential for ↑ antiplatelet effect

H *Ginkgo biloba* / Potential for ↑ antiplatelet effect

H *Ginseng* / Potential for ↑ antiplatelet effect

H *Grapeseed extract* / Potential for ↑ antiplatelet effect

HOW SUPPLIED
Capsules: 0.5 mg, 1 mg

DOSAGE
• **CAPSULES**
Thrombocythemia.
Initial: 0.5 mg 4 x/day or 1 mg twice a day. Maintain for one week or more. **Then,** adjust to lowest effective dose to maintain platelet count less than 600,000/mcL. Can increase the dose by 0.5 mg or less/day in any 1 week. **Maximum dose:** 10 mg/day or 2.5 mg in single dose. Most respond at a dose of 1.5 to 3 mg/day.

NURSING CONSIDERATIONS
ASSESSMENT
1. Document etiology, onset, and duration of thrombocythemia.
2. Note any CAD, liver or renal dysfunction; document cardiovascular assessment and monitor closely.
3. Monitor VS, CBC, liver and renal function; check platelets every 2 days during first week and then weekly thereafter until stabilized.
4. Determine if pregnant.

CLIENT/FAMILY TEACHING
1. Take exactly as directed. Keep all F/U visits to monitor labs and assess drug response.
2. Drug is used to lower platelet counts. Increases usually occur within 4 days after therapy stopped.
3. Practice reliable contraception; may cause fetal harm.
4. Report any palpitations, fever/chills, SOB, dizziness, chest/abdominal pain, or unusual bleeding.

OUTCOMES/EVALUATE
Reduction in platelet counts; ↓ risk of thrombosis

Anistreplase
(an-ih-**STREP**-layz)

A

CLASSIFICATION(S):
Thrombolytic enzyme
PREGNANCY CATEGORY: C
Rx: Eminase

ACTION/KINETICS
Prepared by acylating human plasma derived from lys-plasminogen and purified streptokinase derived from group C beta-hemolytic streptococci. When prepared, anistreplase is an inactive derivative of a fibrinolytic enzyme although the compound can still bind to fibrin. Anistreplase is activated by deacylation and subsequent release of the anisoyl group in the blood stream. The production of plasmin from plasminogen occurs in both the blood stream and the thrombus leading to thrombolysis. Lyses thrombi obstructing coronary arteries and reduces the size of infarcts. **t ½:** 70–120 min.

USES
Management of AMI in adults, for lysis of thrombi obstructing coronary arteries, reduction of infarct size, improvement of ventricular function, and reduction of mortality. Initiate treatment as soon as possible after the onset of symptoms of AMI.

CONTRAINDICATIONS
Use in active internal bleeding; within 2 months of intracranial or intraspinal surgery; recent trauma, including cardiopulmonary resuscitation; history of CVA; intracranial neoplasm; arteriovenous malformation or aneurysm; known bleeding diathesis; severe, uncontrolled hypertension; severe allergic reactions to streptokinase.

SPECIAL CONCERNS
Use with caution in nursing mothers. Safety and effectiveness have not been determined in children.
NOTE: Because the risks of anistreplase therapy may be increased in the following conditions, benefit versus risk must be assessed prior to use: Within 10 days of major surgery (e.g., CABG, obstetric

A

delivery, organ biopsy, previous puncture of noncompressible vessels); cerebrovascular disease; within 10 days of GI or GU bleeding; within 10 days of trauma including cardiopulmonary resuscitation; SBP > 180 mm Hg or DBP > 110 mm Hg; likelihood of left heart thrombus (e.g., mitral stenosis with atrial fibrillation); SBE; acute pericarditis; hemostatic defects including those secondary to severe hepatic or renal disease; pregnancy; clients older than 75 years of age; diabetic hemorrhagic retinopathy or other hemorrhagic ophthalmic conditions; septic thrombophlebitis or occluded arteriovenous cannula at seriously infected site; clients on oral anticoagulant therapy; any condition in which bleeding constitutes a significant hazard or would be difficult to manage due to its location.

SIDE EFFECTS
Bleeding: Including at the puncture site (most common), nonpuncture site hematoma, hematuria, hemoptysis, *GI hemorrhage, intracranial bleeding,* gum/mouth hemorrhage, epistaxis, anemia, eye hemorrhage. **CV:** *Arrhythmias,* conduction disorders, hypotension; *cardiac rupture,* chest pain, emboli (causal relationship to use of anistreplase unknown). **Allergic:** *Anaphylaxis, bronchospasm, angioedema,* urticaria, itching, flushing, rashes, eosinophilia, delayed purpuric rash which may be associated with arthralgia, ankle edema, mild hematuria, GI symptoms, and proteinuria. **GI:** N&V. **Hematologic:** Thrombocytopenia. **CNS:** Agitation, dizziness, paresthesia, tremor, vertigo. **Respiratory:** Dyspnea, lung edema. **Miscellaneous:** Chills, fever, headache, shock.

LABORATORY TEST CONSIDERATIONS
↑ Transaminase levels, thrombin time, activated PTT, and PT. ↓ Plasminogen and fibrinogen.

DRUG INTERACTIONS
↑ Risk of bleeding or hemorrhage if used with heparin, oral anticoagulants, vitamin K antagonists, aspirin, or dipyridamole.

HOW SUPPLIED
Powder for injection, lyophilized: 30 units

DOSAGE
IV only: 30 units over 2–5 min into an IV line or vein as soon as possible after onset of symptoms.

NURSING CONSIDERATIONS
ADMINISTRATION/STORAGE
IV 1. To reconstitute, slowly add 5 mL of sterile water. To minimize foaming, gently roll vial after directing sterile water stream against the side of the vial. Do not shake.
2. The reconstituted solution should be colorless to pale yellow without particulate matter or discoloration.
3. Do not further dilute the reconstituted solution before administration. Give IV over 2-5 min.
4. Do not add reconstituted solution to any infusion fluids; do not add any other medications to the vial or syringe.
5. Discard if not administered within 30 min of reconstitution.

ASSESSMENT
1. Note any history and/or evidence of excessive bleeding.
2. Take a full drug history, noting any aspirin, anticoagulant, or vitamin K antagonist use.
3. Note resistance to the effects of anistreplase, which may be observed if given between 5 days and 12 months after a previous dose, after streptokinase therapy, or after a streptococcal infection.
4. Increased antistreptokinase antibody levels between 5 days and 6 months after anistreplase or streptokinase administration may increase the risk of allergic reactions.
5. Obtain baseline hematologic parameters, type and cross, coagulation studies, cardiac marker panel, and renal function studies.
6. Assess neuro status and monitor closely during/following therapy.

INTERVENTIONS
1. Avoid invasive procedures to minimize bleeding potential. Post bleeding precautions sign.
2. If an arterial puncture is necessary following use of anistreplase, use an upper extremity vessel accessible to compression. Apply 30 min of manual pres-

---

Bold Italic = life threatening side effect   ■ = black box warning   ✦ = Available in Canada

sure followed by application of a pressure dressing. Check puncture site frequently for bleeding.
3. Monitor ECG closely and document any reperfusion arrhythmias.

CLIENT/FAMILY TEACHING
1. Review goals of therapy and inherent risks during acute MI.
2. To be effective, therapy should be instituted as soon as possible after onset of S&S of MI.
3. Expect cardiac scans/imaging post infusion to assess effectiveness.
4. Use caution, risk for bleeding may continue 2-4 days after infusion.
5. Encourage family members to learn CPR.

OUTCOMES/EVALUATE
• Thrombolysis with restoration of blood flow to ischemic cardiac tissue
• ↓ Infarct size; ↓ mortality; Improved ventricular function

Argatroban
(are-**GAT**-roh-ban)

CLASSIFICATION(S):
Anticoagulant, thrombin inhibitor
PREGNANCY CATEGORY: B

ACTION/KINETICS
A synthetic, direct thrombin inhibitor derived from L-arginine. Reversibly binds to the thrombin active site and does not require antithrombin III for antithrombotic activity. Acts by inhibiting thrombin-catalyzed or induced reactions, including fibrin formation; activation of coagulation factors V, VIII, and XIII; protein C; and platelet aggregation. Inhibits both free and clot-associated thrombin. The small molecule provides the needed anticoagulant effect without worsening hypercoagulable states. Has little or no effect on trypsin, Factor Xa, plasmin, and kallikrein. Does not interact with heparin-induced antibodies. Distributes mainly in the extracellular fluid. Steady state reached, by IV infusion, in 1–3 hr and is continued until infusion is stopped. Metabolized in the liver by cytochrome P450 enzymes

(CYP3A4/5). **t ½, terminal:** 39–51 min. Excreted in the feces, primarily through biliary excretion.

USES
(1) Prophylaxis or treatment of thrombosis in heparin-induced thrombocytopenia. (2) Anticoagulant in those with or at risk for heparin-induced thrombocytopenia undergoing percutaneous coronary intervention.

CONTRAINDICATIONS
Overt major bleeding, hypersensitivity to the product or any of its components. Concomitant use of heparin. Lactation.

SPECIAL CONCERNS
Use with caution in hepatic disease and in disease states and circumstances with an increased danger of hemorrhage, including severe hypertension, immediately following lumbar puncture, spinal anesthesia, major surgery (especially the brain, spinal cord, or eye), congenital or acquired bleeding disorders, and GI lesions (e.g., ulcerations). Hemorrhage can occur at any site in the body. Safety and efficacy have not been determined in children less than 18 years of age.

SIDE EFFECTS
Bleeding: Major hemorrhagic events, including GI, GU/hematuria, decreased H&H, multisystem hemorrhage and DIC, limb and below the knee amputation stump, *intracranial hemorrhage, retroperitoneal hemorrhage*. Minor hemorrhagic events, including GI, GU/hematuria, groin, hemoptysis, brachial. Intracranial bleeding in clients with acute MI started on argatroban and streptokinase. **Allergic:** Airway reactions (coughing, dyspnea), rash, bullous eruption, vasodilation. **GI:** Diarrhea, N&V, GERD, abdominal pain, *GI hemorrhage*. **CV:** Hypotension, aortic stenosis, *cardiac arrest, VT, MI, coronary thrombosis, myocardial ischemia, coronary occlusion, arterial thrombosis*, cerebrovascular/vascular disorder, bradycardia, angina pectoris, atrial fibrillation. **Respiratory:** Dyspnea, pneumonia, coughing, lung edema. **GU:** UTI, abnormal renal function. **Miscellaneous:** Fever, pain,

infection, abdominal pain, back pain, chest pain, headache, **sepsis**.

LABORATORY TEST CONSIDERATIONS

Coadministration of argatroban and warfarin produces a combined effect on laboratory measurement of INR. However, concurrent therapy exerts no additional effect on vitamin K-dependent Factor Xa activity, compared with warfarin monotherapy.

OD OVERDOSE MANAGEMENT

Symptoms: Major/minor bleeding events. *Treatment:* Discontinue argatroban or decrease infusion dose. Anticoagulation parameters usually return to baseline within 2–4 hr after discontinuing the drug. Reversal may take longer in hepatic impairment. No specific antidote is available. Provide symptomatic and supportive therapy.

DRUG INTERACTIONS

Concomitant use with antiplatelet drugs, thrombolytics, and other anticoagulants ↑ risk of bleeding (prolongation of PT and INR).

HOW SUPPLIED

Injection: 100 mg/mL

DOSAGE

• **IV INFUSION**

Heparin-induced thrombocytopenia (HIT) or heparin-induced thrombocytopenia and thrombosis syndrome (HITTS).

Adults, initial, without hepatic impairment: 2 mcg/kg/min as a continuous IV infusion. The infusion rate depends on body weight (see package insert). After the initial dose, adjust dose as clinically indicated, not to exceed 10 mcg/kg/min, until the steady state aPTT is 1.5–3 times initial baseline value, not to exceed 100 seconds.

Percutaneous coronary intervention in HIT/HITTS:

Adults, initial: Start a continuous infusion at 25 mcg/kg/min and a bolus of 350 mcg/kg given via a large bore IV line over 3–5 min. Check activated clotting time (ACT) 5–10 min after the bolus dose is completed. If the ACT is greater than 450 seconds, decrease the infusion rate to 15 mcg/kg/min and check the ACT 5–10 min later. Once an ACT between 300 and 450 sec has been reached, continue this infusion for the duration of the procedure. In the event of dissection, impending abrupt closure, thrombus formation during the procedure, or inability to achieve or maintain ACT over 300 sec, give additional bolus doses of 150 mcg/kg and increase the infusion dose to 40 mcg/kg/min. Check ACT after each additional bolus or change in infusion rate.

Impaired hepatic function (for all uses).

Adults, initial, moderate hepatic impairment: 0.5 mcg/kg/min, based on about a 4-fold decrease in argatroban clearance compared with normal hepatic function.

NURSING CONSIDERATIONS

ADMINISTRATION/STORAGE

IV 1. Discontinue all parenteral anticoagulants before giving argatroban.

2. If argatroban is begun after cessation of heparin, allow sufficient time for the effects of heparin on the aPTT to decrease before starting argatroban therapy.

3. To prepare for IV infusion, dilute argatroban in 0.9% NaCl, D5W, or LR injection to a final concentration of 1 mg/mL. Thus, dilute each 2.5 mL vial 100-fold by mixing with 250 mL of diluent.

4. Mix the reconstituted solution by repeated inversion of the diluent bag for 1 min. After preparation, the solution may be briefly hazy due to the formation of microprecipitates. These dissolve rapidly upon mixing.

5. If prepared correctly, the pH of the IV solution is 3.2–7.5.

6. Use of argatroban and warfarin results in prolongation of INR beyond that caused by warfarin alone. Measure INR daily if argatroban and warfarin are given together. Generally, with doses of argatroban of 2 mcg/kg/min or less, argatroban can be discontinued when the INR is greater than 4 on combined therapy. After argatroban is discontinued, repeat INR measurement in 4–6 hr. If the repeat INR is below the desired range, resume argatroban infusion and repeat the procedure daily until the de-

sired therapeutic range on warfarin alone is reached.

7. For doses of argatroban greater than 2 mcg/kg/min, the relationship of INR on warfarin alone to the INR of both drugs given together is less predictable. Thus, temporarily reduce the dose of argatroban to 2 mcg/kg/min. Repeat the INR on argatroban and warfarin 4–6 hr after reducing the argatroban dose and follow the process outlined above for giving argatroban at doses of 2 mcg/kg/min or less.

8. Argatroban is a clear, colorless to pale yellow, slightly viscous solution. Discard vial if the solution is cloudy or an insoluble precipitate is observed.

9. Prepared solutions are stable at 15–30°C (59–85°F) for 24 hr at ambient indoor light. Prepared solutions are stable for 48 hr or less when stored at 2–8°C (36–46°F) in the dark. Do not expose prepared solutions to direct sunlight.

ASSESSMENT

1. Note indications for therapy: thrombosis prophylaxis or treatment.

2. Review history noting any conditions that may preclude drug therapy. Note active bleeding sites/disorders.

3. Stop heparin therapy. Obtain and monitor weight, INR, PT/PTT, CBC, and LFTs. Lower dosage with liver dysfunction.

4. Observe closely for evidence of abnormal bleeding or adverse effects. Perform routine vascular checks.

CLIENT/FAMILY TEACHING

1. Review goals of therapy and potential bleeding risks.

2. Report any unusual oozing or bleeding sites and wet bandages or bedding.

3. Encourage family members to learn CPR.

OUTCOMES/EVALUATE

Inhibition/treatment of thrombus formation with HIT

Aspirin ■ A
(Acetylsalicylic acid, ASA)

(ah-**SEE**-till-sal-ih-**SILL**-ick **AH**-sid)

CLASSIFICATION(S):
Nonsteroidal anti-inflammatory drug, analgesic, antipyretic
PREGNANCY CATEGORY: C
OTC: Gum Tablets: Aspergum. **Caplets/Tablets:** Arthritis Foundation Pain Reliever, Empirin, Genprin, Genuine Bayer Aspirin Caplets and Tablets, Maximum Bayer Aspirin Caplets and Tablets, Norwich Extra Strength. **Tablets,** Chewable: Bayer Children's Aspirin, St. Joseph Adult Chewable Aspirin. **Tablets, Enteric Coated:** Ecotrin Adult Low Strength, Ecotrin Caplets and Tablets, Ecotrin Maximum Strength Caplets and Tablets, Extra Strength Bayer Enteric 500 Aspirin, $\frac{1}{2}$ Halfprin, Halfprin 81, Heartline, Regular Strength Bayer Enteric Coated Caplets. **Tablets, Controlled/Extended Release:** Bayer Low Adult Strength, Extended Release Bayer 8-Hour Caplets.
Rx: Easprin, ZORprin
♣**OTC:** Asaphen, Asaphen E.C., Entrophen, MSD Enteric Coated ASA, Novasen

Aspirin, buffered
PREGNANCY CATEGORY: C
OTC: Caplets: Asprimox, Asprimox Extra Protection for Arthritis Pain, Extra Strength Bayer Plus Caplets. **Caplets/Tablets:** Arthritis Pain Formula, Asprimox Extra Protection for Arthritis Pain, Bayer Buffered Aspirin, Buffered Aspirin, Buffex, Cama Arthritis Pain Reliever, Tri-Buffered Bufferin Caplets and Tablets. **Tablets, Coated:** Adprin-B, Ascriptin, Ascriptin A/D, Ascriptin Extra Strength, Asprimox, Bufferin, Extra-Strength Adprin-B, Magnaprin, Magnaprin Arthritis Strength Cap-

A

tabs. **Tablets, Effervescent:** Alka-Seltzer with Aspirin, Alka-Seltzer with Aspirin (Flavored), Alka-Seltzer Extra Strength with Aspirin.

SEE ALSO *NONSTEROIDAL ANTI-INFLAMMATORY DRUGS*

ACTION/KINETICS

Exhibits antipyretic, anti-inflammatory, and analgesic effects. The antipyretic effect is due to an action on the hypothalamus, resulting in heat loss by vasodilation of peripheral blood vessels and promoting sweating. The anti-inflammatory effects are probably mediated through inhibition of cyclo-oxygenase, which results in a decrease in prostaglandin (implicated in the inflammatory response) synthesis and other mediators of the pain response. The mechanism of action for the analgesic effects of aspirin is not known fully but is partly attributable to improvement of the inflammatory condition. Aspirin also produces inhibition of platelet aggregation by decreasing the synthesis of endoperoxides and thromboxanes—substances that mediate platelet aggregation.

Large doses of aspirin (5 g/day or more) increase uric acid secretion, while low doses (2 g/day or less) decrease uric acid secretion. However, aspirin antagonizes drugs used to treat gout.

Rapidly absorbed after PO administration. Is hydrolyzed to the active salicylic acid, which is 70–90% protein bound. **Blood levels for arthritis and rheumatic disease:** Maintain 150–300 mcg/mL. **Blood levels for analgesic and antipyretic:** 25–50 mcg/mL. **Blood levels for acute rheumatic fever:** 150–300 mcg/mL. Tinnitus occurs at serum levels above 200 mcg/mL and serious toxicity above 400 mcg/mL. **t ½:** aspirin, 15–20 min; salicylic acid, 2–20 hr, depending on the dose. Salicylic acid and metabolites are excreted by the kidney. The bioavailability of enteric-coated salicylate products may be poor. The addition of antacids (buffered aspirin) may decrease GI irritation and increase the dissolution and absorption of such products.

USES

Analgesic: (1) Pain from integumental structures, myalgias, neuralgias, arthralgias, headache, dysmenorrhea, and similar types of pain. (2) Gout. (3) May be effective in less severe postoperative and postpartum pain; pain secondary to trauma and cancer. **Antipyretic, Anti-Inflammatory:** Arthritis, osteoarthritis, SLE, acute rheumatic fever, gout, and many other conditions. Mucocutaneous lymph node syndrome (Kawasaki disease). **Cardiovascular:** Despite the increased risk of GI bleeding, low-dose aspirin should be used for the following CV events:

1. Reduce risk of death and nonfatal stroke in those who have had an ischemic stroke or TIA; also combined with dipyridamole for this purpose.
2. Reduce risk of vascular mortality with suspected acute MI.
3. Reduce the combined risk of recurrent MI and death after an MI or unstable angina.
4. Reduce risk of MI and sudden death in chronic stable angina.
5. Pre-existing need for aspirin following coronary artery bypass grafting, PTCA, or carotid endarterectomy.
6. Used with ticlopidine as adjunctive therapy to reduce development of subacute stent thrombosis.
7. *Investigational:* Reduce risk of heart problems in healthy adults with a small risk of heart attack and no history of CV disease. Includes men over 40 years of age, postmenopausal women, and younger people with risk factors including, smoking, diabetes, hypertension, and high cholesterol.

Chronic use to prevent cataract formation; low doses to prevent toxemia of pregnancy; in pregnant women with inadequate uteroplacental blood flow. Reduce colon cancer mortality (low doses). Low doses of aspirin and warfarin to reduce risk of a second heart attack. In addition to treatment for CV risk factors, may reduce risk of dying from heart attack or stroke significantly.

CONTRAINDICATIONS

Hypersensitivity to salicylates. Clients with asthma, hay fever, or nasal polyps

---

Bold Italic = life threatening side effect   ▪ = black box warning   ✚ = Available in Canada

have a higher incidence of hypersensitivity reactions. Severe anemia, history of blood coagulation defects, in conjunction with anticoagulant therapy. Salicylates can cause congestive failure when taken in the large doses used for rheumatic diseases. Vitamin K deficiency; 1 week before and after surgery. In pregnancy, especially the last trimester as the drug may cause problems in the newborn child or complications during delivery. In children or teenagers with chicken-pox or flu due to possibility of development of Reye's syndrome.

Controlled-release aspirin is not recommended for use as an antipyretic or short-term analgesic because adequate blood levels may not be reached. Also, controlled-release products are not recommended for children less than 12 years of age and in children with fever accompanied by dehydration.

SPECIAL CONCERNS

■Do not use in children or teenagers with chickenpox or flu symptoms due to the possibility of Reye's syndrome, a rare but serious illness.■ Use with caution during lactation and in the presence of gastric or peptic ulcers, in mild diabetes, erosive gastritis, bleeding tendencies, in cardiac disease, and in liver or kidney disease. Aspirin products now carry the following labeling: 'It is especially important not to use aspirin during the last three months of pregnancy unless specifically directed to do so by a doctor because it may cause problems in the newborn child or complications during delivery.' Regular use of NSAID's may diminish the cardioprotective benefit of aspirin.

SIDE EFFECTS

The toxic effects of the salicylates are dose-related.

GI: Dyspepsia, heartburn, anorexia, nausea, occult blood loss, epigastric discomfort, *massive GI bleeding, potentiation of peptic ulcer.* Possible stomach bleeding in those who ingest three or more alcoholic drinks/day. **Allergic:** *Bronchospasm, asthma-like symptoms, anaphylaxis,* skin rashes, angioedema, urticaria, rhinitis, nasal polyps. **Hematologic:** Prolongation of bleeding time, thrombocytopenia, leukopenia, purpura, shortened erythrocyte survival time, decreased plasma iron levels. **Miscellaneous:** Thirst, fever, dimness of vision.

NOTE: Use of aspirin in children and teenagers with flu or chickenpox may result in the development of *Reye's syndrome.* Also, dehydrated, febrile children are more prone to salicylate intoxication.

OD OVERDOSE MANAGEMENT

Symptoms of Mild Salicylate Toxicity (Salicylism): At serum levels between 150 and 200 mcg/mL. **GI:** N&V, diarrhea, thirst. **CNS:** Tinnitus (most common), dizziness, difficulty in hearing, mental confusion, lassitude. **Miscellaneous:** Flushing, sweating, tachycardia. Symptoms of salicylism may be observed with doses used for inflammatory disease or rheumatic fever. **Symptoms of Severe Salicylate Poisoning:** At serum levels over 400 mcg/mL. **CNS:** Excitement, confusion, disorientation, irritability, hallucinations, lethargy, stupor, *coma, respiratory failure, seizures.* **Metabolic:** Respiratory alkalosis (initially), respiratory acidosis and metabolic acidosis, dehydration. **GI:** N&V. **Hematologic:** Platelet dysfunction, hypoprothrombinemia, increased capillary fragility. **Miscellaneous:** *Hyperthermia, hemorrhage, CV collapse, renal failure,* hyperventilation, pulmonary edema, tetany, hypoglycemia (late).

Treatment (Toxicity):

1. If the client has had repeated administration of large doses of salicylates, document and report evidence of hyperventilation or complaints of auditory or visual disturbances (symptoms of salicylism).

2. Severe salicylate poisoning, whether due to overdose or accumulation, will have an exaggerated effect on the CNS and the metabolic system:

• Clients may develop a salicylate jag characterized by garrulous behavior. They may act as if they were inebriated.

• Convulsions and coma may follow.

3. When working with febrile children or the elderly who have been treated with aspirin, maintain adequate fluid in-

take. These clients are more susceptible to salicylate intoxication if they are dehydrated.

4. The following treatment approaches may be considered for treatment of *acute salicylate toxicity:*

• Initially induce vomiting or perform gastric lavage followed by activated charcoal (most effective if given within 2 hr of ingestion).

• Monitor salicylate levels and acid-base and fluid and electrolyte balance. If required, administer IV solutions of dextrose, saline, potassium, and sodium bicarbonate as well as vitamin K.

• Seizures may be treated with diazepam.

• Treat hyperthermia if present.

• Alkaline diuresis will enhance renal excretion. Hemodialysis is effective but should be reserved for severe poisonings.

• If necessary, administer oxygen and artificial ventilation

DRUG INTERACTIONS

ACE inhibitors / ↓ Effect of ACE inhibitors possibly due to prostaglandin inhibition; also, significantly higher mortality rate using doses of aspirin of at least 325 mg/day

Acetazolamide / ↑ CNS toxicity of salicylates; also, ↑ excretion of salicylic acid in alkaline urine

Alcohol, ethyl / ↑ Chance of GI bleeding caused by salicylates

Alteplase, recombinant / ↑ Risk of bleeding

Aminosalicylate / Possible ↑ effect of PAS due to ↓ excretion by kidney or ↓ plasma protein binding

Ammonium chloride / ↑ Effect of salicylates by ↑ renal tubular reabsorption

Antacids / ↓ Salicylate levels in plasma due to ↑ rate of renal excretion

Anticoagulants, oral / ↑ Effect of anticoagulant by ↓ plasma protein binding and plasma prothrombin

Antirheumatics / Both are ulcerogenic and may cause ↑ GI bleeding

Ascorbic acid / ↑ Effect of salicylates by ↑ renal tubular reabsorption

Beta-adrenergic blocking agents / Salicylates ↓ action of beta-blockers, possibly due to prostaglandin inhibition

Charcoal, activated / ↓ Absorption of salicylates from GI tract

Corticosteroids / Both are ulcerogenic; also, corticosteroids may ↓ blood salicylate levels by ↑ breakdown by liver and ↑ excretion

Dipyridamole / Additive anticoagulant effects

H *Feverfew* / Possible ↑ antiplatelet effect

Furosemide / ↑ Risk of salicylate toxicity due to ↓ renal excretion; also, salicylates may ↓ effect of furosemide in clients with impaired renal function or cirrhosis with ascites

H *Garlic* / Possible ↑ antiplatelet effect

H *Ginkgo biloba* / Possible ↑ effect on platelet aggregation

H *Ginseng* / Possible ↓ effect on platelet aggregation

Griseofulvin / ↓ Salicylate levels

Heparin / Inhibition of platelet adhesiveness by aspirin may result in bleeding tendencies

Hypoglycemics, oral / ↑ Hypoglycemia R/T ↓ plasma protein binding and ↓ excretion

Indomethacin / Both are ulcerogenic → ↑ GI bleeding

Insulin / Salicylates ↑ hypoglycemic effect of insulin

Methionine / ↑ Effect of salicylates by ↑ renal tubular reabsorption

Methotrexate / ↑ Methotrexate effect by ↓ plasma protein binding; also, salicylates block drugs' renal excretion

Nitroglycerin / Combination may result in unexpected hypotension

Nizatidine / ↑ Serum levels of salicylates

NSAIDs / Additive ulcerogenic effects; also, aspirin may ↓ serum levels of NSAIDs

Phenytoin / ↑ Phenytoin effect by ↓ plasma protein binding

Probenecid / Salicylates inhibit uricosuric activity of probenecid

Sodium bicarbonate / ↓ Effect of salicylates by ↑ rate of excretion

Spironolactone / Aspirin ↓ diuretic drug effect

Sulfinpyrazone / Salicylates inhibit uricosuric drug activity

---

Sulfonamides / ↑ Sulfonamides effect R/T displacement from plasma proteins
Valproic acid / ↑ Valproic effect R/T ↓ plasma protein binding

HOW SUPPLIED

Acetylsalicylic Acid. *Chew tablet:* 81 mg; *Enteric coated tablet:* 81 mg, 165 mg, 325 mg, 500 mg, 650 mg, 975 mg; *Gum:* 227.5 mg; *Suppository:* 120 mg, 200 mg, 300 mg, 600 mg; *Tablet:* 325 mg, 500 mg; *Tablet, Delayed Release:* 81 mg; *Tablet, Extended Release:* 650 mg, 800 mg. **Acetylsalicylic Acid, Buffered.** *Caplets:* 325 mg; *Tablets:* 325 mg, 500 mg; *Tablets, Coated:* 325 mg, 500 mg; *Tablets, Effervescent:* 325 mg, 500 mg.

DOSAGE

- **CAPLETS, GUM, CHEWABLE TAB-LETS, COATED TABLETS, EFFERVES-CENT TABLETS, ENTERIC-COATED TABLETS, TABLETS, SUPPOSITORIES, TABLETS DELAYED OR EXTENDED RE-LEASE**

Analgesic, antipyretic.
Adults: 325–500 mg q 3 hr, 325–600 mg q 4 hr, or 650–1,000 mg q 6 hr. As an alternative, the adult chewable tablet (81 mg each) may be used in doses of 4–8 tablets q 4 hr as needed. **Pediatric:** 65 mg/kg/day (alternate dose: 1.5 g/m²/day) in divided doses q 4–6 hr, not to exceed 3.6 g/day. Alternatively, the following dosage regimen can be used: **Pediatric, 2–3 years:** 162 mg q 4 hr as needed; **4–5 years:** 243 mg q 4 hr as needed; **6–8 years:** 320–325 mg q 4 hr as needed; **9–10 years:** 405 mg q 4 hr as needed; **11 years:** 486 mg q 4 hr as needed; **12–14 years:** 648 mg q 4 hr.
Arthritis, rheumatic diseases.
Adults: 3.2–6 g/day in divided doses.
Juvenile rheumatoid arthritis.
60–110 mg/kg/day (alternate dose: 3 g/m²/day) in divided doses q 6–8 hr. When initiating therapy at 60 mg/kg/day, dose may be increased by 20 mg/kg/day after 5–7 days and by 10 mg/kg/day after another 5–7 days.
Acute rheumatic fever.
Adults, initial: 5–8 g/day. **Pediatric, initial:** 100 mg/kg/day (3 g/m²/day) for 2 weeks; **then,** decrease to 75 mg/kg/day for 4–6 weeks.

Reduce risk of death and nonfatal stroke following ischemic stroke or TIA
50–325 mg/day.
Reduce risk of vascular mortality in suspected acute MI.
Initial: 160–162.5 mg, **then** daily for 30 days. Consider subsequent prophylactic therapy.
Reduce combined risk of recurrent MI and death in those with a previous MI or unstable angina or to reduce risk of MI and sudden death in those with chronic stable angina.
75–325 mg/day.
Pre-existing need for aspirin following coronary artery bypass grafting, PTCA, carotid endarterectomy.
Dosage varies by procedure.
Kawasaki disease.
Adults: 80–180 mg/kg/day during the febrile period. After the fever resolves, the dose may be adjusted to 10 mg/kg/day.
NOTE: Aspirin Regimen Bayer 81 mg with Calcium contains 250 mg calcium carbonate (10% of RDA) and 81 mg of acetylsalicylic acid for individuals who require aspirin to prevent recurrent heart attacks and strokes.

NURSING CONSIDERATIONS

ADMINISTRATION/STORAGE

1. Enteric-coated tablets or buffered tablets are better tolerated by some.
2. Take with a full glass of water to prevent lodging of the drug in the esophagus.
3. Have epinephrine available to counteract hypersensitivity reactions should they occur. Asthma caused by hypersensitivity reaction to salicylates may be refractory to epinephrine, so antihistamines should also be available for parenteral and PO use.

ASSESSMENT

1. Take a complete drug history and note any evidence of hypersensitivity. Individuals allergic to tartrazine should not take aspirin. Clients who have tolerated salicylates well in the past may suddenly have an allergic or anaphylactoid reaction.
2. If administered for pain, rate and determine the type and pattern of pain, if

A

the pain is unusual, or if it is recurring. Note the effectiveness of aspirin if previously used for pain.

3. Note if client has asthma, hay fever, ulcer disease or nasal polyps.

4. Document age; drug is discouraged in those under 12. Assess for chickenpox or the flu.

5. Test stool and urine for blood; monitor CBC routinely during high-dose and chronic therapy.

6. Determine if diagnostic tests scheduled. Drug causes irreversible platelet effects. Anticipate 4–7 days for the body to replace these once drug discontinued; hence no salicylates one week prior to procedure.

7. Determine any history of peptic ulcers or bleeding tendencies. Obtain bleeding parameters with prolonged use.

8. Review drugs currently prescribed for drug interactions.

9. The therapeutic serum level of salicylate is 150–300 mcg/mL for adult and juvenile rheumatoid arthritis and acute rheumatic fever. Reassure that the higher dosage is necessary for anti-inflammatory effects.

CLIENT/FAMILY TEACHING

1. Take only as directed. To reduce gastric irritation or lodging in the esophagus, administer with meals, milk, a full glass of water, or crackers.

2. Do not take salicylates if product is off-color or has a strange odor. Note expiration date.

3. Report any toxic effects: ringing in the ears, difficulty hearing, dizziness or fainting spells, unusual increase in sweating, severe abdominal pain, or mental confusion.

4. Salicylates potentiate the effects of antidiabetic drugs. Monitor FS and report low sugars.

5. When administering for antipyretic effect, follow temperature administration parameters.

• Obtain temperature 1 hr after administering to assess outcome.

• With marked diaphoresis, dry client, change linens, provide fluids, and prevent chilling.

6. Cardiac clients on large doses should report symptoms of CHF.

7. Tell dentist and other HCPs you are taking salicylates.

8. Before purchasing other OTC preparations, notify provider and note the quantity used per day.

9. Salicylates should be administered to children only upon specific medical recommendation due to increased risk of Reye's syndrome.

10. If child refuses medication or vomits it, consider aspirin suppositories or acetaminophen.

11. Children who are dehydrated and who have a fever are especially susceptible to aspirin intoxication from even small doses. Report any gastric irritation/pain; may be S&S of hypersensitivity or toxicity.

12. Sodium bicarbonate may decrease the serum level of aspirin, reducing its effectiveness.

13. Report any unusual bruising or bleeding. Large doses may increase PT and should be avoided. Aspirin and NSAIDs may interfere with blood-clotting mechanisms (antiplatelet effects) and are usually discontinued 1 week before surgery to prevent increased risk of bleeding.

14. Avoid indiscriminate use; store appropriately.

OUTCOMES/EVALUATE

• Relief of pain/discomfort; Improved joint mobility/function
• ↓ Fever; ↓ Vascular mortality
• ↓ Inflammation
• Prophylaxis of MI/TIA

Atenolol

(ah-**TEN**-oh-lohl)

CLASSIFICATION(S):
Beta-adrenergic blocking agent
PREGNANCY CATEGORY: C
Rx: Tenormin
✤Rx: Apo-Atenol, Gen-Atenolol, Novo-Atenol, Nu-Atenol, PMS-Atenolol, ratio-Atenolol, Rhoxal-atenolol

---

Bold Italic = life threatening side effect   ■ = black box warning   ✤ = Available in Canada

ACTION/KINETICS
Predominantly beta-1 blocking activity. Has no membrane stabilizing activity or intrinsic sympathomimetic activity. Low lipid solubility. **Peak blood levels:** 2–4 hr. **t½:** 6–9 hr. 50% eliminated unchanged in the feces. Geriatric clients have a higher plasma level than younger clients and a total clearance value of about 50% less.

USES
(1) Hypertension (either alone or with other antihypertensives such as thiazide diuretics). (2) Long-term treatment of angina pectoris due to coronary atherosclerosis. (3) Acute MI. *Investigational:* Prophylaxis of migraine, alcohol withdrawal syndrome, situational anxiety, ventricular arrhythmias, prophylactically to reduce incidence of supraventricular arrhythmias in coronary artery bypass graft surgery.

SPECIAL CONCERNS
Dosage not established in children.

HOW SUPPLIED
Injection: 0.5 mg/mL; *Tablet:* 25 mg, 50 mg, 100 mg

DOSAGE————
• **TABLETS**
Hypertension.
Initial: 50 mg/day, either alone or with diuretics; if response is inadequate, 100 mg/day. Doses higher than 100 mg/day will not produce further beneficial effects. Maximum effects usually seen within 1–2 weeks.
Angina.
Initial: 50 mg/day; if maximum response is not seen in 1 week, increase dose to 100 mg/day (some clients require 200 mg/day).
Alcohol withdrawal syndrome.
50–100 mg/day.
Prophylaxis of migraine.
50–100 mg/day.
Ventricular arrhythmias.
50–100 mg/day.
Prior to coronary artery bypass graft surgery.
50 mg/day started 72 hr prior to surgery.

Adjust dosage in cases of renal failure to 50 mg/day if C_{CR} is 15–35 mL/min/1.73 m^2 and to 50 mg every other day if C_{CR} is less than 15 mL/min/1.73 m^2.
• **IV**
Acute myocardial infarction.
Initial: 5 mg over 5 min followed by a second 5-mg dose 10 min later. Begin treatment as soon as possible after client arrives at the hospital. In clients who tolerate the full 10-mg dose, give a 50-mg tablet 10 min after the last IV dose followed by another 50-mg dose 12 hr later. **Then,** 100 mg/day or 50 mg twice a day for 6–9 days (or until discharge from the hospital).

NURSING CONSIDERATIONS

❦ Do not confuse atenolol with albuterol (sympathomimetic) or with timolol (beta-blocker).

ADMINISTRATION/STORAGE
1. For hemodialysis clients, give 25 or 50 mg in the hospital after each dialysis. Give under hospital supervision as significant decreases in BP may occur.
[IV] 2. For IV use, the drug may be diluted in NaCl injection, dextrose injection, or both.
3. If there is any question in using IV atenolol, eliminate IV administration and use tablets, 100 mg once daily or 50 mg twice a day for 7 or more days.

ASSESSMENT
1. Document indications for therapy, type, and onset of symptoms.
2. Note any history of diabetes, pulmonary disease, or cardiac failure.
3. List drugs prescribed to ensure none interact. Assess VS, EKG, and lung sounds.

CLIENT/FAMILY TEACHING
1. Take as directed at the same time each day. May take with food if GI upset occurs.
2. This is a beta blocker that lowers BP, and heart rate, controls angina and may decrease mortality from recurrent MI. With angina, do not stop abruptly; may cause an anginal attack.
3. Report any adverse effects or changes in mood or affect, especially severe depression and/or fatigue.
4. May enhance sensitivity to cold.

5. With initiation of therapy or change in dosage stress importance of returning as scheduled for evaluation of drug response. Keep log of HR and BP at different times during the day for provider review.

OUTCOMES/EVALUATE
- ↓ BP; ↓ HR
- ↓ Frequency of anginal attacks
- Prevention of repeat infarction

Atorvastatin calcium
(ah-**TORE**-vah-**stah**-tin)

CLASSIFICATION(S):
Antihyperlipidemic, HMG-CoA reductase inhibitor
PREGNANCY CATEGORY: X
Rx: Lipitor

SEE ALSO *ANTIHYPERLIPIDEMIC AGENTS— HMG-COA REDUCTASE INHIBITORS.*

ACTION/KINETICS
Undergoes first-pass metabolism by CYP3A4 enzymes to active metabolites. **t ½:** 14 hr. Plasma levels are not affected by renal disease but they are markedly increased with chronic alcoholic liver disease. Metabolized in the liver to active metabolites. Decreases in LDL cholesterol range from 35–40% (10 mg/day) to 50–60% (80 mg/day). Less than 2% excreted in the urine. Greater than 98% bound to plasma proteins.

USES
(1) Adjunct to diet to decrease elevated total and LDL cholesterol, apo-B, and triglyceride levels and to increase HDL cholesterol in primary hypercholesterolemia (including heterozygous familial and nonfamilial) and mixed dyslipidemia (including Frederickson type IIa and IIb). (2) Adjunct to other lipid-lowering treatments to reduce total and LDL cholesterol in homozygous familial hypercholesterolemia. (3) Primary dysbetalipoproteinemia (Frederickson type III) in those not responding adequately to diet. (4) Adjunct to diet to treat elevated serum triglyceride levels (Frederickson type IV). (5) Adjunct to diet to reduce total and LDL cholesterol and apo-B levels in boys and postmenarchal girls 10–17 years of age with heterozygous familial hypercholesterolemia; used after a trial of diet therapy if the following are present: (a) LDL cholesterol remains 190 mg/dL or higher or (b) LDL remains 160 mg/dL or higher AND there is a positive family history of premature CV disease or two or more other CVD risk factors are present. (6) Prophylaxis of CV disease by reducing the risk of MI, revascularization, and angina in adults without clinically evident coronary heart disease but with multiple risk factors (e.g., diabetes, smoking, normal to mildly elevated cholesterol levels) for it.

CONTRAINDICATIONS
Active liver disease or unexplained persistently high LFTs. Use with grapefruit juice. Pregnancy, lactation.

SPECIAL CONCERNS
Safety and efficacy have not been determined in children less than 18 years of age.

SIDE EFFECTS
SEE ALSO *ANTIHYPERLIPIDEMIC AGENTS— HMG-COA REDUCTASE INHIBITORS.*
GI: Altered LFTs (usually within the first 3 months of therapy), flatulence, dyspepsia. **CNS:** Headache, paresthesia, asthenia, insomnia. **Musculoskeletal:** Myalgia, leg pain, back pain, arthritis, arthralgia. **Respiratory:** Sinusitis, bronchitis, pharyngitis, rhinitis. **Miscellaneous:** Infection, rash, pruritus, allergy, influenza, accidental trauma, peripheral edema, chest pain, alopecia.

LABORATORY TEST CONSIDERATIONS
↑ CPK (due to myalgia).

DRUG INTERACTIONS

ADDITIONAL DRUG INTERACTIONS
Antacids / ↓ Atorvastatin plasma levels
Clarithromycin / ↑ Atorvastatin plasma levels; possibility of severe myopathy or rhabdomyolysis
Colestipol / ↓ Atorvastatin plasma levels
Digoxin / ↑ Digoxin levels after 80 mg atorvastatin R/T ↑ digoxin absorption
Diltiazem / ↑ Plasma atorvastatin levels → ↑ risk of myopathy

---

Erythromycin / ↑ Atorvastatin plasma levels; possibility of severe myopathy or rhabdomyolysis
Nefazodone / ↑ RIsk of myopathy
Oral contraceptives / ↑ Plasma levels of norethindrone and ethinyl estradiol
Protease inhibitors (e.g., nelfinavir, ritonavir) / ↑ Atorvastatin levels → ↑ risk of myopathy
Verapamil ↑ Risk of myopathy

HOW SUPPLIED
Tablets: 10 mg, 20 mg, 40 mg, 80 mg

DOSAGE
- **TABLETS**

  Hypercholesterolemia (heterozygous familial and non-familial) and mixed dyslipidemia (Fredrieksen type IIa and IIb).
  Initial: 10–20 mg once daily (40 mg/day for those who require more than a 45% reduction in LDL cholesterol); **then,** a dose range of 10–80 mg once daily may be used. Individualize therapy according to goal of therapy and response.
  Homozygous familial hypercholesterolemia.
  10–80 mg/day. Used as an adjunct to other lipid-lowering treatments.
  Heterozygous familial hypercholesterolemia in children 10–17 years of age.
  Initial: 10 mg/day; **then,** individualize dosage to a maximum of 20 mg/day. Adjust dosage at 4–week or more intervals.
  Prophylaxis of CV disease.
  Adults: 10 mg/day.

NURSING CONSIDERATIONS
ADMINISTRATION/STORAGE
1. Give as a single dose at any time of the day, with or without food.
2. Determine lipid levels within 2–4 weeks; adjust dosage accordingly.
3. For an additive effect, may be used in combination with a bile acid binding resin. Do not use atorvastatin with fibrates.

ASSESSMENT
1. Document indications for therapy, onset and duration of disease, and other agents and measures trialed.
2. Obtain baseline cholesterol profile and LFTs. Monitor LFTs at 6 and 12

weeks after starting therapy and with any dosage change, then semiannually thereafter. If ALT or AST exceed 3 times the normal level, reduce dose or withdraw drug. Assess need for liver biopsy if elevations remain after stopping drug therapy.
3. Review dietary habits, weight, and exercise patterns; identify life-style changes needed.

CLIENT/FAMILY TEACHING
1. These drugs help to lower blood cholesterol and fat levels, which have been proven to promote CAD.
2. Take drug at the same time each day with or without food; avoid alcohol.
3. Continue dietary restrictions of saturated fat and cholesterol, regular exercise and weight loss in the overall goal of lowering cholesterol levels. See dietician for additional dietary recommendations.
4. Report immediately any unexplained muscle pain, weakness, or tenderness, especially if accompanied by fever or malaise.
5. Use UV protection (i.e., sunglasses, sunscreens, clothing/hat) to prevent photosensitivity. Avoid prolonged exposure to direct or artificial sunlight.
6. Practice reliable birth control; may cause fetal damage.
7. Report for lab studies to evaluate effectiveness and need for dosage adjustments.

OUTCOMES/EVALUATE
Reduction in total and LDL cholesterol levels

Atropine sulfate
(**AH**-troh-peen)

CLASSIFICATION(S):
Cholinergic blocking drug
PREGNANCY CATEGORY: C
Rx: Atropair, AtroPen, Atropine Sulfate Ophthalmic, Atropine-1 Ophthalmic, Atropine-Care Ophthalmic, Atropisol Ophthalmic, Isopto Atropine Ophthalmic, Sal-Tropine
✦Rx: Minims Atropine

H = Herbal   IV = Intravenous   ℞ = sound-alike drug

A

SEE ALSO *CHOLINERGIC BLOCKING AGENTS.*

ACTION/KINETICS

Blocks acetylcholine effects on postganglionic cholinergic receptors in smooth muscle, cardiac muscle, exocrine glands, urinary bladder, and the AV and SA nodes in the heart. Ophthalmologically, blocks acetylcholine effects on the sphincter muscle of the iris and the accommodative muscle of the ciliary body. This results in dilation of the pupil (mydriasis) and paralysis of the muscles required to accommodate for close vision (cycloplegia). **Peak effect:** *Mydriasis,* 30–40 min; *cycloplegia,* 1–3 hr. **Recovery:** Up to 12 days. **Duration, PO:** 4–6 hr. **t ½:** 2.5 hr. Metabolized by the liver although 30–50% is excreted through the kidneys unchanged.

USES

PO:
1. Adjunct in peptic ulcer treatment.
2. Relieve pylorospasm, small intestine hypertonicity, and colon hypermotility.
3. Relax biliary and ureteral colic spasm and bronchial spasms.
4. Decrease tone of the detrusor muscle of the urinary bladder in treating urinary tract disorders.
5. Preanesthetic to control salivation and bronchial secretions.
6. Control rhinorrhea of acute rhinitis or hay fever.
7. Has been used for parkinsonism but more effective drugs are available.

Parenteral:
1. Restore cardiac rate and arterial pressure during anesthesia when vagal stimulation, due to intra-abdominal surgical traction, causes a sudden decrease in pulse rate and cardiac action.
2. Decrease degree of AV heart block when increased vagal tone is a major factor in the conduction defect (e.g., due to digitalis).
3. Overcome severe bradycardia and syncope due to hyperactive carotid sinus reflex.
4. Relax upper GI tract and colon during hypertonic radiography.
5. Antidote (with external cardiac massage) for CV collapse from toxicity due

to cholinergic drugs, pilocarpine, physostigmine, or isofluorophate.
6. Treat anticholinesterase poisoning from organophosphates; antidote for mushroom poisoning due to muscarine.
7. Poisoning by susceptible organophosphorus nerve agents having cholinesterase activity; also, poisoning due to organophosphorus or carbamate insecticides.
8. Control the crying and laughing episodes in clients with brain lesions.
9. Treat closed head injuries that cause acetylcholine to be released or be present in CSF, which causes abnormal EEG patterns, stupor, andneurological symptoms.
10. Relieve hypertonicity of uterine muscle.
11. As a preanesthetic or in dentistry to decrease secretions.

Ophthalmologic: Cycloplegic refraction or pupillary dilation in acute inflammatory conditions of the iris and uveal tract. *Investigational:* Treatment and prophylaxis of posterior synechiae; pre- and postoperative mydriasis; treatment of malignant glaucoma.

ADDITIONAL CONTRAINDICATIONS

Ophthalmic use: Infants less than 3 months of age, primary glaucoma or a tendency toward glaucoma, adhesions between the iris and the lens, geriatric clients and others where undiagnosed glaucoma or excessive pressure in the eye may be present, in children who have had a previous severe systemic reaction to atropine.

SPECIAL CONCERNS

Use with caution in infants, small children, geriatric clients, diabetes, hypo- or hyperthyroidism, narrow anterior chamber angle, individuals with Down syndrome.

ADDITIONAL SIDE EFFECTS

Ophthalmologic: Blurred vision, stinging, increased intraocular pressure, contact dermatitis. Long-term use may cause irritation, photophobia, eczematoid dermatitis, conjunctivitis, hyperemia, or edema.

OD OVERDOSE MANAGEMENT

Treatment of Ocular Overdose: Eyes should be flushed with water or normal saline. A topical miotic may be necessary.

HOW SUPPLIED

Autoinjector: 0.5 mg/0.7 mL, 1 mg/0.7 mL, 2 mg/0.7 mL; *Injection:* 0.05 mg/mL, 0.1 mg/mL, 0.3 mg/mL, 0.4 mg/mL, 0.5 mg/mL, 0.8 mg/mL, 1 mg/mL; *Ophthalmic Ointment:* 1%; *Ophthalmic Solution:* 0.5%, 1%; *Tablet:* 0.4 mg

DOSAGE

- **TABLETS**

  Anticholinergic or antispasmodic.

Adults: 0.3–1.2 mg q 4–6 hr. **Pediatric, over 41 kg:** same as adult; **29.5–41 kg:** 0.4 mg q 4–6 hr; **18.2–29.5 kg:** 0.3 mg q 4–6 hr; **10.9–18.2 kg:** 0.2 mg q 4–6 hr; **7.3–10.9 kg:** 0.15 mg q 4–6 hr; **3.2–7.3 kg:** 0.1 mg q 4–6 hr.

  Prophylaxis of respiratory tract secretions and excess salivation during anesthesia.

Adults: 2 mg.

  Parkinsonism.

Adults: 0.1–0.25 mg 4 times per day.

- **IM, IV, SC**

  Anticholinergic.

Adults, IM, IV, SC: 0.4–0.6 mg q 4–6 hr. **Pediatric, SC:** 0.01 mg/kg, not to exceed 0.4 mg (or 0.3 mg/m²).

  Treatment of toxicity from cholinesterase inhibitors.

Adults, IV, initial: 2–4 mg; **then,** 2 mg repeated q 5–10 min until muscarinic symptoms disappear and signs of atropine toxicity begin to appear. **Pediatric, IM, IV, initial:** 1 mg; **then,** 0.5–1 mg q 5–10 min until muscarinic symptoms disappear and signs of atropine toxicity appear.

  Treatment of mushroom poisoning due to muscarine.

Adults, IM, IV: 1–2 mg q hr until respiratory effects decrease.

  Treatment of organophosphate poisoning.

Adults, IM, IV, initial: 1–2 mg; **then,** repeat in 20–30 min (as soon as cyanosis has disappeared). Dosage may be continued for up to 2 days until symptoms improve.

  Arrhythmias.

Pediatric, IV: 0.01–0.03 mg/kg.

  Prophylaxis of respiratory tract secretions, excessive salivation, succinylcho-line- or surgical procedure-induced arrhythmias.

Pediatric, up to 3 kg, SC: 0.1 mg; **7–9 kg:** 0.2 mg; **12–16 kg:** 0.3 mg; **20–27 kg:** 0.4 mg; **32 kg:** 0.5 mg; **41 kg:** 0.6 mg.

- **ATROPEN**

  Organophosphorus or carbamate poisoning.

Adults and children weighing more than 90 lbs (and generally over 10 years of age): 2 mg. **Children weighing 40–90 lbs (generally 4–10 years of age):** 1 mg. **Children weighing 15–40 lbs (generally 6 months–4 years of age):** 0.5 mg.

- **OPHTHALMIC SOLUTION**

  Uveitis.

Adults: 1–2 gtt instilled into the eye(s) up to 4 times per day. **Children:** 1–2 gtt of the 0.5% solution into the eye(s) up to 3 times per day.

  Refraction.

Adults: 1–2 gtt of the 1% solution into the eye(s) 1 hr before refraction. **Children:** 1–2 gtt of the 0.5% solution into the eye(s) twice a day for 1–3 days before refraction.

- **OPHTHALMIC OINTMENT**

Instill a small amount into the conjunctival sac up to 3 times per day.

NURSING CONSIDERATIONS

ADMINISTRATION/STORAGE

1. After instillation of the ophthalmic ointment, compress the lacrimal sac by digital pressure for 1–3 min to decrease systemic effects.

2. Have physostigmine available in the event of overdose.

3. Use the AtroPen Auto-injector as soon as symptoms of organophosphorus or carbamate poisoning appear. In moderate to severe poisoning, use of more than 1 AtroPen may be required until atropinization (e.g., flushing, mydriasis, tachycardia, dry mouth and nose) is achieved.

4. Do not use more than 3 AtroPen injections unless the client is under the supervision of a trained medical provider.

5. In severe poisonings due to organophosphorus nerve agents or carbamate

---

insecticides, it may be desirable to give an anticonvulsant (e.g., diazepam) concomitantly if seizures are suspected in an unconscious client (since classic tonic-clonic jerking may not be seen). Administration of a cholinesterase reactivator (e.g., pralidoxime chloride) may be helpful.

6. See the package insert for AtroPen to determine the number of AtroPen auto-injectors to use based on symptoms observed.

7. Administer AtroPen as follows:

• Snap the grooved end of the plastic sleeve down and over the yellow safety cap. Remove the AtroPen from the plastic sleep. Do not put fingers on the green tip.

• Firmly grasp the AtroPen with the green tip pointed down.

• Pull off the yellow safety cap with the other hand.

• Aim and firmly jab the green tip straight down (a 90° angle) against the outer thigh. The AtroPen device will activate and deliver the drug. It is permissable to inject through clothing but be sure pockets at the injection site are empty. Very thin clients and small children should also be injected into the thigh but before giving the injection, bunch up the thigh to provide a thicker area for injection.

• Hold the auto-injector firmly in place for at least 10 sec to allow the injection to finish.

• Remove the AtroPen and massage the injection site for several seconds. If the needle is not visible, check to be sure the yellow safety cap has been removed; repeat the above steps but press harder.

8. Store the AtroPen auto-injector from 15–30°C (59–86°F). Do not freeze and protect from light.

IV 9. May give by direct IV undiluted or may dilute in up to 10 mL sterile water and administer at 0.6 –1 mg over 1 min.

10. Do not add to any existing IV solution. May give through 3-way stop cock, Y connection, or injection port.

11. Dose is dependent on condition being treated and age of recipient. See drug insert.

12. Store unopened at room temperature 15-30°C (59-86°F) in airtight, light resistant container.

ASSESSMENT

1. Document indications for therapy, onset and characteristics of S&S.

2. Check for any history of glaucoma before ophthalmic administration; may precipitate an acute crisis.

3. Obtain VS and ECG; monitor CV status during IV therapy.

CLIENT/FAMILY TEACHING

1. When used in the eye, vision will be temporarily impaired. Close work, operating machinery, or driving a car should be avoided until drug effects have worn off.

2. Do not blink excessively; wait 5 min before instilling other drops. Stop eye drops and report if eye pain, conjunctivitis, rapid pulse/palpitations or dizziness occurs.

3. Drug impairs heat regulation; avoid strenuous activity in hot environments; wear sunglasses.

4. Males with BPH may experience urinary retention and hesitancy; advise to void before use.

5. Increase fluids and add bulk to diet to ensure hydration and diminish constipating effects.

6. Drug inhibits salivation; use sugarless candies and gums to decrease dry mouth symptoms.

7. Use caution may experience dizziness, confusion, or visual problems. Report all adverse side effects.

OUTCOMES/EVALUATE

• ↑ HR

• Desired pupillary dilatation

• ↓ GI activity; ↓ Salivation

• Reversal of muscarinic effects of anticholinesterase agents

B

Benazepril hydrochloride ■ⓒ

(beh-**NAYZ**-eh-prill)

CLASSIFICATION(S):
Antihypertensive; ACE inhibitor
PREGNANCY CATEGORY: D
Rx: Lotensin

SEE ALSO *ANGIOTENSIN-CONVERTING ENZYME INHIBITORS.*

ACTION/KINETICS
Both supine and standing BPs are reduced with mild-to-moderate hypertension and no compensatory tachycardia. Also an antihypertensive effect in clients with low-renin hypertension. Food does not affect the extent of absorption. Almost completely converted to the active benazeprilat, which has greater ACE inhibitor activity. Is about 37% or more bioavailable. **Onset:** 1 hr. **Duration:** 24 hr. **Peak plasma levels, benazepril:** 30–60 min. **Peak plasma levels, benazeprilat:** 1–2 hr if fasting and 2–4 hr if not fasting. **t ½, benazeprilat:** 10–11 hr. **Peak reduction in BP:** 2–4 hr after dosing. **Peak effect with chronic therapy:** 1–2 weeks. About 20% benazeprilat excreted through the urine and 11–12% excreted in the bile. About 96.7% bound to plasma proteins.

USES
Hypertension, alone or in combination with thiazides.

CONTRAINDICATIONS
Hypersensitivity to benazepril or any other ACE inhibitor.

SPECIAL CONCERNS
■When used in pregnancy during the second and third trimesters, ACE inhibitors can cause injury and even death to the developing fetus. When pregnancy is detected, discontinue the ACE inhibitor as soon as possible.■ Use with caution during lactation. Safety and effectiveness have not been determined in children.

SIDE EFFECTS
CNS: Headache, dizziness, fatigue, anxiety, insomnia, drowsiness, nervousness. **GI:** N&V, constipation, abdominal pain, gastritis, melena, pancreatitis. **CV:** Symptomatic hypotension, postural hypotension, syncope, angina pectoris, palpitations, peripheral edema, ECG changes. **Dermatologic:** Flushing, photosensitivity, pruritus, rash, diaphoresis. **GU:** Decreased libido, impotence, UTI. **Respiratory:** Cough, asthma, bronchitis, dyspnea, sinusitis, bronchospasm. **Neuromuscular:** Paresthesias, arthralgia, arthritis, asthenia, myalgia. **Hematologic:** Occasionally, eosinophilia, leukopenia, neutropenia, decreased hemoglobin. **Miscellaneous:** Angioedema, which may be associated with involvement of the tongue, glottis, or larynx, hypertonia, proteinuria, hyponatremia, infection.

LABORATORY TEST CONSIDERATIONS
↑ Serum creatinine, BUN, serum potassium. ↓ Hemoglobin. ECG changes.

DRUG INTERACTIONS
Diuretics / Excessive ↓ in BP
Lithium / ↑ Serum lithium levels with ↑ risk of lithium toxicity
Potassium-sparing diuretics, potassium supplements / ↑ Risk of hyperkalemia

HOW SUPPLIED
Tablet: 5 mg, 10 mg, 20 mg, 40 mg

DOSAGE
• **TABLETS**
Clients not receiving a diuretic.
Initial: 10 mg once daily; **maintenance:** 20–40 mg/day given as a single dose or in two equally divided doses. Total daily doses greater than 80 mg have not been evaluated.
Clients receiving a diuretic.
Initial: 5 mg/day.
$C_{CR} < 30$ mL/min/1.73 m^2. Start with 5 mg/day; **maintenance:** titrate dose upward until BP is controlled or to a maximum total daily dose of 40 mg.

B

NURSING CONSIDERATIONS
Ⓒ Do not confuse Lotensin with lovastatin (antihyperlipidemic).

ADMINISTRATION/STORAGE
1. Base dosage adjustment on measuring peak (2–6 hr after dosing) and trough responses. Consider increasing the dose or give divided doses if once-daily dosing does not provide an adequate trough response.
2. If BP not controlled by benazepril alone, add a diuretic.
3. If receiving a diuretic, discontinue the diuretic, if possible, 2–3 days before beginning benazepril therapy.

ASSESSMENT
1. Note any previous experience with this class of drugs.
2. Review diet, weight loss, exercise, and life-style changes necessary to control BP.
3. Monitor CBC, electrolytes, renal (especially in geriatric clients) and LFTs. Check urine for protein.

CLIENT/FAMILY TEACHING
1. Take only as directed. May be taken with or without food. Do not chew or crush; swallow tablets whole.
2. May be dizzy, faint or lightheaded during first few days of therapy; use caution.
3. Avoid concomitant administration of potassium-sparing diuretics/supplements; may lead to increased K⁺ levels.
4. Report headache, fatigue, dizziness, drowsiness, mouth sores, rash, sore throat, swelling of hands/feet, chest pain and cough. Use birth control; report if pregnancy suspected.
5. Bring record of BP at different times during the day.

OUTCOMES/EVALUATE
BP control

Betaxolol hydrochloride
(beh-**TAX**-oh-lohl)

CLASSIFICATION(S):
Beta-adrenergic blocking agent

PREGNANCY CATEGORY: C
Rx: Betoptic, Betoptic S, Kerlone

SEE ALSO BETA-ADRENERGIC BLOCKING AGENTS.

ACTION/KINETICS
Inhibits beta-1-adrenergic receptors (beta-2 receptors inhibited at high doses). Has some membrane stabilizing activity but no intrinsic sympathomimetic activity. Low lipid solubility. Reduces the production of aqueous humor, thus reducing IOP. No effect on pupil size or accommodation. **t ½:** 14–22 hr. Metabolized in the liver with most excreted through the urine; about 15% is excreted unchanged.

USES
PO: Hypertension, alone or with other antihypertensive agents (especially thiazide diuretics). **Ophthalmic:** (1) Ocular hypertension. (2) Chronic open-angle glaucoma, alone or in combination with other antiglaucoma drugs.

SPECIAL CONCERNS
Use with caution during lactation. Safety and effectiveness have not been determined in children. Geriatric clients are at greater risk of developing bradycardia.

HOW SUPPLIED
Ophthalmic Solution: 0.5%; *Ophthalmic Suspension:* 0.25%; *Tablet:* 10 mg, 20 mg

DOSAGE
• **TABLETS**
  Hypertension.
Initial: 10 mg once daily either alone or with a diuretic. If desired effect is not reached, may increase dose to 20 mg; doses higher than 20 mg will not increase the therapeutic effect. In geriatric clients the initial dose should be 5 mg/day.

• **OPHTHALMIC SOLUTION, SUSPENSION**
  Ocular hypertension; chronic open-angle glaucoma.
Adults, usual: 1–2 gtt twice a day. If used to replace another drug, continue the drug being used and add 1 gtt of betaxolol twice a day. Discontinue the previous drug the following day. If transferring from several antiglaucoma drugs being used together, adjust one

---

Bold Italic = life threatening side effect   ■ = black box warning   ♣ = Available in Canada

drug at a time at intervals of not less than 1 week. The agents being used can be continued and add 1 gtt betaxolol twice a day. The next day another agent should be discontinued. The remaining antiglaucoma drug dosage can be decreased or discontinued depending on client response.

NURSING CONSIDERATIONS

ADMINISTRATION/STORAGE
1. Full antihypertensive effect usually observed within 7 to 14 days.
2. As PO dose is increased, the HR decreases.
3. Discontinue PO therapy gradually over a 2-week period.
4. Shake ophthalmic suspension well before use.
5. Store ophthalmic products at room temperature not to exceed 30°C (86°F).

ASSESSMENT
1. Note indications for therapy, frequency/characteristics of symptoms, and other agents trialed.
2. Monitor lung sounds, weight, EKG and VS.

CLIENT/FAMILY TEACHING
1. Review appropriate method/indications for therapy; take/use as directed. Do not stop suddenly.
2. Drug may mask S&S of hypoglycemia, and cause increased cold sensitivity.
3. Avoid OTC agents without approval.
4. With HTN, monitor BP and record; report any adverse drug effects.
5. With eye therapy, review instillation procedure. Wear sunglasses and avoid sun exposure; may cause photophobia.
6. Use caution, may cause dizziness or drowsiness. Change positions slowly to prevent sudden drop in BP.
7. Report any SOB, wheezes, confusion, rash, unusual bruising/bleeding, slow pulse, or cold hands/feet.

OUTCOMES/EVALUATE
- ↓ BP (PO)
- ↓ Intraocular pressure (ophthalmic)

Bisoprolol fumarate ©
(**BUY**-soh-**proh**-lol)

B

CLASSIFICATION(S):
Beta-adrenergic blocking agent
PREGNANCY CATEGORY: C
Rx: Zebeta
❧Rx: Monocor

SEE ALSO *BETA-ADRENERGIC BLOCKING AGENTS.*

ACTION/KINETICS
Inhibits beta-1-adrenergic receptors and, at higher doses, beta-2 receptors. No intrinsic sympathomimetic activity and no membrane-stabilizing activity. **t½:** 9–12 hr. Over 90% of PO dose is absorbed. Approximately 50% is excreted unchanged through the urine and the remainder as inactive metabolites; a small amount (less than 2%) is excreted through the feces.

USES
Hypertension alone or in combination with other antihypertensive agents. *Investigational:* Angina pectoris, SVTs, PVCs.

SPECIAL CONCERNS
Use with caution during lactation. Safety and efficacy have not been determined in children. Due to selectivity for beta-1 receptors, it may be used with caution in clients with bronchospastic disease who do not respond to, or who cannot tolerate, other antihypertensive therapy.

HOW SUPPLIED
Tablet: 5 mg, 10 mg

DOSAGE
- **TABLETS**
  Antihypertensive.
Dose must be individualized. **Adults, initial:** 5 mg once daily (in some, 2.5 mg/day may be appropriate). **Maintenance:** If the 5-mg dose is inadequate, the dose may be increased to 10 mg/day and then, if needed, to 20 mg once daily. In impaired renal (C_{CR} < 40 mL/min) or hepatic function (hepatitis or cirrhosis), initially give 2.5 mg with caution in titrating the dose upward.

NURSING CONSIDERATIONS

🖉 Do not confuse Zebeta with DiaBeta (an oral hypoglycemic).

ADMINISTRATION/STORAGE

1. Food does not affect bioavailability; may give without regard to meals.
2. Bisoprolol is not dialyzable so dose adjustments are not required in clients undergoing hemodialysis.
3. Dosage adjustment is not necessary in the elderly.

ASSESSMENT

1. Document indications for therapy, previous agents used, and outcome.
2. Monitor CBC, glucose, electrolytes, renal and LFTs; reduce dose with dysfunction.
3. Once baseline parameters determined, continue to monitor BP in both arms with client lying, sitting, and standing.
4. Document EKG and CXR. Assess lung sounds and note any arrhythmias.

CLIENT/FAMILY TEACHING

1. Take as directed at the same time each day with or without food.
2. Use caution as drug may cause dizziness, and drowsiness. Change positions slowly to avoid sudden drop in low BP.
3. Do not stop suddenly without provider knowledge. Avoid OTC drugs without approval.
4. With diabetes, monitor FS closely. Report any weakness, or fatigue, as drug does not block dizziness and sweating as signs of hypoglycemia.
5. Report any lack of response or adverse side effects.

OUTCOMES/EVALUATE

- ↓ BP; relief of angina
- Stable cardiac rhythm

Bivalirudin
(**by**-val-ih-**ROO**-din)

CLASSIFICATION(S):
Anticoagulant, thrombin inhibitor
PREGNANCY CATEGORY: B
Rx: Angiomax

SEE ALSO *ANTICOAGULANTS.*

ACTION/KINETICS

Direct-acting thrombin inhibitor by binding to both the catalytic site and to the anion-binding exosite of circulating and clot-bound thrombin. Binding to thrombin is reversible. When bound to thrombin, all effects of thrombin are inhibited, including activation of platelets, cleavage of fibrinogen, and activation of the positive amplification reactions of thrombin. Advantages over heparin include activity against clot-bound thrombin, more predictable anticoagulation, and no inhibition by components of the platelet release reaction. **t½, after IV:** 25 min. t½ is increased in clients with renal impairment. Metabolized in the liver with about 20% excreted unchanged in the urine.

USES

As an anticoagulant with aspirin in clients with unstable angina undergoing percutaneous transluminal coronary angioplasty (PTCA).

CONTRAINDICATIONS

Use in active major bleeding, cerebral aneurysm, intracranial hemorrhage. IM use.

SPECIAL CONCERNS

Reduce dose in moderate to severe impaired renal function. Increased risk of hemorrhage with GI ulceration or hepatic disease. Hypertension may increase risk of cerebral hemorrhage. Use with caution following recent surgery or trauma and during lactation. Safety and efficacy not established when used with glycoprotein IIb/IIIa inhibitors, in clients with unstable angina who are not undergoing PTCA, in those with other acute coronary syndromes, or in children.

SIDE EFFECTS

Major side effect is bleeding with possiblity (infrequent) of major hemorrhage, including ***intracranial hemorrhage*** and ***retroperitoneal hemorrhage***. **CV:** Hypotension, hypertension, bradycardia, syncope, vascular anomaly, ***ventricular fibrillation***. **GI:** N&V, dyspepsia, abdominal pain. **CNS:** Headache, insomnia, anxiety, nervousness, cerebral ischemia, confusion, facial pa-

---

Bold Italic = life threatening side effect   ■ = black box warning   ✦ = Available in Canada

ralysis. **Dermatologic:** Hematoma, pain at injection site. **Renal:** Urinary retention, kidney failure, oliguria. **Miscellaneous:** Back pain, pain, pelvic pain, fever, lung edema, infection, *sepsis*.

LABORATORY TEST CONSIDERATIONS
Prolongation of aPTT, activated clotting time, thrombin time, and PT.

OD OVERDOSE MANAGEMENT
Treatment: Discontinue the drug and monitor closely for signs of bleed. No known antidote. Bivalirudin is hemodialyzable.

HOW SUPPLIED
Powder for Injection, lyophilized: 250 mg/vial

DOSAGE
• **IV ONLY**
  Unstable angina undergoing PTCA
Adults: IV bolus dose of 1 mg/kg followed by a 4-hr IV infusion at a rate of 2.5 mg/kg/hr. After the initial 4-hr infusion, an additional IV infusion may be started at a rate of 0.2 mg/kg/hr for up to 20 hr, if needed. Use with aspirin (300–325 mg/day).
Reduce the infusion dose as follows in impaired renal function: 20% in moderate renal impairment (GFR of 30–59 mL/min); 60% in severe renal impairment (GFR of 10–29 mL/min); and, 90% in dialysis-dependent clients.

NURSING CONSIDERATIONS
ADMINISTRATION/STORAGE
IV 1. Initiate just prior to PTCA.
2. To reconstitute, add 5 mL sterile water to each 250 mg vial and gently swirl until material is dissolved. Each reconstituted vial is further diluted in 50 mL of D5W or 0.9% NaCl for a final concentration of 5 mg/mL.
3. Adjust dose according to client weight.
4. If the low-rate infusion (i.e., 0.2 mg/kg/hr) is needed, prepare as follows: reconstitute the 250 mg vial with 5 mL of sterile water and further dilute in 500 mL of D5W or 0.9% NaCl for a final concentration of 0.5 mg/mL.
5. Do not mix with any other medications before administration.
6. The following drugs resulted in haze formation, microparticulate formation, or gross precipitation: Alteplase, amiodarone HCl, amphotericin B, chlorpromazine HCl, diazepam, prochlorperazine edisylate, reteplase, streptokinase, and vancomycin HCl. Do not give in the same IV line with bivalirudin.
7. Do not use if the preparation contains particulate matter.
8. Do not freeze reconstituted or diluted drug.
9. Reconstituted drug may be stored at 2–8°C (36–46°F) for up to 24 hr. Diluted drug (0.5 mg/mL–5 mg/mL) is stable at room temperature for up to 24 hr.

ASSESSMENT
1. Document indications for and method of therapy (bolus/infusion).
2. Note any history of cerebral aneurysm, intracranial hemorrhage, recent GI bleed or surgery. Monitor cardiac and neurologic status during therapy. Report any deficits.
3. Monitor ECG, CBC, bleeding parameters, renal and LFTs; reduce dose with renal dysfunction. Assess carefully for any evidence of bleeding abnormalities.

CLIENT/FAMILY TEACHING
1. Review procedure, and reasons for therapy during PTCA.
2. Report any adverse side effects or unusual bruising or bleeding. New onset SOB, chest pain or edema warrant evaluation. Avoid aspirin or drugs used to treat swelling or pain (NSAIDs).
3. Incorporate life style changes related to smoking cessation, reduction in alcohol use, diet and exercise into daily routine.
4. Avoid jostling or activities that may cause injury. Use electric razor, soft toothbrush and nightlight to prevent injury.
5. Encourage family members to learn CPR.

OUTCOMES/EVALUATE
Anticoagulation during angioplasty

Bosentan ■

(boh-**SEN**-tan)

CLASSIFICATION(S):
Vasodilator, endothelin receptor antagonist
PREGNANCY CATEGORY: X
Rx: Tracleer

ACTION/KINETICS

Bosentan is the first of a new class of drugs. Endothelin-1 (ET-1) is a neurohormone whose effects are mediated by binding to ET_A and ET_B receptors in the endothelium and smooth muscle. ET-1 levels are increased in plasma and lung tissue of clients with pulmonary arterial hypertension. Bosentan is a specific and competitive antagonist at endothelin receptor types ET_A and ET_B. Bosentan is highly bound (> 98%) to plasma proteins. **Maximum plasma levels:** 3–5 hr. Metabolized in the liver to three metabolites, one of which is active. Steady state reached in 3–5 days. Excreted in the bile. **t ½, terminal:** About 5 hr.

USES

To improve exercise ability and decrease the rate of worsening in pulmonary arterial hypertension in those with WHO Class III or IV symptoms. *Investigational:* Improve microcirculatory blood flow in splanchnic organs during septic shock. *NOTE:* Because of potential liver injury and to decrease the chance as much as possible for fetal exposure, bosentan may be prescribed only through the Tracleer Access Program.

CONTRAINDICATIONS

Use in moderate or severe liver abnormalities or elevated aminotransferases >3 times ULN. Pregnancy, use with cyclosporine A or glyburide. Hypersensitivity to bosentan or any component of the medication. Lactation.

SPECIAL CONCERNS

■(1) Potential for serious liver toxicity (See *Administration/Storage*). (2) Likely to produce major birth defects if used during pregnancy. Exclude pregnancy before starting treatment. Because of the possibility of serious liver damage and potential damage to a fetus, the manufacturer has set up the Tracleer Access Program.■ Use with caution in those with mildly impaired liver function. Safety and efficacy have not been determined in children.

SIDE EFFECTS

CV: Flushing, hypotension, palpitations, edema, lower limb edema. **Miscellaneous:** Headache, nasopharyngitis, abnormal liver function, anemia, dyspepsia, fatigue, pruritus.

LABORATORY TEST CONSIDERATIONS

↑ Liver transferases. Dose-related ↓ in H & H.

DRUG INTERACTIONS

Contraceptives, hormonal (oral, injectable, implantation) / Possible contraceptive failure due to ↑ liver metabolism of hormones
Cyclosporine A / ↑ Bosentan trough levels by about 30 fold and steady-state levels by 3–4 fold. ↓ Cyclosporine A levels by about 50%. **Do not give together**
Glyburide / ↓ Glyburide levels by about 40% and bosentan levels by about 30%. Also, ↑ risk of elevated liver aminotransferases. **Do not give together**
Ketoconazole / ↑ Bosentan plasma levels by about 2 fold
Simvastatin (and other statins) / ↓ Plasma statin levels by about 50% R/T ↑ hepatic metabolism
Warfarin / ↓ Plasma warfarin levels and INR

HOW SUPPLIED

Tablets: 62.5 mg, 125 mg

DOSAGE

• TABLETS

Pulmonary arterial hypertension.
Initial: 62.5 mg twice a day for 4 weeks. **Then,** increase to maintenance dose of 125 mg twice a day. In those with a body weight less than 40 kg and who are over 12 years of age, the recommended initial and maintenance doses are 62.5 mg twice a day.

NURSING CONSIDERATIONS

ADMINISTRATION/STORAGE

1. Use the following guidelines for dosage adjustment and monitoring in

clients who develop aminotransferase abnormalities:

• If ALT/AST levels are >3 and 5 or less times ULN, confirm by another aminotransferase test. If confirmed, stop treatment and monitor aminotransferase levels at least every 2 weeks. If levels return to pretreatment values, continue or reintroduce the treatment as appropriate (see below).

• If ALT/AST levels are >5 and 8 or less times ULN, confirm by another aminotransferase test. If confirmed, stop treatment and monitor aminotransferase levels at least every 2 weeks. Once levels return to pretreatment values, consider reintroduction as described below.

• If ALT/AST levels are >8 times ULN, stop treatment and do not consider bosentan reintroduction.

2. If bosentan is reintroduced, begin again with the starting dose. Check aminotransferase levels within 3 days and thereafter.

3. If aminotransferase levels are accompanied by N&V, fever, abdominal pain, jaundice, unusual lethargy or fatigue (i.e., symptoms of liver injury) or increases in bilirubin 2 or more times ULN, stop treatment.

4. To avoid the potential for clinical deterioration after abrupt discontinuation, reduce dose gradually (i.e., 62.5 twice a day for 3–7 days).

ASSESSMENT

1. Note indications for therapy, other agents trialed, when diagnosed, and stage of pulmonary artery hypertension.

2. List drugs currently prescribed to ensure none interact adversely; drug is highly protein bound.

3. Ensure client is not pregnant; perform pregnancy test on all females of childbearing potential.

4. After initial labs, monitor LFTs and pregnancy tests monthly; H&H after 1 and 3 mo and then q 3 mo to assess for any deficiencies. CXR, ABGs, and PFTs as indicated.

CLIENT/FAMILY TEACHING

1. Review bosentan medication guide for safe drug administration. Take twice

a day as directed and increase dosage after 4 weeks upon provider recommendation only.

2. Drug has two significant concerns: potential for serious liver damage and fetal damage. Thus, it is only administered through the Tracleer Access Program @ 1-866-228-3546. All adverse drug reactions should also be reported directly to this number by the provider.

3. Drug is not a cure but may improve clinical symptoms of disease. Report all side effects and any changes in breathing or exercise tolerance.

4. Practice reliable contraception; use an additional form of contraception with the hormonal form as drug will cause major birth defects.

5. Continue all other therapies prescribed by pulmonologist. Keep all scheduled appointments with lab every month and provider as scheduled.

OUTCOMES/EVALUATE

• Improved exercise tolerance

• ↓ Clinical worsening of pulmonary artery hypertension

Bretylium tosylate

(breh-**TILL**-ee-um **TOZ**-ill-ayt)

CLASSIFICATION(S):
Antiarrhythmic, class III
PREGNANCY CATEGORY: C
Rx: Bretylium tosylate in D5W

ACTION/KINETICS

Inhibits catecholamine release at nerve endings by decreasing excitability of the nerve terminal. Initially there is a release of norepinephrine, which may cause tachycardia and a rise in BP; this is followed by a blockade of release of catecholamines. Also increases the duration of the action potential and the effective refractory period, which may assist in reversing arrhythmias. **Peak plasma concentration and effect:** 1 hr after IM. Antifibrillatory effect within a few minutes after IV use. Suppression of ventricular tachycardia and ventricular arrhythmias takes 20–120 min, whereas suppression of PVCs does not occur for 6–9 hr. **Therapeutic serum levels:** 0.5–1.5 mcg/mL. **t ½:** Approximately 5–10 hr. **Duration:** 6–8 hr. From 0 to 8% is protein bound. Up to 90% of drug is excreted unchanged in the urine after 24 hr.

USES
(1) Life-threatening ventricular arrhythmias that have failed to respond to first line antiarrhythmics (e.g., lidocaine). (2) Prophylaxis and treatment of ventricular fibrillation. For short-term use only. *Investigational:* Second-line drug (after lidocaine) for advanced cardiac life support during CPR.

CONTRAINDICATIONS
Severe aortic stenosis, severe pulmonary hypertension.

SPECIAL CONCERNS
Safety and efficacy in children have not been established. Dosage adjustment required in impaired renal function.

SIDE EFFECTS
CV: Hypotension (including postural hypotension), transient hypertension, increased frequency of PVCs, bradycardia, precipitation of anginal attacks, initial increase in arrhythmias, sensation of substernal pressure. **GI:** N&V (especially after rapid IV administration), diarrhea, abdominal pain, hiccoughs. **CNS:** Vertigo, dizziness, lightheadedness, syncope, anxiety, paranoid psychosis, confusion, mood swings. **Miscellaneous:** Renal dysfunction, flushing, hyperthermia, SOB, nasal stuffiness, diaphoresis, conjunctivitis, erythematous macular rash, lethargy, generalized tenderness.

OD **OVERDOSE MANAGEMENT**
Symptoms: Marked hypertension followed by hypotension. *Treatment:* Treat hypertension with nitroprusside or another short-acting IV antihypertensive. Treat hypotension with appropriate fluid therapy and pressor agents such as norepinephrine or dopamine.

DRUG INTERACTIONS
Digoxin / Bretylium may aggravate toxicity due to initial release of norepinephrine
Procainamide, Quinidine / Concomitant use ↓ inotropic effect of bretylium and ↑ hypotension

HOW SUPPLIED
Injection: 50 mg/mL; *Injection in D5W:* 2 mg/mL, 4 mg/mL

DOSAGE
• **IV INFUSION**
Immediate, life-threatening ventricular arrhythmias.
Adults: 5 mg/kg by rapid IV injection of undiluted drug. If ventricular fibrillation persists, iincrease dose to 10 mg/kg and repeat as necessary.
Acute ventricular fibrillation in children.
5 mg/kg/dose IV followed by 10 mg/kg at 15–30 min intervals up to a maximum total dose of 30 mg/kg. **Maintenance:** 5–10 mg/kg/dose q 6 hr.
For continuous suppression of ventricular arrhythmias.
1–2 mg/minute of the diluted solution by continuous IV infusion. Alternatively, infuse 5–10 mg/kg of the diluted solution over more than 8 min q 6 hr.
Other ventricular arrhythmias.
Adults: 5–10 mg/kg of diluted drug by IV infusion over more than 8 min. More rapid infusion may cause N&V. Give subsequent doses at 1 to 2 hr intervals if the arrhythmia persists. **Maintenance:** Give same dose q 6 hr or a constant infusion of 1 to 2 mg/min. **Children:** 5–10 mg/kg/dose q 6 hr.
• **IM**
Other ventricular arrhythmias.
Adults: 5–10 mg/kg of undiluted solution followed, if necessary, by the same dose at 1–2-hr intervals; **then,** give same dosage q 6–8 hr.

NURSING CONSIDERATIONS
ADMINISTRATION/STORAGE
1. For IM, use drug undiluted.
2. Rotate injection sites so that no more than 5 mL of drug is given at any site to avoid atrophy, necrosis, fibrosis, vascular degeneration, or inflammation.
3. Keep supine during therapy; observe for postural hypotension.
4. Start on an oral antiarrhythmic medication as soon as possible.
IV 5. For IV infusion, bretylium is compatible with D5W, 0.9% NaCl, D5/0.45% NaCl, D5/0.9% NaCl, D5/RL, 5% NaHCO₃, 20% mannitol, 1/6 molar sodium lac-

tate, RL, CaCl$_2$ (54.5 mEq/L) in D5W, and KCl (40 mEq/L) in D5W.

6. For direct IV, administer undiluted over 15–30 sec, may repeat in 15–30 min if symptoms persist. May further dilute 500 mg in 50 mL and infuse over 10–30 min.

ASSESSMENT

1. Document indications for therapy, pretreatment ECG, and VS.

2. If taking digitalis, may aggravate digitalis toxicity.

INTERVENTIONS

1. Monitor VS and rhythm strips as dose is titrated on client response.

2. To reduce N&V, administer IV slowly over 10 min while supine. Once infusion complete keep supine until the BP has stabilized.

3. Supervise once ambulation is permitted, may experience lightheadedness and vertigo.

4. Bretylium often causes a fall in supine BP within 1 hr of IV administration. If SBP < 75 mm Hg, anticipate need for pressor agents.

5. If clients develop side effects, stay to reassure and reorient as needed.

CLIENT/FAMILY TEACHING

1. Drug is used to convert abnormal heart ryhthm to a normal rhythm.

2. Do not change positions suddenly; may experience sudden drop in BP causing dizziness.

3. Report any chest pain or SOB immediately.

OUTCOMES/EVALUATE

• Termination of life-threatening ventricular arrhythmia, stable cardiac rhythm

• Serum drug levels (0.5–1.5 mcg/mL)

Bumetanide ■ ⓒ
(byou-**MET**-ah-nyd)

CLASSIFICATION(S):
Diuretic, loop
PREGNANCY CATEGORY: C
Rx: Bumetanide, Bumex
✤Rx: Burinex

SEE ALSO *DIURETICS, LOOP.*

ACTION/KINETICS

Inhibits reabsorption of both sodium and chloride in the proximal tubule and the ascending loop of Henle. Possible activity in the proximal tubule to promote phosphate excretion. **Onset, PO:** 30–60 min. **Peak effect, PO:** 1–2 hr. **Duration, PO:** 4–6 hr (dose-dependent). **Onset, IV:** Several minutes. **Peak effect, IV:** 15–30 min. **Duration, IV:** 3.5–4 hr. **t ½:** 1–1.5 hr. The t ½ decreases from 6 hr at birth to 2.4 hr at one month of age. Metabolized in the liver although 45% excreted unchanged in the urine.

USES

(1) Edema associated with CHF, nephrotic syndrome, hepatic disease. (2) Adjunct to treat acute pulmonary edema. Especially useful in clients refractory to other diuretics. *Investigational:* Treatment of adult nocturia. Not effective in males with prostatic hypertrophy.

CONTRAINDICATIONS

Anuria. Hepatic coma or severe electrolyte depletion until condition improved/corrected. Hypersensitivity to drug. Lactation.

SPECIAL CONCERNS

■Potent diuretic; excess amounts can cause profound diuresis with water and electrolyte depletion. Individualize dosage; monitor carefully.■ Safety and efficacy in children under 18 have not been established. Geriatric clients may be more sensitive to the hypotensive and electrolyte effects and are at greater risk for developing thromboembolic problems and circulatory collapse. SLE may be activated or made worse. Clients allergic to sulfonamides may show cross sensitivity to bumetanide. Sudden changes in electrolyte balance may cause hepatic encephalopathy and coma in clients with hepatic cirrhosis and ascites.

SIDE EFFECTS

Electrolyte and fluid changes: Excess water loss, *dehydration,* electrolyte depletion including hypokalemia, hypochloremia, hyponatremia, hypovolemia, thromboembolism, *circulatory collapse.* **Otic:** Tinnitus, reversible and irreversible hearing impairment, deafness, vertigo (with a sense of fullness in the ears). **CV: *Reduction in blood volume may cause circulatory collapse and vascular thrombosis and embolism, especially in geriatric clients.*** Hypotension, ECG changes, chest pain. **CNS:** Asterixis, encephalopathy with preexisting liver disease, vertigo, headache, dizziness. **GI:** Upset stomach, dry mouth, N&V, diarrhea, GI pain. **GU:** Premature ejaculation, difficulty maintaining erection, renal failure. **Musculoskeletal:** Arthritic pain, weakness, muscle cramps, fatigue. **Hematologic:** Agranulocytosis, thrombocytopenia. **Allergic:** Pruritus, urticaria, rashes. **Miscellaneous:** Sweating, hyperventilation, rash, nipple tenderness, photosensitivity, pain following parenteral use.

LABORATORY TEST CONSIDERATIONS
Alterations in LDH, AST, ALT, alkaline phosphatase, creatinine clearance, total serum bilirubin, serum proteins, cholesterol. Changes in hemoglobin, PT, hematocrit, WBCs, platelet and differential counts, phosphorus, carbon dioxide content, bicarbonate, and calcium. ↑ Urinary glucose and protein, serum creatinine. Also, hyperuricemia, hypochloremia, hypokalemia, azotemia, hyponatremia, hyperglycemia.

OD OVERDOSE MANAGEMENT
Symptoms: Profound loss of water, electrolyte depletion, dehydration, decreased blood volume, ***circulatory collapse (possibility of vascular thrombosis and embolism).*** Symptoms of electrolyte depletion include: anorexia, cramps, weakness, dizziness, vomiting, and mental confusion. *Treatment:* Replace electrolyte and fluid losses and monitor urinary and serum electrolyte levels. Emesis or gastric lavage. Oxygen or artificial respiration may be necessary. General supportive measures.

HOW SUPPLIED
Injection: 0.25 mg /mL; *Tablet:* 0.5 mg, 1 mg, 2 mg

DOSAGE——————————
• **TABLETS**
Adults: 0.5–2 mg once daily; if response is inadequate, a second or third dose may be given at 4–5-hr intervals up to a maximum of 10 mg/day.
• **IV, IM**
Adults: 0.5–1 mg; if response is inadequate, a second or third dose may be given at 2–3-hr intervals up to a maximum of 10 mg/day. Initiate PO dosing as soon as possible.

NURSING CONSIDERATIONS
Do not confuse Bumex with Buprenex (narcotic analgesic).
ADMINISTRATION/STORAGE
1. The recommended PO medication schedule is on alternate days or for 3–4 days with a 1–2-day rest period in between.
2. Bumetanide, at a 1:40 ratio of bumetanide: furosemide, may be ordered if allergic to furosemide.
3. Reserve IV or IM administration for clients in whom PO use is not practical or absorption from the GI tract is impaired.
IV 4. In severe chronic renal insufficiency, a continuous infusion (12 mg over 12 hr) may be more effective and cause fewer side effects than intermittent bolus therapy.
5. Prepare solutions fresh for IM or IV; use within 24 hr.
6. Ampules may be reconstituted with D5W, NSS, or RL solution.
7. Administer IV solutions slowly over 1–2 min.

ASSESSMENT
1. Document indications for therapy and pretreatment findings.
2. Note any sulfonamide allergy; may be cross sensitivity.
3. Monitor electrolytes, I&O, liver and renal function studies; assess for ↓ K+.
4. Review history; note any hearing impairment, lupus, or thromboembolic events. Assess hearing for ototoxicity, especially if receiving other ototoxic drugs.
5. *NOTE:* 1 mg of bumetanide is equivalent to 40 mg of furosemide.
6. Monitor VS. Rapid diuresis may cause dehydration and circulatory collapse (especially in the elderly). Hypotension may occur when administered with antihypertensives.

CLIENT/FAMILY TEACHING

1. Take early in the day to prevent nighttime voidings. With alternate day therapy keep a written record or calendar to ensure proper therapy and no overdosage.

2. Do not perform activities that require mental alertness until drug effects realized. Change positions slowly to prevent sudden drop in BP causing dizziness.

3. Review dietary requirements such as reduced sodium and high potassium; may see dietitian PRN.

4. Record weights; report any sudden weight gain (>3 lbs/day or 5 lbs/week) or evidence of swelling in the hands or feet.

5. Report any unusual side effects.

OUTCOMES/EVALUATE

↓ Peripheral and sacral edema; enhanced diuresis

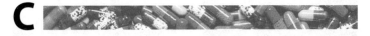

C

Calcium chloride

(**KAL**-see-um **KLOH**-ryd)

CLASSIFICATION(S):

Calcium salt

PREGNANCY CATEGORY: C

SEE ALSO *CALCIUM SALTS.*

USES

(1) Mild hypocalcemia due to neonatal tetany, tetany due to parathyroid deficiency or vitamin D deficiency, and alkalosis. (2) Prophylaxis of hypocalcemia during exchange transfusions. (3) Intestinal malabsorption. (4) Treat effects of serious hyperkalemia as measured by ECG. (5) Cardiac resuscitation after open heart surgery when epinephrine fails to improve weak or ineffective myocardial contractions. (6) Adjunct to treat insect bites or stings to relieve muscle cramping. (7) Depression due to Mg overdosage. (8) Acute symptoms of lead colic. (9) Rickets, osteomalacia. (10) Reverse symptoms of verapamil overdosage.

CONTRAINDICATIONS

Use to treat hypocalcemia of renal insufficiency. IM or SC use.

SPECIAL CONCERNS

Use usually restricted in children due to significant irritation and possible tissue necrosis and sloughing caused by IV calcium chloride.

ADDITIONAL SIDE EFFECTS

Peripheral vasodilation with moderate decreases in BP. Extravasation can cause severe necrosis, sloughing, or abscess formation if given IM or SC.

HOW SUPPLIED

Injection: 100 mg /mL

DOSAGE

- **IV ONLY**

Hypocalcemia, replenish electrolytes.
Adults: 0.5–1 g q 1–3 days (given at a rate not to exceed 13.6–27.3 mg/min).
Pediatric: 25 mg/kg (0.2 mL/kg up to 1–10 mL/kg) given slowly.

Mg intoxication.
0.5 g promptly; observe for recovery before other doses given.

Cardiac resuscitation.
0.5–1 g IV or 0.2–0.8 g injected into the ventricular cavity as a single dose. **Pediatric:** 0.2 mL/kg.

Hyperkalemia.
Sufficient amount to return ECG to normal.

NOTE: The preparation contains 27.2% calcium and 272 mg calcium/g (13.6 mEq/g).

NURSING CONSIDERATIONS

ADMINISTRATION/STORAGE

1. Never administer IM or SC.

IV 2. May give undiluted by IV push.

ASSESSMENT

Note indications for therapy, serum levels, and other agents trialed.

H = Herbal   IV = Intravenous   ℝ = sound-alike drug

OUTCOMES/EVALUATE
- Desired serum calcium levels
- ↓ Mg and potassium levels

Candesartan cilexetil

(**kan**-deh-**SAR**-tan)

CLASSIFICATION(S):
Antihypertensive, angiotensin II receptor blocker

PREGNANCY CATEGORY: C (first trimester), **D** (second and third trimesters)

Rx: Atacand

SEE ALSO *ANGIOTENSIN II RECEPTOR ANTAGONISTS* AND *ANTIHYPERTENSIVE DRUGS.*

ACTION/KINETICS
Is about 15% bioavailable. Is rapidly and completely bioactivated to candesartan by ester hydrolysis during absorption from the GI tract. Food does not affect bioavailability. Effect somewhat less in blacks. **t ½, elimination:** 9 hr. Excreted mainly unchanged in the urine (33%) and feces (67%). Is greater than 99% bound to plasma proteins.

USES
Treat hypertension alone or in combination with other antihypertensive drugs. *Investigational:* Prophylaxis of migraine headaches.

SPECIAL CONCERNS
■If used during the second and third trimesters, drugs that act on the renin-angiotensin system may cause injury or death to the developing fetus. When pregnancy is detected, discontinue candesartan as soon as possible.■ Possibility of fetal and neonatal toxicities in infants born to mothers who took candesartan during pregnancy.

SIDE EFFECTS
GI: N&V, abdominal pain, diarrhea, dyspepsia, gastroenteritis. **CNS:** Headache, dizziness, paresthesia, vertigo, anxiety, depression, somnolence. **CV:** Tachycardia, palpitation; rarely, *angina pectoris, MI.* **Body as a whole:** Fatigue, asthenia, fever, peripheral edema. **Respiratory:** URTI, pharyngitis, rhinitis, bronchitis, coughing, dyspnea, sinusitis, epistaxis. **GU:** Impaired renal function, hematuria. **Dermatologic:** Rash, increased sweating. **Miscellaneous:** Backpain, chest pain, arthralgia, myalgia, angioedema.

LABORATORY TEST CONSIDERATIONS
↑ Creatine phosphatase. Albuminuria, hyperglycemia/triglyceridemia/uricemia.

ADDITIONAL DRUG INTERACTIONS
When used with lithium, serum lithium levels may be increased; monitor carefully.

HOW SUPPLIED
Tablets: 4 mg, 8 mg, 16 mg, 32 mg

DOSAGE
- **TABLETS**
  Hypertension, monotherapy.
Adults, usual initial: 16 mg once daily for monotherapy in those not volume depleted. Can be given once or twice daily in doses from 8 to 32 mg. If BP is not controlled, a diuretic can be added.

NURSING CONSIDERATIONS
ADMINISTRATION/STORAGE
1. Maximum BP reduction is reached within 4 to 6 weeks.
2. Initiate dosage under close supervision in those with possible depletion of intravascular volume (e.g., after a diuretic). Consider giving a lower dose.
3. May give with or without food.
4. If BP is not controlled by candesartan alone, a diuretic may be added.

ASSESSMENT
1. Note disease onset and duration, other agents trialed and outcome.
2. Assess VS, electrolytes, renal and LFTs. Carefully monitor elderly and those with renal dysfunction for desired response and adverse side effects.
3. Ensure adequate hydration, especially with diuretic therapy in renal dysfunction.

CLIENT/FAMILY TEACHING
1. Take as directed with or without food; ensure adequate fluid intake.
2. Practice barrier birth control; report if pregnancy suspected.
3. Continue life style modifications, i.e. diet, regular exercise, stress reduction, no smoking, and moderate alcohol in-

---

Bold Italic = life threatening side effect   ■ = black box warning   ✤ = Available in Canada

take to ensure BP control. Report any adverse effects.

OUTCOMES/EVALUATE
- ↓ BP
- Migraine prophylaxis

Captropil ■
(**KAP**-toe-prill)

CLASSIFICATION(S):
Antihypertensive, ACE inhibitor
PREGNANCY CATEGORY: C (first trimester); **D** (second and third trimesters)
Rx: Capoten
♣Rx: Apo-Capto, Gen-Captopril, Novo-Captoril, Nu-Capto, PMS-Captopril, ratio-Captopril

SEE ALSO *ANGIOTENSIN-CONVERTING ENZYME (ACE) INHIBITORS.*

ACTION/KINETICS
Onset: 30 min or less. **Peak serum levels:** 30–90 min; presence of food decreases absorption by 30–40%. Is 75% or more bioavailable. **Time to peak effect:** 60–90 min. **Duration:** 6–10 hr (dose related). **t½, normal renal function, elimination:** 2 hr; **t½, impaired renal function:** 3.5–32 hr. More than 95% of absorbed dose excreted in urine (40–50% unchanged). 25–30% is bound to plasma proteins.

USES
(1) Antihypertensive, alone or in combination with other antihypertensive drugs, especially thiazide diuretics. May be used as initial therapy for those with normal renal function. *Note:* In clients with impaired renal function, especially those with collagen vascular disease, reserve captopril for hypertensive clients who have either developed unacceptable side effects on other drugs or have failed to respond satisfactorily to drug combinations. (2) In combination with diuretics and digitalis in treatment of CHF. (3) To improve survival following MI in clinically stable clients with LV dysfunction manifested as an ejection fraction of 40% or less; to reduce the incidence of overt heart failure and sub-

sequent hospitilization for CHF in these clients. (4) Treatment of diabetic nephropathy (proteinuria > 500 mg/day) in those with type I insulin-dependent diabetes and retinopathy. *Investigational:* Rheumatoid arthritis, hypertensive crisis, neonatal and childhood hypertension, hypertension related to scleroderma renal crisis, diagnosis of anatomic renal artery stenosis, diagnosis of primary aldosteronism, Raynaud's syndrome, diagnosis of renovascular hypertension, enhance sensitivity and specificity of renal scintigraphy, idiopathic edema, and Bartter's syndrome.

CONTRAINDICATIONS
Use with a history of angioedema related to previous ACE inhibitor use.

SPECIAL CONCERNS
■Can cause injury and even death in the developing fetus if used during the second and third trimesters. Discontinue as soon as possible if pregnancy is detected.■ Use with caution in cases of impaired renal function and during lactation. Use in children only if other antihypertensive therapy has proven ineffective in controlling BP. May cause a profound drop in BP following the first dose or if used with diuretics.

SIDE EFFECTS
Dermatologic: Rash (usually maculopapular) with pruritus and occasionally fever, eosinophilia, and arthralgia. Alopecia, erythema multiforme, photosensitivity, exfoliative dermatitis, *Stevens-Johnson syndrome,* reversible pemphigoid-like lesions, bullous pemphigus, onycholysis, flushing, pallor, scalded mouth sensation. **GI:** N&V, anorexia, constipation or diarrhea, gastric irritation, abdominal pain, dysgeusia, peptic/aphthous ulcers, dyspepsia, dry mouth, glossitis, pancreatitis. **Hepatic:** Jaundice, cholestasis, hepatitis. **CNS:** Headache, dizziness, insomnia, malaise, fatigue, paresthesias, confusion, depression, nervousness, ataxia, somnolence. **CV:** Hypotension, angina, *MI,* Raynaud's phenomenon, chest pain, palpitations, tachycardia, *CVA, CHF, cardiac arrest,* orthostatic hypotension, rhythm disturbances, cerebrovascular insufficiency. **Renal:** Renal insufficiency/failure, pro-

C

teinuria, urinary frequency, oliguria, polyuria, nephrotic syndrome, interstitial nephritis. **Respiratory: *Bronchospasm*,** cough, dyspnea, asthma, ***pulmonary embolism/infarction*.** **Hematologic:** Agranulocytosis, neutropenia, thrombocytopenia, pancytopenia, ***aplastic/hemolytic anemia*. Other:** Decrease/loss of taste perception with weight loss (reversible), angioedema, asthenia, syncope, fever, myalgia, arthralgia, vasculitis, blurred vision, impotence, hyperkalemia, hyponatremia, myasthenia, gynecomastia, rhinitis, eosinophilic pneumonitis.

LABORATORY TEST CONSIDERATIONS
False + test for urine acetone.

OD **OVERDOSE MANAGEMENT**
Symptoms: Hypotension with SBP of <80 mm Hg a possibility. *Treatment:* Volume expansion with NSS (IV) is the treatment of choice to restore BP.

ADDITIONAL DRUG INTERACTIONS
Indomethacin / ↓ 24-hr antihypertensive effects of captopril
Iron salts / ↓ Captopril blood levels; separate administration by at least 2 hr
Probenecid / ↑ captopril blood levels R/T ↓ renal excretion

HOW SUPPLIED
Tablet: 12.5 mg, 25 mg, 50 mg, 100 mg

DOSAGE————————————————

• **TABLETS**
Hypertension.
Adults, initial: 25 mg 2–3 times per day. If unsatisfactory response after 1–2 weeks, increase to 50 mg 2–3 times per day; if still unsatisfactory after another 1–2 weeks, add a thiazide diuretic (e.g., hydrochlorothiazide, 25 mg/day). May increase dose to 100–150 mg 2–3 times per day, not to exceed 450 mg/day.
Accelerated or malignant hypertension.
Stop current medication (except for the diuretic) and initiate captopril at 25 mg 2–3 times per day. May increase dose q 24 hr until a satisfactory response is obtained or the maximum dose reached. Furosemide may be indicated.
Heart failure.
Initial: 25 mg three times per day; **then,** if necessary, increase dose to 50 mg 3 times per day and evaluate re-

sponse. Delay further increases for at least 2 weeks to determine if a satisfactory response has been attained. **Maintenance:** 50–100 mg three times per day for most clients. Do not exceed 450 mg/day.
NOTE: For adults, give an initial dose of 6.25–12.5 mg (0.15 mg/kg 3 times per day in children) 2–3 times per day to clients who are sodium- and water-depleted due to diuretics, who will continue to be on diuretic therapy, and who have renal impairment.
Left ventricular dysfunction after MI.
Therapy may be started as early as 3 days after the MI. **Initial dose:** 6.25 mg; **then,** begin 12.5 mg three times per day and increase to 25 mg three times per day over the next several days. The target dose is 50 mg three times per day over the next several weeks. Other treatments for MI may be used concomitantly (e.g., aspirin, beta blockers, thrombolytic drugs).
Diabetic nephropathy.
25 mg three times per day for chronic use. Other antihypertensive drugs (e.g., beta blockers, centrally-acting drugs, diuretics, vasodilators) may be used with captopril if additional drug therapy is needed to reduce BP.
Hypertensive crisis.
Initial: 25 mg; **then,** 100 mg 90–120 min later, 200–300 mg/day for 2–5 days (then adjust dose). Sublingual captopril, 25 mg, has also been used successfully.
Rheumatoid arthritis.
75–150 mg/day in divided doses.
Severe childhood hypertension.
Initial: 0.3 mg/kg titrated to 6 mg or less given in 2 to 3 divided doses.
NOTE: For all uses, reduce dose in clients with renal impairment.

NURSING CONSIDERATIONS
ADMINISTRATION/STORAGE
1. Do not discontinue without the provider's consent.
2. Give 1 hr before meals.
3. Discontinue previous antihypertensive medication 1 week before starting captopril, if possible.
4. The tablets can be used to prepare a solution of captopril if desired.

Bold Italic = life threatening side effect   ■ = black box warning   ♣ = Available in Canada

ASSESSMENT

1. Note disease onset, other medical conditions, other agents trialed and outcome.
2. Monitor VS, potassium, hematologic, renal, and LFTs.
3. Determine if diuretics or nitrates prescribed; may act synergistically and cause a more pronounced response.
4. Document any ACE intolerance.
5. Determine ability to understand/comply with therapy.
6. Note ejection fraction (at or below 40%) in stable, post-MI clients.
7. Usually very effective with heart failure, diabetes, and arthritis.

INTERVENTIONS

1. Observe for precipitous drop in BP within 3 hr after initial dose if on diuretic therapy and a low-salt diet.
2. If BP falls rapidly, place supine; have saline infusion available.
3. Check for proteinuria monthly for 9 months during therapy and CBC every two weeks for the first 3 months of therapy.
4. Withhold potassium-sparing diuretics; hyperkalemia may result. Hyperkalemia may occur several months after administration of spironolactone and captopril.

CLIENT/FAMILY TEACHING

1. Take 1 hr before meals, on an empty stomach; food interferes with drug absorption.
2. Report any fever, skin rash, sore throat, mouth sores, fast or irregular heartbeat, chest pain, or cough.
3. May develop dizziness, fainting, or lightheadedness; usually disappears once body adjusts to drug. Avoid sudden changes in posture and activities/exercise in hot weather to prevent dizziness/fainting. Consume plenty of fluids to prevent dehydration.
4. Loss of taste may be experienced for the first 2–3 months; report if persists/interferes with nutrition/weight.
5. Carry ID and a list of medications currently prescribed.
6. Call with any questions concerning symptoms or effects of drug therapy; do not stop taking abruptly. Report for regular F/U of BP, electrolytes and urine protein.
7. Insulin-dependent clients may experience hypoglycemia; monitor FS closely.
8. Avoid OTC agents without approval.
9. Practice reliable contraception; report if pregnancy suspected.

OUTCOMES/EVALUATE

- ↓ BP
- Improvement in symptoms of CHF (↓ preload, ↓ afterload)
- Improved mortality post-MI

Carvedilol

(kar-**VAY**-dih-lol)

CLASSIFICATION(S):
Alpha-beta adrenergic blocking agent
PREGNANCY CATEGORY: C
Rx: Coreg

SEE ALSO *ALPHA-1 AND BETA-ADRENERGIC BLOCKING AGENTS.*

ACTION/KINETICS

Has both alpha- and beta-adrenergic blocking activity. Decreases cardiac output, reduces exercise- or isoproterenol-induced tachycardia, reduces reflex orthostatic hypotension, causes vasodilation, and reduces peripheral vascular resistance. Significant beta-blocking activity occurs within 60 min while alpha-blocking action is observed within 30 min. BP is lowered more in the standing than in the supine position. Significantly lowers plasma renin activity when given for at least 4 weeks. Rapidly absorbed after PO administration; significant first-pass effect. **Terminal t ½:** 7–10 hr. Food delays absorption rate. Over 98% is bound to plasma protein. Plasma levels average 50% higher in geriatric compared with younger clients. Extensively metabolized in the liver; metabolites excreted primarily via the bile into the feces.

USES

(1) Essential hypertension used either alone or in combination with other antihypertensive drugs, especially thiazide

diuretics. (2) Mild to severe heart failure of ischemic or cardiomyopathic origin; used with diuretics, ACE inhibitors, and digitalis to increase survival and reduce risk of hospitalization. (3) Reduce CV mortality in clinically stable clients who have survived an acute MI and have a left ventricular ejection fraction of 40% or less (with or without symptomatic heart failure). *Investigational:* Angina pectoris, idiopathic cardiomyopathy.

CONTRAINDICATIONS
Clients with NYHA Class IV decompensated cardiac failure, bronchial asthma, or related bronchospastic conditions, second- or third-degree AV block, SSS (unless a permanent pacemaker is in place), cardiogenic shock, severe bradycardia, drug hypersensitivity. Hepatic impairment. Lactation.

SPECIAL CONCERNS
Use with caution in hypertensive clients with CHF controlled with digitalis, diuretics, or an ACE inhibitor. Use with caution in PVD, in surgical procedures using anesthetic agents that depress myocardial function, in diabetics receiving insulin or oral hypoglycemic drugs, in those subject to spontaneous hypoglycemia, or in thyrotoxicosis. Worsening cardiac failure or fluid retention may occur during up-titration of carvedilol. Signs of hyperthyroidism or hypoglycemia, especially tachycardia, may be masked. Clients with a history of severe anaphylactic reaction to a variety of allergens may be more reactive to repeated challenge while taking beta blockers. Safety and efficacy have not been established in children less than 18 years of age.

SIDE EFFECTS
CV: Bradycardia, postural hypotension, dependent/peripheral edema, AV block, bundle branch block, cerebrovascular disorder, extrasystoles, hyper/hypotension, palpitations, peripheral ischemia, syncope, angina, aggravated angina, *cardiac failure,* myocardial ischemia, tachycardia, CV disorder, fluid overload. **CNS:** Dizziness, headache, somnolence, insomnia, ataxia, hypesthesia, paresthesia, vertigo, depression, nervousness, migraine, neuralgia, paresis, amnesia, confusion, sleep disorder, impaired concentration, abnormal thinking, paranoia, convulsions, emotional lability, hypokinesia. **Body as a whole:** Fatigue, viral infection, rash, allergy, asthenia, malaise, pain, injury, fever, infection, peripheral edema, generalized edema, somnolence, sweating, *sudden death.* **GI:** Diarrhea, abdominal pain, bilirubinemia, N&V, flatulence, dry mouth, anorexia, dyspepsia, melena, periodontitis, increased hepatic enzymes, hepatotoxicity, *GI hemorrhage.* **Respiratory:** Rhinitis, pharyngitis, sinusitis, bronchitis, dyspnea, *asthma, bronchospasm,* pulmonary edema, respiratory alkalosis, dyspnea, respiratory disorder, URTI, coughing, rales. **GU:** UTI, albuminuria, hematuria, frequency of micturition, abnormal renal function, impotence, renal insufficiency, kidney failure. **Dermatologic:** Pruritus, erythematous rash, alopecia, maculopapular rash, psoriaform rash, photosensitivity reaction, exfoliative dermatitis, increased sweating. **Metabolic:** Hypertriglyceridemia, hypercholesterolemia, hyper/hypoglycemia, hypo/hypervolemia, hyperuricemia, weight gain/loss, gout, dehydration, glycosuria, hyponatremia, hypo/hyperkalemia, diabetes mellitus. **Hematologic:** Thrombocytopenia, anemia, leukopenia, pancytopenia, purpura, atypical lymphocytes, *aplastic anemia (rare).* **Musculoskeletal:** Back pain, arthralgia, myalgia, arthritis, muscle cramps. **Otic:** Decreased hearing, tinnitus. **Miscellaneous:** Hot flushes, leg cramps, abnormal vision, blurred vision, decreased hearing, decreased libido, *anaphylactoid reaction.*

LABORATORY TEST CONSIDERATIONS
↑ ALT, AST, BUN, NPN, alkaline phosphatase, GGT, creatinine. ↓ HDL.

OD OVERDOSE MANAGEMENT
Symptoms: Severe hypotension, bradycardia, cardiac insufficiency, *cardiogenic shock, cardiac arrest, generalized seizures,* respiratory problems, bronchospasms, vomiting, lapse of consciousness. *Treatment:* Place client in a supine position, monitor carefully, and treat under intensive care conditions. Continue treatment for a sufficient peri-

od consistent with the 7- to 10-hr drug half-life.
• Gastric lavage or induced emesis shortly after ingestion.
• For excessive bradycardia, atropine, 2 mg IV. If bradycardia is resistant to therapy; use pacemaker therapy.
• To support cardiovascular function, give glucagon, 5–10 mg IV rapidly over 30 sec, followed by a continuous infusion of 5 mg/hr. Sympathomimetics (dobutamine, isoproterenol, epinephrine) may be given.
• For peripheral vasodilation, give epinephrine or norepinephrine with continuous monitoring of circulatory conditions.
• For bronchospasm, give beta sympathomimetics as aerosol or IV or use aminophylline IVPB.
• With seizures, give diazepam or clonazepam slowly IV.

DRUG INTERACTIONS
Antidiabetic agents / ↑ Hypoglycemic effects due to beta blockade
Calcium channel blocking agents / ↑ Risk of conduction disturbances; monitor ECG and BP
Catecholamine-depleting drugs (e.g., reserpine) / Possible hypotension or severe bradycardia
Cimetidine / ↑ Carvedilol AUC by about 30%; no change in C_{max}
Clonidine / Potentiation of BP and heart rate lowering effects
Cyclosporine / ↑ Cyclosporine blood levels R/T ↓ liver breakdown
Digoxin / ↑ Digoxin levels
Diphenhydramine / ↑ Carvedilol plasma levels R/T inhibition of metabolism
Disopyramide / ↓ Disopyramide clearance → sinus bradycardia and hypotension; monitor carefully
Hydroxychloroquine / ↑ Plasma and CV effects of carvedilol R/T inhibition of metabolism
Rifampin / ↓ Plasma carvedilol AUC and C_{max} by about 70%
Selective serotonin reuptake inhibitors (e.g., fluoxetine, paroxetine) / Inhibition of carvedilol metabolism → excessive bradycardia; monitor cardiac function if used together

HOW SUPPLIED
Tablet: 3.125 mg, 6.25 mg, 12.5 mg, 25 mg

DOSAGE
• **TABLETS**
Essential hypertension.
Initial: 6.25 mg twice per day. If tolerated, using standing systolic pressure measured about 1 hr after dosing, maintain dose for 7–14 days. **Then,** increase to 12.5 mg twice per day, if necessary, based on trough BP, using standing systolic pressure 2 hr after dosing. Maintain this dose for 7–14 days; adjust upward to 25 mg twice per day. if necessary and tolerated. Do not exceed 50 mg/day.
Congestive heart failure.
Individualize dose. **Initial:** 3.125 mg twice per day for 2 weeks. If tolerated, increase to 6.25 mg twice per day. Double dose every 2 weeks to the highest tolerated level, up to a maximum of 25 mg twice per day in those weighing less than 85 kg and 50 mg twice per day in those weighing over 85 kg.
Left ventricular dysfunction following MI.
Individualize dose. **Initial:** 6.25 mg twice per day; increase after 3–10 days, based on tolerability, to 12.5 mg twice per day. Increase again to a target dose of 25 mg twice per day. A lower starting dose (3.125 mg twice per day) may be used due to low BP, HR, or fluid retention.
Angina pectoris.
25–50 mg twice per day.
Idiopathic cardiomyopathy.
6.25–25 mg twice per day.

NURSING CONSIDERATIONS
ADMINISTRATION/STORAGE
1. The full antihypertensive effect is seen within 7–14 days.
2. Addition of a diuretic can produce additive effects and exaggerate the orthostatic effect.
3. Fluid retention can be treated with an increase in the dose of diuretics, whether or not heart failure symptoms have worsened.
4. Episodes of dizziness or fluid retention during initiation of therapy can

---

H = Herbal   **IV** = Intravenous   *@* = sound-alike drug

C

usually be managed by discontinuing the drug. This does not preclude subsequent successful titration of or a favorable response to the drug.

5. Reduce the dose if bradycardia (HR less than 55 beats/min) occurs.

ASSESSMENT

1. Document indications for therapy, type/onset of symptoms, other agents trialed, and outcome.

2. Note any history/evidence of bronchospastic conditions, asthma, advanced AV block, or severe bradycardia; drug contraindicated.

3. Obtain baseline VS, EKG, CBC, and renal and LFTs and monitor. Assess lung sounds and for evidence of edema. Note ejection fraction and stress test results.

CLIENT/FAMILY TEACHING

1. Take as prescribed with food to slow absorption and decrease incidence of orthostatic effects.

2. Avoid activities that require mental acuity until drug effects realized.

3. Do not stop abruptly due to beta-blocking activity (especially with ischemic heart disease); call provider.

4. To prevent ↓ BP, sit or lie until symptoms subside; rise slowly from a sitting or lying position. Concomitant therapy with a diuretic may aggravate orthostatic drug effects.

5. Decreased tearing may be noted by contact lens wearers.

6. Dosing adjustments will be made every 7–14 days based on standing SBP measured 1 hr after dosing.

OUTCOMES/EVALUATE

• Desired reduction of BP
• ↓ Progression of CHF
• ↓ Remodeling
• ↓ Mortality

Cholestyramine resin

(koh-less-**TEER**-ah-meen)

CLASSIFICATION(S):

Antihyperlipidemic, bile acid sequestrant

PREGNANCY CATEGORY: B

Rx: Cholestyramine Light, LoCHOLEST, LoCHOLEST Light, Prevalite, Questran, Questran Light

✤**Rx:** Novo-Cholamine, Novo-Cholamine Light, PMS-Cholestyramine, Questran Light

ACTION/KINETICS

Binds sodium cholate (bile salts) in the intestine; thus, the principal precursor of cholesterol is not absorbed due to formation of an insoluble complex, which is excreted in the feces. Decreases cholesterol and LDL and either has no effect or increases triglycerides, VLDL, and HDL. Also, itching is relieved as a result of removing irritating bile salts. The antidiarrheal effect results from the binding and removal of bile acids. **Onset, to reduce plasma cholesterol:** Within 24–48 hr, but levels may continue to fall for 1 yr; **to relieve pruritus:** 1–3 weeks; **relief of diarrhea associated with bile acids:** 24 hr. Cholesterol levels return to pretreatment levels 2–4 weeks after discontinuance. Fat-soluble vitamins (A, D, K) and possibly folic acid may have to be administered IM during long-term therapy because cholestyramine binds these vitamins in the intestine.

USES

(1) Adjunct to reduce elevated serum cholesterol in primary hypercholesterolemia in those who do not respond adequately to diet. (2) Pruritus associated with partial biliary obstruction. (3) Diarrhea due to bile acids. *Investigational:* Antibiotic-induced pseudomembranous colitis (i.e., due to toxin produced by *Clostridium difficile*), digitalis toxicity, treatment of chlordecone (Kepone) poisoning, treatment of thyroid hormone overdose.

CONTRAINDICATIONS

Complete obstruction or atresia of bile duct.

SPECIAL CONCERNS

Use during pregnancy only if benefits outweigh risks. Use with caution during lactation and in children. Long-term effects and efficacy in decreasing cholesterol levels in pediatric clients are not known. Geriatric clients may be more likely to manifest GI side effects as well as adverse nutritional effects. Exercise caution in clients with phenylketonuria as Prevalite contains 14.1 mg phenylalanine per 5.5-g dose.

SIDE EFFECTS
GI: Constipation (may be severe), N&V, diarrhea, heartburn, GI bleeding, anorexia, flatulence, belching, abdominal distention/pain or cramping, loose stools, indigestion, aggravation of hemorrhoids, rectal bleeding or pain, black stools, bleeding duodenal ulcer, peptic ulceration, GI irritation, dysphagia, dental bleeding, hiccoughs, sour taste, pancreatitis, diverticulitis, cholecystitis, cholelithiasis. Fecal impaction in elderly clients. Large doses may cause steatorrhea. **CNS:** Migraine/sinus headaches, dizziness, anxiety, vertigo, insomnia, fatigue, lightheadedness, syncope, drowsiness, femoral nerve pain, paresthesia. **Hypersensitivity:** Urticaria, dermatitis, asthma, wheezing, rash. **Hematologic:** Increased PT, ecchymosis, anemia. **Musculoskeletal:** Muscle or joint pain, backache, arthritis, osteoporosis. **GU:** Hematuria, dysuria, burnt odor to urine, diuresis. **Other:** Bleeding tendencies (due to hypoprothrombinemia). Deficiencies of vitamins A and D. Uveitis, weight loss or gain, osteoporosis, swollen glands, increased libido, weakness, SOB, edema, swelling of hands/feet; hyperchloremic acidosis in children, rash/irritation of the skin, tongue, and perianal area.

LABORATORY TEST CONSIDERATIONS Liver function abnormalities.

OD OVERDOSE MANAGEMENT
Symptoms: GI tract obstruction.

DRUG INTERACTIONS
Anticoagulants, PO / ↓ Anticoagulant effect R/T ↓ GI tract absorption
Aspirin / ↓ Aspirin absorption from GI tract
Clindamycin / ↓ Clindamycin absorption from GI tract
Clofibrate / ↓ Clofibrate absorption from GI tract
Digoxin / ↓ Digitalis effect R/T ↓ GI tract absorption
Furosemide / ↓ Furosemide absorption from GI tract
Gemfibrozil / ↓ Gemfibrozil bioavailability
Glipizide / ↓ Serum glipizide levels
Hydrocortisone / ↓ Hydrocortisone effect R/T ↓ GI tract absorption
Imipramine / ↓ Imipramine absorption from GI tract
Iopanoic acid / Results in abnormal cholecystography
Lovastatin / Effects may be additive
Methyldopa / ↓ Methyldopa absorption from GI tract
Nicotinic acid / ↓ Nicotinic acid absorption from GI tract
Penicillin G / ↓ Penicillin G effect R/T ↓ GI tract absorption
Phenytoin / ↓ Phenytoin absorption from GI tract
Phosphate supplements / ↓ Phosphate absorption from GI tract
Piroxicam / ↑ Piroxicam elimination
Propranolol / ↓ Propranolol effect R/T ↓ GI tract absorption
Tetracyclines / ↓ Tetracycline effects R/T ↓ GI tract absorption
Thiazide diuretics / ↓ Thiazide effects R/T ↓ GI tract absorption
Thyroid hormones, Thyroxine / ↓ Thyroid effects R/T ↓ GI tract absorption
Tolbutamide / ↓ Tolbutamide absorption from GI tract
Troglitazone / ↓ Troglitazone absorption from the GI tract
Ursodiol / ↓ Ursodiol effects R/T ↓ GI tract absorption
Vitamins A, D, E, K / Malabsorption of fat-soluble vitamins
Vitamin C / ↑ Vitamin C absorption
NOTE: These drug interactions may also be observed with colestipol.

HOW SUPPLIED
Powder for Suspension: 4 g/dose, 4 g/5.5 g powder, 4 g/5.7 g powder, 4 g/6.4 g powder, 4 g/9 g powder

DOSAGE
• **POWDER**
Adults, initial: 4 g 1–2 times per day. Dose is individualized. For Prevalite, give 1 packet or 1 level scoopful (5.5 g Prevalite: 4 g anhydrous cholestyramine). **Maintenance:** 2–4 packets or scoopfuls per day (8–16 g anhydrous cholestyramine resin) mixed with 60–180 mL water or noncarbonated

C

beverage. The recommended dosing schedule is twice per day but it can be given in one to six doses per day. Maximum daily dose: 6 packets or scoopfuls (equivalent to 24 g cholestyramine).

NURSING CONSIDERATIONS
ADMINISTRATION/STORAGE
1. Always mix powder with 60–180 mL water or noncarbonated beverage before administering; resin may cause esophageal irritation or blockage. Highly liquid soups or pulpy fruits such as applesauce or crushed pineapple may be used. Do not take in dry form.
2. After placing contents of 1 packet of resin on the surface of 4–6 oz of fluid, allow it to stand without stirring for 2 min, occasionally twirling the glass, and then stir slowly (to prevent foaming) to form a suspension.
3. Avoid inhaling powder; may be irritating to mucous membranes.
4. Cholestyramine may interfere with the absorption of other drugs taken orally; thus, take other drug(s) 1 hr before or 4–6 hr after dosing.

ASSESSMENT
1. Document indications for therapy, symptom type/onset, and other agents trialed.
2. Determine onset of pruritus and note bile acid level with cholestasia.
3. Monitor CBC, cholesterol profile, and liver and renal function studies.
4. Vitamins A, D, E, K, and folic acid will need to be administered in a water-miscible form during long-term therapy.
5. Assess skin and eyes for evidence of jaundice or bile deposits.

CLIENT/FAMILY TEACHING
1. Other prescribed medications should be taken at least 1 hr before or 4-6 hr after taking drug. These drugs interfere with the absorption and desired effects of other medications.
2. Do not take drug in dry form; always spinkle powder on surface of liquid (preferably milk, water or juice) and let stand a few min, then stir and drink. Avoid carbonated beverages as these cause too much foaming. Add extra fluid to bottom of glass and swirl to

ensure entire dose consumed. Take before meals and at bedtime.
3. Review constipating effects of drug and ways to control: daily exercise, fluid intake of 2.5–3 L/day, increased intake of citrus fruits, fruit juices, and high-fiber foods; also, a stool softener may help. If constipation persists, a change in dosage or drug may be indicated.
4. Clients with high cholesterol levels should follow dietary restrictions of fat and cholesterol as well as risk factor reduction such as smoking cessation, alcohol reduction, weight loss, and regular exercise.
5. Report tarry stools or abnormal bleeding as supplemental vitamin K (10 mg/week) may be necessary. CBC, PT, and renal function tests should be done routinely.
6. Itching (pruritus) may subside 1–3 weeks after taking the drug but may return after the medication is discontinued. Corn starch or oatmeal baths may also alleviate symptoms. Report any unusual or intolerable side effects.

OUTCOMES/EVALUATE
- Control of pruritus
- ↓ Serum cholesterol levels
- ↓ Diarrheal stools
- ↓ Bile acid levels

Cilostazol   ■ⓒ
(sih-**LESS**-tah-zohl)

CLASSIFICATION(S):
Antiplatelet drug
PREGNANCY CATEGORY: C
Rx: Pletal

ACTION/KINETICS
Inhibits cellular phosphodiesterase (PDE), especially PDE III. Cilostazol and several metabolites inhibit cyclic AMP PDE III. Suppression of this isoenzyme causes increased levels of cyclic AMP resulting in vasodilation and inhibition of platelet aggregation. Inhibits platelet aggregation caused by thrombin, ADP, collagen, arachidonic acid, epinephrine, and shear stress. High fat meals significantly increase absorption. Significantly

plasma protein bound. Extensively metabolized by the liver with two of the metabolites being active. Primarily excreted through the urine (74%) with the rest in the feces.

USES
Reduce symptoms of intermittent claudication.

CONTRAINDICATIONS
See Black Box Warning in *Special Concerns*. Concurrent use of grapefruit juice. Lactation.

SPECIAL CONCERNS
■Cilostazol and several of its metabolites are phosphodiesterase III inhibitors. Such compounds have caused decreased survival in those with class III-IV CHF. Contraindicated in clients with CHF of any severity.■ Safety and efficacy have not been determined in children.

SIDE EFFECTS
GI: Abnormal stool, diarrhea, dyspepsia, flatulence, N&V, abdominal pain, anorexia, cholelithiasis, colitis, duodenal ulcer, duodenitis, esophageal hemorrhage, esophagitis, gastritis, gastroenteritis, gum hemorrhage, hematemesis, melena, gastric ulcer, periodontal abscess, rectal hemorrhage, stomach ulcer, tongue edema. **CNS:** Headache, dizziness, vertigo, anxiety, insomnia, neuralgia. **CV:** Palpitation, tachycardia, hypertension, angina pectoris, atrial fibrillation/flutter, cerebral infarct, cerebral ischemia, CHF, *heart arrest, hemorrhage,* hypotension, MI, myocardial ischemia, nodal arrhythmia, postural hypotension, supraventricular tachycardia, syncope, varicose veins, vasodilation, ventricular extrasystole or *ventricular tachycardia.* **Respiratory:** Rhinitis, pharyngitis, increased cough, dyspnea, bronchitis, asthma, epistaxis, hemoptysis, pneumonia, sinusitis. **Musculoskeletal:** Back pain, myalgia, asthenia, leg cramps, arthritis, arthralgia, bone pain, bursitis. **Dermatologic:** Rash, dry skin, furunculosis, skin hypertrophy, urticaria. **GU:** Hematuria, UTI, cystitis, urinary frequency, vaginal hemorrhage, vaginitis. **Hematologic:** Anemia, ecchymosis, iron deficiency anemia, polycythemia, purpura. **Ophthalmic:** Amblyopia, blindness, conjunctivitis, diplopia, eye hemorrhage, retinal hemorrhage. **Miscellaneous:** Infection, peripheral edema, hyperesthesia, paresthesia, flu syndrome, ear pain, tinnitus, chills, facial edema, fever, generalized edema, malaise, neck rigidity, pelvic pain, *retroperitoneal hemorrhage,* diabetes mellitus.

LABORATORY TEST CONSIDERATIONS
↑ GGT, creatinine. Albuminuria, hyperlipemia, hyperuricemia.

OD OVERDOSE MANAGEMENT
Symptoms: Severe headache, diarrhea, hypotension, tachycardia, possible cardiac arrhythmias. *Treatment:* Observe client carefully and provide symptomatic treatment.

DRUG INTERACTIONS
Diltiazem, erythromycin, grapefruit juice, itraconazole, ketoconazole, macrolide antibiotics, and omeprazole inhibit liver enzymes that breakdown cilostazol, resulting in ↑ plasma levels. Reduce dose of these drugs if used concomitantly.

HOW SUPPLIED
Tablets: 50 mg, 100 mg

DOSAGE
- **TABLETS**
  Intermittent claudication.
  100 mg twice a day taken 30 min or more before or 2 hr after breakfast and dinner. Consider a dose of 50 mg twice a day during coadministration of diltiazem, erythromycin, itraconazole, or ketoconazole.

NURSING CONSIDERATIONS
℮ Do not confuse Pletal with Plavix (also an antiplatelet drug).

ADMINISTRATION/STORAGE
The dosage of cilostazol may be reduced or discontinued without platelet hyperaggregability.

ASSESSMENT
1. Determine onset and characteristics of symptoms. Measure distance walked before pain elicited.
2. List drugs currently prescribed to ensure none interact. Determine any history or evidence of CV disease or CHF.
3. Monitor CBC, and for liver or renal dysfunction. Document ABIs.

H = Herbal   IV = Intravenous   ℮ = sound-alike drug

4. Assess extent/amount/duration of nicotine use.

CLIENT/FAMILY TEACHING
1. Take 30 min before or 2 hr after meals. Avoid consuming grapefruit juice.
2. Read the patient package insert carefully before starting therapy and each time therapy is renewed.
3. May experience headaches, GI upset, dizziness, or runny nose; report if bothersome.
4. Do not smoke; enroll in formal smoking cessation program.
5. Continue to walk past the point of severe pain before resting, then resume walking to improve symptoms and distance able to walk before pain recurs.
6. Beneficial effects may be seen in 2 to 4 weeks, but up to 12 weeks may be needed before evident.

OUTCOMES/EVALUATE
• Increased walking distance without pain
• ↓ S&S intermittent claudication

Clonidine hydrochloride

(**KLOH**-nih-deen)

CLASSIFICATION(S):
Antihypertensive, centrally-acting
PREGNANCY CATEGORY: C
Rx: Catapres, Catapres-TTS-1, -2, and -3, Duraclon
✤**Rx:** Apo-Clonidine, Dixarit, Novo-Clonidine, Nu-Clonidine

SEE ALSO *ANTIHYPERTENSIVE AGENTS.*

ACTION/KINETICS
Stimulates alpha-adrenergic receptors of the CNS, which results in inhibition of the sympathetic vasomotor centers and decreased nerve impulses. Thus, bradycardia and a fall in both SBP and DBP occur. Plasma renin levels are decreased, while peripheral venous pressure remains unchanged. Few orthostatic effects. Although NaCl excretion is markedly decreased, potassium excretion remains unchanged. To relieve spasticity, it decreases excitatory amino acids by central presynaptic α–receptor agonism. Tolerance to the drug may develop. **Onset, PO:** 30–60 min; **transdermal:** 2–3 days. **Peak plasma levels, PO:** 3–5 hr; **transdermal:** 2–3 days. **Maximum effect, PO:** 2–4 hr. **Duration, PO:** 12–24 hr; **transdermal:** 7 days (with system in place). **t ½:** 12–16 hr. Approximately 50% excreted unchanged in the urine; 20% excreted through the feces. The transdermal dosage form contains the following levels of drug: Catapres-TTS-1 contains 2.5 mg clonidine (surface area 3.5 cm²), with 0.1 mg released daily; Catapres-TTS-2 contains 5 mg clonidine (surface area 7 cm²), with 0.2 mg released daily; and Catapres-TTS-3 contains 7.5 mg clonidine (surface area 10.5 cm²), with 0.3 mg released daily.

Epidural use causes analgesia at presynaptic and postjunctional alpha-2-adrenergic receptors in the spinal cord due to prevention of pain signal transmission to the brain. **t ½, distribution, epidural:** 19 min; **elimination:** 22 hr.

USES
Oral, Transdermal: (1) Alone or with a diuretic or other antihypertensives to treat mild to moderate hypertension. (2) Treat spasticity. *Investigational:* Alcohol withdrawal, atrial fibrillation, attention deficit hyperactivity disorder, constitutional growth delay in children, cyclosporine-associated nephrotoxicity, diabetic diarrhea, Gilles de la Tourette's syndrome, hyperhidrosis, hypertensive emergencies, mania, menopausal flushing, opiate detoxification, diagnosis of pheochromocytoma, postherpetic neuralgia, psychosis in schizophrenia, reduce allergen-induced inflammatory reactions in extrinsic asthma, restless leg syndrome, facilitate smoking cessation, ulcerative colitis.
Epidural: With opiates for severe pain in cancer clients not relieved by opiate analgesics alone. Most effective for neuropathic pain.

CONTRAINDICATIONS
Epidurally: Presence of an injection site infection, clients on anticoagulant therapy, in bleeding diathesis, administration above the C4 dermatome. For ob-

---

Bold Italic = life threatening side effect   ■ = black box warning   ✤ = Available in Canada

stetic, postpartum, or perioperative pain.

SPECIAL CONCERNS

Use with caution during lactation and in the presence of severe coronary insufficiency, recent MI, cerebrovascular disease, or chronic renal failure. Safe use in children not established; when used for attention deficit disorder, even one extra dose can be harmful. Geriatric clients may be more sensitive to the hypotensive effects; a decreased dosage may also be necessary in these clients due to age-related decreases in renal function. For children, restrict epidural use to severe intractable pain from malignancy that is unresponsive to epidural or spinal opiates or other analgesic approaches.

SIDE EFFECTS

CNS: Drowsiness (common), sedation, confusion, dizziness, headache, fatigue, malaise, nightmares, nervousness, restlessness, anxiety, mental depression, increased dreaming, insomnia, hallucinations, delirium, agitation. **GI:** Dry mouth (common), constipation, anorexia, N&V, parotid pain, weight gain, hepatitis, parotitis, ileus, pseudo-obstruction, abdominal pain. **CV:** CHF, severe hypotension, Raynaud's phenomenon, abnormalities in ECG, palpitations, tachycardia/bradycardia, postural hypotension, conduction disturbances, sinus bradycardia, *CVA*. **Dermatologic:** Urticaria, skin rashes, sweating, *angioneurotic edema,* pruritus, thinning of hair, alopecia, skin ulcer. **GU:** Impotence, urinary retention, decreased sexual activity, loss of libido, nocturia, difficulty in urination, UTI. **Respiratory:** Hypoventilation, dyspnea. **Musculoskeletal:** Muscle or joint pain, leg cramps, weakness. **Other:** Gynecomastia, increase in blood glucose (transient), increased sensitivity to alcohol, chest pain, tinnitus, hyperaesthesia, pain, infection, thrombocytopenia, syncope, blurred vision, withdrawal syndrome, dryness of mucous membranes of nose; itching, burning, dryness of eyes; skin pallor, fever. *NOTE:* When used for ADHD in children, can cause serious side effects, including bradycardia, hypotension, and respiratory depression.

Transdermal products: Localized skin reactions, pruritus, erythema, allergic contact sensitization and contact dermatitis, localized vesiculation, hyperpigmentation, edema, excoriation, burning, papules, throbbing, blanching, generalized macular rash.

NOTE: Rebound hypertension may be manifested if clonidine is withdrawn abruptly.

LABORATORY TEST CONSIDERATIONS

Transient ↑ blood glucose, serum phosphatase, and serum CPK. Weakly + Coombs' test. Electrolyte imbalance.

OD OVERDOSE MANAGEMENT

Symptoms: Hypotension, bradycardia, respiratory and CNS depression, hypoventilation, hypothermia, apnea, miosis, agitation, irritability, lethargy, *seizures, cardiac conduction defects, arrhythmias,* transient hypertension, diarrhea, vomiting. *Treatment:* Maintain respiration; perform gastric lavage followed by activated charcoal. Mg sulfate may be used to hasten the rate of transport through the GI tract. IV atropine sulfate (0.6 mg for adults; 0.01 mg/kg for children). Epinephrine, or dopamine to treat persistent bradycardia. IV fluids and elevation of the legs are used to reverse hypotension; if unresponsive to these measures, dopamine (2–20 mcg/kg/min) may be used. To treat hypertension, diazoxide, IV furosemide, or an alpha-adrenergic blocking drug may be used.

DRUG INTERACTIONS

Alcohol / ↑ Depressant effects

Beta-adrenergic blocking agents / Paradoxical hypertension; also, ↑ severity of rebound hypertension following clonidine withdrawal

CNS depressants / ↑ CNS depressant effect

Levodopa / ↓ Levodopa effect

Local anesthetics / Epidural clonidine → prolonged duration of epidural local anesthetics

Mirtazapine / Loss of BP control → antagonism of α–2 adrenergic receptors

Prazosin / ↓ Clonidine antihypertensive effect

Narcotic analgesics / Potentiation of clonidine hypotensive effect

Tolazoline / Blocks antihypertensive effect

Tricyclic antidepressants / Blocks antihypertensive effect

Verapamil / ↑ Risk of AV block and severe hypotension

HOW SUPPLIED

Film, Extended Release, Transdermal: 0.1 mg/24 hr, 0.2 mg/24 hr, 0.3 mg/24 hr; *Injection:* 0.1 mg/mL, 0.5 mg/mL; *Tablet:* 0.1 mg, 0.2 mg, 0.3 mg

DOSAGE

• TABLETS

Hypertension.

Initial: 0.1 mg twice a day; **then,** increase by 0.1–0.2 mg/day until desired response is attained; **maintenance:** 0.2–0.6 mg/day in divided doses (maximum: 2.4 mg/day). Tolerance necessitates increased dosage or concomitant administration of a diuretic. Gradual increase of dosage after initiation minimizes side effects. **Pediatric:** 0.05–0.4 mg once a day.

NOTE: In hypertensive clients unable to take PO medication, clonidine may be administered sublingually at doses of 0.2–0.4 mg/day.

Treat spasticity.

Adults and children: 0.1–0.3 mg; given in divided doses.

Alcohol withdrawal.

0.3–0.6 mg q 6 hr.

Atrial fibrillation.

0.075 mg 1–2 times per day with or without digoxin.

Attention deficit hyperactivity disorder.

0.005 mg/kg/day for 8 weeks.

Constitutional growth delay in children.

0.038–0.15 mg/m^2/day.

Diabetic diarrhea.

0.1–0.6 mg q 12 hr.

Gilles de la Tourette syndrome.

0.15–0.2 mg/day.

Hyperhidrosis.

0.25 mg 3–5 times per day.

Hypertensive urgency (diastolic > 120 mm Hg).

Initial: 0.1–0.2 mg; **then,** 0.050–0.1 mg q hr to a maximum of 0.8 mg.

Menopausal flushing.

0.1–0.4 mg/day.

Withdrawal from opiate dependence.

0.015–0.016 mg/kg/day.

Diagnosis of pheochromocytoma.

0.3 mg/day.

Postherpetic neuralgia.

0.2 mg/day.

Psychosis in schizophrenia.

Less than 0.9 mg/day.

Reduce allergen-induced inflammation in extrinsic asthma.

0.15 mg for 3 days or 0.075 mg/1.5 mL saline by inhalation.

Restless leg syndrome.

0.1–0.3 mg/day, up to 0.9 mg/day.

Facilitate cessation of smoking.

0.15–0.75 mg/day for 3–10 weeks.

Ulcerative colitis.

0.3 mg 3 times per day.

• TRANSDERMAL

Hypertension.

Initial: Use 0.1-mg system; **then,** if after 1–2 weeks adequate control has not been achieved, can use another 0.1-mg system or a larger system. The antihypertensive effect may not be seen for 2–3 days. The system should be changed q 7 days.

Treat spasticity.

Adults and children: 0.1–0.3 mg; apply patch q 7 days.

Cyclosporine-associated nephrotoxicity.

0.1–0.2 mg/day.

Diabetic diarrhea.

0.3 mg/24 hr patch (1 or 2 patches/week).

Menopausal flushing.

0.1 mg/24-hr patch.

Facilitate cessation of smoking.

0.2 mg/24-hr patch.

• EPIDURAL INFUSION

Analgesia.

Initial: 0.03 mg/hr. Dose may then be titrated up or down, depending on pain relief and side effects.

NURSING CONSIDERATIONS

€ Do not confuse Catapres with Cataflam (a nonsteroidal anti-inflammatory drug) or with Combipres (combination antihypertensive drug). Do not confuse clonidine with Klonopin (an anticonvulsant).

Bold Italic = life threatening side effect   ■ = black box warning   ✦ = Available in Canada

ADMINISTRATION/STORAGE

1. It may take 2–3 days to achieve effective blood levels using the transdermal system. Therefore, reduce any prior drug dosage gradually.

2. Clients with severe hypertension may require other antihypertensive drug therapy in addition to transdermal clonidine.

3. If the drug is to be discontinued, do so gradually over a period of 2–4 days.

4. Do not use a preservative when given epidurally.

5. Store injection at controlled room temperature. Discard any unused portion.

ASSESSMENT

1. Document indications for therapy, onset, type of symptoms, and previous treatments.

2. Obtain baseline CBC, liver and renal function studies. Promote periodic eye exams.

3. Note occupation; drug may interfere with the ability to work.

4. List drugs currently prescribed to prevent any interactions. With propranolol, observe for a paradoxical hypertensive response. With tolazoline or TCA, be aware that these may block the antihypertensive action of clonidine; clonidine dosage may need to be increased

5. Tolerance may develop with long term use; an increased dose or addition of a diuretic may improve response.

6. Note evidence of alcohol, drug, or nicotine addiction. These agents usually work well for BP control in this group of clients (especially the once-a-week patch).

7. Initially, monitor BP closely. BP decreases occur within 30–60 min after administration and may persist for 8 hr. Note any fluctuations to determine whether to use clonidine alone or concomitantly with a diuretic. A stable BP reduces orthostatic effects with postural changes.

8. Patch (transdermal) may take 2-3 days to exert effects and therefore oral therapy may be needed during this time. Assess skin sites for rash or itching and change sites weekly.

CLIENT/FAMILY TEACHING

1. With the transdermal system, apply to a hairless area of skin, such as upper arm or torso. Change the system q 7 days and use a different site with each application.

2. If taken PO, take last dose of the day at bedtime to ensure overnight control of BP. Keep a log of BP and HR.

3. Do not engage in activities that require mental alertness, such as operating machinery or driving a car; may cause drowsiness.

4. Do not change regimen or discontinue drug abruptly. Withdrawal should be gradual to prevent rebound hypertension.

5. Record weight daily, in the morning, in clothing of the same weight, to determine if there is edema caused by sodium retention. Any fluid retention should disappear after 3–4 days. Change positions slowly to prevent any sudden drop in BP and associated dizziness.

6. Clonidine may reduce the effect of levodopa; report any increase in the S&S of Parkinson's disease previously controlled with levodopa.

7. Report any depression (may be precipitated by drug), especially with history of mental depression.

OUTCOMES/EVALUATE

- ↓ BP; ↓ menopausal S&S
- Control of withdrawal symptoms
- Control of neuropathic pain

Clopidogrel bisulfate ©

(kloh-**PID**-oh-grel)

CLASSIFICATION(S):

Antiplatelet drug

PREGNANCY CATEGORY: B

Rx: Plavix

ACTION/KINETICS

Inhibits platelet aggregation by inhibiting binding of adenosine diphosphate (ADP) to its platelet receptor and subsequent ADP-mediative activation of glycoprotein GPIIb/IIIa complex. Modifies receptor irreversibly; thus, platelets are affected for remainder of their lifespan. Also inhibits platelet aggregation caused by agonists other than ADP by blocking amplification of platelet activation by released ADP. Rapidly absorbed from GI tract; food does not affect bioavailability. **Peak plasma levels:** About 1 hr. Extensively metabolized in liver; about 50% excreted in urine and 46% in feces. **t ½, elimination:** 8 hr.

USES

(1) Reduction of MI, stroke, and vascular death in clients with atherosclerosis documented by recent stroke, MI, or established peripheral arterial disease. (2) Acute coronary syndrome (unstable angina and non-Q wave MI), including those on medical management and those managed with percutaneous coronary intervention (with or without stent) or CABG; clopidogrel has been shown to decrease the rate of a combined endpoint of cardiovascular death, MI, or stroke as well as the rate of a combined endpoint of cardiovascular death, MI, stroke, or refractory ischemia.

CONTRAINDICATIONS

Lactation. Active pathological bleeding such as peptic ulcer or intracranial hemorrhage.

SPECIAL CONCERNS

Use with caution in those at risk of increased bleeding from trauma, surgery, or other pathological conditions. Safety and efficacy have not been determined in children.

SIDE EFFECTS

CV: Edema, hypertension, syncope, palpitations, atrial fibrillation, *intracranial hemorrhage, major/life-threatening bleeding, retroperitoneal hemorrhage, hemorrhage of operative wound, cardiac failure, pulmonary hemorrhage,* ocular hemorrhage. **GI:** Abdominal pain, dyspepsia, diarrhea, N&V, hemorrhage, ulcers (peptic, gastric, duodenal), *perforated hemorrhagic gastritis, hemorrhagic upper GI ulcer.* **Hepatic:** Infectious hepatitis, fatty liver. **CNS:** Headache, dizziness, depression, hypesthesia, neuralgia, paresthesia, vertigo, anxiety, insomnia. **Body as a whole:** Chest pain, accidental injury, flu-like symptoms, pain, fatigue, asthenia, fever, allergic reactions, ischemic necrosis, generalized edema, leg cramps, gout. **Respiratory:** URTI, dyspnea, rhinitis, bronchitis, coughing, pneumonia, sinusitis, hemothorax. **Hematologic:** Purpura, thrombotic thrombocytopenic purpura (rare), epistaxis, hematoma, anemia, hemarthrosis, hemoptysis, thrombocytopenia, *aplastic anemia,* hypochromic anemia, neutropenia, agranulocytosis, granulocytopenia, leukemia, leukopenia. **Musculoskeletal:** Arthralgia, back pain, arthritis, arthrosis. **Dermatologic:** Disorders of skin/appendages, rash, pruritus, eczema, skin ulceration, bullous eruption, erythematous rash, maculopapular rash, urticaria. **GU:** UTI, cystitis, menorrhagia, abnormal renal function, acute renal failure. **Hypersensitivity:** Angioedema, bronchospasm, *anaphylaxis.* **Ophthalmic:** Cataract, conjunctivitis.

LABORATORY TEST CONSIDERATIONS

Hypercholesterolemia, hematuria, bilirubinemia, hyperuricemia. ↑ Hepatic enzymes, NPN. ↓ Platelets, neutrophils. Prolonged bleeding time.

LABORATORY TEST CONSIDERATIONS

↑ Hepatic enzymes, NPN. ↓ Platelets, neutrophils. Prolonged bleeding time. Hypercholesterolemia, hematuria, bilirubinemia, hyperuricemia.

DRUG INTERACTIONS

CYP2C9 substrates / At high concentrations clopidogrel inhibits CYP2C9; caution should be used when these drug are coadministered.

[H] *Evening primrose oil* / Potential for ↑ antiplatelet effect

[H] *Feverfew* / Potential for ↑ antiplatelet effect

[H] *Garlic* / Potential for ↑ antiplatelet effect

[H] *Ginger* / Potential for ↑ antiplatelet effect

[H] *Ginkgo biloba* / Potential for ↑ antiplatelet effect

[H] *Grapeseed extract* / Potential for ↑ antiplatelet effect

NSAIDs / ↑ Risk of occult blood loss *Warfarin* / Clopidogrel prolongs bleeding time; safety of use with warfarin not established

HOW SUPPLIED

Tablets: 75 mg

DOSAGE

* **TABLETS**

  Recent MI, stroke, or established peripheral arterial disease.

  Adults: 75 mg once daily with or without food.

Bold Italic = life threatening side effect   ■ = black box warning   ✦ = Available in Canada

Acute coronary syndrome.
Initial: Single 300 mg loading dose; **then,** 75 mg once daily. Initiate and continue aspirin (75–325 mg once daily).

NURSING CONSIDERATIONS

℞ Do not confuse Plavix with Pletal (also an antiplatelet drug) or Paxil (antidepressant).

ADMINISTRATION/STORAGE
Dosage adjustment not necessary for geriatric clients or with renal disease.

ASSESSMENT
1. Document atherosclerotic event (MI, stroke) or established peripheral arterial disease requiring therapy.
2. Assess for any active bleeding as with ulcers or intracranial bleeding.
3. List all drugs prescibed/consumed especially OTC i.e., NSAIDS, ASA, herbals.

CLIENT/FAMILY TEACHING
1. Take exactly as directed; may take without regard to food. Food will lessen chance of stomach upset.
2. May cause dizziness or drowsiness.
3. Avoid OTC agents especially aspirin, aspirin-containing products, or NSAIDs unless prescribed.
4. Report any unusual bruising or bleeding; advise all providers of prescribed therapy.
5. Drug should be discontinued 7 days prior to elective surgery.

OUTCOMES/EVALUATE
- Inhibition of platelet aggregation
- Reduction of atherosclerotic events

Colesevelam hydrochloride
(**koh**-leh-**SEV**-eh-lam)

CLASSIFICATION(S):
Antihyperlipidemic, bile acid sequestrant
PREGNANCY CATEGORY: B
Rx: WelChol

ACTION/KINETICS
Binds bile acids, including glycocholic acid (the major bile acid in humans), in the intestine, impeding their reabsorption. As the bile acid pool becomes depleted, the hepatic enzyme, cholesterol 7-α-hydroxylase, is upregulated which increases the conversion of cholesterol to bile acids. This causes an increased demand for cholesterol in liver cells, resulting in the effects of both increasing transcription and activity of the cholesterol biosynthetic enzyme (HMG-CoA) reductase and increasing the number of hepatic LDL receptors. The result is an increased clearance of LDL cholesterol from the blood, thus lowering serum LDL cholesterol levels. Is not absorbed from the GI tract. Maximum response achieved within 2 weeks.

USES
Given alone or with an HMG-CoA reductase inhibitor, in addition to diet and exercise, to reduce elevated LDL cholesterol in those with primary hypercholesterolemia (Fredrickson Type IIa).

CONTRAINDICATIONS
Use in bowel obstruction.

SPECIAL CONCERNS
Use with caution in clients with triglyceride levels greater than 300 mg/dL and in those with a susceptibility to vitamin K or fat soluble vitamin deficiencies. Safety and efficacy have not been established in children or for use in clients with dysphagia, swallowing disorders, severe GI motility disorders, or major GI tract surgery.

SIDE EFFECTS
GI: Flatulence, constipation, diarrhea, nausea, dyspepsia. **Respiratory:** Sinusitis, rhinitis, increased cough, pharyngitis. **Body as a whole:** Infection, headache, pain, back pain, abdominal pain, flu syndrome, accidental injury, asthenia, myalgia.

DRUG INTERACTIONS
Give consideration to monitoring drug levels or effects when giving other drugs for which alterations in blood levels could have clinical significance on safety or efficacy.

HOW SUPPLIED
Tablet: 625 mg

DOSAGE
- **TABLETS**
  Primary hypercholesterolemia.

Monotherapy, initial: Three tablets twice a day with meals or 6 tablets once per day with a meal. Can be increased to 7 tablets, depending on desired effect. **Combination therapy:** Three tablets twice a day with meals or 6 tablets once per day with a meal. Doses of 4–6 tablets per day can be taken safely with a HMG-CoA reductase inhibitor or when the 2 drugs are dosed apart.

NURSING CONSIDERATIONS

ADMINISTRATION/STORAGE
Store at room temperature and protect from moisture.

ASSESSMENT
1. Note indications for therapy, other agents trialed and the outcome.
2. Prior to starting therapy, secondary causes of hypercholesterolemia (e.g., poorly controlled diabetes, hypothyroidism, nephrotic syndrome, dysproteinemias, obstructive liver disease, other drug therapy, alcholism) should be ruled out.
3. Obtain a 12 hr fasting lipid profile prior to therapy; assess total-C, HDL/LDL-C, and Triglycerides. Avoid/monitor carefully if Triglycerides > 300. Periodically assess serum cholesterol as outlined in the National Cholesterol Education Program guidelines to confirm a favorable initial and chronic response.
4. Determine if client suffers from vitamin K or fat soluble vitamin deficiency, bowel, GI motility or swallowing dysfunction, or major GI tract surgery as these may preclude therapy.

CLIENT/FAMILY TEACHING
1. Take as directed with a liquid and a low fat/low cholesterol meal.
2. Continue to make lifestyle changes that lower coronary risk factors such as smoking cessation, reduction in alcohol intake, low fat/low cholesterol diet, regular daily exercise, weight loss, and reduction in stress.
3. Practice reliable birth control; stop drug and report if pregnancy suspected.
4. Consume foods high in bulk and fiber, report if constipation occurs, may require a stool softener.

5. Report any adverse effects and have labs drawn as ordered.

OUTCOMES/EVALUATE
Reduced LDL cholesterol levels

Colestipol hydrochloride
(koh-**LESS**-tih-poll)

CLASSIFICATION(S):
Antihyperlipidemic, bile acid sequestrant
PREGNANCY CATEGORY: B
Rx: Colestid

ACTION/KINETICS
An anion exchange resin that binds bile acids in the intestine, forming an insoluble complex excreted in the feces. The loss of bile acids results in increased oxidation of cholesterol to bile acids and a decrease in LDL and serum cholesterol. Does not affect (or may increase) triglycerides or HDL and may increase VLDL. Not absorbed from the GI tract. **Onset:** 1–2 days; **maximum effect:** 1 month. Return to pretreatment cholesterol levels after discontinuance of therapy: 1 month.

USES
As adjunctive therapy in hyperlipoproteinemia (types IIA and IIB) to reduce serum cholesterol in clients who do not respond adequately to diet. *Investigational:* Digitalis toxicity.

CONTRAINDICATIONS
Complete obstruction or atresia of bile duct.

SPECIAL CONCERNS
Use during pregnancy only if benefits outweigh risks. Use with caution during lactation and in children. Children may be more likely to develop hyperchloremic acidosis although dosage has not been established. Clients over 60 years of age may be at greater risk of GI side effects and adverse nutritional effects.

SIDE EFFECTS
GI: Constipation (may be severe and accompanied by fecal impaction), N&V, diarrhea, heartburn, GI bleeding, anorex-

---

ia, flatulence, steatorrhea, abdominal distention/cramping, bloating, loose stools, indigestion, rectal bleeding/pain, black stools, hemorrhoidal bleeding, *bleeding duodenal ulcer, peptic ulceration,* ulcer attack, GI irritation, dysphagia, dental bleeding/caries, hiccoughs, sour taste, pancreatitis, diverticulitis, cholecystitis, cholelithiasis. **CV:** Chest pain, angina, tachycardia (rare). **CNS:** Migraine or sinus headache, anxiety, vertigo, dizziness, lightheadedness, insomnia, fatigue, tinnitus, syncope, drowsiness, femoral nerve pain, paresthesia. **Hematologic:** Ecchymosis, anemia, beeding tendencies due to hypoprothrombinemia. **Allergic:** Urticaria, dermatitis, asthma, wheezing, rash. **Musculoskeletal:** Backache, muscle/joint pain, arthritis. **Renal:** Hematuria, burnt odor to urine, dysuria, diuresis. **Miscellaneous:** Uveitis, fatigue, weight loss or gain, increased libido, swollen glands, SOB, edema, weakness, swelling of hands/feet, osteoporosis, calcified material in biliary tree and gall bladder, hyperchloremic acidosis in children.

DRUG INTERACTIONS

See *Cholestyramine.* Also, colestipol ↓ bioavailability of diltiazem if colestipol is given with, 1 hr before, or 4 hr after diltiazem.

HOW SUPPLIED

Granules: 5 g/dose, 5 g/7.5 g powder; *Tablet:* 1 g

DOSAGE————————————

• GRANULES
Antihyperlipidemic.
Adults, initial: 5 g 1–2 times per day; **then,** can increase 5 g/day at 1–2-month intervals. **Total dose:** 5–30 g/day given once or in two to three divided doses.

• TABLETS
Adults, initial: 2 g 1–2 times per day. Dose can be increased by 2 g, once or twice daily, at 1–2-month intervals. **Total dose:** 2–16 g/day given once or in divided doses.

NURSING CONSIDERATIONS

ADMINISTRATION/STORAGE

1. If compliance is good and side effects acceptable but the desired effect is not obtained with 2–16 g/day using tablets, consider combined therapy or alternative treatment.
2. Granules are available in an orange-flavored product.

ASSESSMENT

Note indications for therapy, other agents trialed and the outcome. Assess dietary patterns and exercise regimes.

CLIENT/FAMILY TEACHING

1. Take 30 min before meals, preferably with the evening meal, since cholesterol synthesis is increased during the evening hours. Take other drugs 1 hr before or 4 hr after to reduce interference with absorption.
2. Never take dose in dry form. Always mix granules with 90 mL or more of fruit juice, milk, water, carbonated beverages, applesauce, soup, cereal, or pulpy fruit before administering to disguise unpalatable taste and to prevent resin from causing esophageal irritation or blockage.
3. Rinse glass with a small amount of fluid and swallow to ensure the total amount of the drug is taken.
4. Tablets should be swallowed whole one at a time (i.e., they should not be cut, crushed, or chewed); may be taken with plenty of water or other fluids.
5. Consume adequate amounts of fluids, fruits, and fiber to diminish constipating drug effects. Report adverse effects and have blood monitored.
6. Continue to follow dietary restrictions of fat and cholesterol, regular exercise program, smoking cessation, and weight reduction in the overall goal of cholesterol reduction.
7. Serum cholesterol level will return to pretreatment levels within 1 month if drug is discontinued.

OUTCOMES/EVALUATE

↓ LDL-cholesterol levels

D

Dalteparin sodium

(**DAL**-tih-**pair**-in)

CLASSIFICATION(S):
Anticoagulant, low molecular weight heparin
PREGNANCY CATEGORY: B
Rx: Fragmin

SEE ALSO HEPARINS, LOW MOLECULAR WEIGHT.

ACTION/KINETICS
Peak plasma levels: 4 hr. **t ½, SC:** 3–5 hr. t ½ increased in those with chronic renal insufficiency requiring hemodialysis.

USES
(1) Prevent deep vein thrombosis (DVT) in clients undergoing hip replacement or abdominal surgery who are at risk for thromboembolic complications (i.e., pulmonary embolism). High risk includes obesity, general anesthesia more than 30 min, malignancy, history of DVT or pulmonary embolism, age 40 and over. (2) Prevent DVT in those who are at risk for thromboembolic complications (which may lead to pulmonary embolism) due to severely restricted mobility during acute illness. (3) Prevent ischemic complications due to blood clot formation in life-threatening unstable angina and non-Q-wave MI in clients on concurrent aspirin therapy. *Investigational:* Prophylaxis of DVT in those undergoing moderate or high risk surgery, orthopedic surgery, hip fracture surgery, neurosurgery, in clients with ischemic stroke, in those with impaired mobility, in general medical clients (i.e., cancer, bed rest, heart failure, severe lung disease), or in pregnant clients at risk for thromboembolic complications.

SPECIAL CONCERNS
See also *Heparins, Low Molecular Weight.* ■(1) When spinal/epidural anesthesia or spinal puncture is used, those anticoagulated or scheduled to be anticoagulated with low molecular weight heparins or heparinoids to prevent thromboembolic complications are at risk of developing a spinal or epidural hematoma that can result in long-term or permanent paralysis. Risk is increased using indwelling epidural catheters for giving analgesics or by the concurrent use of drugs affecting hemastasis, such as NSAIDs, platelet inhibitors, or other anticoagulants. Risk also appears to increase by traumatic or repeated spinal or epidural puncture. (2) Frequently monitor for signs and symptoms of neurological impairment. If observed, immediate treatment is required. (3) The physician should consider potential benefits vs risk before neuraxial intervention in clients anticoagulated or to be anticoagulated for thromboprophylaxis.■ The multiple dose vial contains benzyl alcohol that has been associated with a fatal 'gasping syndrome' in premature infants.

SIDE EFFECTS
CV: *Hemorrhage,* hematoma at injection site, wound hematoma, reoperation due to bleeding, postoperational transfusions. **Hematologic:** Thrombocytopenia. **Hypersensitivity:** Allergic reactions, including pruritus, rash, fever, injection site reaction, bullous eruption, skin necrosis (rare), *anaphylaxis.* **Miscellaneous:** Pain at injection site.

HOW SUPPLIED
Injection: 2,500 international units/0.2 mL; 5,000 international units/0.2 mL; 7,500 international units/0.3 mL; 10,000 international units/mL; 25,000 international units/mL

DOSAGE
• **SC ONLY**
  Prevention of DVT in abdominal surgery.

Adults: 2,500 international units each day starting 1–2 hr prior to surgery and repeated once daily for 5–10 days postoperatively. High-risk clients: 5,000 international units the night before surgery and repeated once daily for 5–10 days. In malignancy: 2,500 international units 1–2 hr before surgery followed by 2,500 international units 12 hr later and 5,000 international units once daily for 5–10 days.

Prevention of DVT following hip replacement surgery.

Adults: 2,500 international units within 2 hr before surgery with a second dose of 2,500 international units in the evening on the day of surgery (six or more hr after the first dose). If surgery occurs in the evening, omit the second dose on the day of surgery. On the first postoperative day, give 5,000 international units once daily for 5–10 days. Alternatively, can give 5,000 international units the evening before surgery, followed by 5,000 international units once daily for 5–10 days, starting the evening of the day of surgery.

Medical clients during acute illness.

In those with severely restricted mobility during acute illness, give 5,000 international units once daily for up to 12 to 14 days.

Prevent ischemic complications in unstable angina/non-Q-wave MI.

Adults: 120 international units/kg, not to exceed 10,000 international units q 12 hr with concurrent PO aspirin (75–165 mg/day). Continue treatment until client is clinically stabilized (usually 5–8 days).

Systemic anticoagulation.

200 international units/kg SC daily or 100 international units twice a day

NURSING CONSIDERATIONS

ADMINISTRATION/STORAGE

1. Available in single-dose prefilled syringes affixed with a 27-gauge × ½-inch needle.
2. Before withdrawing the drug, inspect the vial visually for particulate matter or discoloration.

3. Do not mix with other infusions or injections unless compatibility data are known.
4. To ensure delivery of the full dose, do not expel the air bubble from the prefilled syringe before injection. Give by deep SC injection while the client is sitting or lying down. May be injected in a U-shaped area around the navel, the upper outer side of the thigh, or the upper outer quadrant of the buttock. Vary the injection site daily.
5. When the area around the navel or thigh is used, use the thumb and forefinger to lift up a skin fold while giving the injection. Insert the entire length of the needle at a 45–90° angle.
6. Store the drug at controlled room temperature of 20–25°C (68–77°F). After the first penetration of the rubber stopper, store the multidose vials at room temperature for up to 2 weeks. Discard any unused drug after 2 weeks.

ASSESSMENT

1. Determine any sensitivity to heparin or pork products.
2. Note indications for therapy and any evidence of active major bleeding, bleeding disorders, or thrombocytopenia. Monitor CBC with platelets, urinalysis, and FOB during therapy.
3. List criteria for inclusion (i.e., over 40, obese, prolonged general anesthesia, additional risk factors).

CLIENT/FAMILY TEACHING

1. Review indications for therapy and self-administration technique.
2. Give by deep SC injection while sitting or lying down. May give in a U-shape area around the navel, the upper outer side of the thigh, or the upper outer quadrangle of the buttock. Change/rotate the injection site daily.
3. If the area around the navel or thigh is used, a fold of skin must be lifted, using the thumb and forefinger, while giving the injection.
4. Insert the entire length of the needle at a 45–90-degree angle.
5. Avoid OTC ASA containing products. Use electric razor and soft toothbrush to prevent tissue trauma.

6. Report any unusual bruising/bleeding or hemorrhage. Therapy may last for 5–10 days.

OUTCOMES/EVALUATE

Post-operative DVT prophylaxis

Danaparoid sodium ∎

(dah-**NAP**-ah-royd)

CLASSIFICATION(S):
Anticoagulant, glycosaminoglycan
PREGNANCY CATEGORY: B
Rx: Orgaran
✤Rx: Orgaran-DVT, Orgaran-HIT

ACTION/KINETICS

A low molecular weight sulfated glycosaminoglycan obtained from porcine mucosa. Prevents fibrin formation in the coagulation pathway via thrombin generation inhibition by anti-Xa and anti-IIa effects. Minimal effect on clotting assays, fibrinolytic activity, or bleeding time. 100% bioavailable with SC use. **t ½:** About 24 hr. Excreted primarily through the kidneys.

USES

Prophylaxis of postoperative deep vein thrombosis (DVT) in clients undergoing elective hip replacement surgery. *Investigational:* Disseminated intravascular coagulation, diabetic nephropathy, ischemic stroke or thromboembolic complications of hemorrhagic stroke, treatment measure for DVT, routine anticoagulant therapy in those requiring hemodialysis. Also, to treat thromboembolism, hemofiltration during CV operations, in pregnant clients at increased risk for thrombosis.

CONTRAINDICATIONS

Use in hemophilia, idiopathic thrombocytopenic purpura, active major bleeding state (including hemorrhagic stroke in the acute phase), and type II thrombocytopenia associated with a positive in vitro test for antiplatelet antibody in the presence of danaparoid. Hypersensitivity to pork products. IM use.

SPECIAL CONCERNS

∎(1) When spinal/epidural anesthesia or spinal puncture is used, those anticoagulated or scheduled to be anticoagulated with low molecular weight heparins or heparinoids to prevent thromboembolic complications are at risk of developing a spinal or epidural hematoma that can result in long-term or permanent paralysis. Risk is increased using indwelling epidural catheters for giving analgesics or by the concurrent use of drugs affecting hemostasis, such as NSAIDs, platelet inhibitors, or other anticoagulants. Risk also appears to increase by traumatic or repeated spinal or epidural puncture. (2) Frequently monitor for signs and symptoms of neurologic impairment. If observed, immediate treatment is required. (3) The physician should consider potential benefits vs risk before neuraxial intervention in clients anticoagulated or to be anticoagulated for thromboprophylaxis.∎ Cannot be dosed interchangeably (unit for unit) with either heparin or low molecular weight heparins. Use with extreme caution in disease states where there is an increased risk of hemorrhage, including severe uncontrolled hypertension, acute bacterial endocarditis, congenital or acquired bleeding disorders, active ulcerative and angiodysplastic GI disease, nonhemorrhagic stroke, postoperative indwelling epidural catheter use, and shortly after brain, spinal, or ophthalmologic surgery. Use with caution during lactation and in those with severely impaired renal function. Use with caution in clients receiving oral anticoagulants or platelet inhibitors. Safety and efficacy have not been determined in children.

SIDE EFFECTS

CV: *Intraoperative blood loss, postoperative blood loss.* **GI:** N&V, constipation. **CNS:** Insomnia, headache, dizziness. **Dermatologic:** Rash, pruritus. **GU:** UTI, urinary retention. **Miscellaneous:** Fever, pain at injection site, peripheral edema, joint disorder, edema, asthenia, anemia, pain, infection.

Bold Italic = life threatening side effect   ∎ = black box warning   ✤ = Available in Canada

OD OVERDOSE MANAGEMENT
Symptoms: Bleeding disorders, including hemorrhage. *Treatment:* Protamine sulfate partially neutralizes the anti-Xa activity of the drug; however, there is no evidence that protamine sulfate will reduce severe non-surgical bleeding. For serious bleeding, discontinue danaparoid and give blood or blood product transfusions as needed.

HOW SUPPLIED
Injection: 750 anti-Xa units/0.6 mL.

DOSAGE
- **SC ONLY**
  Prophylaxis of DVT in hip replacement surgery.

Adults: 750 anti-Xa units twice a day SC, beginning 1 to 4 hr preoperatively and then not sooner than 2 hr postoperatively. Continue treatment throughout the postoperative period until the risk of deep vein thrombosis has decreased. Average duration of treatment is 7 to 10 days, up to 14 days.

NURSING CONSIDERATIONS

ADMINISTRATION/STORAGE
Protect from light; store at 2–30°C (36–86°F).

ASSESSMENT
1. Note any pork or sulfite sensitivity.
2. Assess for any medical conditions that may preclude drug use (i.e., active hemorrhagic disease, bleeding dyscrasias, etc.).
3. Monitor VS, I&O, CBC, U/A, and renal function studies; note any urinary retention or altered VS.

CLIENT/FAMILY TEACHING
1. Drug is used to prevent the formation of blood clots, especially in the legs. Usually given 1-4 hr before surgery, then 2 hr after surgery, and then twice a day for 7 to 10 days.
2. To administer, lie down and grasp a fold of skin on the abdomen between the thumb and forefinger. Insert the entire length of the needle straight in; use a 25- to 26-gauge needle to minimize tissue trauma. Hold the skin fold throughout the injection; do not rub or massage area after administration; rotate sites with each injection.

3. Alternate administration between the left and right anterolateral and posterolateral abdominal walls.
4. Avoid OTC ASA containing products. Use electric razor and soft toothbrush to prevent tissue trauma.
5. Report any unusual chestpain bruising/bleeding, acute SOB, itching, rash, chest pain, and swelling.

OUTCOMES/EVALUATE
Post-operative DVT prophylaxis

Desirudin ■
(DEH-sih-rue-din)

CLASSIFICATION(S):
Antithrombin drug
PREGNANCY CATEGORY: C
Rx: Iprivask

ACTION/KINETICS
A specific inhibitor of free circulating and clot-bound human thrombin. Desirudin prolongs the clotting time of human plasma by increasing aPTT. One molecule of desirudin binds to 1 molecule of thrombin, thereby blocking the thrombogenic activity of thrombin. As a result, all thrombin-dependent coagulation assays are affected. Thrombin time may exceed 200 seconds, even at low plasma desirudin levels; thus, this test is unsuitable for routine monitoring of desirudin therapy. At therapeutic serum levels, the drug has no effect on factors IXa, Xa, kallikrein, plasmin, tissue plasminogen activator, or activated protein. **Maximum plasma levels:** 1– 3 hr. Primarily metabolized and eliminated by the kidney with about 40–50% excreted unchanged. **$t\frac{1}{2}$, elimination:** 2–3 hr after SC use.

USES
Prophylaxis of DVT that may lead to pulmonary embolism in clients undergoing elective hip replacement surgery.

CONTRAINDICATIONS
IM use. Known hypersensitivity to natural or recombinant hirudins and in those with active bleeding and/or irreversible coagulation disorders.

H = Herbal   **IV** = Intravenous   @ = sound-alike drug

SPECIAL CONCERNS

■(1) When neuraxial anesthesia (epidural/spinal anesthesia) or spinal puncture is employed, clients anticoagulated or scheduled to be anticoagulated with selective thrombin inhibitors, such as desirudin, may be at risk of developing an epidural or spinal hematoma which can result in long-term or permanent paralysis. (2) The risk of the above events may be increased by the use of indwelling spinal catheters for administration of analgesia or by the concomitant use of drugs affecting hemostasis, such as NSAIDs, platelet inhibitors, or other anticoagulants. The risk appears to be increased by traumatic or repeated epidural or spinal puncture. (3) Frequently monitor clients for signs and symptoms of neurological impairment. If neurological compromise is noted, urgent treatment is required. (4) The physician should consider the potential benefit versus risk before neuraxial intervention, in clients anticoagulated or to be anticoagulated for thromboprophylaxis.■ Use with caution in clients with increased risks of hemorrage, including those with recent major surgery, organ biopsy, or puncture of a non-compressible vessel within the last month; also, a history of hemorrhagic stroke, intracranial or intraocular bleeding including diabetic retinopathy, recent ischemic stroke, severe uncontrolled hypertension, bacterial endocarditis, congenital or acquired hemostatic disorder (e.g., hemophilia, liver disease), or a history of GI or pulmonary bleeding within the past 3 months. Use with caution in clients with renal impairment, especially in those with moderate and severe renal impairment (C_{CR} less than 60 mL/min/1.74m^2 body surface area and in those with impaired liver function. Risk of side effects may be greater in elderly clients.

SIDE EFFECTS

Hemorrhagic events: Hematomas; hemorrhages, including retroperitoneal, intracranial, intraocular, intraspinal, or in a major prosthetic joint. **CV:** Deep thrombophlebitis, thrombosis, hypotension, CV disorder. **GI:** N&V. **Body as a whole:** Wound secretion, fever, imparied healing. **Miscellaneous:** Injection site mass, anemia, leg edema, decreased hemoglobin, hematuria, dizziness, epistaxis, leg pain, hematemesis, hypersensitivity reactions, including *anaphylaxis*.

OD OVERDOSE MANAGEMENT

Symptoms: Hemorrhagic complications, excessively high aPTT values. *Treatment:* Discontinue desirudin therapy. Effects of desirudin are partially reversed by using thrombin-rich plasma concentrates. aPTT levels can be decreased by IV administration of 0.3 mcg/kg of desmopressin. Institute emergency procedures as appropriate.

DRUG INTERACTIONS

Abciximab / Use with caution with desirudin

Alteplase / ↑ Risk of bleeding

Anticoagulants (heparin, low molecular weight heparins) / Prolongation of aPTT; do not use together

Aspirin / Use with caution with desirudin

Clopidogrel / Use with caution with desirudin

Dextran / ↑ Risk of bleeding

Dipyridamole / Use with caution with desirudin

Glucocorticoids / ↑ Risk of bleeding

Ketorolac / Use with caution with desirudin

NSAIDs / Use with caution with desirudin

Salicylates / Use with caution with desirudin

Streptokinase / ↑ Risk of bleeding

Sulfinpyrazone / Use with caution with desirudin

Ticlopidine / Use with caution with desirudin

HOW SUPPLIED

Powder for injection, lyophilized: 15 mg

DOSAGE

- **SC**

    Prophylaxis of DVT during hip replacement surgery.

Initial: 15 mg q 12 hr with the initial dose given up to 5–15 min before surgery, but after induction of regional block anesthesia (if used). May be given up to 12 days (average is 9–12 days).

NURSING CONSIDERATIONS

ADMINISTRATION/STORAGE

1. Dosage must be reduced in renal insufficiency as follows:

- If C_{CR} is between 31 and 60 mL/min/1.73 m², begin therapy at 5 mg SC q 12 hr. Monitor aPTT and serum creatinine at least daily. If aPTT exceeds 2 times control, interrupt therapy until the value returns to less than 2 times control and resume therapy at a reduced dose guided by the initial degree of aPTT abnormality.
- If C_{CR} is less than 31 mL/min/1.73 m², begin therapy at 1.7 mg SC q 12 hr. Monitor aPTT and serum creatinine at least daily. If aPTT exceeds 2 times control, interrupt therapy until the value returns to less than 2 times control and consider further dose reductions guided by the initial degree of aPTT abnormality.

2. Reconstitute under sterile conditions. Reconstitute each vial with 0.5 mL of provided diluent (mannitol, 3%, in water for injection). Shake the vial gently until the drug is fully reconstituted.

3. Once reconstituted, each 0.5 mL contains 15.75 mg of desirudin.

4. Use the reconstituted solution immediately, although it is stable for up to 24 hr when stored at room temperature and protected from light. Discard any unused solution. Do not mix with other injections, solvents, or infusions.

5. To administer SC, use a 26- or 27-gauge ½- inch needle. Withdraw the entire reconstituted solution (15.75 mg/0.5 mL) into the syringe and inject the total volume (will deliver 15 mg).

6. Clients should be sitting or lying down; give the injection by deep SC. Alternate administration between the left and right anterolateral and left and right posterolateral thigh or abdominal wall.

7. Introduce the whole length of the needle into a skin fold held between the thumb and forefinger; hold the skin fold throughout the injection.

8. Desirudin can not be used interchangeably with other hirudins as they differ in their manufacturing process and specfic biolobical activity.

9. Protect from light. Store unopened vials from 15–30°C (59–86°F).

Diazoxide IV
(dye-az-**OX**-eyed)

D

CLASSIFICATION(S):
Antihypertensive, direct-acting
PREGNANCY CATEGORY: C
Rx: Hyperstat IV

SEE ALSO *ANTIHYPERTENSIVE AGENTS* AND *DIAZOXIDE ORAL.*

ACTION/KINETICS
Exerts a direct action on vascular smooth muscle to cause arteriolar vasodilation and decreased peripheral resistance. **Onset:** 1–5 min. **Time to peak effect:** 2–5 min. **Duration** (variable): usual, 3–12 hr. Excreted through the kidney (50% unchanged).

USES
May be the drug of choice for hypertensive crisis (malignant and nonmalignant hypertension) in hospitalized adults and children. Often given concomitantly with a diuretic. Especially suitable for clients with impaired renal function, hypertensive encephalopathy, hypertension complicated by LV failure, and eclampsia. Ineffective for hypertension due to pheochromocytoma.

CONTRAINDICATIONS
Hypersensitivity to drug or thiazide diuretics. Treatment of compensatory hypertension due to aortic coarctation or AV shunt. Dissecting aortic aneurysm.

SPECIAL CONCERNS
A decrease in dose may be necessary in geriatric clients due to age-related decreases in renal function. If given prior to delivery, fetal or neonatal hyperbilirubinemia, thrombocytopenia, or altered carbohydrate metabolism may result. Use with caution during lactation and in clients with impaired cerebral or cardiac circulation.

SIDE EFFECTS
CV: Hypotension (may be severe enough to cause shock), sodium and

water retention, especially in clients with impaired cardiac reserve, *atrial or ventricular arrhythmias, cerebral or myocardial ischemia,* marked ECG changes with possibility of *MI,* palpitations, bradycardia, SVT, chest discomfort or nonanginal chest tightness. **CNS:** Cerebral ischemia manifested by unconsciousness, *seizures,* paralysis, confusion, numbness of the hands. Headache, dizziness, weakness, drowsiness, lightheadedness, somnolence, lethargy, euphoria, weakness of short duration, apprehension, anxiety, malaise, blurred vision. **Respiratory:** Tightness in chest, cough, dyspnea, choking sensation. **GI:** N&V, diarrhea, anorexia, parotid swelling, change in taste sense, salivation, dry mouth, ileus, constipation, acute pancreatitis (rare). **Other:** Hyperglycemia (may be serious enough to require treatment), sweating, flushing, sensation of warmth, transient neurologic findings due to alteration in regional blood flow to the brain, hyperosmolar coma in infants, tinnitus, hearing loss, retention of nitrogenous wastes, acute pancreatitis, back pain, increased nocturia, lacrimation, hypersensitivity reactions, papilledema, hirsutism, decreased libido. Pain, cellulitis without sloughing, warmth or pain along injected vein, phlebitis at injection site, extravasation.

LABORATORY TEST CONSIDERATIONS
False + or ↑ uric acid.

OD OVERDOSE MANAGEMENT
Symptoms: Hypotension, excessive hyperglycemia. *Treatment:* Use the Trendelenburg position to reverse hypotension.

DRUG INTERACTIONS
Anticoagulants, oral / ↑ Anticoagulant effect R/T ↓ plasma protein binding
Nitrites / ↑ Hypotensive effect
Phenytoin / ↓ Anticonvulsant effect of phenytoin
Sulfonylureas / Destablization of the client → hyperglycemia
Thiazide diuretics / ↑ Hyperglycemic, hyperuricemic, and antihypertensive diazoxide effect
Vasodilators, peripheral / ↑ Hypotensive effect

HOW SUPPLIED
Injection: 15 mg/mL
DOSAGE
• **IV PUSH (30 SEC OR LESS)**
Hypertensive crisis.
Adults: 1–3 mg/kg up to a maximum of 150 mg; may be repeated at 5–15-min intervals until adequate BP response obtained. Drug may then be repeated at 4–24-hr intervals for 4–5 days or until oral antihypertensive therapy can be initiated. **Pediatric:** 1–3 mg/kg (30–90 mg/m²) using the same dosing intervals as adults.

Repeated use can result in sodium and water retention; therefore, a diuretic may be needed to avoid CHF and for maximum reduction of BP.

NURSING CONSIDERATIONS
ADMINISTRATION/STORAGE
IV 1. Do not administer IM or SC. Medication is highly alkaline.
2. Ensure patency and inject rapidly (30 sec) undiluted into a peripheral vein to maximize response.
3. Assess site for signs of irritation or extravasation. If extravasation occurs, apply ice packs.
4. Protect from light, heat, and freezing.
5. Have a sympathomimetic drug, such as norepinephrine, available to treat severe hypotension should it occur.
6. Protect ampules from light and store between 2–30°C (36–86°F).
ASSESSMENT
1. Assess for sensitivity to thiazide diuretics, sulfa drugs, or diazoxide.
2. With diabetics, can cause serious elevations in blood sugar levels. Note complaints of sweating, flushing, or evidence of hyperglycemia.
3. Obtain uric acid level and assess for evidence of hyperuricemia.
4. Monitor VS/BP frequently until stabilized, then hourly until crisis resolved. Obtain final BP upon arising, prior to ambulation. Keep recumbent during and for 30 min after injection to avoid orthostatic hypotension; for 8–10 hr if furosemide is also administered. Assess for CHF and monitor electrolytes.

CLIENT/FAMILY TEACHING

Drug is injected IV to rapidly lower BP in a monitored environment when other measures fail or a rapid reduction is needed.

OUTCOMES/EVALUATE

Reduction in BP during hypertensive crisis

Digoxin

(dih-**JOX**-in)

CLASSIFICATION(S):

Cardiac glycoside

PREGNANCY CATEGORY: A

Rx: Digitek, Digoxin Injection Pediatric, Lanoxicaps, Lanoxin

♣Rx: Digoxin Injection C.S.D., Digoxin Pediatric Injection C.S.D.

ACTION/KINETICS

Digoxin increases the force and velocity of myocardial contraction (positive inotropic effect) by increasing the refractory period of the AV node and increasing total peripheral resistance. This effect is due to inhibition of sodium/potassium–ATPase in the sarcolemmal membrane, which alters excitation–contraction coupling. Inhibiting sodium/potassium–ATPase results in increased calcium influx and increased release of free calcium ions within the myocardial cells, which then potentiate the contractility of cardiac muscle fibers. Digoxin also decreases the rate of conduction and increases the refractory period of the AV node due to an increase in parasympathetic tone and a decrease in sympathetic tone. Clinical effects are not seen until steady-state plasma levels are reached. The initial dose of digoxin is larger (loading dose) and is traditionally referred to as the *digitalizing dose;* subsequent doses are referred to as *maintenance doses.* **Onset: PO,** 0.5–2 hr; **time to peak effect:** 2–6 hr. **Duration:** Over 24 hr. **Onset, IV:** 5–30 min; **time to peak effect:** 1–4 hr. **Duration:** 6 days. **t ½:** 30–40 hr. **Therapeutic serum level:** 0.5–2.0 ng/mL. From 20% to 25% is protein bound. Serum levels above 2.5 ng/mL indicate toxicity. Fifty percent to 70% is excreted unchanged by the kidneys. Bioavailability depends on the dosage form: tablets (60–80%), capsules (90–100%), and elixir (70–85%). Thus, changing dosage forms may require dosage adjustments.

USES

(1) CHF, including that due to venous congestion, edema, dyspnea, orthopnea, and cardiac arrhythmia. May be drug of choice for CHF because of rapid onset, relatively short duration, and ability to be administered PO or IV. (2) Control of rapid ventricular contraction rate in clients with atrial fibrillation or flutter. (3) Slow HR in sinus tachycardia due to CHF. (4) SVT. (5) Prophylaxis and treatment of recurrent paroxysmal atrial tachycardia with paroxysmal AV junctional rhythm. (6) Cardiogenic shock (value not established).

CONTRAINDICATIONS

Ventricular fibrillation or tachycardia (unless congestive failure supervenes after protracted episode not due to digitalis), in presence of digoxin toxicity, hypersensitivity to cardiac glycosides, beriberi heart disease, certain cases of hypersensitive carotid sinus syndrome.

SPECIAL CONCERNS

Use with caution in clients with ischemic heart disease, acute myocarditis, hypertrophic subaortic stenosis, hypoxic or myxedemic states, Adams-Stokes or carotid sinus syndromes, cardiac amyloidosis, or cyanotic heart and lung disease, including emphysema and partial heart block. Those with carditis associated with rheumatic fever or viral myocarditis are especially sensitive to digoxin-induced disturbances in rhythm. Electric pacemakers may sensitize the myocardium to cardiac glycosides. Also use with caution and at reduced dosage in elderly, debilitated clients, pregnant women and nursing mothers, and newborn, term, or premature infants who have immature renal and hepatic function and in reduced renal and/or hepatic function.

The half-life of digoxin is prolonged in the elderly; anticipate smaller drug doses. Be especially alert to cardiac ar-

D

rhythmias in children. This sign of toxicity occurs more frequently in children than in adults.

SIDE EFFECTS
Digoxin is extremely toxic and has caused death even in clients who have received the drug for long periods of time. There is a narrow margin of safety between an effective therapeutic dose and a toxic dose. Overdosage caused by the cumulative effects of the drug is a constant danger in therapy. Digoxin toxicity is characterized by a wide variety of symptoms, which are hard to differentiate from those of the cardiac disease itself.

One of the most serious side effects of digoxin is hypokalemia. This may lead to cardiac arrhythmias, muscle weakness, hypotension, and respiratory distress. Other agents causing hypokalemia reinforce this effect and increase the chance of digitalis toxicity. Such reactions may occur in clients who have been on digoxin maintenance for a long time. **CV:** Changes in the rate, rhythm, and irritability of the heart and the mechanism of the heartbeat. Extrasystoles, bigeminal pulse, coupled rhythm, ectopic beat, and other forms of arrhythmias have been noted. *Death most often results from ventricular fibrillation.* Discontinue digoxin in adults when pulse rate falls below 60 beats/min. All cardiac changes are best detected by the ECG, which is also most useful in clients suffering from intoxication. *Acute hemorrhage.* **GI:** Anorexia, N&V, excessive salivation, epigastric distress, abdominal pain, diarrhea, bowel necrosis. Clients on digoxin therapy may experience two vomiting stages. The first is an early sign of toxicity and is a direct effect of digoxin on the GI tract. Late vomiting indicates stimulation of the vomiting center of the brain, which occurs after the heart muscle has been saturated with digoxin. **CNS:** Headaches, fatigue, lassitude, irritability, malaise, muscle weakness, insomnia, stupor. Psychotomimetic effects (especially in elderly or arteriosclerotic clients or neonates) including disorientation, confusion, depression, aphasia, delirium, hallucinations, and, rarely, *convulsions.* **Neuromuscular:** Neurologic pain involving the lower third of the face and lumbar areas, paresthesia. **Visual disturbances:** Blurred vision, flickering dots, white halos, borders around dark objects, diplopia, amblyopia, color perception changes. **Hypersensitivity (5–7 days after starting therapy):** Skin reactions (urticaria, fever, pruritus, facial and *angioneurotic edema*). **Other:** Chest pain, coldness of extremities.

LABORATORY TEST CONSIDERATIONS
May ↓ PT. Alters tests for 17-ketosteroids and 17-hydroxycorticosteroids.

OD OVERDOSE MANAGEMENT
The relationship of digoxin levels to symptoms of toxicity varies significantly from client to client; thus, it is not possible to identify digoxin levels that would define toxicity accurately. *Symptoms (Toxicity):* **GI:** Anorexia, N&V, diarrhea, abdominal discomfort, or pain. **CNS:** Blurred, yellow, or green vision and halo effect; headache, weakness, drowsiness, mental depression, apathy, restlessness, disorientation, confusion, *seizures,* EEG abnormalities, delirium, hallucinations, neuralgia, psychosis. **CV:** VT, unifocal or multiform PVCs (especially in bigeminal or trigeminal patterns), paroxysmal/nonparoxysmal nodal rhythms, AV dissociation, accelerated junctional rhythm, excessive slowing of the pulse, *AV block (may proceed to complete block),* atrial fibrillation, *ventricular fibrillation (most common cause of death).* **Children:** Visual disturbances, headache, weakness, apathy, and psychosis occur but may be difficult to recognize. **CV:** Conduction disturbances, supraventricular tachyarrhythmias (e.g., *AV block*), atrial tachycardia with or without block, nodal tachycardia, unifocal or multiform ventricular premature contractions, ventricular tachycardia, sinus bradycardia (especially in infants).
Treatment in Adults:
• Discontinue drug, admit to ICU for continuous ECG monitoring.
• If serum potassium is below normal, KCl should be administered in divided PO doses totaling 3–6 g (40–80 mEq).

Potassium should not be used when severe or complete heart block is due to digoxin and not related to tachycardia.

• *Atropine:* A dose of 0.01 mg/kg IV to treat severe sinus bradycardia or slow ventricular rate due to secondary AV block.

• *Cholestyramine, colestipol, activated charcoal:* To bind digitalis in the intestine, thus preventing enterohepatic recirculation.

• *Digoxin immune FAB:* See drug entry. Given in approximate equimolar quantities as digoxin, it reverses S&S of toxicity, often with improvement within 30 min.

• *Lidocaine:* A dose of 1 mg/kg given over 5 min followed by an infusion of 15–50 mcg/kg/min to maintain normal cardiac rhythm.

• *Phenytoin:* For atrial or ventricular arrhythmias unresponsive to potassium, can give a dose of 0.5 mg/kg at a rate not exceeding 50 mg/min (given at 1–2 hr intervals). The maximum dose should not exceed 10 mg/kg/day.

• *Countershock:* A direct-current countershock can be used *only as a last resort.* If required, initiate at low voltage levels.

Treatment in Children: Give potassium in divided doses totaling 1–1.5 mEq/kg (if correction of arrhythmia is urgent, a dose of 0.5 mEq/kg/hr can be used) with careful monitoring of the ECG. The potassium IV solution should be dilute to avoid local irritation although IV fluid overload must be avoided. Digoxin immune FAB may also be used.

Digoxin is not removed effectively by dialysis, by exchange transfusion, or during cardiopulmonary bypass as most of the drug is found in tissues rather than the circulating blood.

DRUG INTERACTIONS

The following drugs increase serum digoxin levels, leading to possible toxicity: Aminoglycosides, amiodarone, anticholinergics, atorvastatin, benzodiazepines, captopril, diltiazem, dipyridamole, erythromycin, esmolol, flecainide, hydroxychloroquine, ibuprofen, indomethacin, itraconazole, nifedipine, quinidine, quinine, telmisartan, tetracyclines, tolbutamide, verapamil.

Albuterol / ↑ Digoxin binding to skeletal muscle

H *Aloe* / Potential for ↑ digoxin effect R/T aloe-induced hypokalemia

Amiloride / ↓ Digoxin inotropic effects

Aminoglycosides / ↓ Digoxin effect R/T ↓ GI tract absorption

Aminosalicylic acid / ↓ Digoxin effect R/T ↓ GI tract absorption

Amphotericin B / ↑ K depletion caused by digoxin; ↑ risk of digitalis toxicity

Antacids / ↓ Digoxin effect R/T ↓ GI tract absorption

Beta blockers / Complete heart block possible

H *Buckthorn bark/berry* / Potential for ↑ digoxin effect R/T to buckthorn-induced hypokalemia

Calcium preparations / Cardiac arrhythmias following parenteral calcium

H *Cascara sagrada bark* / Potential for ↑ digoxin effect R/T to cascara-induced hypokalemia

Chlorthalidone / ↑ K and Mg loss with ↑ chance of digitalis toxicity

Cholestyramine / Binds digoxin in the intestine and ↓ its absorption

Colestipol / Binds digoxin in the intestine and ↓ its absorption

Disopyramide / May alter effect of digoxin

H *Ephedra* / ↑ Chance of cardiac arrhythmias

Ephedrine / ↑ Chance of cardiac arrhythmias

Epinephrine / ↑ Chanceof cardiac arrhythmias

Ethacrynic acid / ↑ K and Mg loss with ↑ chance of digitalis toxicity

Fluoxetine / Possible ↑ serum digoxin levels

Furosemide / ↑ K and Mg loss with ↑ chance of digoxin toxicity

H *German chamomile flower* / Potential for ↑ digoxin effect R/T to chamomile-induced hypokalemia

H *Ginseng* / ↑ Digoxin levels

Glucose infusions / Large infusions of glucose may cause ↓ in serum potassium and ↑ chance of digoxin toxicity

Grapefruit juice / ↑ Digoxin bioavailability; do not take digoxin with grapefruit juice

H *Hawthorn* / Potentiation of digoxin effect

Hypoglycemic drugs / ↓ Effect of digitalis glycosides due to ↑ breakdown by liver

H *Iceland moss* / Potential for ↑ digoxin effect R/T to iceland moss-induced hypokalemia

H *Indian snakeroot* / ↑ Risk of bradycardia

H *Ivy leaf* / Potential for ↑ digoxin effect R/T to ivy leaf-induced hypokalemia

Levothyroxine / ↓ Serum levels and therapeutic digoxin effect

H *Licorice* / Potential for ↑ digoxin effect R/T to licorice-induced hypokalemia

H *Marshmallow root* / Potential for ↑ digoxin effect R/T to marshmallow root-induced hypokalemia

Methimazole / ↑ Chance of toxic effects of digitalis

Metoclopramide / ↓ Digoxin effect R/T ↓ GI tract absorption

Muscle relaxants, nondepolarizing / ↑ Risk of cardiac arrhythmias

Penicillamine / ↓ Serum digoxin levels.

Propranolol / Potentiates digitalis-induced bradycardia

H *Rhubarb root* / Potential for ↑ digoxin effect R/T to rhubarb root-induced hypokalemia

H *St. John's wort* / ↓ Digoxin plasma levels R/T ↑ renal excretion

H *Sarsaparilla root* / Potential for ↑ absorption of digoxin

H *Senna pod/leaf* / Potential for ↑ digoxin effect R/T to senna-induced hypokalemia

Spironolactone / Either ↑ or ↓ toxic effects of digoxin

Succinylcholine / ↑ Chance of cardiac arrhythmias

Sulfasalazine / ↓ Digoxin effect of R/T ↓ GI tract absorption

Sympathomimetics / ↑ Chance of cardiac arrhythmias

Thiazides / ↑ K and Mg loss with ↑ chance of digoxin toxicity

Thioamines / ↑ Effect and toxicity of digoxin

Thyroid / ↓ Digoxin effect

Triamterene / ↑ Digoxin effects

HOW SUPPLIED

Capsule: 0.05 mg, 0.1 mg, 0.2 mg; *Elixir, Pediatric:* 0.05 mg/mL; *Injection:* 0.1 mg/mL, 0.25 mg/mL; *Tablet:* 0.125 mg, 0.25 mg

DOSAGE

• **CAPSULES**

Digitalization: Rapid.

Adults: 0.4–0.6 mg initially followed by 0.1–0.3 mg q 6–8 hr until desired effect achieved.

Digitalization: Slow.

Adults: A total of 0.05–0.35 mg/day divided in two doses for a period of 7–22 days to reach steady-state serum levels. **Pediatric.** Digitalizing dosage is divided into three or more doses with the initial dose being about one-half the total dose; doses are given q 4–8 hr. **Children, 10 years and older:** 0.008–0.012 mg/kg. **5–10 years:** 0.015–0.03 mg/kg. **2–5 years:** 0.025–0.035 mg/kg. **1 month–2 years:** 0.03–0.05 mg/kg. **Neonates, full-term:** 0.02–0.03 mg/kg. **Neonates, premature:** 0.015–0.025 mg/kg.

Maintenance.

Adults: 0.05–0.35 mg once or twice daily. **Premature neonates:** 20–30% of total digitalizing dose divided and given in two to three daily doses. **Neonates to 10 years:** 25–35% of the total digitalizing dose divided and given in two to three daily doses.

• **ELIXIR, TABLETS**

Digitalization: Rapid.

Adults: A total of 0.75–1.25 mg divided into two or more doses each given at 6–8-hr intervals.

Digitalization: Slow.

Adults: 0.125–0.5 mg/day for 7 days. **Pediatric.** (Digitalizing dose is divided into two or more doses and given at 6–8-hr intervals.) **Children, 10 years and older, rapid or slow:** Same as adult dose. **5–10 years:** 0.02–0.035 mg/kg. **2–5 years:** 0.03–0.05 mg/kg. **1 month–2 years:** 0.035–0.06 mg/kg. **Premature and newborn infants to 1 month:** 0.02–0.035 mg/kg.

Bold Italic = life threatening side effect   ■ = black box warning   ♣ = Available in Canada

Maintenance.
Adults: 0.125–0.5 mg/day. **Pediatric:** One-fifth to one-third the total digitalizing dose daily. *NOTE:* An alternate regimen (referred to as the "small-dose" method) is 0.017 mg/kg/day. This dose causes less toxicity.

• **IV**
Digitalization.
Adults: Same as tablets. **Maintenance:** 0.125–0.5 mg/day in divided doses or as a single dose. **Pediatric:** Same as tablets.

NURSING CONSIDERATIONS
ADMINISTRATION/STORAGE
1. Measure liquids precisely, using a calibrated dropper or syringe.
2. Obtain written parameters indicating the pulse rates, both high and low, at which cardiac glycosides are to be held; changes in rate or rhythm may indicate toxicity.
3. Lanoxicaps gelatin capsules are more bioavailable than tablets. Thus, the 0.05-mg capsule is equivalent to the 0.0625-mg tablet; the 0.1- mg capsule is equivalent to the 0.125-mg tablet, and the 0.2-mg capsule is equivalent to the 0.25-mg tablet.
4. Differences in bioavailability have been noted between products; monitor clients when changing from one product to another.
5. If switching from tablets or elixir to liquid filled capsules or parenteral route expect reduction in dosage as the absorption if much higher with the capsules and parenteral form.
6. Protect from light.
IV 7. Give IV injections over 5 min (or longer) either undiluted or diluted fourfold or greater with sterile water for injection, 0.9% NaCl, RL injection, or D5W.
ASSESSMENT
For clients starting on a digitalizing dose:
1. Document type, onset, and characteristics of symptoms. If administered for heart failure, note causes; ensure that failure not solely related to diastolic dysfunction as drug's positive inotropic effect may increase cardiac out-flow obstruction with hypertrophic cardiomyopathy.
2. Note any drugs prescribed that would adversely interact with digoxin and monitor; diuretics may increase toxicity.
3. Assess for hyper/hypothyroidism; hypothyroid clients are sensitive to glycosides while hyperthyroid clients may require a higher dose of drug.
4. Monitor CBC, serum electrolytes, calcium, Mg, liver and renal function tests. Reduce dose with renal dysfunction.
5. Obtain ECG; note rhythm/rate.
6. Document cardiopulmonary findings; note presence of S3, JVD, HJR, displaced PMI, HR above 100 bpm, rales, peripheral edema, DOE, PND, and echo, MUGA, and/or cardiac catheterization findings. Note NYHA Classification based on client symptoms.
7. Elderly clients must be observed for early S&S of toxicity (N&V, anorexia, confusion, and visual disturbances) because their rate of drug elimination is slower.
INTERVENTIONS
For clients being digitalized and for clients on a maintenance dose of digoxin:
1. During digitalization, monitor closely.
2. Observe monitor for bradycardia and/or arrhythmias, count apical rate for at least 1 min before administering the drug. Obtain written parameters (e.g., HR > 60 bpm) for drug administration.
• Document adult HR below 50 bpm and hold drug. Report if an arrhythmia (irregular pulse) or any sudden increase or decrease in pulse rate, pulse deficit, and changes in rhythm occurs.
• If child's HR is 90–110 bpm or if an arrhythmia is present, withhold drug and report.
3. Anticipate more than once daily dosing in most children (up to age 10) due to higher metabolic activity.
4. With co-worker simultaneously take the apical and radial pulse for 1 min, and report pulse deficit (e.g., the wrist rate is less than the apical rate); may indicate an adverse drug reaction.

H = Herbal   IV = Intravenous   ℂ = sound-alike drug

5. Monitor weights and I&O. Weight gain may indicate edema. Adequate intake will help prevent cumulative toxic drug effects.

6. If taking non-potassium-sparing diuretics as well as digoxin, will need potassium supplements. Provide the most palatable preparation available. (Liquid potassium preparations are usually bitter.)

7. If gastric distress experienced, use an antacid. Antacids containing Al or Mg and kaolin/pectin mixtures should be given 6 hr before or 6 hr after dose of cardiac glycoside to prevent decreased therapeutic effects.

8. When given to newborns, use a cardiac monitor to identify early evidence of toxicity: excessive slowing of sinus rate, sinoatrial arrest, or prolonged PR interval.

9. Monitor digoxin levels periodically and assess for symptoms of toxicity; draw specimenmore than 6 hr after last dose. Have digoxin antidote available (digoxin immune FAB) for severe toxicity.

10. Use caution; digoxin withdrawal may worsen heart failure.

CLIENT/FAMILY TEACHING

1. Take after meals to lessen gastric irritation.

2. Do not take with grapefruit juice.

3. Maintain a written record of pulse rates and weights; review guidelines for withholding medication and reporting abnormal pulse rates.

4. Do not change brands; different preparations have variations in bioavailability and could cause toxicity or loss of effect.

5. Follow directions carefully for taking the medication. If one dose of drug is accidentally missed, do not double up on the next dose.

6. Report any adverse effects or toxic drug symptoms: Anorexia, N&V, abdominal pain and diarrhea are often early symptoms due to the toxic effects on the GI tract and CTZ stimulation. Disorientation, agitation, visual disturbances, changes in color perception, irregular heart beat and hallucinations may also occur.

7. Maintain a sodium-restricted diet. Read labels and review foods low in sodium; consult dietitian for assistance in food selection, meal planning, and preparation.

8. Consult provider before taking any other medications, whether prescribed or OTC, because drug interactions occur frequently with cardiac glycosides.

9. Report any persistent cough, difficulty breathing, or swelling (S&S of CHF).

10. Identify community health agencies to assist in maintaining health.

11. Return for scheduled follow-up visits and lab tests.

OUTCOMES/EVALUATE

• Stable cardiac rate and rhythm, improved breathing patterns, ↓ severity of S&S of CHF, improved CO, improved activity tolerance, ↓ weight, and improved diuresis

• Serum drug levels within therapeutic range (e.g., digoxin 0.5–2.0 ng/mL)

Digoxin Immune Fab (Ovine)

CLASSIFICATION(S):
Antidote for digoxin poisoning
PREGNANCY CATEGORY: C
Rx: Digibind, DigiFab

ACTION/KINETICS

Digoxin immune Fab are antibodies that bind to digoxin making them unavailable to bind at their site of action. In cases of digoxin toxicity, the antibodies bind to digoxin and the complex is excreted through the kidneys. As serum levels of digoxin decrease, digoxin bound to tissue is released into the serum to maintain equilibrium and this is then bound and excreted. The net result is a decrease in both tissue and serum digoxin. **Onset:** Less than 1 min. Improvement in signs of toxicity occurs within 30 min. **t ½:** 15–20 hr (after IV administration). Each vial contains either 38 mg or 40 mg of pure digoxin immune Fab, which will bind approximately 0.5 mg digoxin.

D

USES
Life-threatening digoxin toxicity or overdosage. Symptoms of toxicity include severe sinus bradycardia, second- or third-degree heart block which does not respond to atropine, ventricular tachycardia, and ventricular fibrillation.

NOTE: Cardiac arrest can be expected if a healthy adult ingests more than 10 mg digoxin or a healthy child ingests more than 4 mg. Also, steady-state serum concentrations of digoxin greater than 10 ng/mL or potassium concentrations greater than 5 mEq/L as a result of digoxin therapy require use of digoxin immune Fab.

SPECIAL CONCERNS
Use with caution during lactation. Use in infants only if benefits outweigh risks. Clients sensitive to products of sheep origin may also be sensitive to digoxin immune Fab. Skin testing may be appropriate for high-risk clients.

SIDE EFFECTS
CV: Worsening of CHF or low CO, atrial fibrillation (all due to withdrawal of the effects of digoxin). **Other:** Hypokalemia. Rarely, hypersensitivity reactions occur, including fever and *anaphylaxis.*

HOW SUPPLIED
Injection: 38 mg/vial (Digibind), 40 mg/vial (DigiFab)

DOSAGE————————
* **IV**

Dosage depends on the serum digoxin concentration. A large dose has a faster onset but there is an increased risk of allergic or febrile reactions. The package insert should be carefully consulted.

Acute ingestion of an unknown amount of digoxin.
Adults and children: Twenty vials (760 mg Digibind or 800 mg DigiFab). In small children, monitor the amount of overload.

Toxicity during chronic therapy.
Adults: Six vials (228 mg of Digibind or 240 mg DigiFab) is usually enough to reverse most cases of toxicity. **Children, less than 20 kg:** A single vial (38 mg Digibind or 40 mg DigiFab) should be sufficient.

NURSING CONSIDERATIONS
ADMINISTRATION/STORAGE
IV 1. The dose of antidote estimated based on ingested digoxin dffers significantly from that calculated based on the serum digoxin levels. Errors in amount of antidote required may result from inaccurate estimates of the amount of digitalis ingested or absorbed from nonsteady-state serum digitalis concentrations. Also, inaccurate serum digitalis level measurements are a possible source of error.

2. To calculate the dose (in # of vials) of the antidote for acute ingestion of a known amount of digitalis, divide the total digitalis body load (in mg) by 0.5 (i.e., amount of digitalis bound/vial). The total body load (mg) will be about equal to the amount ingested in mg for digoxin capsules.

3. To estimate the number of vials for adults when a steady-state serum digoxin level is known, multiply the serum digoxin concentration in ng/mL times the weight in kg and then divide by 100.

4. Reconstitute lyophilized material with 4 mL of sterile water for injection to give a concentration of 10 mg/mL (DigiFab) or 9.5 mg/mL (Digibind). If small doses required (e.g., in infants), Digibind or DigiFab can be further diluted (34 mL sterile isotonic saline when using Digibind or 36 mL sterile isotonic saline for DigiFab) for a concentration of 1 mg/mL.

5. Administer over a 30-min period through a 0.22-μm membrane filter; may use bolus injection if immediate danger of cardiac arrest.

6. Use reconstituted antibody immediately. May store up to 4 hr at 2–8°C (36–46°F). Unreconstituted vials of Digibind can be stored at up to 30°C (86°F) for a total of 30 days. Do not freeze DigiFab.

7. If acute digoxin ingestion results in severe symptoms and serum concentration is not known, 800 mg (20 vials) of digoxin immune Fab may be given. Monitor for volume overload in small children.

H = Herbal   IV = Intravenous   ℚ = sound-alike drug

D

8. Administer to infants with a tuberculin syringe.

ASSESSMENT
1. Determine amount, time of drug ingestion, and serum digoxin level.
2. If previous reaction suspected or high-risk client, perform skin testing: Prepare a 10-mL solution (0.1 mL of drug in 9.9 mL NSS). Administer 0.1 mL intradermally or perform a scratch test by placing 1 drop of solution on the skin and making a scratch through the drop with a sterile needle; assess site in 20 min. *Do not* use if reaction is positive: urticarial wheal with erythematous surrounding skin.
3. Do not administer to those with known allergy to sheep proteins.
4. Monitor VS and cardiac rhythm. Assess for electrolyte imbalance; note hypokalemia or evidence of CHF.
5. Wait several days for redigitalization to ensure complete elimination of Digibind. Levels will take 5–7 days to stabilize following treatment, although improvement in S&S of toxicity should be evident in 30 min.

CLIENT/FAMILY TEACHING
Drug is used to reverse the effects of too high a concentration of digoxin in the body. Should take effect in a couple of hours but digoxin levels will not show changes until about 2 days later. Report any chest pain, dizziness, or breathing difficulty.

OUTCOMES/EVALUATE
- Resolution of digoxin toxicity
- Controlled cardiac rhythm

Diltiazem hydrochloride   ©

(dill-**TIE**-ah-zem)

CLASSIFICATION(S):
Calcium channel blocker
PREGNANCY CATEGORY: C
Rx: Capsules, Extended-Release:
Cardizem CD, Cardizem SR, CartiaXT, Dilacor XR, Diltia XT, Diltiazem HCl Extended Release, Taztia XT, Tiazac. **Injection:** Cardizem. **Tablets:** Cardizem. **Tablets, Extended-Release:** Cardizem LA.

✝**Rx:** Apo-Diltiaz Injectable, Apo-Diltiaz CD, Apo-Diltiaz SR, Gen-Diltiazem, Novo-Diltiazem, Novo-Diltiazem CD, Novo-Diltiazem SR, Nu-Diltiaz, Nu-Diltiaz-CD, ratio-Diltiazem CD, Rhoxal-Diltiazem CD

SEE ALSO *CALCIUM CHANNEL BLOCKING AGENTS.*

ACTION/KINETICS
Decreases SA and AV conduction and prolongs AV node effective and functional refractory periods. Also decreases myocardial contractility and peripheral vascular resistance. Slight decrease in HR. **Tablets: Onset,** 30–60 min; **time to peak plasma levels:** 2–3 hr; **t ½, first phase:** 20–30 min; **second phase:** about 3–4.5 hr (5–8 hr with high and repetitive doses); **duration:** 4–8 hr. **Extended-Release Capsules: Onset,** 2–3 hr; **time to peak plasma levels:** 6–11 hr; **t ½:** 5–7 hr; **duration:** 12 hr. **Therapeutic serum levels:** 0.05–0.2 mcg/mL. 70–80% protein bound. Metabolized to desacetyldiltiazem, which manifests 25–50% of the activity of diltiazem. Excreted through both the bile and urine.

USES
PO: (1) Angina pectoris due to coronary artery spasm. (2) Chronic stable angina (classic effort-associated angina). (3) Hypertension (extended- or sustained-release only). **Parenteral:** (1) Temporary control of rapid ventricular rate in atrial fibrillation or flutter. (2) Rapid conversion of paroxysmal SVT to sinus rhythm (including AV nodal re-entrant tachycardias and reciprocating tachycardias associated with an extranodal accessory pathway such as Wolff-Parkinson-White syndrome or short PR syndrome). *Investigational:* Prophylaxis of reinfarction of nonQ wave MI; tardive dyskinesia, Raynaud's syndrome.

CONTRAINDICATIONS
Hypotension or cardiogenic shock. Second- or third-degree AV block and sick sinus syndrome except in presence of a functioning ventricular pacemaker.

Bold Italic = life threatening side effect   ■ = black box warning   ✝ = Available in Canada

Acute MI, pulmonary congestion. IV diltiazem with IV beta-blockers. Atrial fibrillation or atrial flutter associated with an accessory bypass tract (e.g., as in W-P-W syndrome or PR syndrome). Ventricular tachycardia. Use of Cardizem LyoJect Syringe in newborns (due to presence of benzyl alcohol). Lactation.

SPECIAL CONCERNS

Safety and effectiveness in children have not been determined. The half-life may be increased in geriatric clients. Use with caution in hepatic disease and in CHF. Abrupt withdrawal may cause an increase in the frequency and duration of chest pain. Use with beta blockers or digitalis is usually well tolerated, although the effects of coadministration cannot be predicted (especially in clients with left ventricular dysfunction or cardiac conduction abnormalities).

SIDE EFFECTS

CV: AV block, bradycardia, CHF, hypotension, syncope, palpitations, peripheral edema, **arrhythmias,** angina, tachycardia, **abnormal ECG, ventricular extrasystoles.** **GI:** N&V, diarrhea, constipation, anorexia, abdominal discomfort, cramps, dry mouth, dysgeusia. **CNS:** Weakness, nervousness, dizziness, lightheadedness, headache, depression, psychoses, hallucinations, disturbances in sleep, somnolence, insomnia, amnesia, abnormal dreams. **Dermatologic:** Rashes, dermatitis, pruritus, urticaria, erythema multiforme, **Stevens-Johnson syndrome.** **Other:** Photosensitivity, joint pain or stiffness, flushing, nasal or chest congestion, dyspnea, SOB, nocturia/polyuria, sexual difficulties, weight gain, paresthesia, tinnitus, tremor, asthenia, gynecomastia, gingival hyperplasia, petechiae, ecchymosis, purpura, bruising, hematoma, leukopenia, double vision, epistaxis, eye irritation, thirst, alopecia, **bundle branch block,** abnormal gait, hyperglycemia.

LABORATORY TEST CONSIDERATIONS

↑ Alkaline phosphatase, CPK, LDH, AST, ALT.

ADDITIONAL DRUG INTERACTIONS

Amiodarone / Possible cardiotoxicity with bradycardia and ↓ CO

Amlodipine / ↑ Plasma amlodipine levels possibly R/T ↓ liver metabolism
Anesthetics / ↑ Risk of depression of cardiac contractility, conductivity, and automaticity as well as vascular dilation
Buspirone / ↑ Buspirone effects
Carbamazepine / ↑ Diltiazem effect R/T ↓ liver breakdown
Cimetidine / ↑ Diltiazem bioavailability
Colestipol / ↓ Diltiazem bioavailability when colestipol given 1 hr before or 4 hr after diltiazem R/T ↓ diltiazem absorption
Cyclosporine / ↑ Cyclosporine effect → possible renal toxicity
Digoxin / Possible ↑ serum digoxin levels
HMG-CoA reductase inhibitors / ↑ Plasma levels of HMG-CoA reductase inhibitors
Imipramine / ↑ Serum levels
Lithium / ↑ Risk of neurotoxicity
Methylprednisolone / ↑ Pharmacologic and toxicologic effects of methylprednisolone
Moricizine / ↑ Moricine levels and ↓ diltiazem levels
Quinidine / ↑ Therapeutic and toxic effects of quinidine
Ranitidine / ↑ Diltiazem bioavailability
Sirolimus / ↑ Plasma sirolimus levels
Tacrolimus / ↑ Tacrolimus levels → ↑ toxicity
Theophyllines / ↑ Risk of pharmacologic and toxicologic theophylline effects

HOW SUPPLIED

Capsule, Extended Release: 60 mg, 90 mg, 120 mg, 180 mg, 240 mg, 300 mg, 360 mg, 420 mg; *Capsule, Sustained Release:* 60 mg, 90 mg, 120 mg; *Injection:* 5 mg/mL; *Powder for Injection:* 25 mg; *Tablet:* 30 mg, 60 mg, 90 mg, 120 mg; *Tablet, Extended-Release:* 120 mg, 180 mg, 240 mg, 300 mg, 360 mg, 420 mg

DOSAGE

• **TABLETS (IMMEDIATE RELEASE)**
Angina.

Individualize dose. **Adults, initial:** 30 mg 4 times a day before meals and at bedtime; **then,** increase gradually to total daily dose of 180–360 mg (given in three to four divided doses). Increments may be made q 1–2 days until the optimum response is attained.

- **TABLETS (EXTENDED-RELEASE)**
  Hypertension.
Individualize dose. **Adults, initial, monotherapy:** 180–240 mg once daily; some may respond to lower doses. May be titrated to a maximum dose of 540 mg/day. Schedule dosage adjustments accordingly as maximum effect usually seen within 14 days.
  Angina.
Individualize dose. **Adults, initial:** 180 mg; **then,** may increase dose at intervals of 7–14 days if adequate response not obtained. Doses above 360 mg appear not to have any additional benefit.
- **CAPSULES, EXTENDED-RELEASE**
  Angina.
Cardizem CD and Cartia XT: Adults, initial: 120 or 180 mg once daily. Up to 480 mg/day may be required. Dosage adjustments should be carried out over a 7–14-day period.
Dilacor XR and Diltia XT: Adults, initial: 120 mg once daily; **then,** dose may be titrated, depending on the needs of the client, up to 480 mg once daily. Titration may be carried out over a 7–14-day period.
Tiazac: Adults, initial: 120–180 once daily. Some may respond to higher doses up to 540 mg once daily. When necessary, carry out titration over 7–14 days.
  Hypertension.
Cardizem CD and Cartia XT: Adults, initial: 180–240 mg once daily. Some respond to lower doses. Maximum antihypertensive effect usually reached within 14 days. Usual range is 240–360 mg once daily.
Dilacor XR and Diltia XT: Adults, initial: 180–240 mg once daily.Clients 60 years and older may respond to a lower dose of 120 mg. Usual range is 180–480 mg once daily. The dose may be increased to 540 mg/day with little or no increased risk of side effects. May be used alone or in combination with other antihypertensive drugs, such as diuretics
Tiazac: Adults, initial: 120–240 mg once daily. Maximum effect usually reached by 14 days of therapy; thus, schedule dosage adjustments accord-

ingly. Usual range is 120–540 mg once daily. May be used alone or with other antihypertensive drugs.
- **CAPSULES, SUSTAINED-RELEASE CARDIZEM SR:**
Adults, initial: 60–120 mg twice a day; **then,** when maximum antihypertensive effect is reached (approximately 14 days), adjust dosage to a range of 240–360 mg/day. May be used alone or in combination with other antihypertensive drugs, such as diuretics
- **IV BOLUS**
  Atrial fibrillation/flutter; paroxysmal SVT.
Adults, initial: 0.25 mg/kg (average 20 mg) given over 2 min; **then,** if response is inadequate, a second dose may be given after 15 min. The second bolus dose is 0.35 mg/kg (average 25 mg) given over 2 min. Subsequent doses should be individualized. Some clients may respond to an initial dose of 0.15 mg/kg (duration of action may be shorter).
- **CONTINUOUS IV INFUSION**
  Atrial fibrillation/flutter.
Adults, initial: For continuous reduction of HR (up to 24 hr) for those with atrial fibrillation/flutter, begin an IV infusion immediately after the IV bolus dose. Initial infusion rate is 10 mg/hr; may be increased in 5 mg increments to 15 mg/hr. Infusion longer than 24 hr at a dose of 15 mg/hr is not recommended.

NURSING CONSIDERATIONS
℮ Do not confuse Cardizem with Cardene (also a calcium channel blocker).
ADMINISTRATION/STORAGE
1. Sublingual nitroglycerin may be taken concomitantly for acute angina. Diltiazem may also be taken together with long-acting nitrates.
2. Clients treated with diltiazem alone or in combination with other medications may be switched safely to once daily extended-release diltiazem capsules or tablets at the nearest equivalent total daily dose. However, subsequent titration to a higher or lower dose may be necessary and should be initated if needed.

Bold Italic = life threatening side effect ■ = black box warning ✦ = Available in Canada

3. Use with beta blockers or digitalis is usually well tolerated, but the combined effects cannot be predicted, especially with cardiac conduction abnormalities or LV dysfunction.

IV 4. May be administered by direct IV over 2 min or as an infusion (see *Dosage*). For IV infusion, drug may be mixed with NSS, D5W, or D5/0.45% NaCl.

5. Do not mix Cardizem LyoJect or Cardizem Monovial with any other drugs in the same container.

6. Do not give diltiazem injection, Cardizem LyoJect, and Cardizem Monovial in the same IV line.

7. The infusion may be maintained for up to 24 hr; beyond 24 hr is not recommended.

8. The injection should be refrigerated at 2–8°C (36–46°F). May be stored at room temperature for 1 month; then, discard remaining solution.

9. Store Cardizem LyoJect and Cardizem Monovial at room temperature (15–20°C; 59–86°F). Do not freeze. Reconstituted drug is stable for 24 hr at controlled room temperature. Discard any unused portion of Cardizem LyoJect.

ASSESSMENT

1. Document indications for therapy, symptom onset, and any previous treatments.

2. Note any edema or CHF; review ECG for evidence of AV block.

3. Monitor renal and LFTs; reduce dose with impaired function.

4. Drug half-life may be prolonged in elderly; monitor closely.

CLIENT/FAMILY TEACHING

1. Take the extended-release capsules on an empty stomach. Do not open, chew, or crush; should be swallowed whole.

2. Use caution; may cause drowsiness/ dizziness.

3. Rise slowly from a lying to a sitting and standing position; may cause ↓ BP.

4. Report persistent and bothersome side effects including headaches, constipation, unusual tiredness, or weakness.

5. Continue carrying short-acting nitrites (nitroglycerin) at all times and use as directed. Avoid prolonged sun exposure and use precaution if necessary to prevent photosensitivy reaction.

6. Continue diet (low fat and low Na), regular exercise, and decreased caffeine; stop tobacco and alcohol. Decrease fluid and sodium intake to control swelling.

OUTCOMES/EVALUATE

• ↓ Frequency and intensity of vasospastic anginal attacks

• ↓ BP; stable cardiac rhythm

Dipyridamole

(dye-peer-**ID**-ah-mohl)

CLASSIFICATION(S):
Anticoagulant, platelet adhesion inhibitor

PREGNANCY CATEGORY: B

Rx: Persantine, Persantine IV

✦Rx: Apo-Dipyridamole FC, Dipyridamole for Injection, Novo-Dipiradol

ACTION/KINETICS

In higher doses may act by several mechanisms, including inhibition of red blood cell uptake of adenosine, itself an inhibitor of platelet reactivity; inhibition of platelet phosphodiesterase, which leads to accumulation of cAMP within platelets; direct stimulation of release of prostacyclin or prostaglandin D_2; and/or inhibition of thromboxane A_2 formation. Dipyridamole prolongs platelet survival time in clients with valvular heart disease and has maintained platelet count in open heart surgery. Also causes coronary vasodilation which may be due to inhibition of adenosine deaminase in the blood, thus allowing accumulation of adenosine which is a potent vasodilator. Vasodilation may also be caused by delaying the hydrolysis of cyclic 3′,5′-adenosine monophosphate as a result of inhibition of the enzyme phosphodiesterase. Incompletely absorbed from the GI tract. **Peak plasma levels, after PO:** 75 min.

t ½, after PO: initial, 40 min; **terminal,** 10–12 hr. Metabolized in the liver and mainly excreted in the bile. Significantly bound to plasma proteins.

USES

PO. (1) As an adjunct to coumarin anticoagulants in preventing post-operative thromboembolic complications of cardiac valve replacement. (2) Use with aspirin to prevent myocardial reinfarction and reduction of post MI mortality (combination therapy does not appear to be any more beneficial than use of aspirin alone). **IV.** As an alternative to exercise in thallium myocardial perfusion imaging for the evaluation of CAD in those who cannot exercise adequately. *NOTE:* Not effective for the treatment of acute episodes of angina and is not a substitute for the treatment of angina pectoris.

SPECIAL CONCERNS

Use with caution in hypotension and during lactation. Safety and efficacy have not been determined in children less than 12 years of age.

SIDE EFFECTS

• **AFTER PO USE. GI:** GI intolerance, N&V, diarrhea.
CNS: Dizziness, headache, syncope. **CV:** Peripheral vasodilation, flushing. Rarely, angina pectoris or aggravation of angina pectoris (usually at the beginning of therapy). **Miscellaneous:** Weakness, rash, pruritus.
• **AFTER IV USE.**
Most common side effects (1% or greater) are listed. GI: Nausea, dyspepsia. **CNS:** Headache, dizziness, paresthesia, fatigue. **CV:** Chest pain, angina pectoris, ECG abnormalities (ST-T changes, extrasystoles, tachycardia), precipitation of acute myocardial ischemia in clients with CAD, hypotension, flushing, blood pressure lability, hypertension. **Miscellaneous:** Dyspnea, unspecified pain.

OD OVERDOSE MANAGEMENT
Symptoms: Hypotension of short duration. *Treatment:* Use of a vasopressor may be beneficial. Due to the high percentage of protein binding of dipyridamole, dialysis is not likely to be beneficial.

DRUG INTERACTIONS

Digoxin / ↑ Digoxin bioavailability
H *Evening primrose oil* / Potential for ↑ antiplatelet effect
H *Feverfew* / Potential for ↑ antiplatelet effect
H *Garlic* / Potential for ↑ antiplatelet effect
H *Ginger* / Potential for ↑ antiplatelet effect
H *Ginkgo biloba* / Potential for ↑ antiplatelet effect
H *Ginseng* / Potential for ↑ antiplatelet effect
H *Grapeseed extract* / Potential for ↑ antiplatelet effect

HOW SUPPLIED

Injection: 5 mg/mL; *Tablets:* 25 mg, 50 mg, 75 mg.

DOSAGE

• **TABLETS**
Adjunct in prophylaxis of thromboembolism after cardiac valve replacement.
Adults: 75–100 mg 4 times per day as an adjunct to warfarin therapy. Do not give aspirin concomitantly.
Prevention of thromboembolic complications in other thromboembolic disorders.
Adults: 150–400 mg/day in combination with another platelet-aggregation inhibitor (e.g., aspirin) or an anticoagulant.
• **IV**
Adjunct to thallium myocardial perfusion imaging.
Adjust the dose according to body weight. Recommended dose is 0.142 mg/kg/min infused over 4 min. Total dose should not exceed 60 mg.

NURSING CONSIDERATIONS

ADMINISTRATION/STORAGE

IV 1. When used IV, to prevent irritation, dilute the injection in at least a 1:2 ratio with D5W, 0.45% NaCl, or 0.9% NaCl injection. The total volume should be 20 to 50 mL.
2. With imaging, give thallium-201 within 5 min after the IV injection.
3. Do not mix with other drugs in the same syringe or infusion container.

ASSESSMENT

1. Document indications for therapy, type, onset, and characteristics of symptoms.
2. List all drugs currently prescribed to ensure none interact unfavorably.
3. Document mental status, skin color, and cardiopulmonary findings.
4. Monitor VS, ECG, CBC, PT, PTT, and INR.

CLIENT/FAMILY TEACHING

1. Drug helps prevent clots by inhibiting platelet stickiness; may also decrease frequency of chest pain and increase exercise tolerance. May take several months of therapy before effects evident.
2. Avoid alcohol and tobacco due to hypotensive vasoconstrictive effects and use of any other unprescribed drugs including aspirin without approval.
3. May cause dizziness and lightheadedness; use caution and change positions slowly to minimize ↓ BP.
4. Try small frequent meals if nausea or gastric distress is experienced.
5. Report any increased chest pain, rash, fainting or severe headaches.

OUTCOMES/EVALUATE

- CAD evaluation with imaging
- Prevention of thromboembolism

Dobutamine hydrochloride ©

(doh-**BYOU**-tah-meen)

CLASSIFICATION(S):
Sympathomimetic direct-acting
PREGNANCY CATEGORY: B
Rx: Dobutrex

SEE ALSO *SYMPATHOMIMETIC DRUGS.*

ACTION/KINETICS

Stimulates beta-1 receptors (in the heart), increasing cardiac function, CO, and SV, with minor effects on HR. Decreases afterload reduction although SBP and pulse pressure may remain unchanged or increase (due to increased CO). Also decreases elevated ventricular filling pressure and helps AV node conduction. **Onset:** 1–2 min. **Peak effect:** 10 min. **t ½:** 2 min. **Therapeutic plasma levels:** 40–190 ng/mL. Metabolized by the liver and excreted in urine.

USES

Short-term treatment of cardiac decompensation in adults secondary to depressed contractility due to organic heart disease or cardiac surgical procedures. *Investigational:* Congenital heart disease in children undergoing diagnostic cardiac catheterization.

CONTRAINDICATIONS

Idiopathic hypertrophic subaortic stenosis.

SPECIAL CONCERNS

Safe use during childhood or after AMI not established.

SIDE EFFECTS

CV: Marked increase in HR, BP, and **ventricular ectopic activity,** precipitous drop in BP, premature ventricular beats, anginal and nonspecific chest pain, palpitations. **Hypersensitivity:** Skin rash, pruritus of the scalp, fever, eosinophilia, **bronchospasm. Other:** Nausea, headache, SOB, fever, phlebitis, and local inflammatory changes at the injection site.

OD OVERDOSE MANAGEMENT

Symptoms: Excessive alteration of BP, anorexia N&V, tremor, anxiety, palpitations, headache, SOB, anginal and nonspecific chest pain, **myocardial ischemia, ventricular fibrillation or tachycardia.** *Treatment:* Reduce the rate of administration or discontinue temporarily until the condition stabilizes. Establish an airway, ensuring oxygenation and ventilation. Initiate resuscitative measures immediately. Treat severe ventricular tachyarrhythmias with propranolol or lidocaine.

ADDITIONAL DRUG INTERACTIONS

Concomitant use with nitroprusside causes ↑ CO and ↓ PAWP.

HOW SUPPLIED

Injection: 12.5 mg/mL

DOSAGE

- **IV INFUSION**

Adults, individualized, usual: 2.5–15 mcg/kg/min (up to 40 mcg/kg/min). Rate of administration and duration of therapy depend on response of client, as determined by HR, presence of ectopic activity, BP, and urine flow.

NURSING CONSIDERATIONS

℃ Do not confuse dobutamine with dopamine (also a sympathomimetic).

ADMINISTRATION/STORAGE

[IV] 1. Reconstitute solution according to manufacturer directions; takes place in two stages.

2. Before administration, the solution is diluted further according to the fluid needs of the client. This more dilute solution should be used within 24 hr. Solutions that can be used for further dilution include D5W, D5/0.45% NaCl injection, D5/0.9% NaCl injection, D10W, Isolyte M with D5W injection, RL injection, D5/RL, Normosol-M in D5W, 20% Osmitrol in water for injection, 0.9% NaCl injection, and sodium lactate injection.

3. The more concentrated solution may be refrigerated for 48 hr or stored at room temperature for 6 hr. After dilution (in glass or Viaflex containers), the solution is stable for 24 hr at room temperature. Dilute solutions may darken; does not affect potency when used within designated time spans.

4. Drug is incompatible with alkaline solutions. Do not give with agents or diluents containing both sodium bisulfite and ethanol. Is physically incompatible with hydrocortisone sodium succinate, cefazolin, cefamandole, neutral cephalothin, penicillin, sodium ethacrynate, and heparin sodium.

5. Drug is compatible when given through same tubing with dopamine, lidocaine, tobramycin, verapamil, nitroprusside, KCl, and protamine sulfate.

6. Give using an electronic infusion device. Carefully reconstitute and calculate dosage according to weight and desired response.

ASSESSMENT

Note indications for therapy; ensure adequately hydrated prior to infusion.

INTERVENTIONS

1. Monitor CVP to assess vascular volume and cardiac pumping efficiency. Normal range 5–10 cm water (1–7 mm Hg). Elevated CVP may indicate disruption of CO, as in pump failure or pulmonary edema; low CVP may indicate hypovolemia.

2. Monitor PAWP to assess the pressures in the left atrium and ventricle and to measure the efficiency of CO; usual range is 6–12 mm Hg.

3. Monitor ECG and BP continuously during drug administration; review written parameters for SBP and titrate infusion.Drug increases AV node conduction causing those with AFib to develop rapid ventricular rate; have digoxin available to give in this event.

4. Record I&O.

5. Monitor glucose in diabetics; increased insulin may be needed.

CLIENT/FAMILY TEACHING

Drug is administered IV to improve cardiac function thus increasing BP and improving urine output. Report any chest pain, increased SOB, headaches, or IV site pain.

OUTCOMES/EVALUATE

- ↑ CO; ↑ urine output
- SBP > 90 mm Hg

Dofetilide ∎
(doh-**FET**-ih-lyd)

CLASSIFICATION(S):
Antiarrhythmic
PREGNANCY CATEGORY: C
Rx: Tikosyn

SEE ALSO *ANTIARRHYTHMIC DRUGS.*

ACTION/KINETICS

Acts by blocking the cardiac ion channel carrying the rapid component of the delayed rectifier potassium currents. Blocks only I_{Kr} with no significant block of other repolarizing potassium currents (e.g., I_{Ks}, I_{K1}). No effect on sodium channels or adrenergic receptors. Dofetilide increases the monophasic action potential duration due to delayed repolarization. **Maximum plasma levels:** 2–3 hr during fasting. Steady state plasma levels reached in 2–3 days. Metabolized in the liver and excreted in

---

the urine. **t ½, terminal:** About 10 hr. Women have lower oral clearances than men.

USES

(1) Conversion of atrial fibrillation or atrial flutter to normal sinus rhythm. (2) Maintenance of normal sinus rhythm in clients witih atrial fibrillation/atrial flutter of more than 1 week duration and who have been converted to normal sinus rhythm. Reserve for those in whom atrial fibrillation/atrial flutter is highly symptomatic due to life-threatening ventricular arrhythmias. *NOTE:* Available only to hospitals and prescribers who receive dosing and treatment initiation education through the *Tikosyn* education program.

CONTRAINDICATIONS

Congenital or acquired long QT syndromes, in those with a baseline QT interval greater than 440 msec (500 msec in clients with ventricular conduction abnormalities), severe renal impairment (C_{CR} less than 20 mL/min). Concomitant use of verapamil, cimetidine, trimethoprim (alone or with sulfamethoxazole), ketoconazole, prochlorperazine, megestrol. Lactation.

SPECIAL CONCERNS

■(1) To minimize risk of induced arrhythmia, place clients started or restarted on dofetilide in a facility that can determine creatinine clearance and provide continuous ECG monitoring and cardiac resuscitation for a minimum of 3 days. (2) Drug is available only to hospitals and prescribers who have received appropriate dofetilide dosing and treatment initiation education.■ There is a greater risk of dofetilide-induced TdP (type of ventricular tachycardia) in female clients than in male clients. Use with caution in severe hepatic impairment. Use with drugs that prolong the QT interval has not been studied with dofetilide use; therefore, do not use bepridil, certain macrolide antibiotics, phenothiazines, or TCAs with dofetilide. Safety and efficacy have not been determined in children less than 18 years of age.

SIDE EFFECTS

CV: Ventricular arrhythmias (especially TdP type ventricular tachycardia), *torsades de pointes,* angina pectoris, atrial fibrillation, hypertension, palpitation, supraventricular tachycardia, ventricular tachycardia, bradycardia, cerebral ischemia, *CVA, MI, heart arrest, ventricular fibrillation,* AV block, bundle branch block, heart block. **CNS:** Headache, dizziness, insomnia, anxiety, paresthesia. **GI:** Nausea, diarrhea, abdominal pain. **Respiratory:** Respiratory tract infection, dyspnea, increased cough. **Miscellaneous:** Chest pain, flu syndrome, accidental injury, back pain, rash, arthralgia, asthenia, pain, peripheral edema, sweating, UTI, angioedema, edema, facial paralysis, flaccid paralysis, liver damage, paralysis, *sudden death,* syncope.

OD OVERDOSE MANAGEMENT

Symptoms: Excessive prolongation of QT interval. *Treatment:* Symptomatic and supportive. Initiate cardiac monitoring. Can use charcoal slur but is effective only when given within 15 min of dofetilide. To treat TdP or overdose, may give isoproterenol infusion, with or without cardiac pacing. IV Mg sulfate may be useful to manage TdP. Monitor until QT interval returns to normal.

DRUG INTERACTIONS

Amiloride / Possible ↑ dofetilide levels
Amiodarone / Possible ↑ dofetilide levels
Cannabinoids / Possible ↑ dofetilide levels
Cimetidine / ↑ Risk of arrhythmia (TdP) R/T ↓ liver metabolism of dofetilide
Digoxin / ↑ Risk of torsades de pointes
Diltiazem / Possible ↑ dofetilide levels
Grapefruit juice / Possible ↑ dofetilide levels
Ketoconazole / ↑ Risk of arrhythmia (TdP) R/T ↓ liver metabolism of dofetilide
Macrolide antibiotics / Possible ↑ dofetilide levels
Megestrol / Possible ↑ dofetilide levels → arrhythmias
Metformin / Possible ↑ dofetilide levels
Nefazadone / Possible ↑ dofetilide levels

Norfloxacin / Possible ↑ dofetilide levels

Potassium-depleting diuretics / Hypokalemia or hypomagnesemia may occur, → ↑ potential for torsades de pointes

Prochlorperazine / Possible ↑ dofetilide levels → arrhythmias

Quinine / Possible ↑ dofetilide levels

Triamterene / Possible ↑ dofetilide levels

Trimethoprim or Trimethoprim/Sulfamethoxazole / ↑ Risk of arrhythmia (TdP) R/T ↓ liver metabolism of dofetilide

Verapamil / Possible ↑ dofetilide levels → arrhythmias

Zafirlukast / Possible ↑ dofetilide levels

HOW SUPPLIED

Capsules: 125 mcg, 250 mcg, 500 mcg

DOSAGE————————

- **CAPSULES**

  Conversion of atrial fibrillation/flutter; maintenance of normal sinus rhythm.

The dosing for dofetilide must be undertaken using the following steps:

1. Before giving the first dose, determine the QTc using an average of 5–10 beats. If the QTc is greater than 440 msec (500 msec in those with ventricular conduction abnormalities), dofetilide is contraindicated. Also, do not use if the heart rate is less than 60 bpm.

2. Before giving the first dose, calculate the C_{CR} using the following formulas:

Males: (Weight [kg] x [140 - age])/(72 x serum creatinine [mg/dL])

Females: 0.84 x male value

3. Determine the starting dose of dofetilide as follows: **C_{CR} greater than 60 mL/min:** 500 mcg twice per day; **C_{CR} 40–60 mL/min:** 250 mcg twice per day; **C_{CR} 20–less than 40 mL/min:** 125 mcg twice per day; **C_{CR} less than 20 mL/min:** DO NOT USE DOFETILIDE; CONTRAINDICATED IN THESE CLIENTS. The maximum daily dose is 500 mcg twice per day.

4. Give the adjusted dose based on C_{CR} and begin continuous ECG monitoring.

5. At 2–3 hr after giving the first dofetilide dose, determine the QTc. If the QTc has increased by more than 15% compared with the baseline established in Step 1 or if the QTc is 500 msec (550 msec in those with ventricular conduc-

tion abnormalities), adjust subsequent dosing as follows: If the starting dose based on C_{CR} is 500 mcg twice per day, the adjusted dose (for QTc prolongation) is 250 mcg twice a day. If the starting dose is 250 mcg twice per day, the adjusted dose (for QTc prolongation) is 125 mcg twice per day. If the starting dose is 125 mcg twice per day, the adjusted dose (for QTc prolongation) is 125 mcg once daily.

6. At 2–3 hr after each subsequent dose of dofetilide, determine QTc for in-hospital doses 2 through 5. No further down titration of dofetilide based on QTc is recommended. Discontinue if at any time after the second dose of dofetilide, the QTc is greater than 500 msec (550 msec in those with ventricular conduction abnormalities).

7. Continuously monitor by ECG for a minimum of 3 days or for a minimum of 12 hr after electrical or pharmacologic conversion to normal sinus rhythm, whichever time is greater.

NURSING CONSIDERATIONS

ADMINISTRATION/STORAGE

1. Therapy must be started (and, if necessary, reinitiated) in a setting where continuous ECG monitoring and personnel trained in the management of serious ventricular arrhthymias are available for a minimum of 3 days.

2. Do not discharge clients within 12 hr of electrical or pharmacologic conversion to normal sinus rhythm.

3. Prior to electrical or pharmacologic cardioversion, anticoagulate clients with atrial fibrillation according to usual medical practices. Anticoagulants may be continued after cardioversion. Correct hypokalemia before starting dofetilide therapy.

4. Re-evaluate renal function q 3 months or as warranted. Discontinue dofetilide if the QTc is greater than 500 msec (550 msec in those with ventricular conduction abnormalities) and monitor carefully until QTc returns to baseline levels. If renal function decreases, adjust the dose as directed under *Dosage.*

Bold Italic = life threatening side effect   ■ = black box warning   ✦ = Available in Canada

5. The highest dose of 500 mcg twice a day is the most effective. However, the risk of torsades de pointes is increased. Thus, a lower dose may be used. If at any time the lower dose is increased, the client must be hospitalized for 3 days. Previous tolerance of higher doses does not eliminate the need for hospitalization.

6. Do not consider electrical conversion if the client does not convert to normal sinus rhythm within 24 hr after starting dofetilide.

7. Withdraw previous antiarrhythmic drug therapy before starting dofetilide therapy; during withdrawal, carefully monitor for a minimum of 3 plasma half-lives. Do not initiate dofetilide following amiodarone therapy until amiodarone plasma levels are less than 0.3 mcg/mL or until amiodarone has been withdrawn for 3 or more months.

8. Protect capsules from moisture and humidity. Dispense in tight containers.

ASSESSMENT

1. Identify arrhythmia and duration. Note any S&S associated with arrhythmia. Monitor ECG strips continously for at least three day after starting for evidence of prolonged QT interval which requires reduction in dose or stopping therapy.

2. Note drugs prescribed to ensure none interact. Do not give within 3 mo of amiodarone therapy unless level below 0.3 mcg/mL. Avoid use of drugs that prolong the QT interval.

3. Monitor electrolytes, renal and LFTs; avoid use with dysfunction. Low K and Mg can increase risk of torsades de pointes.

4. Drug is available only through the Tikosyn Dosing Program with provider education.

CLIENT/FAMILY TEACHING

1. Take exactly as prescribed without regard to food or meals; avoid grapefruit juice.

2. Do not double the next dose if a dose is missed. Take next dose at usual time.

3. Report any change in prescriptions or OTC/supplement use. Inform all providers especially if hospitalized or pre-

scribed a new medication for any condition. Do not take any interacting drugs for at least two day, after stopping dofetilide, to allow for drug to get out of system.

4. Do not use OTC tagamet may use zantac, pepcid, axid and prevacid for acid indigestion or ulcer therapy.

5. Reports any adverse effects including diarrhea, sweating, vomiting, loss of thirst or appetite to provider immediately.

6. Read the package insert prior to use. Drug adherence is imperative with this therapy. Must report as scheduled for ECG evaluation and report any adverse effects to ensure no serious drug related complications.

OUTCOMES/EVALUATE

• Conversion of atrial fibrillation/flutter to NSR

• Maintenance of NSR once converted

Dopamine hydrochloride @

(**DOH**-pah-meen)

CLASSIFICATION(S):
Sympathomimetic, direct- and indirect-acting
PREGNANCY CATEGORY: C

SEE ALSO *SYMPATHOMIMETIC DRUGS.*

ACTION/KINETICS

Dopamine is the immediate precursor of epinephrine in the body. Exogenously administered, it produces direct stimulation of beta-1 receptors and variable (dose-dependent) stimulation of alpha receptors (peripheral vasoconstriction). Will cause a release of norepinephrine from its storage sites. These actions result in increased myocardial contraction, CO, and SV, as well as increased renal blood flow and sodium excretion. Exerts little effect on DBP and induces fewer arrhythmias than are seen with isoproterenol. **Onset:** 5 min. **Duration:** 10 min. **t ½:** 2 min. Does not cross the blood-brain barrier. Metabolized in liver and excreted in urine.

USES
Cardiogenic shock due to MI, trauma, endotoxic septicemia, open heart surgery, renal failure, and chronic cardiac decompensation (as in CHF). Clients most likely to respond include those in whom urine flow, myocardial function, and BP have not deteriorated significantly. Best responses are observed when the time is short between onset of symptoms of shock and initiation of dopamine and volume correction. *Investigational:* COPD, CHF, respiratory distress syndrome in infants.

ADDITIONAL CONTRAINDICATIONS
Pheochromocytoma, uncorrected tachycardia, ventricular fibrillation, or arrhythmias. Pediatric clients.

SPECIAL CONCERNS
Use with caution during lactation. Safety and efficacy have not been established in children. Dosage may have to be adjusted in geriatric clients with occlusive vascular disease.

ADDITIONAL SIDE EFFECTS
CV: Ectopic heartbeats, tachycardia, anginal pain, palpitations, vasoconstriction, hypotension, hypertension. Infrequently: Aberrant conduction, bradycardia, widened QRS complex. **Other:** Dyspnea, N&V, headache, mydriasis. Infrequently: Piloerection, azotemia, polyuria. High doses may cause mydriasis and ventricular arrhythmia. Extravasation may result in necrosis and sloughing of surrounding tissue.

OD OVERDOSE MANAGEMENT
Symptoms: Extravasation. *Treatment:* To prevent sloughing and necrosis, infiltrate as soon as possible with 10–15 mL of 0.9% NaCl solution containing 5–10 mg phentolamine using a syringe with a fine needle. Infiltrate liberally throughout the ischemic area.

ADDITIONAL DRUG INTERACTIONS
Anesthetics, halogenated hydrocarbon / Sensitization of myocardium to dopamine → serious arrhythmias
Diuretics / Additive or potentiating effect
Guanethidine / Partial or total reversal of antihypertensive effect of guanethidine
MAO inhibitors / ↑ Pressor response to dopamine → hypertension

Oxytocic drugs / Possible severe persistent hypertension
Phenytoin / Possible seizures, severe hypotension, and bradycardia
Propranolol / ↓ Effect of dopamine
Tricyclic antidepressants / Possible ↓ dopamine pressor effect

HOW SUPPLIED
Injection: 40 mg/mL, 80 mg/mL, 160 mg/mL

DOSAGE
• **IV INFUSION**
Shock.
Initial: 2–5 mcg/kg/min; **then,** increase in increments of 1–4 mcg/kg/min at 10–30-min intervals until desired response is obtained.
Severely ill clients.
Initial: 5 mcg/kg/min; **then,** increase rate in increments of 5–10 mcg/kg/min up to 20–50 mcg/kg/min as needed.
NOTE: Dopamine is a potent drug. Be sure to dilute the drug before administration. The drug should not be given as a bolus dose.

NURSING CONSIDERATIONS
ℂ Do not confuse dopamine with dobutamine (also a sympathomimetic).

ADMINISTRATION/STORAGE
IV 1. Must be diluted before use—see package insert.
2. For reconstitution use dextrose or saline solutions: 200 mg/250 mL for a concentration of 0.8 mg/mL or 800 mcg/mL; 400 mg/250 mL for a concentration of 1.6 mg/mL or 1,600 mcg/mL. Alkaline solutions such as 5% NaHCO₃, oxidizing agents, or iron salts will inactivate drug.
3. Dilute just prior to administration, solution stable for 24 hr at room temperature; protect from light.
4. To prevent fluid overload, may use more concentrated solutions with higher doses.
5. Administer using an electronic infusion device. Carefully reconstitute and calculate dosage.
6. When discontinuing, gradually decrease dose; sudden cessation may cause marked hypotension.

Bold Italic = life threatening side effect   ■ = black box warning   ♣ = Available in Canada

ASSESSMENT
Note indications for therapy; ensure adequate hydration prior to infusion.

INTERVENTIONS
1. Monitor VS, I&O, and ECG; titrate infusion to maintain SBP as ordered.
2. Be prepared to monitor CVP and PAWP. Report ectopy, palpitations, anginal pain, or vasoconstriction.

CLIENT/FAMILY TEACHING
Drug is administered IV to improve cardiac function thus increasing BP and improving urine output. Report any chest pain, increased SOB, headaches, or IV site pain.

OUTCOMES/EVALUATE
- SBP > 90; ↑ urine output
- Improved organ perfusion

Doxazosin mesylate ©
(dox-**AYZ**-oh-sin)

CLASSIFICATION(S):
Antihypertensive, peripherally-acting
PREGNANCY CATEGORY: B
Rx: Cardura
❋**Rx:** Apo-Doxazosin, Cardura-1, -2, -4, Gen-Doxazosin, Novo-Doxazosin, ratio-Doxazosin

ACTION/KINETICS
Blocks the alpha-1 (postjunctional) adrenergic receptors resulting in a decrease in systemic vascular resistance and a corresponding decrease in BP. **Peak plasma levels:** 2–3 hr. **Peak effect:** 2–6 hr. Significantly bound (98%) to plasma proteins. Metabolized in the liver to active and inactive metabolites, which are excreted through the feces and urine. **t ½:** 22 hr.

USES
(1) Hypertension, alone or in combination with diuretics, calcium channel blockers, ACE inhibitors, or beta blockers. (2) BPH, both urinary outflow obstruction and obstructive and irritative symptoms. May be used in BPH clients whether hypertensive or normotensive.

CONTRAINDICATIONS
Clients allergic to prazosin or terazosin.
SPECIAL CONCERNS
Use with caution during lactation, in impaired hepatic function, or in those taking drugs known to influence hepatic metabolism. Safety and effectiveness have not been demonstrated in children. Due to the possibility of severe hypotension, do not use the 2-, 4-, and 8-mg tablets for initial therapy.
SIDE EFFECTS
CV: Dizziness (most frequent), syncope, vertigo, lightheadedness, edema, palpitation, arrhythmia, postural hypotension, tachycardia, peripheral ischemia. **CNS:** Fatigue, headache, paresthesia, kinetic disorders, ataxia, somnolence, nervousness, depression, insomnia. **Musculoskeletal:** Arthralgia, arthritis, muscle weakness, muscle cramps, myalgia, hypertonia. **GU:** Polyuria, sexual dysfunction, urinary incontinence, urinary frequency. **GI:** Nausea, diarrhea, dry mouth, constipation, dyspepsia, flatulence, abdominal pain, vomiting. **Respiratory:** Rhinitis, epistaxis, dyspnea. **Miscellaneous:** Fatigue or malaise, rash, pruritus, flushing, urticaria, abnormal vision, conjunctivitis, eye pain, tinnitus, chest pain, asthenia, facial edema, generalized pain, slight weight gain.
OD OVERDOSE MANAGEMENT
Symptoms: Hypotension. *Treatment:* IV fluids.
HOW SUPPLIED
Tablet: 1 mg, 2 mg, 4 mg, 8 mg
DOSAGE
- **TABLETS**
  Hypertension.
Adults: initial, 1 mg once daily at bedtime; **then,** depending on the response (client's standing BP both 2–6 hr and 24 hr after a dose), the dose may be increased to 2 mg/day. A maximum of 16 mg/day may be required to control BP.
  Benign prostatic hyperplasia.
Initial: 1 mg once daily. **Maintenance:** Depending on the urodynamics and symptoms, dose may be increased to 2 mg daily and then 4–8 mg once daily (maximum recommended dose). The recommended titration interval is 1–2 weeks.

NURSING CONSIDERATIONS
€ Do not confuse Cardura with Ridaura (gold-containing anti-inflammatory).

ADMINISTRATION/STORAGE
1. To minimize the possibility of severe hypotension, limit initial dosage to 1 mg/day.
2. Increasing the dose higher than 4 mg/day increases the possibility of severe syncope, postural dizziness, vertigo, and postural hypotension.

ASSESSMENT
1. Note indications for therapy, other agents trialed. Explore experience/allergy to prazosin or terazosin; a quinazoline derivative.
2. Assess supine and standing BP at 2 to 6 hr and 24 hr after dosing. Check ECG for arrhythmia.
3. With BPH, score severity.

CLIENT/FAMILY TEACHING
1. Take once daily; do not stop abruptly. May take first dose at bedtime to minimize side effects.
2. Record BP and weight; note swelling of hands/feet. Dosage may be increased every two weeks for high BP and every 1 to 2 weeks for prostate enlargement.
3. Rise slowly to a sitting position before attempting to stand to prevent ↓ BP. This may occur 2–6 hr after a dose.
4. Driving and hazardous tasks should be avoided for 24 hr after first dose until effects are evident; may experience dizziness and fainting.
5. Report adverse effects or if S&S do not improve after several weeks of therapy as drug dosage may need adjustment.

OUTCOMES/EVALUATE
• ↓ BP
• ↓ S&S of BPH/nocturia list

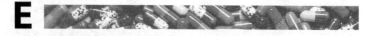

E

Enalapril maleate ■ €
(en-**AL**-ah-prill)

CLASSIFICATION(S):
Antihypertensive, ACE inhibitor
PREGNANCY CATEGORY: D
Rx: Enalaprilat, Vasotec

SEE ALSO ANGIOTENSIN-CONVERTING ENZYME INHIBITORS.

ACTION/KINETICS
Converted in the liver by hydrolysis to the active metabolite, enalaprilat. The parenteral product is enalaprilat injection. About 60% bioavailable after PO. **Onset, PO:** 1 hr; **IV:** 15 min. **Time to peak action, PO:** 4–6 hr; **IV:** 1–4 hr. **Duration, PO:** 24 hr or more; **IV:** About 6 hr. Approximately 50–60% is protein bound. **t ½, enalapril, PO:** 1.3 hr; **IV:** 15 min. **t ½, enalaprilat, PO:** 11 hr. Excreted through the urine (half unchanged) and feces; over 90% of enalaprilat is excreted through the urine.

USES
PO: (1) Alone or in combination with other antihypertensives (especially thiazide diuretics) for the treatment of hypertension. Hypertension in children. (2) In combination with digitalis and diuretic in acute and chronic CHF. (3) Asymptomatic left ventricular dysfunction in clinically stable asymptomatic clients. **IV:** Treatment of hypertension when PO is not practical. *Investigational:* Hypertension related to scleroderma renal crisis. Enalaprilat may be used for hypertensive emergencies (effect is variable).

SPECIAL CONCERNS
■When used during the second and third trimesters of pregnancy, injury and even death can result in the developing fetus. When pregnancy is detected, discontinue as soon as possible.■ Use with caution during lactation. Safe-

---

ty and effectiveness have not been determined in children.

SIDE EFFECTS

CV: Palpitations, hypotension, chest pain, angina, **CVA, MI,** orthostatic hypotension, disturbances in rhythm, tachycardia, **cardiac arrest,** orthostatic effects, atrial fibrillation, tachycardia, bradycardia, Raynaud's phenomenon. **GI:** N&V, diarrhea, abdominal pain, alterations in taste, anorexia, dry mouth, constipation, dyspepsia, glossitis, ileus, melena, stomatitis. **CNS:** Insomnia, headache, fatigue, dizziness, paresthesias, nervousness, sleepiness, ataxia, confusion, depression, vertigo, abnormal dreams. **Hepatic:** Hepatitis, hepatocellular or cholestatic jaundice, pancreatitis, elevated liver enzymes, hepatic failure. **Respiratory:** Bronchitis, cough, dyspnea, bronchospasm, URI, pneumonia, pulmonary infiltrates, asthma, **pulmonary embolism and infarction, pulmonary edema. Renal:** Renal dysfunction, oliguria, UTI, transient increases in creatinine and BUN. **Hematologic:** Rarely, neutropenia, thrombocytopenia, bone marrow depression, decreased H&H in hypertensive or CHF clients. Hemolytic anemia, including hemolysis, in clients with G6PD deficiency. **Dermatologic:** Rash, pruritus, alopecia, flushing, erythema multiforme, exfoliative dermatitis, photosensitivity, urticaria, increased sweating, pemphigus, **Stevens-Johnson syndrome,** herpes zoster, **toxic epidermal necrolysis. Other:** Angioedema, asthenia, impotence, blurred vision, fever, arthralgia, arthritis, vasculitis, eosinophilia, tinnitus, syncope, myalgia, muscle cramps, rhinorrhea, sore throat, hoarseness, conjunctivitis, tearing, dry eyes, loss of sense of smell, hearing loss, peripheral neuropathy, anosmia, myositis, flank pain, gynecomastia.

ADDITIONAL DRUG INTERACTIONS

Rifampin may ↓ the effects of enalapril. Do not discontinue without first reporting to the provider.

HOW SUPPLIED

Tablet: 2.5 mg, 5 mg, 10 mg, 20 mg; *Injection:* 1.25 mg/mL (as enalaprilat)

DOSAGE

- **TABLETS (ENALAPRIL)**
  Antihypertensive in clients not taking diuretics.
  Initial: 5 mg/day; **then,** adjust dosage according to response (range: 10–40 mg/day in one to two doses).
  Antihypertensive in clients taking diuretics.
  Initial: 2.5 mg. Since hypotension may occur following the initiation of enalapril, the diuretic should be discontinued, if possible, for 2–3 days before initiating enalapril. If BP is not maintained with enalapril alone, diuretic therapy may be resumed.
  Hypertension in children.
  Initial: 0.08 mg/kg, up to 5 mg, once daily. Adjust dose depending on response. Do not give to neonates and children with a GFR <30 mL/min/1.73 m^2.
  Adjunct with diuretics and digitalis in heart failure.
  Initial: 2.5 mg 1–2 times per day; **then,** depending on the response, 2.5–20 mg/day in two divided doses. Dose should not exceed 40 mg/day. Dosage must be adjusted in clients with renal impairment or hyponatremia.
  In clients with impaired renal function.
  Initial: 5 mg/day if C$_{CR}$ ranges between 30 and 80 mL/min and serum creatinine is less than 3 mg/dL; 2.5 mg/day if C$_{CR}$ is less than 30 mL/min and serum creatinine is more than 3 mg/dL and in dialysis clients on dialysis days.
  Renal impairment or hyponatremia.
  Initial: 2.5 mg/day if serum sodium is less than 130 mEq/L and serum creatinine is more than 1.6 mg/dL. The dose may be increased to 2.5 mg twice a day and then 5 mg twice a day or higher if required; dose is given at intervals of 4 or more days. Maximum daily dose is 40 mg.
  Asymptomatic LV dysfunction following MI.
  2.5 mg twice a day, titrated as tolerated to the daily dose of 20 mg in divided doses.
- **IV (ENALAPRILAT)**
  Hypertension.

1.25 mg over a 5-min period; repeat q 6 hr.

Antihypertensive in clients taking diuretics.
Initial: 0.625 mg over 5 min; if an adequate response is seen after 1 hr, administer another 0.625-mg dose. Thereafter, 1.25 mg q 6 hr. In those taking diuretics, start with 0.625 mg enalaprilat over 5 min; if there is an inadequate effect after 1 hr, repeat the 0.625 mg dose. Give additional doses of 1.25 mg q 6 hr.

Clients with impaired renal function.
Give enalaprilat, 1.25 mg q 6 hr for clients with a C_{CR} more than 30 mL/min and an initial dose of 0.625 mg for clients with a C_{CR} less than 30 mL/min. If there is an adequate response, an additional 0.625 mg may be given after 1 hr; thereafter, additional 1.25-mg doses can be given q 6 hr. For dialysis clients, the initial dose is 0.625 mg q 6 hr.

NURSING CONSIDERATIONS

Do not confuse enalapril with Anafranil (an antidepressant) or with Eldepryl (an antiparkinson drug).

ADMINISTRATION/STORAGE
1. To convert from IV to PO therapy in clients on a diuretic, begin with 2.5 mg/day for clients responding to a 0.625-mg IV dose. Thereafter, 2.5 mg/day may be given.
2. Use lower dose if receiving diuretics or with impaired renal function.
3. A 1 mg/mL suspension may be prepared for use in children (see instructions in the labeling).
4. Carefully select the dosage of all enalapril products in the geriatric client due to decreased renal function with advancing age.
IV 5. To convert from PO to IV therapy in clients not on a diuretic, use the recommended IV dose (i.e., 1.25 mg every 6 hr). To convert from IV to PO therapy, begin with 5 mg/day.
6. Following IV administration, first dose peak effect may take 4 hr (whether or not on a diuretic). For subsequent doses, the peak effect is usually within 15 min.

7. Give enalaprilat as a slow IV infusion (over 5 min) either alone or diluted up to 50 mL with an appropriate diluent. Any of the following can be used: D5W, D5/RL, McGaw Isolyte E, 0.9% NaCl, D5/ 0.9% NaCl.
8. When used initially for heart failure, observe for at least 2 hr after the initial dose and until BP has stabilized for an additional hour. If possible, reduce dose of diuretic.
9. Store below 30°C (86°F).

ASSESSMENT
1. Document indications for therapy, presenting symptoms, other agents trialed, and the outcome.
2. Record ECG, VS, and weight.
3. Monitor CBC, electrolytes, liver and renal function studies. Reduce dose with impaired renal function.

CLIENT/FAMILY TEACHING
1. Use caution, may cause orthostatic effects and dizziness.
2. Maintain a healthy diet; limit intake of caffeine; avoid alcohol, salt substitutes, or high Na and high K foods.
3. Report any weight loss that may result from the loss of taste or rapid weight gain that may result from fluid overload.
4. Any persistent dry cough, flu-like symptoms, rash, or unusual side effects should be reported immediately.

OUTCOMES/EVALUATE
- ↓ BP
- ↓ Preload and afterload with CHF

Enoxaparin ■
(ee-**nox**-ah-**PAIR**-in)

CLASSIFICATION(S):
Anticoagulant, low molecular weight heparin
PREGNANCY CATEGORY: B
Rx: Lovenox
✦**Rx:** Lovenox HP

SEE ALSO *HEPARINS, LOW MOLECULAR WEIGHT.*

ACTION/KINETICS
t ½, elimination: 4.5 hr after single SC dose, 7 hr after repeated dosing. Elimi-

nation may be delayed in the elderly. **Duration:** 12 hr following a 40-mg dose. Excreted mainly through the urine.

USES

(1) Acute (in the hospital) and extended (at home for up to three weeks) prophylaxis of DVT, which may lead to pulmonary embolism, after hip or knee replacement surgery or abdominal surgery in those at risk for thromboembolic complications, including severely restricted mobility due to acute illness. (2) With warfarin for inpatient treatment of DVT with and without pulmonary embolism; with warfarin for outpatient treatment of DVT without pulmonary embolism. (3) With aspirin to prevent ischemic complications of unstable angina and non-Q-wave MI. Can be used in geriatric clients.

CONTRAINDICATIONS

Hypersensitivity to enoxaparin, heparin, pork products and in those with active major bleeding or in those with thrombocytopenia associated with a positive in vitro test for anti-platelet antibody in the presence of enoxaparin sodium.

SPECIAL CONCERNS

■(1) When spinal/epidural anesthesia or spinal puncture is used, those anticoagulated or scheduled to be anticoagulated with low molecular weight heparins or heparinoids to prevent thromboembolic complications are at risk of developing a spinal or epidural hematoma that can result in long-term or permanent paralysis. Risk is increased using indwelling epidural catheters for giving analgesics or by the concurrent use of drugs affecting hemostasis, such as NSAIDs, platelet inhibitors, or other anticoagulants. Risk also appears to increase by traumatic or repeated spinal or epidural puncture. (2) Frequently monitor for signs and symptoms of neurological impairment. If observed, immediate treatment is required. (3) The physician should consider potential benefits vs risk before neuraxial intervention in clients anticoagulated or to be anticoagulated for thromboprophylaxis.■ Use with caution during pregnancy.

SIDE EFFECTS

Hematologic: Thrombocytopenia, thrombocythemia, *hemorrhage,* hypochromic anemia, ecchymosis. **At site of injection:** Mild local irritation, pain, hematoma, erythema. **GI:** Nausea. **CNS:** Confusion. **Miscellaneous:** Fever, pain, edema, peripheral edema, spinal hematoma.

HOW SUPPLIED

Injection: 30 mg/0.3 mL, 40 mg/0.4 mL, 60 mg/0.6 mL, 80 mg/0.8 mL, 100 mg/1 mL, 120 mg/0.8 mL, 150 mg/1 mL, 300 mg/3 mL

DOSAGE——————

- **SC ONLY**

Prophylaxis of DVT in hip or knee replacement.

Adults: 30 mg q 12 hr with the initial dose given within 12–24 hr after surgery (providing hemostasis has been established) for 7–10 days (usually), up to 14 days. For hip replacement, a dose of 40 mg once daily may be considered; give 9–15 hr before surgery and continue for 3 weeks.

Prophylaxis of DVT in abdominal surgery.

Adults: 40 mg once daily, with the initial dose given 2 hr prior to surgery. Give for 7–10 days, up to 12 days.

Prophylaxis of DVT for medical clients during acute illness.

40 mg once daily for 6–11 days (up to 14 days has been well tolerated.

Treatment of DVT without pulmonary embolism for outpatients.

1 mg/kg SC q 12 hr.

Treatment of DVT with or without pulmonary embolism for inpatients.

1 mg/kg SC q 12 hr or 1.5 mg/kg SC once daily at the same time each day.

NOTE: For both in- and outpatients, initiate warfarin within 72 hr of enoxaparin. Continue enoxaparin for a minimum of 5 days and until an INR of 2–3 is reached (average duration is 7 days; up to 17 days has been well tolerated).

Unstable angina/Non-Q-wave MI.

1 mg/kg q 12 hr with PO aspirin (100–325 mg once/day). Usual duration for enoxaparin is 2–8 days, up to 12.5 days.

Note: For clients with a C_{CR} less than

E

E

30 mL/min, the dose is 30 mg once daily for DVT prophylaxis in abdominal surgery, hip or knee replacement surgery, or medical clients during acute illness. The dose is 1 mg/kg once daily for prophylaxis of ischemic complications of unstable angina and non-Q-wave MI (when used with aspirin), inpatient treatment of acute DVT with or without pulmonary embolism (when used with warfarin), or outpatient treatment of acute DVT without pulmonary embolism (when given with warfarin).

NURSING CONSIDERATIONS

ADMINISTRATION/STORAGE

1. Consider adjusting dose for low weight (< 45 kg) clients and those with a C_{CR} < 30 mL/min.
2. Use a tuberculin sysringe or equivalent to assure withdrawal of the appropriate volume of drug.
3. Give only by deep SC when client is lying down; do *not* give IM.
4. Continue treatment throughout the postsurgical period until the risk of DVT has decreased.
5. Do not mix with other injections or infusions.
6. Discard any unused solution.
7. Do *not* interchange (unit for unit) with unfractionated heparin or other low molecular weight heparins as they differ in their manufacturing process, molecular weight distribution, anti-Xa and anti-IIa activities, units, and dosage.
8. The injection is clear and colorless to pale yellow; store at temperatures < 25°C (<77°F). Do not freeze.

ASSESSMENT

1. Note indications for therapy, clinical presentation, any S&S of pulmonary embolism or DVT.
2. Assess for any history of heparin or pork product sensitivity or disorders that may preclude drug therapy.
3. Document baseline hematologic parameters, liver function, and coagulation studies. If normal coagulation, monitor platelet counts. Drug may cause significant, nonsymptomatic increases in SGOT and SGPT.
4. Monitor VS; observe for early S&S of bleeding. Any unexplained fall in hematocrit or BP should lead to a search for a bleeding site. Those with spinal or epidural anesthesia should have neuro assessments regularly.
5. Assess clients with renal dysfunction and the elderly closely. Report any evidence of a thromboembolic event.

CLIENT/FAMILY TEACHING

1. Clients may self-inject only if their provider determines that it is appropriate and with medical follow-up if needed. Lie down during self-administration; use prefilled syringes and administer at the same time each day.
2. Alternate administration between the left and right anterolateral and posterolateral abdominal wall.
3. Introduce the entire length of the needle into a skin fold held between the thumb and forefinger; hold throughout the injection. To minimize bruising, do not rub the site.
4. May experience mild discomfort, irritation, and hematoma at injection site. Report any unusual bruising, bleeding or weakness. Practice reliable contraception.
5. Avoid OTC agents that contain aspirin; use electric razor to shave, a soft toothbrush and a nightlight to prevent falls and potential bleeding.

OUTCOMES/EVALUATE

• DVT prophylaxis post surgery
• Thromboembolic occurrence/recurrence prophylaxis

Ephedrine sulfate
(eh-**FED**-rin)

CLASSIFICATION(S):
Sympathomimetic, direct- and indirect-acting
PREGNANCY CATEGORY: C
OTC: Systemic: Ephedrine Sulfate (capsule). **Nasal Decongestant:** Pretz-D
Rx: Systemic: Ephedrine Sulfate (Injection)

SEE ALSO *SYMPATHOMIMETIC DRUGS.*

ACTION/KINETICS

Releases norepinephrine from synaptic storage sites. Has direct effects on alpha, beta-1, and beta-2 receptors, causing increased BP due to arteriolar constriction and cardiac stimulation, bronchodilation, relaxation of GI tract smooth muscle, nasal decongestion, mydriasis, and increased tone of the bladder trigone and vesicle sphincter. It may also increase skeletal muscle strength, especially in myasthenia clients. Significant CNS effects include stimulation of the cerebral cortex and subcortical centers. Hepatic glycogenolysis is increased, but not as much as with epinephrine. More stable and longer-lasting than epinephrine. Rapidly and completely absorbed following parenteral use. **Onset, IM:** 10–20 min; **PO:** 15–60 min; **SC:** > 20 min. **Duration, IM, SC:** 30–60 min; **PO:** 3–5 hr. **t ½, elimination:** About 3 hr when urine is at a pH of 5 and about 6 hr when urinary pH is 6.3. Excreted mostly unchanged through the urine (rate dependent on urinary pH—increased in acid urine).

USES

PO: Temporary relief of shortness of breath, tightness of chest, and wheezing due to bronchial asthma. **Parenteral:** (1) Allergic disorders, including bronchial asthma. (2) Vasopressor in shock. **Nasal:** (1) Nasal congestion due to the common cold, hay fever, or other upper respiratory allergies. (2) Nasal congestion associated with sinusitis. (3) Promote nasal or sinus drainage. *Investigational:* Narcolepsy, depression (to enhance physical and mental energy).

ADDITIONAL CONTRAINDICATIONS

Angle closure glaucoma, anesthesia with cyclopropane or halothane, thyrotoxicosis, diabetes, obstetrics where maternal BP is greater than 130/80. Lactation.

SPECIAL CONCERNS

Geriatric clients may be at higher risk to develop prostatic hypertrophy. May cause hypertension resulting in intracranial hemorrhage or anginal pain in clients with coronary insufficiency or ischemic heart disease.

ADDITIONAL SIDE EFFECTS

CNS: Nervousness, shakiness, confusion, delirium, hallucinations. Anxiety and nervousness following prolonged use. **CV:** Precordial pain, *excessive doses may cause hypertension sufficient to result in cerebral hemorrhage*. **GU:** Difficult and painful urination, urinary retention in males with prostatism, decrease in urine formation. **Miscellaneous:** Pallor, respiratory difficulty, hypersensitivity reactions. **Abuse:** Prolonged abuse can cause an anxiety state, including symptoms of paranoid schizophrenia, tachycardia, poor nutrition and hygiene, dilated pupils, cold sweat, and fever.

ADDITIONAL DRUG INTERACTIONS

Alpha-adrenergic blockers / Antagonism of vasoconstricting and hypertensive effects of ephedrine
Dexamethasone / ↓ Dexamethasone effect
Diuretics / Diuretics ↓ response to sympathomimetics
Furazolidone / ↑ Pressor effect → possible hypertensive crisis and intracranial hemorrhage
Guanethidine / ↓ Guanethidine effect by displacement from its action site
Halothane / Serious arrhythmias R/T sensitization of myocardium to sympathomimetics by halothane
MAO Inhibitors / ↑ Pressor effect → possible hypertensive crisis and intracranial hemorrhage
Methyldopa / Effect of ephedrine ↓ in methyldopa-treated clients
Oxytocic drugs / Severe persistent hypertension

HOW SUPPLIED

Capsule: 25 mg; *Injection:* 50 mg/mL; *Nasal Spray:* 0.25%

DOSAGE

• CAPSULES

Bronchial asthma, systemic nasal decongestant.

Adults and children over 12 years of age: 12.5–25 mg q 4 hr, not to exceed 150 mg in 24 hr. **Children, less than 12 years:** Consult a provider.

• SC, IM, SLOW IV

Bronchial asthma.

Adults: 25–50 mg SC or IM; or, 5–25 mg by slow IV repeated q 5–10 min, if needed. **Children:** 0.5–0.75 mg/kg (16.7–25 mg/m^2) SC, IM, or IV q 4–6 hr.
Vasopressor.
Adults: 25–50 mg (IM or SC) or 5–25 mg (by slow IV push) repeated at 5- to 10-min intervals, if necessary. Absorption following IM is more rapid than following SC use. **Pediatric (IM):** 16.7 mg/m^2 q 4–6 hr.

• **NASAL SPRAY (0.25%)**
   Nasal decongestant.
Adults and children over 12 years: 2–3 sprays in each nostril no more than q 4 hr. **Children, 6–11 years:** 1 or 2 sprays in each nostril no more than q 4 hr. Do not use topically for more than 3 or 4 consecutive days. Do not use in children under 6 years of age unless ordered by provider.

NURSING CONSIDERATIONS
ADMINISTRATION/STORAGE
1. Tolerance may develop; however, temporary cessation of therapy restores the original drug response.
[IV] 2. May administer 10 mg IV undiluted over at least 1 min.
3. Use only clear solutions and discard any unused solution with IV therapy. Protect against exposure to light; drug is subject to oxidation.

ASSESSMENT
1. Document indications for therapy and symptom characteristics.
2. Assess mental status and pulmonary function; monitor ECG and VS. If administered for hypotension, monitor BP until stabilized.
3. If used for prolonged periods, assess for drug resistance. Rest without medication for 3–4 days, then resume to regain response.

CLIENT/FAMILY TEACHING
1. Notify provider if SOB is unrelieved by medication and accompanied by chest pain, dizziness, or palpitations. Report any elevated or irregular pulse.
2. Review proper method for nasal instillation.
3. Avoid activities that require mental alertness until drug effects realized. Do not take within 2 hr of bedtime; may cause insomnia.
4. With males, report any difficulty or pain with voiding; may be drug-induced urinary retention.
5. Report any signs of depression, lack of interest in personal appearance, complaints of insomnia or anorexia or decreased effectiveness. Tolerance may occur within 1-2 months.
6. Avoid OTC drugs and alcohol.

OUTCOMES/EVALUATE
• Improved airway exchange
• ↓ Nasal congestion/mucus
• ↑ BP
• Control of narcolepsy

Epinephrine
(ep-ih-**NEF**-rin)

CLASSIFICATION(S):
Sympathomimetic, direct-acting
PREGNANCY CATEGORY: C
OTC: Aerosol: Primatene Mist.
Rx: Injection: Ana-Guard, EpiPen, EpiPen Jr., Sus-Phrine.

Epinephrine bitartrate
PREGNANCY CATEGORY: C
OTC: Aerosol: AsthmaHaler Mist.

Epinephrine borate
PREGNANCY CATEGORY: C
Rx: Ophthalmic Solution: Epinal.

Epinephrine hydrochloride
PREGNANCY CATEGORY: C
OTC: Solution for Inhalation: AsthmaNefrin, MicroNefrin, Nephron, S-2 Inhalant.
Rx: Injection: Adrenalin Chloride.
Ophthalmic Solution: Glaucon.
Solution for Inhalation: Adrenalin Chloride.
✤**Rx:** Vaponefrin

Bold Italic = life threatening side effect   ■ = black box warning   ✤ = Available in Canada

SEE ALSO *SYMPATHOMIMETIC DRUGS.*

ACTION/KINETICS

Causes marked stimulation of alpha, beta-1, and beta-2 receptors, causing sympathomimetic stimulation, pressor effects, cardiac stimulation, bronchodilation, and decongestion. It crosses the placenta but not the blood-brain barrier. **Extreme caution must be taken never to inject 1:100 solution intended for inhalation—injection of this concentration has caused death. SC: Onset,** 5–10 min; **duration:** 4–6 hr. **Inhalation: Onset,** 1–5 min; **duration:** 1–3 hr. **IM, Onset:** variable; duration: 1–4 hr. Ineffective when given PO.

USES

Inhalation: (1) Temporary relief of shortness of breath, tightness of chest, and wheezing due to bronchial asthma. (2) Postintubation and infectious croup. (3) MicroNefrin is used for chronic obstructive lung disease, chronic bronchitis, broncheolitis, bronchial asthma, and other peripheral airway diseases.

Injection: (1) Relieve respiratory distress in bronchial asthma, during acute asthma attacks, and for reversible bronchospasm in chronic bronchitis, emphysema, and other obstructive pulmonary diseases. (2) Severe acute anaphylactic reactions, including anaphylactic shock and cardiac arrest, to restore cardiac rhythm. (3) Allergic reactions caused by bees, wasps, hornets, yellow jackets, bumble bees, and fire ants; severe allergic reactions or anaphylaxis caused by allergy injections; allergic reactions due to exposure to pollens, dusts, molds, foods, drugs, and exercise. (4) Severe, life-threatening asthma attacks with wheezing, dyspnea, and inability to breathe. (5) Vasopressor in shock. (6) Infiltration of tissue to delay absorption of drugs, including local anesthetics.

Ophthalmic: (1) Hemostatic during ocular surgery; treatment of conjunctival congestion during surgery; to induce mydriasis during surgery; treat ocular hypertension during surgery. (2) Adjunct in the treatment of open-angle glaucoma (may be used with miotics, beta blockers, hyperosmotic agents, or carbonic anhydrase inhibitors). (3) To produce mydriasis; to treat conjunctivitis.

Topical: Control bleeding.

NOTE: Autoinjectors are available for emergency self-administration of first aid for anaphylactic reactions due to insect stings or bites, foods, drugs, and other allergens as well as idiopathic or exercise-induced anaphylaxis.

ADDITIONAL CONTRAINDICATIONS

Narrow-angle glaucoma. Use when wearing soft contact lenses (may discolor lenses). Aphakia. Lactation.

SPECIAL CONCERNS

May cause anoxia in the fetus. Safety and efficacy of ophthalmic products have not been determined in children; administer parenteral epinephrine to children with caution. Syncope may occur if epinephrine is given to asthmatic children. Administration of the SC injection by the IV route may cause severe or fatal hypertension or cerebrovascular hemorrhage. Epinephrine may temporarily increase the rigidity and tremor of parkinsonism. Use with caution and in small quantities in the toes, fingers, nose, ears, and genitals or in the presence of peripheral vascular disease as vasoconstriction-induced tissue sloughing may occur.

ADDITIONAL SIDE EFFECTS

CV: *Fatal ventricular fibrillation, cerebral or subarachnoid hemorrhage,* obstruction of central retinal artery. *A rapid and large increase in BP may cause aortic rupture, cerebral hemorrhage, or angina pectoris.* **GU:** Decreased urine formation, urinary retention, painful urination. **CNS:** Anxiety, fear, pallor. Parenteral use may cause or aggravate disorientation, memory impairment, psychomotor agitation, panic, hallucinations, *suicidal or homicidal tendencies,* schizophrenic-type behavior. **Miscellaneous:** Prolonged use or overdose may cause elevated serum lactic acid with severe metabolic acidosis. **At injection site:** Bleeding, urticaria, wheal formation, pain. Repeated injections at the same site may cause necrosis from vascular constriction. **Ophthalmic:**

Transient stinging or burning when administered, conjunctival hyperemia, brow ache, headache, blurred vision, photophobia, allergic lid reaction, ocular hypersensitivity, poor night vision, eye ache, eye pain. Prolonged ophthalmic use may cause deposits of pigment in the cornea, lids, or conjunctiva. When used for glaucoma in aphakic clients, reversible cystoid macular edema may occur.

ADDITIONAL DRUG INTERACTIONS
Alpha-adrenergic blocking agents / Antagonism of vasocontrictor and hypertensive effects
Antihistamines / Epinephrine effects potentiated
Beta-adrenergic blocking agents / Possible initial hypertension followed by bradycardia
Diuretics / ↓ Vascular response
Ergot alkaloids / Reversal of epinephrine pressor effects
General anesthetics (halothane, cyclopropane) / ↑ Sensitivity of myocardium to epinephrine → arrhythmias
Levothyroxine / Potentiation of epinephrine effects
Nitrites / Reversal of epinephrine pressor effects
Phenothiazines / Reversal of epinephrine pressor effects

HOW SUPPLIED
Epinephrine: *Autoinjector:* 0.15 mg (0.15 mL), 0.3 mg (0.3 mL); *Aerosol:* 0.2 mg/inh; *Injection:* 1:200 (5 mg/mL), 1:1000 (1 mg/mL), 1:2000 (0.5 mg/mL), 1:10,000 (0.1 mg/mL).
Epinephrine bitartrate: *Aerosol:* 0.35 mg/inh.
Epinephrine borate: *Solution:* 0.5%, 1%.
Epinephrine hydrochloride: *Injection:* 1:1000 (1 mg/mL); *Nasal Solution:* 0.1%; *Solution for Inhalation:* 1:100, 1:1000; *Ophthalmic solution:* 0.1%, 1%, 2%; *Solution for Inhalation (Racenephrine HCl):* 2.25%

DOSAGE
• **INHALATION AEROSOL**
Bronchodilation.
Adults and children 4 years and older, initial: 1 inhalation; **then,** wait 1 min or more—if no relief, use once more. Do not reuse for 3 or more hr.
• **NEBULIZATION**
Bronchodilation.
Adults and children 4 years and older (for AsthmaNefrin, 12 years and older). *Hand pump nebulizer:* place 0.5 mL (about 8–10 drops) of racemic epinephrine placed into the reservoir. Place the nebulizer nozzle into the partially opened mouth and squeeze the bulb 1–3 times. Inhale deeply. Give 2–3 additional inhalations if relief does not occur within 2–3 min. Can use 4–6 times per day but no more often than q 3 hr. *Aerosol nebulizer:* Add 0.5 mL (about 10 drops) of racemic epinephrine to 3 mL of diluent or 0.2–0.4 mL (about 4–8 drops) of MicroNefrin to 4.6–4.8 mL water. Give for 15 min q 3–4 hr.
• **SC, IM**
Bronchodilation
Adults, initial: 0.2–1 mL (0.2–1 mg) of the 1:1000 solution SC or IM q 4 hr. **Infants and children (except premature infants and full-term newborns):** 0.01 mL/kg or 0.3 mL/m² (0.1 mg/kg or 0.3 mg/m²) SC. Do not exceed 0.5 mL (0.5 mg) in a single pediatric dose. Can repeat q 20 min to 4 hr, if necessary. The dose of Ana-Guard is as follows. **Adults and children over 12 years:** 0.3 mL; **6–12 years old:** 0.2 mL; **2–6 years old:** 0.15 mL; **infants to 2 years old:** 0.05–0.1 mL. Give a second dose after 10 min if symptoms are not noticeably improved.
• **IV**
Bronchodilation, hypersensitivity reactions.
Adults: 0.1–0.25 mg (1–2.5 mL) of the 1:10,000 solution injected slowly. **Infants:** 0.05 mg; may be repeated at 20–30 min intervals to manage asthma attacks. **Neonates:** 0.01 mg/kg.
NOTE: If the client is intubated, the IV dose of epinephrine can be given via the endotracheal tube directly into the bronchial tree as it is rapidly absorbed through the lung capillary bed.
• **AUTOINJECTOR, IM**
First aid for anaphylaxis.
The autoinjectors deliver a single dose of epinephrine of either 0.15 mg for

---

Bold Italic = life threatening side effect   ■ = black box warning   ✦ = Available in Canada

those weighing 15–30 kg or 0.3 mg for those weighing more than 30 kg. In cases of a severe reaction, repeat injections may be necessary.

Vasopressor.

Adults, IM or SC, initial: 0.5 mg repeated q 5 min if needed; **then,** give 0.025–0.050 mg IV q 5–15 min as needed. **Adults, IV, initial:** 0.1–0.25 mg given slowly. May be repeated q 5–15 min as needed. Or, use IV infusion beginning with 0.001 mg/min and increasing the dose to 0.004 mg/min if needed. **Pediatric, IM, SC:** 0.01 mg/kg, up to a maximum of 0.3 mg repeated q 5 min if needed. **Pediatric, IV:** 0.01 mg/kg/5–15 min if an inadequate response to IM or SC administration is observed.

Cardiac stimulant.

Adults, intracardiac or IV: 0.1–1 mg repeated q 5 min if needed. **Pediatric, intracardiac or IV:** 0.005–0.01 mg/kg (0.15–0.3 mg/m²) repeated q 5 min if needed; this may be followed by IV infusion beginning at 0.0001 mg/kg/min and increased in increments of 0.0001 mg/kg/min up to a maximum of 0.0015 mg/kg/min.

Adjunct to local anesthesia.

Adults and children: 0.1–0.2 mg in a 1:200,000–1:20,000 solution.

Adjunct with intraspinal anesthetics.

Adults: 0.2–0.4 mg added to the anesthetic spinal fluid.

- **SOLUTION**

Antihemorrhagic, mydriatic.

Adults and children, intracameral or subconjunctival: 0.01–0.1% solution.

Topical antihemorrhagic.

Adults and children: 0.002–0.1% solution.

Nasal decongestant.

Adults and children over 6 years of age: Apply 0.1% solution as drops or spray or with a sterile swab as needed.

- **BORATE OPHTHALMIC SOLUTION, HYDROCHLORIDE OPHTHALMIC SOLUTION**

Glaucoma.

Adults: 1–2 gtt into affected eye(s) 1–2 times per day. Determine frequency of use by tonometry. Dosage has not been established in children.

NURSING CONSIDERATIONS

ADMINISTRATION/STORAGE

1. Briskly massage site of SC or IM injection to hasten drug action. Do not expose drug to heat, light, or air, as this causes deterioration.

2. Discard solution if reddish brown and after expiration date.

3. With sodium bisulfite as a preservative in the topical preparation, slight stinging may occur after administration.

4. Do not use the topical preparation in children under 6 years of age.

5. Ophthalmic use may result in discomfort, which decreases over time.

6. The ophthalmic preparation is not for injection.

7. If the ophthalmic glaucoma product is used with a miotic, instill miotic 2-10 min prior.

8. Keep the ophthalmic product tightly sealed and protected from light. Store at 2–4°C (36–75°F). Discard solution if it becomes discolored or contains a precipitate.

9. *Never administer* 1:100 solution IV; use the 1:1,000 solution.

10. Use a tuberculin syringe to measure. Parenteral doses are small and drug is potent, thus errors in measurement may be disastrous.

11. For direct IV administration to adults, the drug must be well diluted as a 1:1,000 solution; inject quantities of 0.05–0.1 mL of solution cautiously taking about 1 min for each injection; note response (BP and pulse). Dose may be repeated several times if necessary. May be further diluted in D5W or NSS.

ASSESSMENT

1. Assess for sulfite sensitivity.

2. Document indications for therapy; describe type/onset of symptoms and anticipated results.

3. Assess cardiopulmonary function.

4. During IV therapy, continuously monitor ECG, BP, and pulse until desired effect achieved. Then take VS every 2–5 min until stabilized; once stable, monitor BP q 15–30 min.

5. Note any symptoms of shock such as cold, clammy skin, cyanosis, and loss of consciousness.

E

CLIENT/FAMILY TEACHING

1. Take as directed. Review method for administration carefully. When prescribed for anaphylaxis, administer autoinjector immediately and seek medical care. Check expiration dates.

2. Report any increased restlessness, chest pain, heart fluttering, SOB, lack of response, adverse effects, or insomnia as dosage adjustment may be necessary. May elevate blood sugar.

3. Limit intake of caffeine (colas, coffee, tea, and chocolate); avoid OTC drugs without approval.

4. Rinse mouth and inhaler after use. If also prescribed steroid inhaler take bronchodilator first and wait at least 5 min before administering steroid inhaler so air passages are open and receptive.

5. Nasal application may sting slightly. Nasal OTC products may work initially but with prolonged use exacerbate symptoms.

6. Ophthalmic solution may burn initially and a brow headache may occur; this should subside. Remove contact lenses; may stain lens.

7. Use caution when performing activities that require careful vision; ophthalmic solution may diminish visual fields, cause double vision, and alter night vision.

8. Discard any discolored or precipitated solutions.

OUTCOMES/EVALUATE

- Restoration of cardiac activity
- Improved CO with EC bypass
- ↓ IOP
- Reversal of S&S of anaphylaxis
- Improved airway exchange
- Hemostasis with ocular surgery

Eplerenone

(eh-**PLEH**-reh-none)

PREGNANCY CATEGORY: B
Rx: Inspra

ACTION/KINETICS

Binds to the mineralocorticoid receptor and blocks binding of aldosterone. Aldosterone increases BP through induction of sodium reabsorption and other mechanisms. Thus, by blocking aldosterone binding, sodium is not reabsorbed and BP decreases. **Peak plasma levels:** About 1.5 hr. **Steady state:** Reached in 2 days. Absorption not affected by food. Metabolized primarily via CYP3A4 in the liver. About two-thirds excreted in the urine and one-third in the feces. **t ½, terminal:** 4–6 hr. About 50% bound to plasma proteins.

USES

(1) Hypertension, alone or in combination with other antihypertensive drugs. (2) Improve survival of stable clients with left ventricular systolic dysfunction (ejection fraction of 40% or less) and clinical evidence of CHF after an acute MI. *Investigational:* Alone or in combination with an angiotensin-converting enzyme inhibitor for reducing left ventricular hypertrophy. As adjunctive therapy in diabetic hypertension with microalbuminuria.

CONTRAINDICATIONS

Serum potassium greater than 5.5 mEq/L at initiation, type 2 diabetes with microalbuminuria, serum creatinine greater than 2 mg/dL in males or greater than 1.8 mg/dL in females, C_{CR} less than 30 mL/min. Also, clients concurrently taking potassium supplements, potassium-sparing diuretics (e.g., amiloride, spironolactone, triamterene), or strong inhibitors of CYP 450 3A4 drugs (clarithromycin, ketoconazole, itraconazole, nefazodone, nelfinavir, ritonavir, troleandomycin). Lactation

SPECIAL CONCERNS

Safety and efficacy have not been determined in children.

SIDE EFFECTS

Hyperkalemia is the primary risk; can result in decreased renal function and serious, sometimes *fatal arrhythmias.* **GI:** Diarrhea, abdominal pain. **GU:** Mastodynia in males, abnormal vaginal bleeding, gynecomastia (males). **Miscellaneous:** Dizziness, coughing, fatigue, flu-like symptoms.

LABORATORY TEST CONSIDERATIONS

↑ ALT, BUN, uric acid, serum creatinine. Hyponatremia, hypercholesterolemia,

---

albuminuria, hypertriglyceridemia, hyperkalemia.

DRUG INTERACTIONS

ACE inhibitors / ↑ Risk of hyperkalemia
Angiotensin II antagonists / ↑ Risk of hyperkalemia
CYP3A4 inhibitors (itraconazole, ketoconazole) / Up to a 5-fold increase in eplerenone exposure
Lithium / Potential lithium toxicity; monitor serum lithium levels
NSAIDs / Potential ↓ antihypertensive effect and severe hyperkalemia
H *St. John's wort* / About a 30% ↓ in eplerenone AUC.

HOW SUPPLIED

Tablets: 25 mg, 50 mg

DOSAGE

- **TABLETS**
  Hypertension.

Initial: 50 mg once daily. If inadequate response, increase dose to 50 mg twice a day. Higher doses are not recommended as no greater effect is noted and there is an increased risk of hyperkalemia. For clients taking weak CYP3A4 inhibitors (erythromycin, fluconazole, saquinavir, verapamil), reduce starting dose to 25 mg once daily.

  CHF post MI.

Initial: 25 mg once daily; titrate to target dose of 50 mg once daily, preferable within 4 weeks, as tolerated. Adjust dose as follows based on serum potassium. **Less than 5 mEq/L potassium:** Increase dose from 25 mg every other day to 25 mg daily to 50 mg daily; **Serum potassium from 5–5.4 mEq/L:** Maintain dosage; no adjustment; **Serum potassium, 5.5–5.9 mEq/L:** Decrease dose from 50 mg daily to 25 mg daily to 25 mg every other day to withholding the drug; **Serum potassium, 6 mEq/L or greater:** Withhold drug.

NURSING CONSIDERATIONS

ADMINISTRATION/STORAGE
Store from 15–30°C (59–86°F).

ASSESSMENT
1. Note indications for therapy, symptom characteristics, and other agents trialed.
2. List drugs prescribed to ensure none interact.

3. Assess BP, serum K+, renal, and LFTs. With post MI heart failure, note LV ejection fraction and systolic dysfunction.

CLIENT/FAMILY TEACHING
1. Take as directed with or without food. Do not take with grapefruit juice and avoid all supplements containing potassium.
2. Keep log of BP and HR for provider review.
3. Avoid activities that require mental alertness until drug effects realized.
4. Report as scheduled for F/U. Continue lifestyle changes that help control BP, i.e., weight loss, regular daily exercise, tobacco/alcohol cessation, stress/salt reduction.
5. Avoid OTC meds and ETOH.

OUTCOMES/EVALUATE
↓ BP ↓ Mortality post MI with CHF

Epoprostenol sodium
(eh-poh-**PROST**-en-ohl)

CLASSIFICATION(S):
Vasodilator, peripheral
PREGNANCY CATEGORY: B
Rx: Flolan

SEE ALSO *ANTIHYPERTENSIVE AGENTS.*

ACTION/KINETICS
Acts by direct vasodilation of pulmonary and systemic arterial vascular beds and by inhibition of platelet aggregation. IV infusion in clients with pulmonary hypertension results in increases in cardiac index and SV and decreases in pulmonary vascular resistance, total pulmonary resistance, and mean systemic arterial pressure. Is rapidly hydrolyzed at the neutral pH of the blood as well as by enzymatic degradation. Metabolites are less active than the parent compound. **t ½:** 6 min.

USES
Long-term IV treatment of primary pulmonary hypertension (including those with scleroderma spectrum of the disease who do not respond to conventional therapy) in NYHA Class III and Class IV clients.

CONTRAINDICATIONS

Chronic use in those with CHF due to severe LV systolic dysfunction and in those who develop pulmonary edema during dosing.

SPECIAL CONCERNS

Abrupt withdrawal or sudden large decreases in the dose may cause rebound pulmonary hypertension. Use caution in dose selection in the elderly due to the greater frequency of decreased hepatic, renal, or cardiac function, as well as concomitant disease or other drug therapy. Use with caution during lactation. Safety and efficacy not determined in children.

SIDE EFFECTS

Those occurring during acute dosing. **CV:** Flushing, hypotension, bradycardia, tachycardia. **GI:** N&V, abdominal pain, dyspepsia. **CNS:** Headache, anxiety, nervousness, agitation, dizziness, hypesthesia, paresthesia. **Miscellaneous:** Chest pain, musculoskeletal pain, dyspnea, back pain, sweating.

Those occurring as a result of the drug delivery system.

Due to the chronic indwelling catheter: Local infection, pain at the injection site, sepsis, infections.

Those occurring during chronic dosing.

CV: Flushing, tachycardia. **GI:** N&V, diarrhea. **CNS:** Headache, anxiety, nervousness, tremor, dizziness, hypesthesia, hyperesthesia, paresthesia. **Musculoskeletal:** Jaw pain, myalgia, nonspecific musculoskeletal pain. **Miscellaneous:** Flu-like symptoms, chills, fever, sepsis.

OD OVERDOSE MANAGEMENT

Symptoms: Flushing, headache, hypotension, tachycardia, nausea, vomiting, diarrhea. *Treatment:* Reduce dose of epoprostenol.

DRUG INTERACTIONS

Anticoagulants / Possible ↑ risk of bleeding
Antiplatelet drugs / Possible ↑ risk of bleeding
Diuretics / Additional ↓ in BP
Vasodilators / Additional ↓ in BP

HOW SUPPLIED

Powder for reconstitution: 0.5 mg, 1.5 mg

DOSAGE

- **CHRONIC IV INFUSION**
  Pulmonary hypertension.
Acute dosing: The initial chronic infusion rate is first determined. The mean maximum dose that did not elicit dose-limiting pharmacologic effects was 8.6 ng/kg/min. **Continuous chronic infusion, initial:** 4 ng/kg/min less than the maximum-tolerated infusion rate determined during acute dosing. If the maximum-tolerated infusion rate is less than 5 ng/kg/min, start the chronic infusion at one-half the maximum-tolerated infusion rate. **Dosage adjustments:** Changes in the chronic infusion rate are based on persistence, recurrence, or worsening of the symptoms of primary pulmonary hypertension. If symptoms require an increase in infusion rate, increase by 1–2 ng/kg/min at intervals (at least 15 min) sufficient to allow assessment of the clinical response. If a decrease in infusion rate is necessary, gradually make 2-ng/kg/min decrements every 15 min or longer until the dose-limiting effects resolve. Avoid abrupt withdrawal or sudden large reductions in infusion rates.

NURSING CONSIDERATIONS

ADMINISTRATION/STORAGE

IV 1. Chronic administration is delivered continuously by a permanent indwelling central venous catheter and an ambulatory infusion pump (see package insert for requirements for the infusion pump). Unless contraindicated, give therapy to decrease the risk of pulmonary thromboembolism or systemic embolism.

2. Do not dilute reconstituted solutions or administer with other parenteral solutions or medications.

3. Check package insert carefully to make 100 mL of a solution with the appropriate final concentration of drug and for infusion delivery rates for doses equal to or less than 16 ng/kg/min based on client weight, drug delivery

rate, and concentration of solution to be used.

4. Protect unopened vials from light and store at 15–25°C (59–77°F). Protect reconstituted solutions from light and refrigerate at 2–8°C (36–46°F) for no more than 40 hr.

5. Do not freeze reconstituted solutions; discard any solution refrigerated for more than 48 hr.

6. A single reservoir of reconstituted solution can be given at room temperature for 8 hr; alternatively, it can be used with a cold pouch and given for up to 24 hr. Do not expose solution to sunlight.

ASSESSMENT

1. Perform a full cardiopulmonary assessment. Based on symptoms, determine NYHA functional class (III or IV). Note other agents used and outcome.

2. Determine mental status and ability to handle medication preparation and IV administration; or identify someone in the home that can and is willing to perform this function on a regular basis. Initiate home infusion referral.

3. Determine that a permanent indwelling central venous catheter is available for continuous ambulatory delivery once dosing completed.

4. Assess central venous access site for any evidence of infection, discharge, odor, erythema, or swelling.

5. Consult manufacturer's guidelines for dosage and delivery rate based on client weight for acute dosing.

6. Monitor cardiopulmonary response during therapy. Drug helps reduce RV and LV afterload and increases CO and SV.

CLIENT/FAMILY TEACHING

1. Drug helps reduce work of the heart thus improving symptoms of SOB, fatigue, and exercise intolerance.

2. Administered continously through an indwelling catheter to the heart by a portable external infusion pump; may be needed for years to help control symptoms.

3. Proper site care, pump maintenance (troubleshooting and care) and accurate reconstitution for prescribed drug concentration; proper storage, light protection, pouch filling, pump settings, and port care are imperative to safe therapy. Review written guidelines for all the above regularly. Call with questions or problems.

4. When drug is reconstituted and administered at room temperature, the pump must be programmed to administer pouch contents in 8 hr, whereas if drug is reconstituted and refrigerated at 2–8°C (36–46°F) may be administered in cold pouch over 24 hr.

5. Side effects that indicate excessive dosing and require a reduction in dosage and reporting include tachycardia, headache, N&V, diarrhea, hypotension.

6. Brief interruptions in therapy may cause rapid deterioration in condition. Report loss of effect, worsening of condition or any S&S of infusion site infection.

OUTCOMES/EVALUATE

- Improvement in exercise capacity
- ↓ Dyspnea and fatigue with pulmonary hypertension

Eprosartan mesylate

(eh-proh-**SAR**-tan)

CLASSIFICATION(S):

Antihypertensive, angiotensin II receptor blocker

PREGNANCY CATEGORY: C (first trimester), **D** (second and third trimesters)

Rx: Teveten

ACTION/KINETICS

Acts by blocking the vasoconstrictor and aldosterone-secreting effects of angiotensin II by blocking selectively the binding of angiotensin II to angiotensin II receptors located in the vascular smooth muscle and adrenal gland. About 13% bioavailable. **Peak plasma levels:** 1–2 hr. Food delays absorption. $t\frac{1}{2}$, **terminal:** 5–9 hr. Excreted mostly unchanged in both the feces (about 90%) and urine (about 7%). Significantly bound (about 98%) to plasma protein.

USES

Hypertension, alone or with other anti-hypertensives (diuretics, calcium channel blockers).

SPECIAL CONCERNS

■Use during the second and third trimesters of pregnancy can cause injury and even death to the fetus. When pregnancy is detected, discontinue as soon as possible.■ Symptomatic hypotension may be seen in clients who are volume- and/or salt-depleted (e.g., those taking diuretics). Safety and efficacy have not been determined in children.

SIDE EFFECTS

GI: Abdominal pain, diarrhea, dyspepsia, anorexia, constipation, dry mouth, esophagitis, flatulence, gastritis, gastroenteritis, gingivitis, nausea, periodontitis, toothache, vomiting. **CNS:** Depression, headache, dizziness, anxiety, ataxia, insomnia, migraine, neuritis, nervousness, paresthesia, somnolence, tremor, vertigo. **CV:** Angina pectoris, bradycardia, abnormal ECG, extrasystoles, atrial fibrillation, hypotension, tachycardia, palpitations, peripheral ischemia. **Respiratory:** URTI, sinusitis, bronchitis, chest pain, rhinitis, pharyngitis, coughing, asthma, epistaxis. **Musculoskeletal:** Arthralgia, myalgia, arthritis, aggravated arthritis, arthrosis, skeletal pain, tendonitis, back pain. **GU:** UTI, albuminuria, cystitis, hematuria, frequent micturition, polyuria, renal calculus, urinary incontinence. **Metabolic:** Diabetes mellitus, gout. **Body as a whole:** Viral infection, injury, fatigue, alcohol intolerance, asthenia, substernal chest pain, peripheral edema, dependent edema, fatigue, fever, hot flushes, flu-like symptoms, malaise, rigors, pain, leg cramps, herpes simplex. **Hematologic:** Anemia, purpura, leukopenia, neutropenia, thrombocytopenia. **Dermatologic:** Eczema, furunculosis, pruritus, rash, maculopapular rash, increased sweating. **Ophthalmic:** Conjunctivitis, abnormal vision, xerophthalmia. **Otic:** Otitis externa, otitis media, tinnitus.

LABORATORY TEST CONSIDERATIONS

↑ ALT, AST, creatine phosphokinase, BUN, creatinine, alkaline phosphatase. ↓ Hemoglobin. Glycosuria, hypercholesterolemia, hyperglycemia, hyperkalemia, hypokalemia, hyponatremia.

HOW SUPPLIED

Tablets: 400 mg, 600 mg

DOSAGE

* **TABLETS**
  Hypertension.
  Adults, initial: 600 mg once daily as monotherapy in clients who are not volume-depleted. Can be given once or twice daily with total daily doses ranging from 400–800 mg.

NURSING CONSIDERATIONS

ADMINISTRATION/STORAGE

1. If the antihypertensive effect using once daily dosing is inadequate, a twice-a-day regimen at the same total daily dose or an increase in dose may be more effective.
2. Maximum BP reduction may not occur for 2–3 weeks.
3. May be used in combination with thiazide diuretics or calcium channel blockers if additional BP lowering effect is needed.
4. Discontinuing treatment does not lead to a rapid rebound increase in BP.

ASSESSMENT

1. Document disease onset, symptoms, and other agents trialed.
2. Correct volume depletion if evident. Monitor BP, CBC, K+, sodium, microalbumin, renal, and LFTs.

CLIENT/FAMILY TEACHING

1. Take as directed once or twice daily with or without food.
2. Continue life style modifications, i.e., regular exercise, weight loss, smoking/alcohol cessation, low fat/salt diet for BP control.
3. Practice reliable birth control. Report if pregnant.
4. Immediately report any lip, tongue or facial swelling as well as any fever or sore throat. Report any persistent dry cough.
5. Keep a record of BP readings and bring to F/U visits.

OUTCOMES/EVALUATE

↓ BP; control of HTN

Bold Italic = life threatening side effect   ■ = black box warning   ♣ = Available in Canada

Eptifibatide

(**ep**-tih-**FY**-beh-tide)

CLASSIFICATION(S):
Antiplatelet drug, glycoprotein IIb/IIIa inhibitor
PREGNANCY CATEGORY: B
Rx: Integrilin

ACTION/KINETICS
Reversibly inhibits platelet aggregation by preventing the binding of fibrinogen, von Willebrand factor, and other adhesive ligands to GP IIb/IIIa. Immediately effective after IV use. **t ½, elimination:** 2.5 hr. Drug and metabolites are excreted through kidneys.

USES
(1) Treatment of acute coronary syndrome (unstable angina or non-Q-wave MI), including those to be managed medically and those undergoing percutaneous coronary intervention. (2) Treatment of those undergoing percutaneous coronary intervention, including those undergoing intracoronary stenting.

CONTRAINDICATIONS
History of bleeding diathesis or evidence of active abnormal bleeding within the past 30 days. Severe hypertension (systolic BP > 200 mm Hg or diastolic BP > 110 mm Hg) inadequately controlled. Major surgery within the past 6 weeks, history of stroke within 30 days or any history of hemorrhagic stroke, current or planned use of another parenteral GP IIb/IIIa inhibitor, platelet count less than 100,000/mm³, dependency on renal dialysis. Serum creatinine of 2.0 mg/dL or more (for the 180 mcg/kg bolus and the 2 mcg/kg/min infusion) or 4.0 mg/dL or more (for the 135 mcg/kg bolus and the 0.5 mcg/kg/min infusion). Lactation.

SPECIAL CONCERNS
Bleeding is the most common complication; there is a greater risk in older clients. Use with caution when used with other drugs that affect hemostasis, including thrombolytics, oral anticoagulants, NSAIDs, dipyridamole, ticlopidine,

and clopidogrel. Use with caution during lactation. Safety and efficacy have not been determined in children.

SIDE EFFECTS
CV: Major bleeding, including *intracranial hemorrhage,* bleeding from the femoral artery access site, and bleeding that leads to decreases in hemoglobin greater than 5 g/dL. Minor bleeding, including spontaneous gross hematuria, spontaneous hematemesis, or blood loss with a hemoglobin decrease of more than 3 g/dL. Oropharyngeal (especially gingival), genitourinary, GI, and retroperitoneal bleeding. Hypotension. **Hypersensitivity/allergy:** *Anaphylaxis,* other allergic S&S.

DRUG INTERACTIONS
Possible additive effects when used with thrombolytics, anticoagulants, or other antiplatelet drugs.
H *Evening primrose oil* / Potential for ↑ antiplatelet effect
H *Feverfew* / Potential for ↑ antiplatelet effect
H *Garlic* / Potential for ↑ antiplatelet effect
H *Ginger* / Potential for ↑ antiplatelet effect
H *Ginkgo biloba* / Potential for ↑ antiplatelet effect
H *Ginseng* / Potential for ↑ antiplatelet effect
H *Grapeseed extract* / Potential for ↑ antiplatelet effect

HOW SUPPLIED
Injection: 0.75 mg/mL, 2 mg/mL

DOSAGE
• **IV**
   Acute coronary syndrome.
Adults, inital: IV bolus of 180 mcg/kg as soon as possible following diagnosis, followed by a continuous infusion of 2 mcg/kg/min until hospital discharge or initiation of coronary artery bypass surgery, up to 72 hr. If percutaneous coronary intervention will be undertaken, consider decreasing the infusion rate to 0.5 mcg/kg/min at the time of the procedure. Continue the infusion for an additional 20–24 hr after the procedure, allowing for up to 96 hr of therapy. Clients weighing > 121 kg have received a maximum bolus of 22.6 mg

(11.3 mL of the 2 mg/mL injection) followed by a maximum rate of 15 mg (20 mL of the 0.75 mg/mL injection)/hr.

Percutaneous coronary intervention.
Adults, in those with a serum creatinine <2 mg/dL: IV bolus of 180 mcg/kg given immediately before initiation of PCI followed by a continuous infusion of 2 mcg/kg/min and a second bolus dose of 180 mcg/kg 10 min after the first bolus. This is followed by a continuous infusion until hospital discharge or for up to 18–24 hr, whichever comes first. A minimum of 12 hr of infusion is recommended. Give those weighing more than 121 kg a maximum of 22.6 mg/bolus followed by a maximum infusion rate of 7.5 mg/hr. **Adults, in those with a serum creatinine between 2 and 4 mg/dL:** IV bolus of 180 mcg/kg given immediately before initiation of PCI, immediately followed by a continuous infusion of 1 mcg/kg/min and a second 180 mcg/kg bolus given 10 min after the first. Give those weighing more than 121 kg a maximum of 22.6 mg/bolus followed by a maximum infusion rate of 7.5 mg/hr.

NURSING CONSIDERATIONS

ADMINISTRATION/STORAGE
IV 1. In those undergoing CABG surgery, discontinue prior to surgery.
2. Aspirin has been used with eptifibatide with the following possible doses. In acute coronary syndrome, aspirin, 160–325 mg initially and daily thereafter. In PCI, aspirin, 160–325 mg 1–24 hr prior to intervention and daily thereafter.
3. The following heparin doses are recommended. In acute coronary syndrome, achieve a target aPTT of 50–70 sec during medical management. If the weight is 70 or more kg, give a 5,000 unit heparin bolus followed by infusion of 1,000 unit/hr. If the weight is less than 70 kg, give a 60 unit/kg bolus followed by infusion of 12 unit/kg/hr. For PCI, achieve a target ACT of 200–300 sec. Give heparin, 60 unit/kg, as a bolus initially in those not treated with heparin within 6 hr prior to PCI. Give additional boluses during PCI to maintain

ACT within target. Do not give heparin infusion after the PCI.
4. Inspect the vial for particulate matter or discoloration before use.
5. May be given in the same IV line as alteplase, atropine, dobutamine, heparin, lidocaine, meperidine, metoprolol, midazolam, morphine, nitroglycerin, or verapamil; do not give in same line as furosemide.
6. May be given in the same IV line with 0.9% NaCl or D5/NSS; may also contain up to 60 mEq/L of KCl.
7. Withdraw the bolus dose from the 10-mL vial and give by IV push over 1–2 min. Immediately following the bolus dose, start the continuous infusion. If using an infusion pump, give undiluted directly from the 100-mL vial by spiking the 100-mL vial with a vented infusion set. Center the spike within the circle on the stopper top.
8. Store vials at 2–8°C (36–46°F). Protect from light until use. Discard any portion left in the vial.

ASSESSMENT
1. Determine onset, duration, and characteristics of symptoms.
2. Note any conditions that would preclude therapy: recent CVA or surgery, platelets < 100,000/mm^3, uncontrolled BP, abnormal bleeding or history of bleeding diathesis, hemorrhagic stroke, renal failure, or dialysis.
3. Monitor ECG, bleeding times, liver and renal function studies.
4. Stop drug prior to CABG surgery.
5. Used in conjunction with aspirin and heparin; review dosing guidelines.
6. Assess femoral artery access site for evidence of bleeding. Stop heparin and eptifibatide therapy if unable to stop bleeding with pressure.

CLIENT/FAMILY TEACHING
1. Review risks associated with therapy. Drug is a blood thinner used to prevent clot formation with unstable angina and non-Q-wave MI.
2. Bleeding is the most common side effect of drug therapy; usually occurs at graft site but may also occur as GU, GI, oropharyngeal, or retroperitoneal bleeding. Report any unusual bleeding or other adverse side effects.

---

3. Family should learn CPR.

OUTCOMES/EVALUATE
- Inhibition of platelet aggregation
- ↓ Death/MI with acute coronary syndrome

Esmolol hydrochloride ©

(**EZ**-moh-lohl)

CLASSIFICATION(S):
Beta-adrenergic blocking agent
PREGNANCY CATEGORY: C
Rx: Brevibloc, Brevibloc Double Strength

SEE ALSO *BETA-ADRENERGIC BLOCKING AGENTS.*

ACTION/KINETICS
Preferentially inhibits beta-1 receptors. Rapid onset (< 5 min) and a short duration of action. Has no membrane-stabilizing or intrinsic sympathomimetic activity. Low lipid solubility. **t ½:** 9 min. Rapidly metabolized by esterases in RBCs.

USES
(1) Supraventricular tachycardia in those with atrial fibrillation or atrial flutter in perioperative, postoperative, or other emergent situations when short-term control is needed. (2) Noncompensatory sinus tachycardia when rapid heart rate requires intervention. (3) Tachycardia and hypertension during induction and tracheal intubation, during surgery, on emergence from anesthesia, and postoperatively.

SPECIAL CONCERNS
Dosage has not been established in children.

ADDITIONAL SIDE EFFECTS
Dermatologic: Inflammation at site of infusion, flushing, pallor, induration, erythema, burning, skin discoloration, edema. **Other:** Urinary retention, midscapular pain, asthenia, changes in taste.

ADDITIONAL DRUG INTERACTIONS
Digoxin / ↑ Digoxin blood levels
Morphine / ↑ Esmolol blood levels

HOW SUPPLIED
Injection: 10 mg/mL, 20 mg/mL, 250 mg/mL

DOSAGE
- **IV INFUSION**
  SVT.
  Initial: 500 mcg/kg/min for 1 min; **then,** 50 mcg/kg/min for 4 min. If after 5 min an adequate effect is not achieved, repeat the loading dose followed by a maintenance infusion of 100 mcg/kg/min for 4 min. This procedure may be repeated, increasing the maintenance infusion by 50 mcg/kg/min increments (for 4 min) until the desired HR or lowered BP is approached. **Then,** omit the loading infusion and reduce incremental infusion rate from 50 to 25 mcg/kg/min or less. The interval between titrations may be increased from 5 to 10 min.
  Once the HR has been controlled, the client may be transferred to another antiarrhythmic agent. Reduce the infusion rate of esmolol by 50% 30 min after the first dose of the alternative antiarrhythmic agent. If satisfactory control is observed for 1 hr after the second dose of the alternative agent, the esmolol infusion may be stopped.
  Intraoperative and postoperative tachycardia and hypertension.
  Immediate control: 80 mg (about 1 mg/kg) bolus dose over 30 sec followed by 150 mcg/kg/min for 1 min followed by a 4-min maintenance infusion of 50 mcg/kg/min. If an adequate effect is not seen in 5 min, repeat the same loading dose and follow with a maintenance infusion of 100 mcg/kg/min.
  Gradual control: Dosing schedule is the same as for supraventricular tachycardia (SVT).

NURSING CONSIDERATIONS
© Do not confuse Brevibloc with Brevital (a barbiturate).

ADMINISTRATION/STORAGE
Ⅳ 1. Infusions may be necessary for 24–48 hr.
2. Not for direct IV push administration.
3. Do not dilute concentrate with sodium bicarbonate.

H = Herbal   Ⅳ = Intravenous   © = sound-alike drug

4. To minimize irritation and thrombophlebitis, do not infuse concentrations greater than 10 mg/mL.

5. Diluted esmolol (concentration of 10 mg/mL) is compatible with D5W, D5/RL, D5/Ringer's injection, D5/0.9% NaCl, D5/0.45% NaCl, 0.45% NaCl, RL, KCl (40 mEq/L) in D5W, and 0.9% NaCl.

ASSESSMENT

1. Note indications for therapy, type, onset, and characteristics of S&S.

2. Document and monitor CP assessments, ECG, and VS. Assess for hypotension or bradycardia.

3. Administer in a monitored environment; wean using guidelines.

OUTCOMES/EVALUATE

- Suppression of SVT
- Restoration of stable rhythm

Ethacrynate sodium   ■ ©

(eth-ah-**KRIH**-nayt)

CLASSIFICATION(S):
Diuretic, loop
PREGNANCY CATEGORY: B
Rx: Edecrin Sodium

Ethacrynic acid

(eth-ah-**KRIH**-nik)

PREGNANCY CATEGORY: B
Rx: Edecrin

SEE ALSO *DIURETICS, LOOP.*

ACTION/KINETICS

Inhibits the reabsorption of sodium and chloride in the loop of Henle; it also decreases reabsorption of sodium and chloride and increases potassium excretion in the distal tubule. Also acts directly on the proximal tubule to enhance excretion of electrolytes. Large quantities of sodium and chloride and smaller amounts of potassium and bicarbonate ion are excreted during diuresis. **Onset, PO:** 30 min; **IV:** Within 5 min. **Peak, PO:** 2 hr; **IV:** 15–30 min. **Duration, PO:** 6–8 hr. **IV:** 2 hr. **t ½, after**

PO: 60 min. Metabolites are excreted through the urine. Diuresis and electrolyte loss are more pronounced with ethacrynic acid than with thiazide diuretics. Is often effective in clients refractory to other diuretics. Careful monitoring of the diuretic effects is necessary.

USES

Of value with resistance to less potent diuretics. (1) CHF, acute pulmonary edema, edema associated with nephrotic syndrome, ascites due to idiopathic edema, lymphedema, malignancy. (2) Short-term use for ascites as a result of malignancy, lymphedema, or idiopathic edema. (3) Short-term use in pediatric clients (except infants) with congenital heart disease. *Investigational.* **Ethacrynic acid:** Single injection into the eye to treat glaucoma (effective for a week or more). **Ethacrynate sodium:** Hypercalcemia, bromide intoxication, and with mannitol in ethylene glycol poisoning.

CONTRAINDICATIONS

Pregnancy (usually), lactation, use in neonates. Anuria and severe renal damage.

SPECIAL CONCERNS

■Potent diuretic; excess amounts can lead to a profound diuresis with water and electrolyte depletion. Careful medical supervision is required; individualize dosage.■ Geriatric clients may be more sensitive to the usual adult dose. Use with caution in diabetics and in those with hepatic cirrhosis (who are particularly susceptible to electrolyte imbalance). Monitor gout clients carefully. Safety and efficacy of oral use in infants and IV use in children have not been established.

SIDE EFFECTS

Electrolyte imbalance: Hypokalemia/natremia, hypochloremic alkalosis, hypomagnesemia/calcemia. **GI:** Anorexia, nausea, vomiting, diarrhea (may be sudden, watery, profuse diarrhea), acute pancreatitis, abdominal discomfort/pain, jaundice, *GI bleeding or hemorrhage,* dysphagia. **Hematologic:** Severe neutropenia, thrombocytopenia, *agranulocytosis,* rarely Henoch-Schoenlein purpura in clients with rheumatic heart disease. **CNS:** Apprehension, con-

---

Bold Italic = life threatening side effect   ■ = black box warning   ✤ = Available in Canada

fusion, vertigo, headache. **Body as a whole:** Fever, chills, fatigue, malaise. **Otic:** Sense of fullness in the ears, tinnitus, irreversible hearing loss. **Miscellaneous:** Hematuria, acute gout, abnormal LFTs in seriously ill clients on multiple drug therapy including ethacrynic acid, blurred vision, rash, local irritation and pain following parenteral use, hyperuricemia/glycemia.

Ethacrynic acid may cause death in critically ill clients refractory to other diuretics. These include (a) clients with severe myocardial disease who also received digitalis and who developed acute hypokalemia with fatal arrhythmias and (b) those with severely decompensated hepatic cirrhosis with ascites, with or without encephalopathy, who had electrolyte imbalances. Death is due to intensification of the electrolyte effect.

OD OVERDOSE MANAGEMENT

Symptoms: Profound water loss, electrolyte depletion (causes dizziness, weakness, mental confusion, vomiting, anorexia, lethargy, cramps), dehydration, reduction of blood volume, *circulatory collapse (possibility of vascular thrombosis and embolism).* *Treatment:* Replace electrolytes and fluid and monitor urine output and serum electrolyte levels. Induce emesis or perform gastric lavage. Artificial respiration and oxygen may be needed. Treat other symptoms.

HOW SUPPLIED

Ethacrynate Sodium: *Powder for injection:* 50 mg/vial. **Ethacrynic Acid:** *Tablet:* 25 mg, 50 mg

DOSAGE

ETHACRYNATE SODIUM

• **IV**

Adults: 50 mg (base) (or 0.5–1 mg/kg); may be repeated in 2–4 hr, although only one dose is usually needed. A single 100-mg dose IV has also been used.

ETHACRYNIC ACID

• **TABLETS**

Adults, initial: 50–200 mg/day in single or divided doses to produce a gradual weight loss of 1–2 lb/day. The dose can be increased by 25–50 mg/day if needed. **Maintenance:** Usually 50–200 mg (up to a maximum of 400 mg) daily

may be required in severe, refractory edema. If used with other diuretics, the initial dose should be 25 mg with increments of 25 mg. **Pediatric, initial:** 25 mg/day; can increase by 25 mg/day if needed. **Maintenance:** Adjust dose to needs of client. Dosage for infants has not been determined.

NURSING CONSIDERATIONS

E

℮ Do not confuse Edecrin with Eulexin (an antineoplastic).

ADMINISTRATION/STORAGE

1. Administer tablets after meals.

2. Due to local pain and irritation, do not give SC or IM.

3. Ammonium chloride or arginine chloride may be prescribed for those at a higher risk of developing metabolic acidosis.

IV 4. Reconstitute powder for injection by adding 50 mL of D5W or NaCl injection.

5. Administer intermittent IV slowly over a 30-min period, given either directly or through IV tubing. For direct IV, may give at a rate of 10 mg/min.

6. When reconstituted with D5W injection, the resulting solution may be hazy or opalescent; do not use. Do not mix solution with whole blood or its derivatives.

7. If a second IV injection is necessary, use a different site to prevent thrombophlebitis.

8. Use reconstituted solutions within 24 hr; discard any unused solution.

ASSESSMENT

1. Document indications for therapy, other agents trialed, and outcome.

2. Note any diabetes or cirrhosis; establish lack of anuria.

3. Monitor electrolytes, CBC, liver and renal function studies. With prolonged therapy, obtain a hearing test.

INTERVENTIONS

1. Monitor VS, I&O, and weight. Note excessive diuresis or weight loss; electrolyte imbalance may occur quickly.

2. With rapid excessive diuresis, assess for pain in calves, pelvic area, or the chest; rapid hemoconcentration may cause thromboembolic effects.

H = Herbal   IV = Intravenous   ℮ = sound-alike drug

3. Drug should be withdrawn if severe, watery diarrhea presents. Test for occult blood in urine and stools.

4. Observe for vestibular disturbances. Do not administer concomitantly with any other ototoxic agent. Hearing loss is most common following high or rapid IV dosing.

5. Monitor serum K^+ levels; assess need for supplemental potassium.

6. Since drug has such a profound effect on sodium excretion, dietary salt restriction is not necessary; if sodium is restricted, hyponatremia may result.

CLIENT/FAMILY TEACHING

1. Take as directed upon awakening to ensure sleep not interrupted.

2. Change positions slowly to prevent any sudden drop in BP and associated dizziness.

3. Monitor weight, I&O, and BP; report any excessive weight gain, SOB, swelling of hands or feet or other adverse effects or lack of response.

OUTCOMES/EVALUATE

- Enhanced diuresis
- ↓ Edema (↑ weight loss)
- ↓ Abdominal girth R/T ascites

Ezetimibe

(eh-**ZET**-eh-myb)

CLASSIFICATION(S):
Antihyperlipidemic agents, HMG-CoA reductase inhibitors
PREGNANCY CATEGORY: C
Rx: Zetia

ACTION/KINETICS
Reduces total cholesterol, LDL cholesterol, Apo B, and triglycerides as well as increases HDL cholesterol. Acts by inhibiting the absorption of cholesterol from the small intestine, leading to a decrease in the delivery of cholesterol to the liver. This complements the mechanism of action of HMG-CoA reductase inhibitors. Has no effect on the fat-soluble vitamins A, D, and E. After PO administration, is rapidly conjugated to the active phenolic glucuronide in the small intestine and liver. **Peak plas-** ma **ezetimibe levels:** 4–12 hr. Ezetimibe-glucuronide is bound greater than 90% to plasma proteins. **t ½, parent drug and active metabolite:** 22 hr. Mainly excreted through the feces with smaller amounts through the urine.

USES
(1) Primary hypercholesterolemia, either as monotherapy or combination therapy with HMG-CoA reductase inhibitors. (2) With atorvastatin or simvastatin for homozygous familial hypercholesterolemia. (3) As adjunctive therapy to diet for homozygous sitosterolemia.

CONTRAINDICATIONS
Use with HMG-CoA reductase inhibitors in pregnant and nursing women and in active liver disease or unexplained persistent elevations in serum transaminases. As monotherapy in moderate to severe hepatic insufficiency and during lactation. Use in children less than 10 years of age.

SPECIAL CONCERNS
If used with HMG-CoA reductase inhibitors, be aware of contraindications, special concerns, and side effects of these drugs as well.

SIDE EFFECTS
GI: Diarrhea, abdominal pain. **CNS:** Headache, dizziness. **Musculoskeletal:** Myalgia, back pain, arthralgia, possible myopathy or rhabdomyolysis. **Respiratory:** URTI, sinusitis, pharyngitis, coughing. **Miscellaneous:** Chest pain, fatigue, viral infection.

LABORATORY TEST CONSIDERATIONS
↑ Liver enzymes greater than or equal to 3 times ULN.

DRUG INTERACTIONS
Antacids / ↓ Ezetimibe C_{max} after both Mg- and Ca-containing antacids; no effect on AUC
Cholestyramine / ↓ Ezetimibe AUC probably due to ↓ absorption
Cyclosporine / ↑ Total ezetimibe levels; monitor carefully
Fenofibrate/Gemfibrozil / ↑ Total ezetimibe level

HOW SUPPLIED
Tablet: 10 mg

DOSAGE

TABLETS

Primary hypercholesterolemia, homozygous familial hypercholesterolemia, homozygous sitosterolemia.
10 mg once daily with or without food.

NURSING CONSIDERATIONS

ADMINISTRATION/STORAGE

1. Place client on a standard cholesterol-lowering diet before therapy and for duration of treatment.
2. May be given with a HMG-CoA reductase inhibitor for an incremental effect. Dose of both drugs can be given at the same time.
3. Give at least 2 hr before or at least 4 hr after giving a bile acid sequestrant.
4. Store from 15–30°C (59–86°F) protected from moisture.

ASSESSMENT

1. Note indications for therapy: placque stability or elevated TG/LDL cholesterol in CAD and other agents trialed.
2. Monitor CBC, cholesterol profile, liver and renal function studies. Schedule LFTs at the beginning of therapy and semiannually for the first year of therapy. Special attention should be paid to elevated serum transaminase levels.
3. List all medications prescribed to ensure none interact unfavorably. Identify and list risk factors.

4. Assess level of adherence to weight reduction, exercise, and cholesterol-lowering diet and BP or BS control. Note any alcohol abuse or liver dysfunction.

CLIENT/FAMILY TEACHING

1. Take daily as directed. Avoid taking with antacids; reduces drug effect.
2. A low-cholesterol diet must be followed during drug therapy. Consult dietitian for assistance in meal planning and food preparation.
3. Report any S&S of infections, unexplained muscle pain, tenderness/weakness (especially if accompanied by fever or malaise), surgery, trauma, or metabolic disorders. Report as scheduled for lab tests, eye exam, and F/U.
4. Review importance of following a low-cholesterol diet, regular exercise, low alcohol consumption, and not smoking in the overall plan to reduce serum cholesterol levels and inhibit progression of CAD.
5. Not for use during pregnancy; use barrier contraception.
6. Drug acts by inhibiting cholesterol absorption in the small intestine. May experience GI upset and muscle and back pains.

OUTCOMES/EVALUATE

↓ Total cholesterol, LDL cholesterol and triglycerides ↑ HDL cholesterol

---

F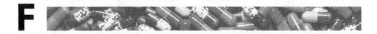

Felodipine

(feh-**LOHD**-ih-peen)

CLASSIFICATION(S):
Calcium channel blocker
PREGNANCY CATEGORY: C
Rx: Plendil
✦Rx: Renedil

SEE ALSO *CALCIUM CHANNEL BLOCKING AGENTS.*

ACTION/KINETICS

Onset after PO: 120–300 min. **Peak plasma levels:** 2.5–5 hr. Moderate increase in HR and moderate decrease in peripheral resistance. No effect on the QRS complex, PR interval, or QT interval with no effect to a slight decrease on myocardial contractility. **t ½, elimination:** 11–16 hr. Metabolized in the liver with 70% excreted in the urine and 10% excreted in the feces. Over 99% bound to plasma protein.

USES
Hypertension, alone or with other antihypertensives. *Investigational:* Raynaud's syndrome, CHF.

CONTRAINDICATIONS
Lactation.

SPECIAL CONCERNS
Use with caution in clients with CHF or compromised ventricular function, especially in combination with a beta-adrenergic blocking agent. Use with caution in impaired hepatic function or reduced hepatic blood flow. May cause a greater hypotensive effect in geriatric clients. Safety and effectiveness have not been determined in children.

SIDE EFFECTS
CV: Significant hypotension, syncope, angina pectoris, peripheral edema, palpitations, AV block, *MI, arrhythmias,* tachycardia. **CNS:** Dizziness, lightheadedness, headache, nervousness, sleepiness, irritability, anxiety, insomnia, paresthesia, depression, amnesia, paranoia, psychosis, hallucinations. **Body as a whole:** Asthenia, flushing, muscle cramps, pain, inflammation, warm feeling, influenza. **GI:** Nausea, abdominal discomfort, cramps, dyspepsia, diarrhea, constipation, vomiting, dry mouth, flatulence. **Dermatologic:** Rash, dermatitis, urticaria, pruritus. **Respiratory:** Rhinitis, rhinorrhea, pharyngitis, sinusitis, nasal and chest congestion, SOB, wheezing, dyspnea, cough, bronchitis, sneezing, respiratory infection. **Miscellaneous:** Anemia, gingival hyperplasia, sexual difficulties, epistaxis, back pain, facial edema, erythema, urinary frequency or urgency, dysuria.

ADDITIONAL DRUG INTERACTIONS
Barbiturates / ↓ Effect of felodipine
Carbamazepine / ↓ Felodipine effects
Cimetidine / ↑ Bioavailability of felodipine
Cyclosporine / ↑ Pharmcologic and toxic effects of felodipine; ↑ cyclosporine levels and toxicity
Digoxin / ↑ Peak plasma levels of digoxin
Erythromycins / ↑ Erythromycin effects; monitor CV status closely
Fentanyl / Possible severe hypotension or ↑ fluid volume
Grapefruit juice / ↑ Plasma levels of felodipine R/T ↓ liver breakdown
Itraconazole / ↑ Felodipine serum levels
Nelfinavir / Possible leg edema and orthostatic hypotension
Oxcarbazepine / ↓ Felodipine effects
Phenytoin / ↓ Effects of felodipine
Ranitidine / ↑ Bioavailability of felodipine

HOW SUPPLIED
Tablet, Extended Release: 2.5 mg, 5 mg, 10 mg

DOSAGE
- **TABLETS, EXTENDED RELEASE**
  Hypertension.
Initial: 5 mg once daily (2.5 mg in clients over 65 years of age and in those with impaired liver function); **then:** adjust dose according to response, usually at 2-week intervals with the usual dosage range being 2.5–10 mg once daily. Doses greater than 10 mg increase the rate of peripheral edema and other vasodilatory side effects.

NURSING CONSIDERATIONS

ADMINISTRATION/STORAGE
Bioavailability is not affected by food. It is increased more than twofold when taken with doubly concentrated grapefruit juice as compared with water or orange juice.

ASSESSMENT
1. Document onset of symptoms, other agents used, and outcome.
2. Note history of heart failure or compromised ventricular function. Assess heart, lungs, and EKG.
3. List drugs currently prescribed; note any potential interactions.
4. During dosage adjustments, monitor BP closely in clients over 65 or with impaired hepatic function.

CLIENT/FAMILY TEACHING
1. Swallow tablets whole; do not chew or crush. Avoid taking with grapefruit juice.
2. Do not stop abruptly; abrupt withdrawal may increase frequency and duration of chest pain.
3. Avoid activities that require mental alertness until effects are realized.

Bold Italic = life threatening side effect   ■ = black box warning   ✚ = Available in Canada

4. Rise slowly from a lying position and dangle feet before standing to minimize postural effects.

5. Report any headaches, flushing or extremity swelling. Keep a written record of BP and HR for review.

6. Practice frequent oral hygiene to minimize incidence and severity of drug-induced gingival hyperplasia.

OUTCOMES/EVALUATE

Control of hypertension

Fenofibrate

(**fee**-noh-**FY**-brayt)

CLASSIFICATION(S):

Antihyperlipidemic

PREGNANCY CATEGORY: C

Rx: Lofibra, Tricor

♣Rx: Fenofibrate: Apo-Fenofibrate, Apo-Feno-Micro, Nu-Fenofibrate. **Fenofibrate Microcoated:** Lipidil Supra. **Fenofibrate Micronized:** Gen-Fenofibrate Micro, Lipidil Micro, Novo-Fenofibrate Micronized, PMS-Fenofibrate Micro

ACTION/KINETICS

Is converted to the active fenofibric acid, which lowers plasma triglycerides. Probable mechanism is to inhibit triglyceride synthesis, resulting in a reduction of VLDL released into the circulation, and by stimulating catabolism of triglyceride-rich lipoprotein. Also increases urinary excretion of uric acid. Well absorbed; absorption is increased when given with food. **Peak plasma levels:** 6–8 hr; **steady-state plasma levels:** within 5 days. **t ½:** : 20 hr with once daily dosing. Fenofibric acid and an inactive metabolite are excreted through the urine. Highly bound to plasma proteins.

USES

(1) Adjunctive therapy to diet to reduce elevated LDL-C, total-C, triglycerides, and Apo B and to increase HDL-C in adults with primary hypercholesterolemia or mixed dyslipidemia (Fredrickson Types IIa and II b). (2) Adjunctive therapy to diet to treat adults with hypertriglyceridemia (Fredrickson Types IV

and V hyperlipidemia). *Investigational:* Polymetabolic syndrome X, hyperuricemia.

CONTRAINDICATIONS

Hepatic or severe renal dysfunction (including primary biliary cirrhosis), those with unexplained, persistent abnormal liver function, and preexisting gallbladder disease. Lactation.

SPECIAL CONCERNS

Due to similarity to clofibrate and gemfibrozil, side effects, including death, are possible. Safety and efficacy have not been determined in children.

SIDE EFFECTS

GI: Pancreatitis, cholelithiasis, dyspepsia, N&V, diarrhea, abdominal pain, dry mouth, constipation, flatulence, eructation, hepatitis, cholecystitis, hepatomegaly, gastroenteritis, rectal disorder, esophagitis, gastritis, colitis, tooth disorder, anorexia, GI disorder, duodenal/peptic ulcer, rectal hemorrhage, fatty liver deposit. **CNS:** Decreased libido, dizziness, increased appetite, insomnia, paresthesia, depression, vertigo, anxiety, hypertonia, nervousness, neuralgia, somnolence. **CV:** Angina pectoris, hypertension, vasodilation, coronary artery disorder, abnormal ECG, ventricular extrasystoles, *MI,* peripheral vascular disorder, migraine, varicose vein, CV disorder, hypotension, palpitation, vascular disorder, arrhythmia, phlebitis, tachycardia, extrasystoles, atrial fibrillation. **Dermatologic:** Rash, pruritus, eczema, herpes zoster, urticaria, acne, sweating, fungal dermatitis, skin disorder, alopecia, contact dermatitis, herpes simplex, maculopapular rash, nail disorder, skin ulcer. **Respiratory:** Rhinitis, respiratory disorder, cough, sinusitis, allergic pulmonary alveolitis, pharyngitis, bronchitis, dyspnea, asthma, pneumonia, laryngitis. **GU:** Polyuria, vaginitis, prostatic disorder, dysuria, abnormal kidney function, urolithiasis, gynecomastia, unintended pregnancy, vaginal moniliasis, cystitis. **Hematologic:** Anemia, leukopenia, ecchymosis, eosinophilia, lymphadenopathy, thrombocytopenia. **Musculoskeletal:** Myopathy, myositis, arthralgia, myalgia, myasthenia, rhabdomyolysis, arthritis, tenosynovitis, joint disorder, arthrosis, leg cramps, bursitis. **Hypersensitivity:** Severe skin rashes, urticaria. **Ophthalmic:** Eye irritation, blurred vision, conjunctivitis, eye floaters, eye disorder, amblyopia, cataract, refraction disorder. **Body as a whole:** Infections, pain, headache, asthenia, fatigue, flu syndrome, photosensitivity, malaise, allergic reaction, fever, weight gain/loss. **Miscellaneous:** Back pain, chest pain, cyst, hernia, accidental injury, diabetes mellitus, gout, edema, peripheral edema.

LABORATORY TEST CONSIDERATIONS
↑ AST, ALT, CPK, creatinine, blood urea. Initial ↓ hemoglobin, hematocrit, WBCs. Hypoglycemia, hyperuricemia. Abnormal LFTs.

DRUG INTERACTIONS
Anticoagulants / Potentiation of coumarin anticoagulants (prolongation of PT)
Bile acid sequestrants / ↓ Absorption of fenofibrate due to binding
Cyclosporine / ↑ Risk of nephrotoxicity
HMG-CoA reductase inhibitors / Possibility of rhabdomyolysis, myopathy, and acute renal failure

HOW SUPPLIED
Capsules, Micronized (Lofibra): 67 mg, 134 mg, 200 mg; *Tablets (Tricor):* 54 mg, 160 mg

DOSAGE

- **CAPSULES, TABLETS**
  Hypertriglyceridemia.
Initial: 54–160 mg/day of the tablets or 67–200 mg/day of the capsules given with meals to optimize bioavailability. Then, individualize based on client response. Increase, if necessary, at 4–8–week intervals. If C_{CR} is less than 50 mL/min, start with 54–67 mg/day; increase dose only after evaluation of effects on renal function and triglyceride levels. In the elderly, limit the initial dose to 54 mg/day.
  Primary hypercholesterolemia or mixed hyperlipidemia.
Initial: 160 mg/day of the tablets or 200 mg/day of the capsules.

NURSING CONSIDERATIONS
ADMINISTRATION/STORAGE
1. Place clients on an appropriate triglyceride-lowering diet before starting

fenofibrate and continue during treatment.
2. Withdraw therapy after 2 months if response is not adequate with the maximum daily dose.

ASSESSMENT
1. Note indications for therapy, other agents trialed, and cardiac risk factors.
2. Control BP, BS and assess renal and LFTs; avoid drug with severe dysfunction.
3. Monitor lipids, CBC, renal and LFTs; if ALT or AST > 3 times normal, discontinue therapy. Reduce dosage with C_{CR} < 50 mL/min.

CLIENT/FAMILY TEACHING
1. Take as directed with meals.
2. Continue to follow diet prescribed for triglyceride reduction as well as a regular exercise program, smoking cessation and alcohol reduction.
3. Report skin rash, GI upset, persistent abdominal pain, or muscle pain, tenderness, fatigue, GU dysfunction or weakness.
4. Avoid therapy with pregnancy and breastfeeding.
5. Report as scheduled for regular liver function tests and triglyceride levels. Drug therapy should be reevaluated after 2 months if desired lipid reduction is not evident with maximum dose therapy.
6. Advise to take 1 or more hr before or 4–6 hr after a bile acid binding resin to avoid decreased absorption.

OUTCOMES/EVALUATE
↓ Triglyceride levels ↓ ASHD

Fenoldopam mesylate
(feh-**NOL**-doh-pam)

CLASSIFICATION(S):
Treatment of hypertension emergency
PREGNANCY CATEGORY: B
Rx: Corlopam

ACTION/KINETICS
Rapid-acting vasodilator that is an agonist for D_1-like dopamine receptors and α_2-adrenoreceptors. Causes vasodi-

lation in coronary, renal, mesenteric, and peripheral arteries; vascular beds do not respond uniformly. **t ½, elimination:** About 5 min in mild to moderate hypertensives. **Steady-state levels:** About 20 min. Metabolized in liver and most is excreted in urine.

USES
Hypertensive emergencies.

CONTRAINDICATIONS
Use with beta-blockers or in those with sulfite sensitivity.

SPECIAL CONCERNS
Use with caution during lactation and in those with glaucoma or intraocular hypertension. Safety and efficacy have not been determined in children.

SIDE EFFECTS
CV: Tachycardia, hypotension, flushing, ST-T abnormalities, postural hypotension, extrasystoles, palpitations, bradycardia, *heart failure, ischemic heart disease, MI,* angina pectoris. **Body as a whole:** Headache, sweating, back pain, non-specific chest pain, pyrexia, limb cramp. **CNS:** Nervousness, anxiety, insomnia, dizziness. **GI:** N&V, abdominal pain or fullness, constipation, diarrhea. **Respiratory:** Nasal congestion, dyspnea, upper respiratory disorder. **Hematologic:** Leukocytosis, bleeding. **Miscellaneous:** Reaction at injection site, UTI, oliguria.

LABORATORY TEST CONSIDERATIONS
↑ Creatinine, BUN, serum glucose, transaminase, LDH. Hypokalemia.

HOW SUPPLIED
Injection concentrate: 10 mg/mL

DOSAGE
• **CONSTANT IV INFUSION**
Hypertensive emergency.
Rate of infusion is individualized according to body weight and to desired speed and extent of effect. See package insert for table of infusion rates. Doses range from 0.025 mcg/kg/min–0.3 mcg/kg/min for a body weight of 40 kg to 0.094 mcg/kg/min–1.13mcg/kg/min for a body weight of 150 kg.

NURSING CONSIDERATIONS

ADMINISTRATION/STORAGE
[IV] 1. Do not use a bolus dose.
2. Most of the effect of a given infusion is reached in 15 min.

3. Initial dose is titrated up or down no more often than every 15 min, and less frequently as desired BP is approached. Recommended increments for titration are 0.05–0.1 mcg/kg/min.
4. Initial doses of 0.03–0.1 mcg/kg/min have been associated with less reflex tachycardia than higher doses (> 0.3 mcg/kg/min).
5. Administer using a calibrated mechanical infusion pump that can deliver desired infusion rate accurately.
6. Infusion may be discontinued abruptly or tapered gradually prior to discontinuation.
7. Transition to PO therapy can be started any time after BP is stablized during fenoldopam infusion.
8. Dilute ampule concentrate in 0.9% NaCl or D5W injection for a final concentration of 40 mcg/mL (i.e., add 4 mL of the concentrate to 1,000 mL; 2 mL of the concentrate to 500 mL; or, 1 mL of the concentrate to 250 mL). Each mL of concentrate contains 10 mg of drug. Each ampule is for single use only.
9. Store ampules at 2–30°C (36–86°F).
10. Diluted solution is stable under normal light and temperature for 24 hr or less. Discard any diluted solution that is not used within 24 hr.

ASSESSMENT
1. Document clinical presentation, onset, characteristics of symptoms, and any evidence of neurologic involvement/changes.
2. Note any glaucoma, sulfite sensitivity, or intraocular hypertension. List drugs prescribed to ensure none interact unfavorably; avoid use with beta–blockers.
3. Monitor VS, ECG, electrolytes, liver and renal function studies. Obtain weight.
4. Assess for physical conditions that may have precipitated event; evaluate life-style changes needed and continue medications to control BP.

CLIENT/FAMILY TEACHING
Drug is administered by IV infusion to help lower very high blood pressure readings quickly.

OUTCOMES/EVALUATE
Reduction in BP with hypertensive crisis

Flecainide acetate ■
(fleh-**KAY**-nyd)

CLASSIFICATION(S):
Antiarrhythmic, Class IC
PREGNANCY CATEGORY: C
Rx: Tambocor

SEE ALSO *ANTIARRHYTHMIC DRUGS.*
ACTION/KINETICS
The antiarrhythmic effect is due to a local anesthetic action, especially on the His-Purkinje system in the ventricle. Drug decreases single and multiple PVCs and reduces the incidence of ventricular tachycardia. **Peak plasma levels:** 3 hr.; **steady state levels:** 3–5 days. **Effective plasma levels:** 0.2–1 mcg/mL (trough levels). **t ½:** 20 hr (12–27 hr). Approximately 30% is excreted in urine unchanged. Metabolized by the cytochrome P450 2D6 isoenzyme system. Impaired renal function decreases rate of elimination of unchanged drug and prolongs the half-life. Food or antacids do not affect absorption. Forty percent is bound to plasma protein.

USES
(1) Life-threatening arrhythmias manifested as sustained ventricular tachycardia. (2) Prevention of paroxysmal atrial fibrillation associated with disabling symptoms and paroxysmal supraventricular tachycardias (PSVT), including atrioventricular nodal reentrant tachycardia, atrioventricular reentrant tachycardia, and other supraventricular tachycardias of unspecified mechanism associated with disabling symptoms in those without structural heart disease. *NOTE:* Not recommended in those with less severe ventricular arrhythmias even if clients are symptomatic.

CONTRAINDICATIONS
Cardiogenic shock, preexisting second- or third-degree AV block, RBBB when associated with bifascicular block (unless pacemaker is present to maintain cardiac rhythm). Recent MI. Chronic atrial fibrillation. Frequent PVCs and symptomatic nonsustained ventricular arrhythmias. Lactation.

SPECIAL CONCERNS
■(1) Flecainide was included in the National Heart Lung and Blood Institutes Cardiac Arrhythmia Suppression Trail. An excessive mortality or non-fatal cardiac arrest rate was seen in those treated with flecainide compared with that seen in those assigned to a carefully matched placebo-control group. The average duration of treatment with felcainide in the study was 10 months. (2) The applicability of this study to other populations is uncertain. However, it is advisable to consider the risks of Class IC agents (including flecainide), coupled with the lack of any evidence of improved survival, generally unacceptable in those without life-threatening ventricular arrhythmias, even if the clients are experiencing unpleasant, but not life-threatenidng, symptoms or signs. (3) Ventricular tachycardia was noted (0.4%) in clients treated with PO flecainide for paroxysmal atrial fibrillation. Flecainide is not recommended for use in those with chronic atrial fibrillation. Case reports of ventricular proarrhythmic effects in those treated with flecainide for atrial fibrillation/flutter have included increased PVCs, ventricular tachycardia, ventricular fibrillation, and death. (4) As with other Class I drugs, those treated with flecainide for atrial flutter have been reported with a 1:1 atrioventricular conduction due to slowing the atrial rate. A paradoxical increase in the ventricular rate may also occur in those with atrial fibrillation who receive flecainide. Concomitant negative chronotropic therapy, such as digoxin or beta-blockers, may lower the risk of this complication.■ Use with caution in SSS, in clients with a history of CHF or MI, in disturbances of potassium levels, in clients with permanent pacemakers or temporary pacing electrodes, renal and liver impairment. Safety and efficacy in children less than 18 years of age are not established. The incidence of proarrhythmic effects may be increased in geriatric clients.

SIDE EFFECTS
CV: *New or worsened ventricular arrhythmias, increased risk of death in*

---

clients with non-life-threatening cardi-ac arrhythmias, new or worsened CHF, palpitations, chest pain, sinus bradycardia, sinus pause, sinus arrest, *ventricular fibrillation, ventricular tachycardia that cannot be resuscitated,* second- or third-degree AV block, nonfatal cardiac arrest, tachycardia, hypertension, hypotension, bradycardia, angina pectoris. **CNS:** Dizziness, faintness, syncope, lightheadedness, neuropathy, unsteadiness, headache, fatigue, paresthesia, paresis, hypoesthesia, insomnia, anxiety, twitching, weakness, neuropathy, malaise, vertigo, depression, *seizures,* euphoria, confusion, depersonalization, apathy, morbid dreams, speech disorders, stupor, amnesia, weakness, somnolence. **GI:** Nausea, constipation, abdominal pain, vomiting, anorexia, dyspepsia, dry mouth, diarrhea, flatulence, change in taste. **Ophthalmic:** Blurred vision, difficulty in focusing, spots before eyes, diplopia, photophobia, eye pain, nystagmus, eye irritation, photophobia. **Hematologic:** Leukopenia, thrombocytopenia. **GU:** Decreased libido, impotence, urinary retention, polyuria. **Musculoskeletal:** Asthenia, tremor, ataxia, arthralgia, myalgia. **Dermatologic:** Skin rashes, urticaria, exfoliative dermatitis, pruritus, alopecia. **Other:** Edema, dyspnea, fever, *bronchospasm,* flushing, increased sweating, tinnitus, swollen mouth, lips, and tongue.

OD **OVERDOSE MANAGEMENT**
Symptoms: Lengthening of PR interval; increase in QRS duration, QT interval, and amplitude of T wave; decrease in HR and contractility; conduction disturbances; hypotension; *respiratory failure* or *asystole. Treatment:* Charcoal will remove unabsorbed drug up to 90 min after drug ingestion. Administration of dopamine, dobutamine, or isoproterenol. Artificial respiration. Intra-aortic balloon pumping, transvenous pacing (to correct conduction block). Acidification of the urine may be beneficial, especially in those with an alkaline urine. Due to the long duration of action of the drug, treatment measures

may have to be continued for a prolonged period of time.

DRUG INTERACTIONS
Acidifying agents / ↑ Renal excretion of flecainide → ↓ bioavailability
Alkalinizing agents / ↓ Renal excretion of flecainide → ↑ bioavailability
Amiodarone / ↑ Plasma levels of flecainide
Cimetidine / ↑ Flecainide plasma levels and half-life
Digoxin / ↑ Digoxin plasma levels
Disopyramide / Additive negative inotropic effects; do not use together unless benefits outweigh risks
Propranolol / Additive negative inotropic effects; also, ↑ plasma levels of both drugs
Ritonavir / Significant ↑ serum flecainide levels; do not use together
Smoking (Tobacco) / ↑ Plasma clearance of flecainide
Verapamil / Additive negative inotropic effects

HOW SUPPLIED
Tablet: 50 mg, 100 mg, 150 mg

DOSAGE————————————
• **TABLETS**
  Sustained ventricular tachycardia.
Initial: 100 mg q 12 hr; **then,** increase by 50 mg twice a day q 4 days until effective dose reached. **Usual effective dose:** 150 mg q 12 hr, not to exceed 400 mg/day.
  PSVT, PAF.
Initial: 50 mg q 12 hr; **then,** dose may be increased in increments of 50 mg twice a day q 4 days until effective dose reached. Maximum recommended dose for those with paroxysmal supraventricular arrhythmias: 300 mg/day. NOTE: For PAF clients, increasing the dose from 50 to 100 mg twice a day may increase efficacy without a significant increase in side effects.
  NOTE: For clients with a C_{CR} less than 35 mL/min/1.73 m^2, the starting dose is 100 mg once daily (or 50 mg twice a day). For less severe renal disease, the initial dose may be 100 mg q 12 hr.

F

NURSING CONSIDERATIONS
ADMINISTRATION/STORAGE

1. For most situations, start therapy in a hospital setting (especially in clients with symptomatic CHF, sustained ventricular arrhythmias, compensated clients with significant myocardial dysfunction, or sinus node dysfunction).

2. In renal impairment, increase the dose at intervals greater than 4 days. Monitor for adverse toxic effects.

3. Most clients treated successfully had trough plasma levels between 0.2 and 1 mcg/mL. The chance of toxic effects increases if the trough plasma levels exceed 1 mcg/mL.

4. If being transferred to flecainide from another antiarrhythmic, allow at least two to four plasma half-lives to elapse for the drug being discontinued before initiating flecainide therapy.

5. Dosing at 8-hr intervals may benefit some.

6. If flecainide is given with amiodarone, reduce the usual flecainide dose by 50% and monitor closely for side effects.

7. To minimize toxicity, reduce dose once arrhythmia controlled.

ASSESSMENT

1. Document physical assessment findings i.e. heart, lungs, JVD, weight. Review history, echocardiograms, and ECGs for evidence of CHF, ventricular arrhythmias, sinus node dysfunction, or abnormal EF.

2. Monitor VS, ECG, CXR, electrolytes, renal and LFTs. Assess ECG for increased arrhythmias or AV block. Preexisting hypo/hyperkalemia may alter drug effects; correct. Monitor for labile BP.

3. Concomitant administration with disopyramide, propranolol, or verapamil will promote negative inotropic (depressant) effects.

4. Check pacing thresholds of clients with pacemakers; adjust before and 1 week following drug therapy.

5. Obtain urinary pH to detect alkalinity or acidity. Alkalinity decreases renal excretion and acidity increases renal excretion, affecting rate of drug elimination.

CLIENT/FAMILY TEACHING

1. Take at the dose and frequency prescribed. Report changes in elimination.

2. Report any bruising or increased bleeding tendencies, dyspnea, edema, or chest pain.

3. Keep appointments so that drug effectiveness can be monitored carefully.

4. Report adverse CNS effects, such as dizziness, visual disturbances, headaches, nausea, or depression.

5. Change positions slowly from lying to standing to prevent drop in BP. Avoid hazardous activities until drug effects realized.

OUTCOMES/EVALUATE

- Termination of lethal ventricular arrhythmias; stable cardiac rhythm
- Therapeutic serum (trough) drug levels (0.2–1.0 mcg/mL)

Fluvastatin sodium
(flu-vah-**STAH**-tin)

CLASSIFICATION(S):
Antihyperlipidemic, HMG-CoA reductase inhibitor
PREGNANCY CATEGORY: X
Rx: Lescol, Lescol XL

SEE ALSO *ANTIHYPERLIPIDEMIC AGENTS—HMG-COA REDUCTASE INHIBITORS.*

ACTION/KINETICS

98% absorbed. Absolute bioavailability: 24%. Undergoes extensive first-pass metabolism by CYP2C9. Metabolized in the liver with 90% excreted through the feces and 5% through the urine. **t½:** Less than 3 hr for immediate-release and about 9 hr for extended release. Greater than 98% bound to plasma protein.

USES

(1) Adjunct to diet for the reduction of elevated total and LDL cholesterol, apo-B, and triglyceride levels in clients with primary hypercholesterolemia (heterozygous familial and nonfamilial) and mixed dyslipidemia (Fredrickson type IIa and IIb) whose response to diet and other nondrug measures has been inadequate. The lipid-lowering effects of

fluvastatin are enhanced when it is combined with a bile-acid binding resin or with niacin. (2) To slow the progression of coronary atherosclerosis in coronary heart disease. (3) Reduce the risk of undergoing coronary revascularization procedures in those with coronary heart disease.

SPECIAL CONCERNS

Use with caution in clients with severe renal impairment.

SIDE EFFECTS

Side effects listed are those most common with fluvastatin. A complete list of possible side effects is provided under *Antihyperlipidemic Agents—HMG-CoA Reductase Inhibitors.* **GI:** N&V, diarrhea, abdominal pain or cramps, constipation, flatulence, dyspepsia, tooth disorder. **Musculoskeletal:** Myalgia, back pain, arthralgia, arthritis. **CNS:** Headache, dizziness, insomnia. **Respiratory:** URI, rhinitis, cough, pharyngitis, sinusitis. **Miscellaneous:** Rash, pruritus, fatigue, influenza, allergy, accidental trauma.

LABORATORY TEST CONSIDERATIONS

↑ Serum transaminases.

ADDITIONAL DRUG INTERACTIONS

Alcohol / ↑ Fluvastatin absorbed

Cimetidine / Significant ↑ in fluvastatin C_{max} and AUC

Diclofenac / ↑ Mean diclofenac C_{max} and AUC

Digoxin / ↑ Digoxin C_{max} and slight ↑ digoxin urinary clearance

Glyburide / ↑ Glyburide C_{max}, AUC, and $t^{1/2}$ and ↑ fluvastatin C_{max} and AUC

Omeprazole / Significant ↑ in fluvastatin C_{max} and AUC

Phenytoin / ↑ Fluvastatin C_{max} and AUC; minimal ↑ phenytoin Cmax and AUC

Ranitidine / Significant ↑ in fluvastatin C_{max} and AUC

Rifampin / ↑ Fluvastatin C_{max} and AUC and ↑ plasma clearance

Warfarin / ↑ INR

HOW SUPPLIED

Capsule: 20 mg, 40 mg; *Tablet, Extended-Release:* 80 mg

DOSAGE————————————

• **CAPSULES, TABLETS**

Hypercholesterolemia and mixed dyslipidemia. Antihyperlipidemic to slow progression of coronary atherosclerosis. Secondary prevention of coronary events.

For those requiring LDL cholesterol reduction to 25% or more, **Adults, initial:** 40 mg as one capsule or 80 mg as one tablet once daily in the evening. Or, 80 mg in divided doses using the 40 mg capsule twice a day. For those requiring LDL cholesterol reduction to less than 25%, **Adults, initial:** 20 mg. **Dose range:** 20–80 mg/day.

Slow progression of coronary atherosclerosis in coronary heart disease.

40 mg twice a day, initiated shortly after a first percutaneous coronary intervention procedure.

NURSING CONSIDERATIONS

ADMINISTRATION/STORAGE

1. Maximum reductions of LDL cholesterol are usually seen within 4 weeks; order periodic lipid determinations during this time, with dosage adjusted accordingly.

2. To avoid fluvastatin binding to a bile-acid binding resin (if given together), give the fluvastatin at bedtime and the resin at least 2 hr before.

3. Dispense in tight containers and protect from light.

ASSESSMENT

1. Review risk factors. Attempt to change/modify as many as possible. Note total cholesterol profile.

2. Monitor LFTs prior to starting treatment, 6-8 weeks into therapy, 3 months later, then yearly if stable; 12 weeks after a dose increase.

3. Evaluate on a standard cholesterol-lowering diet before giving fluvastatin unless client has metabolic syndrome, increased risk factors, HTN with microalbuminuria or diabetes. Continue diet during treatment.

CLIENT/FAMILY TEACHING

1. May be taken with or without food but is usually consumed with the evening meal.

2. Drugs are used to lower blood cholesterol and fat levels, which have been proven to promote CAD.

3. Practice reliable contraception; report if pregnancy suspected or desired.
4. Must continue risk factor reduction, dietary restrictions of saturated fat and cholesterol, and regular exercise programs in addition to drug therapy in the overall goal of lowering cholesterol levels and CHD.
5. Report any muscle pain or weakness, especially with fever or severe fatigue, or other adverse effects. Keep scheduled lab visits.
6. Avoid alcohol consumption.

OUTCOMES/EVALUATE
↓ Triglycerides, LDL, and total cholesterol levels

Fondaparinux sodium ■

(**fon**-dah-**PAIR**-in-uks)

CLASSIFICATION(S):
Anticoagulant, antithrombin
PREGNANCY CATEGORY: B
Rx: Arixtra

ACTION/KINETICS
Antithrombotic action is due to antithrombin III (ATIII)-mediated selective inhibition of Factor Xa. By selectively binding to ATIII, fondaparinux potentiates the innate neutralization of Factor Xa by ATIII. Neutralization of Factor Xa interrupts the blood coagulation cascade and thus inhibits thrombin formation and thrombus development. Does not inactivate thrombin (activated Factor II), has no known effect on platelet function, and does not affect fibrinolytic activity or bleeding time. Rapidly and completely absorbed following SC administration. **Maximum levels:** 2 hr. Does not significantly bind to plasma proteins or RBCs. Excreted unchanged in the urine. $t\frac{1}{2}$, **elimination:** 17–21 hr. Elimination is prolonged in the elderly, in those with renal impairment, and in those weighing less than 50 kg. Anticoagulant effect may last for 2–4 days after discontinuation in clients with nor-

mal renal function and even longer in those with renal impairment.

USES
(1) Prophylaxis of deep vein thrombosis in clients undergoing hip fracture surgery, hip replacement surgery, or knee replacement surgery. May be used for up to 60 days in clients undergoing hip fracture surgery. (2) With warfarin to treat acute DVT. (3) With warfarin to treat acute pulmonary embolism when initial therapy is started in the hospital.

CONTRAINDICATIONS
IM use. In those with severe renal impairment (C_{CR} <30 mL/min) or with body weight <50 kg needing prophylactic therapy and undergoing hip-fracture or knee-replacement surgery (due to increased risk for major bleeding episodes). In those with active major bleeding, bacterial endocarditis, thrombocytopenia associated with a positive in vitro test for antiplatelet antibody in the presence of fondaparinux, or with known sensitivitiy to fondaparinux.

SPECIAL CONCERNS
■ (1) When epidural/spinal anesthesia is used, clients anticoagulated or scheduled to be anticoagulated with low molecular weight heparins, heparinoids, or fondaparinux for prevention of thromboembolic complications are at risk of developing an epidural or spinal hematoma that can cause long-term or permanent paralysis. The risk of such events is increased by the use of indwelling epidural catheters for administration of analgesia or by the comcomitant use of drugs affecting hemostasis, such as NSAIDs, platelet inhibitors, or other anticoagulants. The risk also seems to be increased by traumatic or repeated epidural or spinal puncture. (2) Frequently monitor clients for signs and symptoms of neurologic impairment. If neurologic compromise is noted, urgent treatment is necessary. (3) Consider the potential benefit vs risk before neuraxial intervention in clients anticoagulated or to be anticoagulated for thromboprophylaxis.■ The risk of hemorrhage increases with increasing renal impairment. Use with caution during lactation, in moderate renal impair-

ment (C_{CR} 30–50 mL/min), in the elderly, in those with a history of heparin-induced thrombocytopenia, in those with a bleeding diathesis, uncontrolled arterial hypertension, history of recent GI ulceration, diabetic retinopathy, and hemorrhage. Use with extreme caution in conditions with increased risk of hemorrhage, including congenital or acquired bleeding disorders, active ulcerative and angiodysplastic GI disease, hemorrhagic stroke, in those treated concomitantly with platelet inhibitors, or shortly after brain, spinal, or ophthalmologic surgery. Safety and efficacy have not been determined in children.

SIDE EFFECTS
Bleeding. The most common side effect is *bleeding complications* which include intracranial, cerebral, retroperitoneal, intra-ocular, pericardial, or spinal bleeding, bleeding in the adrenal gland, or reoperation due to bleeding. **CV:** Edema, hypotension, post-operative hemorrhage. **GI:** N&V, constipation, diarrhea, dyspepsia. **CNS:** Insomnia, dizziness, confusion, headache. **GU:** UTI, urinary retention. **Dermatologic:** Hematoma, purpura, rash, bullous eruption. **Miscellaneous:** Thrombocytopenia; injection site bleeding, rash, pruritus; anemia, fever, increased wound drainage, pain.

LABORATORY TEST CONSIDERATIONS
↑ AST, ALT. Hypokalemia.

HOW SUPPLIED
Injection: 2.5 mg/0.5 mL

DOSAGE
• **SC**
  Prophylaxis of DVT in hip fracture, hip or knee replacement surgery.
Adults, initial: 2.5 mg given 6–8 hr after surgery. Administration before 6 hr after surgery has been associated with an increased risk of major bleeding. **Duration:** Give 2.5 mg once daily for 5–9 days (up to 11 days has been tolerated).
  Treatment of actue DVT without pulmonary embolism and of acute pulmonary embolism.
Adults: 5 mg/day for clients weighing less than 50 kg, 7.5 mg for those weighing 50–100 kg, and 10 mg for those over 100 kg. Continue therapy for at least 5 days and until an INR of 2.0–3.0 is achieved with warfarin sodium.

NURSING CONSIDERATIONS
ADMINISTRATION/STORAGE
1. Stop therapy if major bleeding occurs or coagulation indicators change unexpectedly.
2. Drug is provided in a single dose, prefilled syringe affixed with an automatic needle protection system.
3. Can not be used interchangeably (unit for unit) with heparin, low molecular weight heparins, or heparinoids as they differ in the manufacturing process, anti-Xa and anti-IIa activity, units, and dosage.
4. To avoid loss of drug with the prefilled syringe, do not expel the air bubble from the syringe before injection.
5. Do not mix with other injections or infusions.
6. Give in the fatty tissue, alternating injection sites (i.e., between the left and right anterolateral or the left and right posterolateral abdominal wall).
7. Store between 15–30°C (59–86°F). Keep out of the reach of children.

ASSESSMENT
1. Note condition(s) requiring therapy, onset, and estimated duration of therapy.
2. Assess for any conditions that may affect therapy (i.e. age, weight, history of GI ulcerations, diabetic retinopathy, uncontrolled HTN, bleeding diathesis/disorders, hemorrhage, or heparin induced thrombocytopenia).
3. Monitor all sites, incisions, and orifices for bleeding. Assess mobility and adherence to exercise program.
4. Assess carefully for S&S of neurologic impairment; anticoagulated clients undergoing epidural/spinal anesthesia may sustain a spinal/epidural hematoma which could result in paralysis.
5. Monitor CBC, INR, K+, renal and LFTs.

CLIENT/FAMILY TEACHING
1. Drug is used to prevent the formation of blood clots in those extremities that have compromised functioning due to a surgical procedure. Clots may enter the circulation and be transported

to the lung causing a pulmonary embolus which can be lethal.

2. Review guidelines for the appropriate SC method of administration and demonstrate for provider. Start with proper skin prep, pinching and holding a fold of skin for the injection, injecting the solution, removing the syringe, and discarding into a designated container. The syringe has a retractable needle to prevent punctures. Rotate sites to prevent hardening of the tissues.

3. Store prefilled syringes and used syringes safely out of reach and dispose of properly.

4. Report any adverse side effects as well as extremity pain, chest pain, SOB, or any other unusual symptoms.

5. Avoid OTC agents including aspirin, NSAIDs and other agents without provider approval. Keep all F/U visits to evaluate incision site, response to therapy, recovery, and labs.

OUTCOMES/EVALUATE

DVT(blood clot) prevention in those undergoing hip fracture repair or hip/knee replacements

Fosinopril sodium ■ⓒ

(foh-**SIN**-oh-prill)

CLASSIFICATION(S):
Antihypertensive, ACE inhibitor
PREGNANCY CATEGORY: D
Rx: Monopril

SEE ALSO ANGIOTENSIN-CONVERTING ENZYME INHIBITORS.

ACTION/KINETICS
About 36% bioavailable. **Onset:** 1 hr. **Time to peak serum levels:** About 3 hr. Metabolized in the liver to the active fosinoprilat. **Peak effect:** 2–6 hr. **t ½:** 12 hr for fosinoprilat (prolonged in impaired renal function) following IV administration. **Duration:** 24 hr. Approximately 50% excreted through the urine and 50% in the feces. Food decreases the rate, but not the extent, of absorption of fosinopril. Over 99% bound to plasma proteins.

USES
(1) Alone or in combination with other antihypertensive agents (especially thiazide diuretics) to treat hypertension. (2) Treat CHF as adjunctive therapy when added to conventional therapy, including diuretics with or without digoxin.

CONTRAINDICATIONS
Use during lactation.

SPECIAL CONCERNS
■When used during the second and third trimesters of pregnancy, injury and even death can result in the developing fetus. When pregnancy is detected, discontinue as soon as possible.■

SIDE EFFECTS
CV: Orthostatic hypotension, chest pain, hypotension, palpitations, angina pectoris, *CVA, MI,* rhythm disturbances, TIA, tachycardia, *hypertensive crisis,* claudication, bradycardia, hypertension, conduction disorder, *sudden death, cardiorespiratory arrest, shock.* **CNS:** Headache, dizziness, fatigue, confusion, memory disturbance, depression, behavior change, tremors, drowsiness, mood change, insomnia, vertigo, sleep disturbances. **GI:** N&V, diarrhea, abdominal pain, constipation, dry mouth, dysphagia, taste disturbance, abdominal distention, flatulence, heartburn, appetite changes, weight changes. **Hepatic:** Hepatitis, pancreatitis, hepatomegaly, *hepatic failure.* **Respiratory:** Cough, sinusitis, dyspnea, URI, *bronchospasm,* asthma, pharyngitis, laryngitis, tracheobronchitis, abnormal breathing, sinus abnormalities. **Hematologic:** Leukopenia, eosinophilia, decreases in hemoglobin (mean of 0.1 g/dL) or hematocrit, neutropenia. **Dermatologic:** Diaphoresis, photosensitivity, flushing, exfoliative dermatitis, pruritus, rash, urticaria. **Body as a whole:** Angioedema, muscle cramps, fever, syncope, influenza, cold sensation, pain, myalgia, arthralgia, arthritis, edema, weakness, musculoskeletal pain. **GU:** Decreased libido, sexual dysfunction, renal insufficiency, urinary frequency, abnormal urination, kidney pain. **Miscellaneous:** Paresthesias, tinnitus, gout, lymphadenopathy, rhinitis, epistaxis, vision disturbances, eye irrita-

tion, swelling/weakness of extremities, abnormal vocalization, pneumonia, muscle ache.

LABORATORY TEST CONSIDERATIONS
↑ Serum potassium. Transient ↓ H&H. False low measurement of serum digoxin levels with DigiTab RIA Kit for Digoxin.

HOW SUPPLIED
Tablet: 10 mg, 20 mg, 40 mg

DOSAGE
- **TABLETS**
  Hypertension.
Adults: Initial: 10 mg once daily; **then,** adjust dose depending on BP response at peak (2–6 hr after dosing) and trough (24 hr after dosing) blood levels. **Maintenance:** Usually 20–40 mg/day, although some clients manifest beneficial effects at doses up to 80 mg, **Children, 6 to 16 years:** ≥50 kg: 5 to 10 mg once daily as monotherapy.
  In clients taking diuretics.
Discontinue diuretic 2–3 days before starting fosinopril. If diuretic cannot be discontinued, use an initial dose of 10 mg fosinopril.
  Congestive heart failure.
Initial: 10 mg once daily; **then,** following initial dose, observe the client for at least 2 hr for the presence of hypotension or orthostasis (if either is present, monitor until BP stabilizes). An initial dose of 5 mg is recommended in heart failure with moderate to severe renal failure or in those who have had significant diuresis. Increase the dose over several weeks, not to exceed a maximum of 40 mg daily (usual effective range is 20–40 mg once daily).

NURSING CONSIDERATIONS
Ⓒ Do not confuse Monopril with minoxidil (an antihypertensive).

ADMINISTRATION/STORAGE
1. If antihypertensive effect decreases at the end of the dosing interval with once-daily dosing, consider twice a day administration.
2. If also taking a diuretic, discontinue the diuretic 2–3 days prior to beginning fosinopril therapy. If BP is not controlled, restart the diuretic. If the diuret-

ic cannot be discontinued, give an initial dose of 10 mg fosinopril.
3. Do not adjust the dose of fosinopril in renal insufficiency except as noted in *Dosage.*

ASSESSMENT
Note other agents trialed and outcome. Monitor BP, CBC, electrolytes, microalbumin, liver, and renal function studies.

CLIENT/FAMILY TEACHING
1. Take as directed with or without food. BP control does not exceed 24 hr; take at same time(s) each day.
2. May initially cause dizziness and light-headedness so use care. Avoid dehydration and use caution in hot weather and with increased exercise. Monitor and record BP at different times during the day.
3. Avoid OTC agents without provider approval; also salt substitutes containing potassium should be avoided.
4. Change positions slowly to avoid sudden drop in BP.
5. Use reliable contraception. Stop drug and report if pregnancy suspected.
6. Report any adverse side effects especially S&S infection, sore throat, swelling of hands and feet, chest pain, SOB, mouth sores, unusual bruising/bleeding, or irregular heart beat.
7. Continue life style changes aimed at controlling BP: salt restriction, regular exercise, weight reduction, and smoking and alcohol cessation.

OUTCOMES/EVALUATE
Control of BP

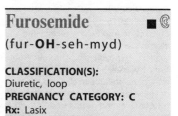

Furosemide   ∎Ⓒ
(fur-**OH**-seh-myd)

CLASSIFICATION(S):
Diuretic, loop
PREGNANCY CATEGORY: C
Rx: Lasix
🍁**Rx:** Apo-Furosemide, Lasix Special

SEE ALSO *DIURETICS, LOOP.*

ACTION/KINETICS

Inhibits the reabsorption of sodium and chloride in the proximal and distal tubules as well as the ascending loop of Henle; this results in the excretion of sodium, chloride, and, to a lesser degree, potassium and bicarbonate ions. The resulting urine is more acid. Diuretic action is independent of changes in clients' acid-base balance. Has a slight antihypertensive effect. **Onset: PO, IM:** 30–60 min; **IV:** 5 min. **Peak: PO, IM:** 1–2 hr; **IV:** 20–60 min. **t ½:** About 2 hr after PO use. **Duration: PO, IM:** 6–8 hr; **IV:** 2 hr. Metabolized in the liver and excreted through the urine. May be effective for clients resistant to thiazides and for those with reduced GFRs.

USES

(1) Edema associated with CHF, nephrotic syndrome, hepatic cirrhosis, and renal disease (2) IV for acute pulmonary edema. (3) PO to treat hypertension alone or in combination with other antihypertensive agents.

CONTRAINDICATIONS

Anuria, hypersensitivity to furosemide, lactation.

SPECIAL CONCERNS

■Furosemide is a potent diuretic. Excess amounts can lead to profound diuresis with water and electrolyte depletion. Careful medical attention is needed; individualize dosage.■ Use with caution in premature infants and neonates due to prolonged half-life in these clients (dosing interval must be extended). Geriatric clients may be more sensitive to the usual adult dose. Allergic reactions may be seen in clients who show hypersensitivity to sulfonamides. Never use with ethacrynic acid.

SIDE EFFECTS

Electrolyte and fluid effects: Fluid and electrolyte depletion leading to dehydration, hypovolemia, thromboembolism. Hypokalemia and hypochloremia may cause metabolic alkalosis. Hyperuricemia, azotemia, hyponatremia. **GI:** Nausea, oral and gastric irritation, vomiting, anorexia, diarrhea (especially in children) or constipation, cramps, pancreatitis, jaundice, ischemic hepatitis. **Otic:** Tinnitus, hearing impairment (may

be reversible or permanent), reversible deafness. Usually following rapid IV or IM administration of high doses. **CNS:** Vertigo, headache, dizziness, blurred vision, restlessness, paresthesias, xanthopsia. **CV:** Orthostatic hypotension, thrombophlebitis, chronic aortitis. **Hematologic:** Anemia, thrombocytopenia, neutropenia, leukopenia, *agranulocytosis,* purpura. *Rarely, aplastic anemia.* **Allergic:** Rashes, pruritus, urticaria, photosensitivity, exfoliative dermatitis, vasculitis, erythema multiforme. **Miscellaneous:** Interstitial nephritis, fever, weakness, hyperglycemia, glycosuria, exacerbation of, aggravation of or worsening of SLE, increased perspiration, muscle spasms, urinary bladder spasm, urinary frequency.

Following IV use. Thrombophlebitis, *cardiac arrest.*

Following IM use: Pain and irritation at injection site, *cardiac arrest.* Because this drug is resistant to the effects of pressor amines and potentiates the effects of muscle relaxants, it is recommended that the PO drug be discontinued 1 week before surgery and the IV drug 2 days before surgery.

OD OVERDOSE MANAGEMENT

Symptoms: Profound water loss, electrolyte depletion (manifested by weakness, anorexia, vomiting, lethargy, cramps, mental confusion, dizziness), decreased blood volume, *circulatory collapse (possibly vascular thrombosis and embolism). Treatment:* Replace fluid and electrolytes. Monitor urine electrolyte output and serum electrolytes. Induce emesis or perform gastric lavage. Oxygen or artificial respiration may be needed. Treat symptoms.

ADDITIONAL DRUG INTERACTIONS

Charcoal / ↓ Absorption of furosemide from GI tract
Clofibrate / Enhanced diuretic effect
Hydantoins / ↓ Diuretic effect of furosemide
Propranolol / ↑ Plasma propranolol levels

HOW SUPPLIED

Injection: 10 mg /mL; *Oral Solution:* 10 mg/mL, 40 mg/5 mL; *Tablet:* 20 mg, 40 mg, 80 mg

---

Bold Italic = life threatening side effect   ■ = black box warning   ✦ = Available in Canada

DOSAGE
- **ORAL SOLUTION, TABLETS**
  Edema.

Adults, initial: 20–80 mg/day as a single dose. For resistant cases, dosage can be increased by 20–40 mg q 6–8 hr until desired diuretic response is attained. Maximum daily dose should not exceed 600 mg. **Pediatric, initial:** 2 mg/kg as a single dose; **then,** dose can be increased by 1–2 mg/kg q 6–8 hr until desired response is attained; maximum dose should not exceed 6 mg/kg.
  Hypertension.

Adults, initial: 40 mg twice a day. Adjust dosage depending on response.

- **IV, IM**
  Edema.

Adults, initial: 20–40 mg; if response inadequate after 2 hr, increase dose in 20-mg increments. **Pediatric, initial:** 1 mg/kg given slowly; if response inadequate after 2 hr, increase dose by 1 mg/kg. Doses greater than 6 mg/kg should not be given.
  Antihypercalcemic.

Adults: 80–100 mg for severe cases; dose may be repeated q 1–2 hr if needed.

- **IV**
  Acute pulmonary edema.

Adults: 40 mg slowly over 1–2 min; if response inadequate after 1 hr, give 80 mg slowly over 1–2 min. Concomitant oxygen and digitalis may be used.

NURSING CONSIDERATIONS
Ⓒ Do not confuse Lasix with Lanoxin (a cardiac glycoside).

ADMINISTRATION/STORAGE
1. Give 2–4 days per week.
2. Food decreases the bioavailability of furosemide and ultimately the degree of diuresis.
3. Slight discoloration resulting from light does not affect potency. However, do not dispense discolored tablets or injection.
4. If used with other antihypertensives, reduce the dose of other agents by at least 50% when furosemide is added in order to prevent an excessive drop in BP.
5. Store in light-resistant containers at room temperature (15–30°C, or 59–86°F).
6. In CHF or chronic renal failure, oral and parenteral doses of 2–2.5 g/day (or higher) are well tolerated.
Ⅳ 7. Give IV injections slowly over 1–2 min.
8. Do not mix with solutions with a pH below 5.5. After pH adjustment, furosemide can be mixed with NaCl injection, RL injection, and D5W and infused at a rate not to exceed 4 mg/min, to prevent ototoxicity.
9. A precipitate may form if mixed with gentamicin, netilmicin, or milrinone in either D5W or NSS.

ASSESSMENT
1. Note indications for therapy and other agents trialed. When more than 40 mg/day is required, give in divided doses, i.e., 40 mg PO twice a day (7 a.m. and 3 p.m.)
2. With renal impairment or if receiving other ototoxic drugs, observe for ototoxicity.
3. Assess closely for signs of vascular thrombosis and embolism, particularly in the elderly. With history of gout, monitor uric acid levels.
4. Monitor BP, weight, edema, breath sounds, I&O and electrolytes; observe for S&S of hypokalemia.
5. With rapid diuresis, observe for dehydration and circulatory collapse; monitor BP and pulse.
6. With chronic use, assess for thiamine deficiency; if used with zaroxlyn assess for low phosphate levels.

CLIENT/FAMILY TEACHING
1. Take in the morning on an empty stomach to enhance absorption and to avoid interruption of sleep. May take with food or milk if GI upset. Time administration to participate in social activities and to minimize need to interrupt sleep to void frequently.
2. Immediately report any muscle weakness/cramps, dizziness, ringing in the ears, sore throat, fever, severe abdominal pain, numbness, or tingling.
3. Drug may cause BP drop. Change positions from lying to standing slowly.

Avoid alcohol and do not exercise heavily in hot weather.

4. Refrigerate solution. Sorbitol in the solution may result in diarrhea, especially in children.

5. Consult provider before taking excessive aspirin for any reason. Salicylate intoxication occurs at lower levels than normal because of competition at the renal excretory sites.

6. Use sunscreens and protective clothing when sun exposed to minimize the effects of drug-induced photosensitivity.

7. Management of end stage heart disease requires diligent monitoring, management, and titration on provider and client part; keep all visits and report any changes or adverse effects.

8. Monitor weights; report any gains of > 2 lb per day or > 10 lb per week.

9. Supplement diet with vegetables and fruits that are high in potassium (bananas, oranges, peaches, dried dates) if oral supplements are not prescribed. Those on a salt-restricted diet should not increase salt intake; NSAIDs and alpha blockers may also cause sodium retention.

OUTCOMES/EVALUATE
- Enhanced diuresis
- Resolution of pulmonary edema
- ↓ Dependent edema
- ↓ Serum calcium levels

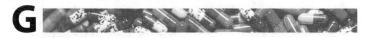

Gemfibrozil ©

(jem-**FIH**-broh-zill)

CLASSIFICATION(S):
Antihyperlipidemic, fibric acid derivative
PREGNANCY CATEGORY: C
Rx: Lopid
♣Rx: Apo-Gemfibrozil, Gen-Gemfibrozil, Novo-Gemfibrozil, Nu-Gemfibrozil, PMS-Gemfibrozil

ACTION/KINETICS
Gemfibrozil, a fibric acid derivative, decreases triglycerides, cholesterol, and VLDL and increases HDL; LDL levels either decrease or do not change. Also, decreases hepatic triglyceride production by inhibiting peripheral lipolysis and decreasing extraction of free fatty acids by the liver. Also, gemfibrozil decreases VLDL synthesis by inhibiting synthesis of VLDL carrier apolipoprotein B as well as inhibits peripheral lipolysis and decreases hepatic extraction of free fatty acids (thus decreasing hepatic triglyceride production). May be beneficial in inhibiting development of atherosclerosis. **Onset:** 2–5 days. **Peak plasma levels:** 1–2 hr; **t ½:** 1.5 hr. Metabolized in the liver with nearly 70% excreted in the urine.

USES
(1) Hypertriglyceridemia (type IV and type V hyperlipidemia) unresponsive to dietary control or in clients who are at risk of pancreatitis and abdominal pain. (2) Reduce risk of coronary heart disease in clients with type IIb hyperlipidemia who have not responded to diet, weight loss, exercise, and other drug therapy.

CONTRAINDICATIONS
Gallbladder disease, primary biliary cirrhosis, hepatic or renal dysfunction. Lactation.

SPECIAL CONCERNS
Safety and efficacy have not been established in children. The dose may have to be reduced in geriatric clients due to age-related decreases in renal function.

SIDE EFFECTS
GI: Cholelithiasis, abdominal or epigastric pain, N&V, diarrhea, dyspepsia, constipation, acute appendicitis, colitis, pancreatitis, cholestatic jaundice, hepatoma. **CNS:** Dizziness, headache, fatigue, vertigo, somnolence, paresthesia,

---

hypesthesia, depression, confusion, syncope, peripheral neuritis, **seizures. CV:** Atrial fibrillation, extrasystole, peripheral vascular disease, **intracerebral hemorrhage. Hematopoietic:** Anemia, leukopenia, eosinophilia, thrombocytopenia, bone marrow hypoplasia. **Musculoskeletal:** Painful extremities, arthralgia, myalgia, myopathy, myositis, myasthenia, rhabdomyolysis, synovitis. **Allergic:** Urticaria, lupus-like syndrome, angioedema, **laryngeal edema,** vasculitis, **anaphylaxis. Dermatologic:** Eczema, dermatitis, pruritus, skin rashes, exfoliative dermatitis, alopecia. **GU:** Impotence, decreased libido, decreased male fertility, impaired renal function, UTI. **Ophthalmic:** Blurred vision, retinal edema, cataracts. **Miscellaneous:** Increased chance of viral and bacterial infections, taste perversion, weight loss.

LABORATORY TEST CONSIDERATIONS
↑ AST, ALT, LDH, CPK, alkaline phosphatase, bilirubin. Hypokalemia, hyperglycemia. Positive antinuclear antibody. ↓ Hemoglobin, WBCs, hematocrit.

OD OVERDOSE MANAGEMENT
Symptoms: Abdominal cramping, N&V, diarrhea, abnormal LFTs, ↑ Serum creatine phosphokinase, joint and muscle pain.

DRUG INTERACTIONS
Anticoagulants, oral / ↑ Anticoagulant effects; adjust dosage
Cyclosporine / ↓ Cyclosporine effect
Lovastatin / Possible rhabdomyolysis
Repaglinide / Significant ↑ repaglinide plasma levels R/T ↓ metabolism by CYP2C8
Rosuvastatin / Two-fold ↑ Rosuvastatin plasma levels
Simvastatin / Possible rhabdomyolysis
Sulfonylureas / ↑ Hypoglycemic effect

HOW SUPPLIED
Tablet: 600 mg

DOSAGE
• **TABLETS**
Adults: 600 mg twice a day 30 min before the morning and evening meal. Dosage has not been established in children. Discontinue if significant improvement not observed within 3 months.

NURSING CONSIDERATIONS
ℭ Do not confuse Lopid with Lorabid (a beta-lactam antibiotic).

ASSESSMENT
1. Document serum HDL and TG levels and note any previous therapy utilized.
2. Monitor CBC and LFTs during therapy; identify risk factors.
3. Assess compliance with therapeutic regimens and life-style changes including restriction of fat in diet, blood sugar control, weight reduction, regular exercise, and avoidance of alcohol.

CLIENT/FAMILY TEACHING
1. Take 30 min before meals.
2. Take as directed; continue to follow prescribed dietary guidelines restricting sugar and CHO, and regular exercise program to reduce risk factors.
3. Use caution when driving or performing other dangerous tasks until drug effects realized; may experience dizziness or blurred vision.
4. Report any unusual bruising or bleeding. If also on anticoagulant therapy, a reduction in anticoagulant may be necessary.
5. Limit intake of alcohol. Report for all F/U lab tests for LFTs and lipid panel.
6. Report any muscle pain/cramps, RUQ abdominal pain or change in stool color or consistency.
7. Report any S&S of gallstones, such as abdominal pain and vomiting.

OUTCOMES/EVALUATE
↓ Serum triglyceride levels ↑ HDL

Guanfacine hydrochloride

(**GWON**-fah-seen)

CLASSIFICATION(S):
Antihypertensive, centrally-acting
PREGNANCY CATEGORY: B
Rx: Tenex

SEE ALSO ANTIHYPERTENSIVE AGENTS.

ACTION/KINETICS
Thought to act by central stimulation of alpha-2 receptors. Causes a decrease in

peripheral sympathetic output and HR resulting in a decrease in BP. May also manifest a direct peripheral alpha-2 receptor stimulant action. **Onset:** 2 hr. **Peak plasma levels:** 1–4 hr. **Peak effect:** 6–12 hr. **t ½:** 12–23 hr. **Duration:** 24 hr. Approximately 50% excreted through the kidneys unchanged.

USES
Hypertension alone or with a thiazide diuretic. *Investigational:* Withdrawal from heroin use, to reduce the frequency of migraine headaches.

CONTRAINDICATIONS
Hypersensitivity to guanfacine. Acute hypertension associated with toxemia. Children less than 12 years of age.

SPECIAL CONCERNS
Use with caution during lactation and in clients with recent MI, cerebrovascular disease, chronic renal or hepatic failure, or severe coronary insufficiency. Geriatric clients may be more sensitive to the hypotensive and sedative effects. Safety and efficacy in children less than 12 years of age have not been determined.

SIDE EFFECTS
GI: Dry mouth, constipation, nausea, abdominal pain, diarrhea, dyspepsia, dysphagia, taste perversion or alterations in taste. **CNS:** Sedation, weakness, dizziness, headache, fatigue, insomnia, amnesia, confusion, depression, vertigo, agitation, anxiety, malaise, nervousness, tremor. **CV:** Bradycardia, substernal pain, palpitations, syncope, chest pain, tachycardia, cardiac fibrillation, CHF, heart block, MI (rare), cardiovascular accident (rare). **Ophthalmic:** Visual disturbances, conjunctivitis, iritis, blurred vision. **Dermatologic:** Pruritus, dermatitis, purpura, sweating, skin rash with exfoliation, alopecia, rash. **GU:** Decreased libido, impotence, urinary incontinence or frequency, testicular disorder, nocturia, acute renal failure. **Musculoskeletal:** Leg cramps, hypokinesia, arthralgia, leg pain, myalgia. **Other:** Rhinitis, tinnitus, dyspnea, paresthesias, paresis, asthenia, edema, abnormal LFTs.

OD OVERDOSE MANAGEMENT
Symptoms: Drowsiness, bradycardia, lethargy, hypotension. *Treatment:* Gastric lavage. Supportive therapy, as needed. The drug is not dialyzable.

DRUG INTERACTIONS
Additive sedative effects when used concomitantly with CNS depressants.

HOW SUPPLIED
Tablet: 1 mg, 2 mg

DOSAGE
• **TABLETS**
  Hypertension.
Initial: 1 mg/day alone or with other antihypertensives; if satisfactory results are not obtained in 3–4 weeks, dosage may be increased by 1 mg at 1–2-week intervals up to a maximum of 3 mg/day in one to two divided doses.
  Heroin withdrawal.
0.03–1.5 mg/day.
  Reduce frequency of migraine headaches.
1 mg/day for 12 weeks.

NURSING CONSIDERATIONS
ADMINISTRATION/STORAGE
1. Divide the daily dose if a decrease in BP is not maintained for over 24 hr; however, the incidence of side effects increases.
2. Adverse effects increase significantly when dose exceeds 3 mg/day.
3. Initiate antihypertensive therapy in clients already taking a thiazide diuretic.
4. Abrupt cessation may result in increases in plasma and urinary catecholamines, symptoms of nervousness and anxiety, and BPs greater than those prior to therapy.

ASSESSMENT
1. Document indications for therapy, onset of symptoms, and any previous agents used and the outcome.
2. Determine the extent of CAD, and note any evidence of renal or liver dysfunction.

CLIENT/FAMILY TEACHING
1. To minimize daytime drowsiness, take at bedtime. Do not perform activities that require mental alertness until drug effects realized.
2. Do not stop drug abruptly; may experience rebound effect. Continue life style changes to ensure BP control, i.e., salt restriction, lipid control, absence of proteinuria, and weight control.

Bold Italic = life threatening side effect   ■ = black box warning   ✦ = Available in Canada

3. Avoid alcohol. May use sugarless gum, ice chips, or sips of water for dry mouth.

4. May cause constipation or skin rash; report if persistent or severe.

5. Avoid OTC cough/cold remedies. Keep record of BP for provider review.

OUTCOMES/EVALUATE
- ↓ BP
- ↓ S&S of heroin withdrawal
- ↓ Migraine headaches

H

Heparin sodium lock flush solution
(HEP-ah-rin)

CLASSIFICATION(S):
Anticoagulant, heparin
PREGNANCY CATEGORY: C
Rx: Heparin I.V. Flush Syringe, Heparin Lock Flush, Hep-Flush 10, Hep-Lock, Hep-Lock U/P

Heparin sodium and sodium chloride
PREGNANCY CATEGORY: C
Rx: Heparin Sodium and 0.45% Sodium Chloride, Heparin Sodium and 0.9% Sodium Chloride

Heparin sodium injection
PREGNANCY CATEGORY: C
✦**Rx:** Hepalean, Hepalean-Lok, Heparin Leo

ACTION/KINETICS
Anticoagulants do not dissolve previously formed clots, but they do forestall their enlargement and prevent new clots from forming. Heparin potentiates the inhibitory action of antithrombin III on various coagulation factors including factors IIa, IXa, Xa, XIa, and XIIa. This occurs due to the formation of a complex with antithrombin III and causing a conformational change in the antithrombin III molecule. Inhibition of factor Xa results in interference with thrombin generation; thus, the action of thrombin in coagulation is inhibited. Heparin also increases the rate of formation of antithrombin III–thrombin complex causing inactivation of thrombin and preventing the conversion of fibrinogen to fibrin. By inhibiting the activation of fibrin-stabilizing factor by thrombin, heparin also prevents formation of a stable fibrin clot. Therapeutic doses of heparin prolong thrombin time, whole blood clotting time, activated clotting time, and PTT. Heparin also decreases the levels of triglycerides by releasing lipoprotein lipase from tissues; the resultant hydrolysis of triglycerides causes increased blood levels of free fatty acids. **Onset: IV,** immediate; **deep SC:** 20–60 min. **Peak plasma levels, after SC:** 2–4 hr. **t ½:** 30–180 min in healthy persons. t ½ increases with dose, severe renal disease, and cirrhosis and in anephric clients and decreases with pulmonary embolism and liver impairment other than cirrhosis. **Metabolism:** Probably by reticuloendothelial system, although up to 50% is excreted unchanged in the urine. Clotting time returns to normal within 2–6 hr.

USES
(1) Pulmonary/peripheral arterial embolism. (2) Prophylaxis and treatment of venous thrombosis and its extension. (3) Atrial fibrillation with embolization. (4) Diagnosis and treatment of DIC. (5) Low doses to prevent DVT and PE in pregnant clients with a history of thromboembolism, urology clients over 40 years of age, clients with stroke or heart failure, AMI or pulmonary infec-

tion, high-risk surgery clients, moderate and high-risk gynecologic clients with no malignancy, neurology clients with extracranial problems, and clients with severe musculoskeletal trauma. (6) Prophylaxis of clotting in blood transfusions, extracorporeal circulation, dialysis procedures, blood samples for lab tests, and arterial and heart surgery. *Investigational:* Prophylaxis of post-MI, CVA, and LV thrombi. By continuous infusion to treat myocardial ischemia in unstable angina refractory to usual treatment. Adjunct to treat coronary occlusion with AMI. Prophylaxis of cerebral thrombosis in evolving stroke.

Heparin lock flush solution: Dilute solutions are used to maintain patency of indwelling catheters used for IV therapy or blood sampling. Not to be used therapeutically.

CONTRAINDICATIONS
Active bleeding, blood dyscrasias (or other disorders characterized by bleeding tendencies such as hemophilia), clients with frail or weakened blood vessels, purpura, thrombocytopenia, liver disease with hypoprothrombinemia, suspected intracranial hemorrhage, suppurative thrombophlebitis, inaccessible ulcerative lesions (especially of the GI tract), open wounds, extensive denudation of the skin, and increased capillary permeability (as in ascorbic acid deficiency). IM use.

Do not administer during surgery of the eye, brain, or spinal cord or during continuous tube drainage of the stomach or small intestine. Use is also contraindicated in subacute endocarditis, shock, threatened abortion, severe hypertension, diverticulitis, colitis, SBE, or hypersensitivity to drug. Premature neonates due to the possibility of a fatal 'gasping syndrome.' Also, regional anesthesia and lumbar block, vitamin K deficiency, leukemia with bleeding tendencies, open wounds or ulcerations, acute nephritis, or impaired hepatic or renal function. In the presence of drainage tubes in any orifice. Alcoholism.

SPECIAL CONCERNS
Use with caution in menstruation, in pregnant women (heparin may cause

hypoprothrombinemia in the infant), during lactation, during the postpartum period, and following cerebrovascular accidents. Geriatric clients may be more susceptible to developing bleeding complications, unusual hair loss, and itching.

SIDE EFFECTS
CV: *Hemorrhage ranging from minor local ecchymoses to major hemorrhagic complications from any organ or tissue.* Higher incidence is seen in women over 60 years of age. Hemorrhagic reactions are more likely to occur in prophylactic administration during surgery than in the treatment of thromboembolic disease. White clot syndrome. **Hematologic:** Thrombocytopenia (both early and late). **Hypersensitivity:** Chills, fever, urticaria are the most common. Rarely, asthma, lacrimation, headache, N&V, rhinitis, *shock, anaphylaxis.* Allergic vasospastic reaction within 6–10 days after initiation of therapy (lasts 4–6 hr) including painful, ischemic, cyanotic limbs. Use a test dose of 1,000 units in clients with a history of asthma or allergic disease. **Miscellaneous:** Hyperkalemia, cutaneous necrosis, osteoporosis (after long-term high doses), delayed transient alopecia, priapism, suppressed aldosterone synthesis. Discontinuance of heparin has resulted in rebound hyperlipemia. **Following IM (usual), SC:** Local irritation, erythema, mild pain, ulceration, hematoma, and tissue sloughing.

LABORATORY TEST CONSIDERATIONS
↑ AST and ALT.

OD OVERDOSE MANAGEMENT
Symptoms: Nosebleeds, hematuria, tarry stools, petechiae, and easy bruising may be the first signs. *Treatment:* Drug withdrawal is usually sufficient to correct heparin overdosage. Protamine sulfate (1%) solution; each mg of protamine neutralizes about 100 USP heparin units.

DRUG INTERACTIONS
Alteplase, recombinant / ↑ Risk of bleeding, especially at arterial puncture sites
Anticoagulants, oral / Additive ↑ PT
Antihistamines / ↓ Effect of heparin

Aspirin / Additive ↑ PT

H *Bromelain* / ↑ Tendency for bleeding

Cephalosporins / ↑ Risk of bleeding R/T additive effect

H *Cinchona bark* / ↑ Anticoagulant effect

Dextran / Additive ↑ PT

Digitalis / ↓ Effect of heparin

Dipyridamole / Additive ↑ PT

H *Feverfew* / Possible additive antiplatelet effect

H *Ginger* / Possible additive antiplatelet effect

H *Ginkgo biloba* / ↑ Effect on blood coagulation

H *Ginseng* / Potential for ↓ effect on platelet aggregation

H *Goldenseal* / Antagonizes action of heparin

Hydroxychloroquine / Additive ↑ PT

Ibuprofen / Additive ↑ PT

Indomethacin / Additive ↑ PT

Insulin / Heparin antagonizes insulin effect

Nicotine / ↓ Effect of heparin

Nitroglycerin / ↓ Effect of heparin

NSAIDs / Additive ↑ PT

Penicillins / ↑ Risk of bleeding R/T possible additive effects

Salicylates / ↑ Risk of bleeding

Streptokinase / Relative resistance to effects of heparin

Tetracyclines / ↓ Effect of heparin

Ticlopidine / Additive ↑ PT

HOW SUPPLIED

Heparin sodium injection: *Injection:* 1,000 units/mL, 2,000 units/mL, 2,500 units/mL, 5,000 units/mL, 7,500 units/mL, 10,000 units/mL, 20,000 units/mL, 40,000 units/mL. **Heparin sodium and sodium chloride:** *Injection:* 200 units/100 mL-0.9% NaCl, 5,000 units/100 mL-0.45%, 10,000 units/100 mL-0.45% NaCl. **Heparin sodium lock flush solution:** 1 units/mL, 10 units/mL, 100 units/mL

DOSAGE————————————

NOTE: Adjusted for each client on the basis of laboratory tests.

• **DEEP SC**
General heparin dosage.
Initial loading dose: 10,000–20,000 units; **maintenance:** 8,000–10,000 units

q 8 hr or 15,000–20,000 units q 12 hr. Use concentrated solution.
Prophylaxis of postoperative thromboembolism.
5,000 units of concentrated solution 2 hr before surgery and 5,000 units q 8–12 hr thereafter for 7 days or until client is ambulatory.

• **INTERMITTENT IV**
General heparin dosage.
Initial loading dose: 10,000 units undiluted or in 50–100 mL saline; **then,** 5,000–10,000 units q 4–6 hr undiluted or in 50–100 mL saline.

• **CONTINUOUS IV INFUSION**
General heparin dosage.
Initial loading dose: 20,000–40,000 units/day in 1,000 mL saline (preceded initially by 5,000 units IV).

• **SPECIAL USES**
Surgery of heart and blood vessels.
Initial, 150–400 units/kg to clients undergoing total body perfusion for open heart surgery. *NOTE:* 300 units/kg may be used for procedures less than 60 min while 400 units/kg is used for procedures lasting more than 60 min. To prevent clotting in the tube system, add heparin to fluids in pump oxygenator.
Extracorporeal renal dialysis.
See instructions on equipment.
Blood transfusion.
400–600 units/100 mL whole blood. 7,500 units should be added to 100 mL 0.9% sodium chloride injection; from this dilution, add 6–8 mL/100 mL whole blood.
Laboratory samples.
70–150 units/10- to 20-mL sample to prevent coagulation.
Heparin lock sets.
To prevent clot formation in a heparin lock set, inject 10–100 units/mL heparin solution through the injection hub in a sufficient quantity to fill the entire set to the needle tip.

NURSING CONSIDERATIONS
ADMINISTRATION/STORAGE
1. Do *not* administer IM.
2. Administer by deep SC injection to minimize local irritation, hematoma, and tissue sloughing and to prolong drug action.

H

• Z-track method: Use any fat roll, but abdominal fat rolls are preferred. Use a ½-in. or ⅝-in. 25- or 27-gauge needle. Grasp skin layer of the fat roll and lift up. Insert needle at about a 45° angle to the skin's fat layer and then administer the medication. Not necessary to aspirate to check if needle is in a blood vessel. Rapidly withdraw the needle while releasing the skin.

• 'Bunch technique' method: Grasp tissue around injection site, creating a tissue roll of about ½ in. in diameter. Insert needle into tissue roll at a 90° angle to the skin surface and inject medication. Not necessary to aspirate. Withdraw needle rapidly when skin is released.

• Do not administer within 2 in. of umbilicus (R/T increased vascularity of area).

3. Do not massage site. Rotate sites of administration.

4. Slight discoloration does not affect potency.

IV 5. Hospitalize for IV therapy.

6. May be diluted in dextrose, NSS, or Ringer's solution and administered over 4–24 hr with an infusion pump.

7. Protect solutions from freezing.

8. Have protamine sulfate, a heparin antagonist, available should excessive bleeding occur.

9. NaCl, 0.9%, is effective in maintaining patency of peripheral (noncentral) intermittent infusion devices and in reducing medical costs. The following procedure is recommended:

• Determine patency by aspirating lock.

• Flush with 2 mL NSS.

• Administer medication therapy. (Flush between drugs.)

• Flush with 2 mL NSS.

• Frequency of flushing to maintain patency when not actively in use varies from every 8 hr to every 24–48 hr.

• This does NOT apply to any central venous access devices. Must use heparin.

ASSESSMENT

1. Note indications for therapy. Identify any bleeding incidents, i.e., bleeding tendencies, family history, or any other incidents of unexplained or active bleeding.

2. Perform test dose (1,000 units SC) on clients with multiple allergies or asthma history.

3. Review drug profile to ensure none interact unfavorably; otherwise, anticipate heparin dosage adjustment.

4. Assess for defects in clotting mechanism or any capillary fragility.

5. Note time frame for therapy (i.e., DVT [initial] 6 months; certain valve replacements—lifetime), and desired INR, PT/PTT and record.

6. Review PMH for conditions that may preclude therapy: alcoholic, chronic GI tract ulcerations, severe renal or liver dysfunction, infections of the endocardium, or PUD which may be a potential site of bleeding. Note any evidence of intracranial hemorrhage.

7. Monitor CBC, PT, PTT, renal, and LFTs.

INTERVENTIONS

1. Post/advise at bedside 'client receiving anticoagulant therapy.'

2. Monitor CBC and PTT closely.

3. Question about bleeding (gums, urine, stools, vomit, bruises). If urine discolored, determine cause, i.e., from drug therapy or hematuria. Indanedione-type anticoagulants turn alkaline urine a red-orange color; acidify urine or test for occult blood.

4. Sudden lumbar pain may indicate retroperitoneal hemorrhage.

5. GI dysfunction may indicate intestinal hemorrhage. Test for blood in urine and feces; check H&H to assess for bleeding.

6. Have protamine sulfate for heparin overdose available (generally for every 100 units of heparin administer 1 mg protamine sulfate IV).

7. Apply pressure to all venipuncture and injection sites to prevent bleeding and hematoma formation.

8. In heparin lock devices, the presence of heparin or NSS may cause lab test interferences.

• To clear flush solution: aspirate and discard 1 mL of fluid from device before withdrawing blood sample.

H

- Inject 1 mL of flush solution into lock after blood samples are drawn.
- With excessively abnormal results, obtain a repeat sample from another site before altering treatment.

9. With SC administration, do not aspirate or massage; administer in lower abdomen and rotate sites.

For Heparin Lock Flush Solution:

1. Aspirate lock to determine patency. Maintain patency: inject 1 mL of flush solution into device diaphragm after each use (maintains catheter patency for up to 24 hr).

2. If administering a drug incompatible with heparin, flush with 0.9% NaCl solution or sterile water for injection before and immediately after incompatible drug administered. Inject another dose of heparin lock flush solution after the final flush.

3. Observe coagulation times carefully with underlying bleeding disorders; ↑ risk for hemorrhage.

4. The presence of heparin or NSS may cause lab test interferences. To clear flush solution:

- Aspirate and discard 1 mL of fluid from device before withdrawing blood sample.
- Inject 1 mL of flush solution into lock after blood samples are drawn.
- With excessively abnormal results, obtain a repeat sample from another site before initiating treatment.

5. Monitor for allergic reactions due to various biologic sources of heparin.

CLIENT/FAMILY TEACHING

1. Review administration technique. Can only be given parenterally. For SC administration inject in lower abdomen. Do not massage after injection. Rotate sites with each dose.

2. Report signs of active bleeding or any excessive menstrual flow; may need to withhold/reduce dosage.

3. Report alterations in GU function, urine color, or any injury.

4. Use an electric razor for shaving and a soft-bristle toothbrush to decrease gum irritation. Hair loss is generally temporary.

5. Arrange furniture to allow open space for unimpeded ambulation and to diminish chances of bumping into objects that may cause bruising/bleeding. Use a night light to illuminate trips to the bathroom. Always wear shoes or slippers.

6. Avoid contact sports and any activities where excessive bumping, bruising or injury may occur.

7. Eat potassium-rich foods (e.g., baked potato, orange juice, bananas, beef, flounder, haddock, sweet potato, turkey, raw tomato). Avoid eating large amounts of vitamin K food (yellow and dark green vegetables).

8. Report increased bruising, bleeding of nose, mouth, gums, mucus or oral secretions, tarry stools, GI upset, SOB, chest pain or difficulty breathing.

9. Avoid alcohol, aspirin, tobacco, and NSAIDs due to increased anticoagulant response.

10. Alert all providers of therapy and wear/carry drug identification.

OUTCOMES/EVALUATE

- PTT: 2–2.5 times the control/normal
- Prevention of thrombus formation
- Clot prophylaxis/treatment
- Indwelling catheter patency

Hydrochlorothiazide

(**hy**-droh-klor-oh-**THIGH**-ah-zyd)

CLASSIFICATION(S):
Diuretic, thiazide
PREGNANCY CATEGORY: B
Rx: Esidrex, Ezide, HydroDIURIL, Hydro-Par, Microzide Capsules, Oretic
✦Rx: Apo-Hydro

SEE ALSO *DIURETICS, THIAZIDE*.

ACTION/KINETICS
Onset: 2 hr. **Peak effect:** 4–6 hr. **Duration:** 6–12 hr. **t ½:** 5.6–14.8 hr.

ADDITIONAL USES
Microzide is available for once-daily, low-dose treatment for hypertension.

SPECIAL CONCERNS
Geriatric clients may be more sensitive to the usual adult dose.

ADDITIONAL SIDE EFFECTS

CV: Allergic myocarditis, hypotension. **Dermatologic:** Alopecia, exfoliative dermatitis, ***toxic epidermal necrolysis,*** erythema multiforme, ***Stevens-Johnson syndrome.*** **Miscellaneous:** ***Anaphylactic reactions, respiratory distress including pneumonitis and pulmonary edema.***

HOW SUPPLIED

Capsule: 12.5 mg; *Oral Solution:* 50 mg/5 mL; *Tablet:* 25 mg, 50 mg, 100 mg

DOSAGE

• CAPSULES, ORAL SOLUTION, TABLETS

Diuretic.

Adults, initial: 25–200 mg/day for several days until dry weight is reached; **then,** 25–100 mg/day or intermittently. Some clients may require up to 200 mg/day.

Antihypertensive.

Adults, initial: 25 mg/day as a single dose. The dose may be increased to 50 mg/day in one to two doses. Doses greater than 50 mg may cause significant reductions in serum potassium. **Pediatric, under 6 months:** 3.3 mg/kg/day in two doses; **up to 2 years of age:** 12.5–37.5 mg/day in two doses; **2–12 years of age:** 37.5–100 mg/day in two doses.

NURSING CONSIDERATIONS

ADMINISTRATION/STORAGE

1. Divide daily doses in excess of 100 mg.
2. Give twice a day at 6–12-hr intervals.
3. When used with other antihypertensives, hydrochlorothiazide dose is usually not more than 50 mg.

ASSESSMENT

1. Note indications for therapy, other agents trialed and the outcome.
2. Assess for glucose intolerance.
3. Monitor BP, weight, uric acid, renal function, microalbumin, and electrolytes; replace potassium as needed.

CLIENT/FAMILY TEACHING

1. Take in the a.m. or as directed, usually with a glass of orange juice. May take with food if GI upset. Report unusual side effects or lack of response.
2. May cause dizziness; change positions slowly and avoid activities that require mental alertness until drug effects realized.
3. Report any swelling of extremities or weight gain of > 2 lb/day.
4. Avoid alcohol, OTC drugs and prolonged sun exposure; may cause delayed (10-14 day) photosensitivity reaction.
5. With diabetes, monitor BS and potassium closely, may cause glucose intolerance.

OUTCOMES/EVALUATE

- ↓ BP
- ↑ Urine output; ↓ edema

Hyoscyamine sulfate

(high-oh-**SIGH**-ah-meen)

CLASSIFICATION(S):
Cholinergic blocking drug
PREGNANCY CATEGORY: C
Rx: Anaspaz, A-Spas S/L, Cystospaz, ED-SPAZ, IB-Stat, Levbid, Levsin, Levsin Drops, Levsin/SL, Levsinex Timecaps, Neosol, NuLev, Symax-SL, Symax-SR

SEE ALSO *CHOLINERGIC BLOCKING AGENTS.*

ACTION/KINETICS

One of the belladonna alkaloids; acts by blocking the action of acetylcholine at the postganglionic nerve endings of the parasympathetic nervous system. **t ½:** 3 ½ hr for tablets, 7 hr for extended-release capsules, and 9 hr for extended-release tablets. Majority of the drug is excreted in the urine unchanged.

USES

(1) To control gastric secretion, visceral spasm, and hypermotility in spastic colitis, spastic bladder, cystitis, pylorospasm, and associated abdominal cramps. (2) Relieve symptoms in functional intestinal disorders (e.g., mild dysenteries and diverticulitis), infant colic, biliary colic. (3) Adjunct to treat peptic ulcer. (4) Irritable bowel syn-

---

Bold Italic = life threatening side effect   ■ = black box warning   ♣ = Available in Canada

drome (e.g., irritable colon, spastic colon, mucous colitis, acute enterocolitis, functional GI disorders). (5) Neurogenic bowel disturbances, including splenic flexure syndrome and neurogenic colon. (6) Reduce pain and hypersecretion in pancreatitis. (7) As a drying agent to relieve symptoms of acute rhinitis. (8) In Parkinsonism to reduce rigidity and tremors and to control associated sialorrhea and hyperhidrosis. (9) Treat poisoning by anticholinesterase agents. (10) Treat cystitis or renal colic. (11) Certain cases of partial heart block associated with vagal activity. (12) Preoperative medication to reduce salivary, tracheobronchial, and pharyngeal secretions. (13) Parenterally to reduce duoendal motility to facilitate the diagnostic radiologic procedure, hypotonic duodenography. May also improve radiologic visibility of the kidneys.

SPECIAL CONCERNS
Heat prostration may occur if the drug is taken in the presence of high environmental temperatures. Use with caution during lactation.

SIDE EFFECTS
See *Cholinergic Blocking Agents.*

HOW SUPPLIED
Capsule, Extended Release: 0.375 mg; *Capsule, Timed Release:* 0.375 mg; *Drops:* 0.125 mg/mL; *Elixir:* 0.125 mg/5 mL; *Injection:* 0.5 mg/mL; *Oral Spray:* 0.125 mg/mL; *Tablet:* 0.125 mg, 0.15 mg; *Tablet, Extended/Sustained Release:* 0.375 mg; *Tablet, Oral Disintegrating:* 0.125 mg; *Tablet, Sublingual:* 0.125 mg

DOSAGE

• **EXTENDED-RELEASE CAPSULES (0.375 MG) OR EXTENDED-RELEASE TABLETS (0.375 MG) OR TIMED RELEASE TABLETS (0.375 MG)**
Adults and children over 12 years of age: 0.375–0.750 mg q 12 hr, not to exceed 1.5 mg in 24 hr.
• **TABLETS (0.125 MG, 0.15 MG); TABLETS, SUBLINGUAL (0.125 MG)**
Adults and children over 12 years of age: 0.125–0.25 mg q 4 hr or as needed, not to exceed 1.5 mg in 24 hr.
• **TABLETS, ORAL DISINTEGRATING**
Adults and children over 12 years: 1 or 2 tablets q 4 hr, up to 12/day or 2

tablets 4 times per day. **Children, 2 to less than 12 years:** ½ –1 tablet q 4 hr, up to 6 per day.
• **ELIXIR (0.125 MG/5 ML)**
Adults and children over 12 years of age: 0.125 mg–0.25 mg (5–10 mL) q 4 hr, not to exceed 1.5 mg (60 mL) in 24 hr. **Children, 2 to 12 years of age: 10 kg:** 1.25 mL (0.031 mg) q 4 hr; **20 kg:** 2.5 mL (0.062 mg) q 4 hr; **40 kg:** 3.75 mL (0.093 mg) q 4 hr; **50 kg:** 5 mL (0.125 mg) q 4 hr.
• **DROPS (0.125 MG/ML)**
Adults and children over 12 years of age: 0.125–0.25 mg (5–10 mL) q 4 hr, not to exceed 1.5 mg (12 mL) in 24 hr. **Children, 2 to 12 years of age:** 0.031–0.125 mg (0.251 mL) q 4 hr or as needed, not to exceed 0.75 mg (6 mL) in 24 hr. **Children, under 2 years of age: 3.4 kg:** 4 drops q 4 hr, not to exceed 24 drops in 24 hr; **5 kg:** 5 drops q 4 hr, not to exceed 30 drops in 24 hr; **7 kg:** 6 drops q 4 hr, not to exceed 36 drops in 24 hr; **10 kg:** 8 drops q 4 hr, not to exceed 48 drops in 24 hr.
• **ORAL SPRAY**
Children, 12 years and younger: 1–2 mL (1 or 2 sprays) q 4 hr as needed, up to 12 mL/day (12 sprays/day).
• **INJECTION (0.5 MG/ML)**
GI disorders.
Adults: 0.25–0.5 mg (0.5–1 mL). Some clients need only one dose while others require doses 2, 3, or 4 times a day at 4 hr intervals.
Diagnostic procedures.
Adults: 0.25–0.5 mg (0.5–1 mL) given IV 5 to 10 min prior to the procedure.
Preanesthetic medication.
Adults and children over 2 years of age: 0.005 mg/kg 30–60 min prior to the time of induction of anesthesia. May also be given at the time the preanesthetic sedative or narcotic is given.
During surgery to reduce drug-induced bradycardia.
Adults and children over 2 years of age: Increments of 0.125 mg (0.25 mL) IV repeated as needed.
Reverse neuromuscular blockade.
Adults and children over 2 years of age: 0.2 mg (0.4 mL) for every 1 mg

neostigmine or equivalent dose of physostigmine or pyridostigmine.

NURSING CONSIDERATIONS

Ⓒ Do not confuse Levbid with Lithobid, Lopid, or Lorabid.

ADMINISTRATION/STORAGE

1. May take hyoscyamine SL tablets sublingually, PO, or chewed. May take hyoscyamine tablets PO or SL.
2. Depending on the use, may give injection SC, IM, or IV.
IV 3. Visually inspect the injectable form for particulate matter/discoloration.

ASSESSMENT

1. Document indications for therapy, type, onset, and characteristics of S&S.
2. List other agents trialed and the outcome. Reduce dose in the elderly.
3. Determine any evidence of glaucoma, bladder neck or GI tract obstruction.
4. Assess elimination/output, abdomen, UGI, CT/US abdomen to R/O pathology.

CLIENT/FAMILY TEACHING

1. Take as prescribed; avoid antacids within 1 hr of taking drug (decreases effectiveness).
2. Do not perform activities that require mental alertness until drug effects realized; dizziness, drowsiness, and blurred vision may occur.
3. Report any loss of symptom control so provider can adjust dose and frequency of administration. Report diarrhea as it may be symptom of intestinal obstruction, especially with a colostomy or ileostomy.
4. Avoid excessive temperatures and activity; drug impairs heat regulation and may decrease perspiration, which may cause fever, heat prostration, or stroke.
5. Males with enlarged prostrate may experience urinary retention/hesitancy; report if persistent or bothersome.
6. Stop drug and report any mental confusion, impaired gait, disorientation, or hallucinations.
7. Avoid alcohol and any other CNS depressants. Use dark glasses when outside to prevent blurred vision.

OUTCOMES/EVALUATE

- ↓ GI motility
- Control of epigastric pain/spasm

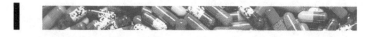

Ibutilide fumarate ■
(ih-**BYOU**-tih-lyd)

CLASSIFICATION(S):
Antiarrhythmic
PREGNANCY CATEGORY: C
Rx: Covert

ACTION/KINETICS

Class III antiarrhythmic agent. Delays repolarization by activation of a slow, inward current (mostly sodium), rather than by blocking outward potassium currents (the way other class III antiarrhythmics act). This results in prolongation in the duration of the atrial and ventricular action potential and refractoriness. Also a dose-related prolongation of the QT interval. High systemic plasma clearance that approximates liver blood flow. **t ½, terminal:** 6 hr. Over 80% is excreted in the urine (with 7% excreted unchanged) and approximately 20% is excreted through the feces. Protein binding is less than 40%

USES

Rapid conversion of atrial fibrillation or atrial flutter of recent onset to sinus rhythm. Base determination of clients to receive ibutilide on expected benefits of maintaining sinus rhythm and whether this outweighs both the risks of the drug and of maintenance therapy. Used in post-cardiac surgery clients.

CONTRAINDICATIONS

Use of certain class Ia antiarrhythmic drugs (e.g., disopyramide, quinidine,

---

Bold Italic = life threatening side effect   ■ = black box warning   ✦ = Available in Canada

procainamide) and certain class III drugs (e.g., amiodarone and sotalol) concomitantly with ibutilide or within 4 hr of postinfusion.

SPECIAL CONCERNS

■(1) May cause potentially fatal arrhythmias, especially sustained polymorphic ventricular tachycardia, usually in association with QT prolongation (torsades de pointes). Arrhythmias can be reversed if treated promptly. (2) It is essential that ibutilide be given in a setting of continuous ECG monitoring and by personnel trained in identification and treatment of acute ventricular arrhythmias, especially polymorphic ventricular tachycardia. (3) Clients with atrial fibrillation of more than 2 to 3 days duration must be adequately anticoagulated, usually for at least 2 weeks. (4) Clients with chronic atrial fibrillation have a strong tendency to revert after conversion to sinus rhythm; treatments to maintain sinus rhythm carry risks. Thus, select clients carefully to be treated with ibutilide, so that the expected benefits of maintaining sinus rhythm outweigh the immediate risks and the risks of maintenance therapy are likely to offer an advantage compared with alternative management.■ Effectiveness has not been determined in clients with arrhythmias of more than 90 days duration. Breast feeding should be discouraged during therapy. Safety and efficacy have not been determined in children less than 18 years of age.

SIDE EFFECTS

CV: *Life-threatening arrhythmias, either sustained or nonsustained polymorphic ventricular tachycardia (torsades de pointes).* Induction/worsening of ventricular arrhythmias. Nonsustained monomorphic ventricular extrasystoles/ventricular tachycardia, sinus tachycardia, SVT, hypo/hypertension, postural hypotension, BBB, AV block, bradycardia, QT-segment prolongation, palpitation, supraventricular extrasystoles, nodal arrhythmia, CHF, *idioventricular rhythm, sustained monomorphic VT.* **Miscellaneous:** Headache, nausea, syncope, renal failure.

OD **OVERDOSE MANAGEMENT**
Symptoms: Increased ventricular ectopy, monomorphic ventricular tachycardia, AV block, nonsustained polymorphic VT. *Treatment:* Treat symptoms.

DRUG INTERACTIONS

Amiodarone / ↑ Risk of prolonged refractoriness
Antidepressants, tricyclic and tetracyclic / ↑ Risk of proarrhythmias
Digoxin / Supraventricular arrhythmias due to ibutilide, may mask cardiotoxicity R/T high digoxin levels
Disopyramide / ↑ Risk of prolonged refractoriness
Histamine H₁ receptor antagonists / ↑ Risk of proarrhythmias
Phenothiazines / ↑ Risk of proarrhythmias
Procainamide / ↑ Risk of prolonged refractoriness
Quinidine / ↑ Risk of prolonged refractoriness
Sotalol / ↑ Risk of prolonged refractoriness

HOW SUPPLIED

IV Solution: 0.1 mg/mL.

DOSAGE

• **IV INFUSION**
 Atrial fibrillation or atrial flutter of recent onset.

Clients weighing 60 kg or more, initial: 1 mg (one vial) infused over 10 min. **Clients weighing less than 60 kg, initial:** 0.01 mg/kg infused over 10 min. If the arrhythmia does not terminate within 10 min after the end of the initial infusion (regardless of the body weight), a second 10-min infusion of equal strength may be given 10 min after completion of the first infusion.

NURSING CONSIDERATIONS

ADMINISTRATION/STORAGE

IV 1. Anticoagulate clients with atrial fibrillation (>2–3 days duration) for at least 2 weeks.
2. May give undiluted or diluted in 50 mL of 0.9% NaCl or D5W. One vial (1 mg) mixed with 50 mL of diluent forms an admixture of approximately 0.017 mg/mL of ibutilide; administer infusion over 10 min.

---

3. Either PVC or polyolefin bags are compatible with drug admixtures.

4. Admixtures with approved diluents are chemically and physically stable for 24 hr at room temperature and for 48 hr if refrigerated.

ASSESSMENT

1. Document onset of arrhythmia and any associated symptoms. Those with AF > 2-3 days require anticoagulation for at least 2 weeks prior to ibutilide therapy.

2. List drugs currently prescribed to ensure none interact unfavorably.

3. Monitor VS, I&O, Mg, and electrolytes, and ECG.

4. Ibutilide must be given in a setting with continuous ECG monitoring and by those trained in the identification/treatment of acute ventricular arrhythmias, especially polymorphic VT.

5. Document conversion to NSR (usually within 30–90 min). Stop drug infusion when arrhythmia terminated or in the event of sustained/nonsustained VT or marked prolongation of QT interval.

6. Observe for at least 4 hr following infusion or until QT interval has returned to baseline. Monitor longer if arrhythmic activity observed.

CLIENT/FAMILY TEACHING

1. Explain the reasons for dosing and why new-onset atrial fibrillation should be terminated (to prevent embolus formation).

2. Review the benefits and possible adverse side effects. Drug can only be given IV, may experience rapid irregular heart beat, headache, and other arrhythmias. Report any chest pain, SOB, numbness or tingling in extremities.

3. Stress the importance of close medical follow-up to determine stability of rhythm.

OUTCOMES/EVALUATE

Conversion of atrial fibrillation to sinus rhythm

Inamrinone lactate

(in-**AM**-rih-nohn)

CLASSIFICATION(S):
Inotropic drug

PREGNANCY CATEGORY: C

ACTION/KINETICS

Causes an increase in CO by increasing the force of contraction of the heart, probably by inhibiting cyclic AMP phosphodiesterase, thereby increasing cellular levels of c-AMP. It reduces afterload and preload by directly relaxing vascular smooth muscle. **Time to peak effect:** 10 min. **t ½, elimination, after rapid IV:** 3.6 hr; **after IV infusion:** 5.8 hr. **Steady-state plasma levels:** 2.4 mcg/mL by maintaining an infusion of 5–10 mcg/kg/min. **Duration:** 30 min–2 hr, depending on the dose. Excreted primarily in the urine both unchanged and as metabolites. Children have a larger volume of distribution and a decreased elimination half-life. *NOTE:* Due to medication errors and confusion with amiodarone, the generic name for amrinone was changed to inamrinone.

USES

Congestive heart failure (short-term therapy in clients unresponsive to digitalis, diuretics, and/or vasodilators). Can be used in digitalized clients.

CONTRAINDICATIONS

Hypersensitivity to inamrinone or bisulfites. Severe aortic or pulmonary valvular disease in lieu of surgery. Acute MI.

SPECIAL CONCERNS

Safety and efficacy have not been established in children. Use with caution during lactation.

SIDE EFFECTS

GI: N&V, abdominal pain, anorexia. **CV:** Hypotension, *supraventricular and ventricular arrhythmias.* **Allergic:** Pericarditis, pleuritis, ascites, allergic reaction to sodium bisulfite present in the product, vasculitis with nodular pulmonary densities, hypoxemia, jaundice. **Other:** Thrombocytopenia, *hepatotoxicity,* fever, chest pain, burning at site of injection.

OD OVERDOSE MANAGEMENT
Symptoms: Hypotension. *Treatment:* Reduce or discontinue drug administration and begin general supportive measures.

DRUG INTERACTIONS
Excessive hypotension when used with disopyramide.

HOW SUPPLIED
Injection: 5 mg/mL

DOSAGE
- IV
  CHF.
Initial: 0.75 mg/kg as a bolus given slowly over 2–3 min; may be repeated after 30 min if necessary. **Maintenance, IV infusion:** 5–10 mcg/kg/min. Do not exceed a daily dose of 10 mg/kg, although up to 18 mg/kg/day has been used in some clients for short periods.

NURSING CONSIDERATIONS
ADMINISTRATION/STORAGE
IV 1. Administer undiluted or diluted in 0.9% or 0.45% saline to a concentration of 1–3 mg/mL. Use diluted solutions within 24 hr.
2. Do not dilute with solutions containing dextrose (glucose) prior to injection. However, the drug may be injected into running dextrose (glucose) infusions through a Y connector or directly into the tubing.
3. Administer loading dose over 2–3 min; may be repeated in 30 min.
4. Solutions should be clear yellow.
5. Do not administer with furosemide; precipitate will form.
6. Protect from light and store at room temperature.

ASSESSMENT
1. Note indications for therapy, other agents trialed and outcome.
2. Obtain baseline VS, CXR, and ECG. Assess electrolytes, BNP, and CBC. Document ejection fraction and pulmonary assessments, noting any new onset S_3, JVD, crackles, or edema.
3. Monitor VS, I&O, weights, and urine output. Document CVP, CO, and PA pressures.
4. Assess for any hypersensitivity reactions, including pericarditis, pleuritis, or ascites.

CLIENT/FAMILY TEACHING
1. Drug is used IV for congestive heart failure in clients who have not responded to the normal treatment with digoxin, diuretics, or vasodilators.
2. Expect frequent monitoring of ECG, BP and heart rate as well as weights. Drug may cause more frequent voiding.
3. Report any increased dizziness, weakness, fatigue, numbness, tingling or swelling of extremities, or pain at IV site.

OUTCOMES/EVALUATE
- ↓ Preload and afterload; ↑ CO, EF
- Improvement in S&S of CHF.

Indapamide
(in-**DAP**-ah-myd)

CLASSIFICATION(S):
Diuretic, thiazide
PREGNANCY CATEGORY: B
Rx: Lozol
✱**Rx:** Apo-Indapamide, Novo-Indapamide, PMS-Indapamide

Indapamide hemihydrate
PREGNANCY CATEGORY: B
✱**Rx:** Gen-Indapamide, Lozide, Nu-Indapamide

SEE ALSO *DIURETICS, THIAZIDES.*

ACTION/KINETICS
Onset: 1–2 weeks after multiple doses. **Peak levels:** 2 hr. **Duration:** Up to 8 weeks with multiple doses. **t ½:** 14 hr. Nearly 100% is absorbed from the GI tract. Excreted through the kidneys (70% with 7% unchanged) and the GI tract (23%).

USES
(1) Alone or in combination with other drugs for treatment of hypertension. (2) Edema in CHF.

SPECIAL CONCERNS
Dosage has not been established in children. Geriatric clients may be more sensitive to the hypotensive and electrolyte effects.

HOW SUPPLIED
Tablet: 1.25 mg, 2.5 mg

DOSAGE
• **TABLETS**
Edema of CHF.
Adults: 2.5 mg as a single dose in the morning. If necessary, may be increased to 5 mg/day after 1 week.
Hypertension.
Adults: 1.25 mg as a single dose in the morning. If the response is not satisfactory after 4 weeks, the dose may be increased to 2.5 mg taken once daily. If the response to 2.5 mg is not satisfactory after 4 weeks, the dose may be increased to 5 mg taken once daily (however, consideration should be given to adding another antihypertensive).

NURSING CONSIDERATIONS
ADMINISTRATION/STORAGE
1. May be combined with other antihypertensive agents if response inadequate. Initially, reduce the dose of other agents by 50%.
2. Doses greater than 5 mg/day do not increase effectiveness but may increase hypokalemia.

ASSESSMENT
1. Document indications for therapy, type, onset, and characteristics of symptoms. Note other agents trialed and the outcome.
2. Monitor BP, weight, I&O, edema, VS, renal function, electrolyes, and uric acid levels.

CLIENT/FAMILY TEACHING
1. Drug is used to remove fluids and lower BP. Take in the morning upon awakening to prevent frequent nighttime voiding.
2. Change positions slowly to prevent sudden drop in BP and dizziness.
3. Follow low sodium diet and choose foods high in potassium (cantalope, broccoli, oranges, grapefruit, bananas, dried fruits, etc). Continue healthy life style by exercising regularly, stop smoking, limit alcohol consumption and strive for weight reduction.
4. Monitor BP and weights; report any gain of more than 2 lbs per day or 10 lbs per week.

5. Avoid prolonged sun exposure and use protection if exposed. Keep all F/U appointments for labs and evaluation.

OUTCOMES/EVALUATE
• ↓ BP
• ↑ Urinary output with ↓ edema

Irbesartan ■
(ihr-beh-**SAR**-tan)

CLASSIFICATION(S):
Antihypertensive, angiotensin II receptor blocker
PREGNANCY CATEGORY: C (first trimester), D (second and third trimesters)
Rx: Avapro

SEE ALSO *ANGIOTENSIN II RECEPTOR ANTAGONISTS AND ANTIHYPERTENSIVE DRUGS.*

ACTION/KINETICS
Rapid absorption after PO use. **Peak plasma levels:** 1.5–2 hr. Is 60–80% bioavailable; food does not affect bioavailability. Effect somewhat less in Blacks. t_{max}: 1.5–2 hr. **$t\frac{1}{2}$, terminal elimination:** 11–15 hr. Metabolized in liver by CYP2C9 and both unchanged drug and metabolites excreted through urine (20%) and feces (80%). Over 90% bound to plasma proteins.

USES
(1) Hypertension, alone or in combination with other antihypertensives. (2) Nephropathy in type 2 diabetics with an elevated serum creatinine and proteinuria (>300 mg/day) in patients with type 2 diabetes and hypertension. Irbesartan reduces the rate of progression of nephropathy as measured by the occurrence of doubling of serum creatinine or end-stage renal disease (need for dialysis or renal transplantation).

CONTRAINDICATIONS
Hypersensitivity to any component of this product.

SPECIAL CONCERNS
■Use during the second and third trimester of pregnancy can cause injury and even death to the fetus. When pregnancy is detected, discontinue as

---

soon as possible.■ Safety and efficacy have not been determined in children less than 6 years of age.

SIDE EFFECTS

GI: Diarrhea, dyspepsia, heartburn, abdominal distension/pain, N&V, constipation, oral lesion, gastroenteritis, flatulence. **CV:** Tachycardia, syncope, orthostatic hypotension, hypotension (especially in volume- or salt-depletion), flushing, hypertension, cardiac murmur, *MI, cardiorespiratory arrest, heart failure, hypertensive crisis, CVA,* angina pectoris, arrhythmias, conduction disorder, TIA. **CNS:** Sleep disturbance, anxiety, nervousness, dizziness, numbness, somnolence, emotional disturbance, depression, paresthesia, tremor. **Musculoskeletal:** Extremity swelling, muscle cramp/ache/weakness, arthritis, musculoskeletal pain, musculoskeletal chest pain, joint stiffness, bursitis. **Respiratory:** Epistaxis, tracheobronchitis, congestion, pulmonary congestion, dyspnea, wheezing, URI, rhinitis, pharyngitis, sinus abnormality. **GU:** Abnormal urination, prostate disorder, UTI, sexual dysfunction, libido change. **Dermatologic:** Pruritus, dermatitis, ecchymosis, facial erythema, urticaria. **Ophthalmic:** Vision disturbance, conjunctivitis, eyelid abnormality. **Otic:** Hearing abnormality, ear infection/pain/abnormality. **Miscellaneous:** Gout, fever, fatigue, chills, facial edema, upper extremity edema, headache, influenza, rash, chest pain.

LABORATORY TEST CONSIDERATIONS

↑ BUN (minor), serum creatinine. ↓ Hemoglobin. Neutropenia.

HOW SUPPLIED

Tablet: 75 mg, 150 mg, 300 mg

DOSAGE

- **TABLETS**

  Hypertension.

  150 mg once daily with or without food, up to 300 mg once daily. Lower initial dose of 75 mg is recommended for clients with depleted intravascular volume or salt. If BP is not controlled by irbesartan alone, hydrochlorothiazide may have an additive effect. Clients not adequately treated by 300 mg irbesartan are unlikely to get benefit from higher dose or twice a day dosing. **Chil**dren, 6–12 years, initial: 75 mg once daily. Titrate those requiring further reduction in BP to 150 mg once daily. **Children, 13–16 years, initial:** 150 mg once daily. Titrate those requiring further reduction in BP to 300 mg once daily.

  Nephropathy in type 2 diabetics.
  Adults: Target dose is 300 mg once daily.

NURSING CONSIDERATIONS

ADMINISTRATION/STORAGE

1. Adjustment of dose is not required in geriatric clients or in hepatic or renal impairment.
2. May be given with other antihypertensive drugs.
3. Store between 15–30°C (59–86°F).

ASSESSMENT

1. Document indications for therapy, onset, duration, characteristics of symptoms, and other agents trialed.
2. If pregnancy is detected, discontinue as soon as possible.
3. Observe infants exposed to an angiotensin II inhibitor in utero for hypotension, oliguria, and ↑ K.
4. Monitor VS, electrolytes, U/A, microalbumin, renal and LFTs.

CLIENT/FAMILY TEACHING

1. Take only as directed. May take with or without food.
2. Avoid tasks that require mental alertness until drug effects realized as it may cause dizziness or drowsiness; change positions slowly to prevent sudden drop in BP.
3. Continue low-fat, low-cholesterol diet, regular exercise, tobacco cessation, salt restriction, and lifestyle changes necessary to maintain lowered BP.
4. Practice reliable contraception. Stop drug and report if pregnancy suspected.

OUTCOMES/EVALUATE

↓ BP; Renal protection in DM.

Isoproterenol hydrochloride

(eye-so-proe-**TER**-e-nole)

CLASSIFICATION(S):
Sympathomimetic
PREGNANCY CATEGORY: C
Rx: Isuprel, Isuprel Mistometer

Isoproterenol sulfate

PREGNANCY CATEGORY: C
Rx: Medihaler-Iso

SEE ALSO *SYMPATHOMIMETIC DRUGS.*

ACTION/KINETICS

Produces pronounced stimulation of both beta-1 and beta-2 receptors of the heart, bronchi, skeletal muscle vasculature, and the GI tract. Has both positive inotropic and chronotropic activity; systolic BP may increase while diastolic BP may decrease. Thus, mean arterial BP may not change or may be decreased. Causes less hyperglycemia than epinephrine, but produces bronchodilation and the same degree of CNS excitation. **Inhalation: Onset,** 2–5 min; **peak effect:** 3–5 min; **duration:** 1–3 hr. **IV: Onset,** immediate; **duration:** less than 1 hr. Partially metabolized; excreted in urine.

USES

Inhalation: Relief of bronchospasms associated with acute and chronic asthma, chronic bronchitis, or emphysema. **Injection:** (1) Bronchospasm during anesthesia. (2) As an adjunct to fluid and electrolyte replacement therapy to treat hypovolemic and septic shock, low cardiac output states, CHF, and cardiogenic shock. (3) Mild or transient heart block that does not require electric shock or pacemaker therapy. (4) For serious episodes of heart block and Adams-Stokes attacks, except when caused by ventricular tachycardia or fibrillation. (5) Cardiac arrest until electric shock or pacemaker therapy is available.

CONTRAINDICATIONS

Tachyarrhythmias, tachycardia, or heart block caused by digitalis intoxication, ventricular arrhythmias that require inotropic therapy, and angina pectoris.

SPECIAL CONCERNS

Use with caution during lactation and in the presence of tuberculosis. Safety and effectiveness have not been determined in children under age 12.

ADDITIONAL SIDE EFFECTS

CV: *Cardiac arrest,* Adams-Stokes attack, hypotension, precordial pain or distress. **CNS:** Hyperactivity, hyperkinesia. **Respiratory:** Wheezing, bronchitis, increase in sputum, *pulmonary/bronchial edema and inflammation, paradoxical airway resistance.* Excessive inhalation causes refractory bronchial obstruction. **Miscellaneous:** Flushing, sweating, swelling of the parotid gland. Sublingual administration may cause buccal ulceration. Side effects of drug are less severe after inhalation.

DRUG INTERACTIONS

Bretylium / Possibility of arrhythmias
Guanethidine / ↑ Pressor response of isoproterenol
Halogenated hydrocarbon anesthetics / Sensitization of the heart to catecholamines → serious arrhythmias
Oxytocic drugs / Possibility of severe, persistent hypertension
Tricyclic antidepressants / Potentiation of pressor effect

HOW SUPPLIED

Isoproterenol Hydrochloride: *Metered dose inhaler (Aerosol):* 103 mcg/inh; *Injection:* 0.02 mg/mL (1:50,000), 0.2 mg/mL (1:5000); *Solution for Inhalation:* 0.5% (1:200), 1% (1:100). **Isoproterenol Sulfate:** *Metered dose inhaler:* 80 mcg/inh

DOSAGE

ISOPROTERENOL HYDROCHLORIDE

- **INHALATION**
  Acute bronchial asthma.
  Hand bulb nebulizer. **Adults and children:** Give 5–15 deep inhalations of the 1:200 solution. Alternatively, in adults, give 3–7 deep inhalations of the 1:100 solution. If no relief occurs after 5–10

Bold Italic = life threatening side effect   ■ = black box warning   ✚ = Available in Canada

min, repeat doses once more. If acute attack recurs, can repeat treatment up to 5 times per day, if necessary. *Metered dose inhaler (aerosol).* One inhalation (103 mcg). Wait 1 min to determine effect before considering a second inhalation. Repeat up to 5 times per day, if necessary.

Bronchospasm in COPD.
Hand bulb nebulizer. Give 5–15 deep inhalations using the 1:200 solution. Severe attacks may require 3–7 inhalations using the 1:100 solution. Wait at least 3–4 hr between doses. *Nebulization by compressed air or oxygen.* Dilute 0.5 mL of the 1:200 solution to 2–2.5 mL with appropriate diluent for a concentration of 1:800 to 1:1,000. Deliver the solution over 10–20 min. May repeat up to 5 times per day. *Intermittent positive pressure breathing.* Dilute 0.5 mL of the 1:200 solution to 2–2.5 mL with water or isotonic saline. Deliver over 15–20 min. May repeat up to 5 times per day. *Metered dose inhaler (aerosol).* 1 or 2 inhalations repeated at no less than 3–4 hr intervals (6–8 times per day). **Children:** For acute bronchospasms, use the 1:200 solution. Do not use more than 0.25 mL of the 1:200 solution for each 10–15 min programmed treatment.

• **IV**
Bronchospasms during anesthesia.
Dilute 1 mL of a 1:5,000 solution to 10 mL with NaCl injection or D5W. **Initial dose:** 0.01–0.02 mg (0.5–1 mL of diluted solution). Repeat when necessary or use a 1:50,000 solution undiluted and give as an initial dose of 0.01–0.02 mg (0.5–1 mL).
Hypovolemic and septic shock.
Start the 1:50,000 solution at the lowest recommended dose and increase the rate of administration gradually, while carefully monitoring.
Heart block, Adams-Stokes attacks, cardiac arrest.
IV injection. Dilute 1 mL of the 1:5,000 solution (0.2 mg) to 10 mL with NaCl or D5W. **Initial dose:** 0.02–0.06 mg (1–3 mL of diluted solution); **then,** 0.01–0.2 mg (0.5–10 mL of diluted solution). *IV infusion.* Dilute 10 mL of the 1:5,000 so-

lution (2 mg) in 500 mL of D5W or dilute 5 mL of the 1:5000 solution (1 mg) in 250 mL of D5W. **Initial dose:** 5 mcg/min (1.25 mL/min of diluted solution).

• **IM**
Heart block, Adams-Stokes attacks, cardiac arrest.
Initial: 0.2 mg (1 mL) of undiluted 1:5,000 solution; **then,** 0.02–1 mg (0.1–5 mL) of undiluted 1:5,000 solution.

• **SC**
Heart block, Adams-Stokes attacks, cardiac arrest.
Initial: 0.2 mg (1 mL) of undiluted 1:5,000 solution; **then,** 0.15–0.2 mg (0.75–1 mL) of undiluted 1:5,000 solution.

• **INTRACARDIAC**
Emergency use in heart block, Adams-Stokes attacks, cardiac arrest.
Give 0.02 mg (0.1 mL) of the undiluted 1:5000 solution.

ISOPROTERENOL SULFATE
• **INHALATION**
Acute bronchial asthma.
Initial: 1 inhalation (80 mcg). If no relief is evident after 2–5 min, a second inhalation may be given. **Maintenance:** 1–2 inhalations 4–6 times per day. Do not give more than 2 inhalations at any one time and no more than 6 inhalations/hr.

NURSING CONSIDERATIONS
ADMINISTRATION/STORAGE
1. Administration to children, except where noted, is the same as that for adults; their smaller ventilatory exchange capacity will permit a proportionally smaller aerosol intake. For their acute bronchospasms, use 1:200 solution.
2. In children, no more than 0.25 mL of the 1:200 solution should be used for each 10–15 min of programmed treatment.
3. Elderly clients usually receive a lower dose.
IV 4. Administer IV in a continuously monitored environment.
5. Do not use the injection if it is pinkish to brownish in color. Protect from light and store at 15–30°C (59–86°F).

ASSESSMENT

1. Document indications for therapy, triggers, characteristics of symptoms.

2. Perform pulmonary assessment; note PFTs and CXRs. Report respiratory problems that worsen after administration; refractory reactions may necessitate drug withdrawal.

3. Identify arrhythmias (especially ventricular) and angina; may preclude drug therapy.

CLIENT/FAMILY TEACHING

1. Review method for inhaler use; a spacer enhances dispersion.

2. Rinse mouth and equipment with water; removes drug residue and minimizes dryness after inhalation.

3. Maintain fluid intake of 2–3 L/day to help liquefy secretions. Reduce intake of caffeine during therapy.

4. Sputum and saliva may appear pink after inhalation therapy; do not become alarmed.

5. With more than one inhalation, wait 2 min before second inhalation. When also taking inhalant glucocorticoids, take isoproterenol first and wait 5 min before using the next inhaler.

6. Do not use more often than prescribed; over use can cause severe cardiac and respiratory problems. Report any chest pain/tightness or increased SOB.

7. Identify parotid gland; withhold drug and report if enlarged.

8. Stop smoking to preserve current level of lung function; enroll in smoking cessation program.

OUTCOMES/EVALUATE

- Improved airway exchange
- ↓ Bronchoconstriction/spasms
- Stable cardiac rhythm

Isosorbide dinitrate ©

(eye-so-**SOR**-byd)

CLASSIFICATION(S):

Coronary vasodilator

PREGNANCY CATEGORY: C

Rx: Dilatrate-SR, Isochron, Isordil, Isordil Tembids, Isordil Titradose, Sorbitrate

✜**Rx:** Apo-ISDN

SEE ALSO *ANTIANGINAL DRUGS - NITRATES/NITRITES.*

ACTION/KINETICS

Sublingual, chewable. Onset: 2–5 min; **duration:** 1–3 hr. **Oral Capsules/Tablets. Onset:** 20–40 min; **duration:** 4–6 hr. **Extended-release. Onset:** up to 4 hr; **duration:** 6–8 hr.

ADDITIONAL USES

Diffuse esophageal spasm. Oral tablets are only for prophylaxis while sublingual and chewable forms may be used to treat angina.

ADDITIONAL CONTRAINDICATIONS

Use to abort acute anginal attacks.

SPECIAL CONCERNS

Use with caution during lactation. Safety and efficacy have not been established in children.

ADDITIONAL SIDE EFFECTS

Vascular headaches occur especially frequently.

ADDITIONAL DRUG INTERACTIONS

Acetylcholine / Acetylcholine effect antagonized

Norepinephrine / Norepinephrine effect antagonized

HOW SUPPLIED

Chew Tablet: 5 mg, 10 mg; *Capsule, Extended Release:* 40 mg; *Tablet:* 5 mg, 10 mg, 20 mg, 30 mg, 40 mg; *Tablet, Extended Release:* 40 mg; *Tablet, Sublingual:* 2.5 mg, 5 mg, 10 mg

DOSAGE

- **TABLETS**
    Antianginal.

Initial: 5–20 mg q 6 hr; **maintenance:** 10–40 mg q 6 hr (usual: 20–40 mg 4 times per day).

- **CHEWABLE TABLETS**
    Antianginal, acute attack.

Initial: 5 mg q 2–3 hr. The dose can be titrated upward until angina is relieved or side effects occur.

    Prophylaxis.

5–10 mg q 2–3 hr.

- **EXTENDED-RELEASE CAPSULES**
    Antianginal.

Bold Italic = life threatening side effect   ■ = black box warning   ✜ = Available in Canada

Initial: 40 mg; **maintenance:** 40–80 mg q 8–12 hr.

- **EXTENDED-RELEASE TABLETS**
  Antianginal.

Initial: 40 mg; **maintenance:** 40–80 mg q 8–12 hr.

- **SUBLINGUAL TABLETS**
  Acute attack.

2.5–5 mg q 2–3 hr as required. The dose can be titrated upward until angina is relieved or side effects occur.

Prophylaxis.

5–10 mg q 2–3 hr.

NURSING CONSIDERATIONS

☜ Do not confuse Isordil with Inderal (a beta-adrenergic blocker).

ASSESSMENT

1. Note indications for therapy; also include onset, location, and characteristics of pain. Rate pain levels.

2. Assess VS and ECG; note stress thallium, catheterization, or IVUS findings as well as CAD history.

CLIENT/FAMILY TEACHING

1. Administer with meals to eliminate or reduce headaches; otherwise, take on an empty stomach to facilitate absorption. Leave product in original container.

2. Tolerance may develop (stay nitrate free for 8-12 hr, usually at night, to prevent tolerance). Short-acting products can be given 2–3 times per day with the last dose no later than 7:00 p.m. The extended-release products can be given once or twice daily at 8:00 a.m. and 2:00 p.m. or as prescribed

3. Review method for administration; do not chew sublingual tablets. None of the products should be crushed or chewed, unless ordered. Do not stop abruptly; may cause heart spasms.

4. Hold chewable tablets in the mouth for 1–2 min; allows absorption through buccal membranes.

5. May take before any stressful activity (sexual activity, exercise).

6. Change positions slowly to avoid sudden drop in BP. Avoid hazardous activities if dizziness occurs and all forms of alcohol.

7. Acetaminophen may assist to relieve drug-induced headaches.

OUTCOMES/EVALUATE

- ↓ Frequency/severity of attacks
- ↑ CO/Exercise tolerance
- Resolution of esophageal spasm

Isosorbide mononitrate ☜

CLASSIFICATION(S):
Coronary vasodilator
PREGNANCY CATEGORY: C
Rx: Imdur, ISMO, Monoket

SEE ALSO *ANTIANGINAL DRUGS - NITRATES/NITRITES* AND *ISOSORBIDE DINITRATE.*

ACTION/KINETICS

Isosorbide mononitrate is the major metabolite of isosorbide dinitrate. The mononitrate is not subject to first-pass metabolism. Bioavailability is nearly 100%. **Onset:** 30–60 min. **t ½:** About 5 hr.

USES

Prophylaxis and treatment of angina pectoris.

CONTRAINDICATIONS

To abort acute anginal attacks. Use in acute MI or CHF.

SPECIAL CONCERNS

Use with caution during lactation and in clients who may be volume depleted or who are already hypotensive. Safety and effectiveness have not been determined in children. The benefits have not been established in acute MI or CHF.

SIDE EFFECTS

CV: Hypotension (may be accompanied by paradoxical bradycardia and increased angina pectoris). **CNS:** Headache, lightheadedness, dizziness. **GI:** N&V. **Miscellaneous:** Possibility of methemoglobinemia.

OD **OVERDOSE MANAGEMENT**

Symptoms: Increased intracranial pressure manifested by throbbing headache, confusion, moderate fever. Also, vertigo, palpitations, visual disturbances, N&V, syncope, air hunger, dyspnea (followed by reduced ventilatory effort), diaphoresis, skin either flushed or cold and clammy, heart block, bradycardia, paralysis, ***coma, seizures, death.***

Treatment: Direct therapy toward an increase in central fluid volume. Do *not* use vasoconstrictors.

DRUG INTERACTIONS
Ethanol / Additive vasodilation
Calcium channel blockers / Severe orthostatic hypotension
Organic nitrates / Severe orthostatic hypotension

HOW SUPPLIED
Tablet: 10 mg, 20 mg; *Tablet, Extended Release:* 30 mg, 60 mg, 120 mg

DOSAGE

• **TABLETS**
Prophylaxis of angina.
20 mg twice a day with the two doses given 7 hr apart, with the first dose upon awakening. A starting dose of 5 mg (one-half of the 10 mg tablet) may be appropriate for clients of particularly small stature; however, increase to at least 10 mg by the second or third day.

• **TABLETS, EXTENDED RELEASE**
Prophylaxis of angina.
Initial: 30 mg or 60 mg once daily; **then,** after several days dosage may be increased to 120 mg. Rarely, 240 mg daily may be needed.

NURSING CONSIDERATIONS

℘ Do not confuse Imdur with Imuran or Inderal.

ADMINISTRATION/STORAGE
The treatment regimen minimizes the development of refractory tolerance.

ASSESSMENT
Note indications for therapy, cardiac history, onset and frequency of occurrence, as well as any triggers. Monitor VS, cardiac status and electrolytes.

CLIENT/FAMILY TEACHING
1. Consume 1–2 L/day of fluids to ensure adequate hydration.
2. Take the extended-release tablet in the morning upon arising as directed. Do not crush or chew; take with a half glass of water.
3. May cause drop in BP. Change positions slowly to prevent dizziness. Do not stop abruptly.
4. Avoid alcohol. Report if chest pain persists/recurs and report adverse effects. Keep all F/U visits and lab and EKG appointments.

OUTCOMES/EVALUATE
Angina prophylaxis

Isradipine
(iss-**RAD**-ih-peen)

CLASSIFICATION(S):
Antihypertensive, calcium channel blocking drug
PREGNANCY CATEGORY: C
Rx: DynaCirc, DynaCirc CR

SEE ALSO *CALCIUM CHANNEL BLOCKING AGENTS.*

ACTION/KINETICS
Binds to calcium channels resulting in the inhibition of calcium influx into cardiac and smooth muscle and subsequent arteriolar vasodilation. Reduced systemic resistance leads to a decrease in BP with a small increase in resting HR. In clients with normal ventricular function, the drug reduces afterload leading to some increase in CO. Causes a slight increase in QT interval and CO and a slight decrease in myocardial contractility. Well absorbed from the GI tract, although it undergoes significant first-pass metabolism. **Peak plasma levels:** 1 ng/mL after 1.5 hr. 95% bound to plasma proteins. **Onset:** 2–3 hr. Food increases the time to peak effect by about 1 hr, although the total bioavailability does not change. Bioavailability increases in those over 65 years of age, those with impaired hepatic function, and those with mild impaired renal function. For the capsules, the antihypertensive effect usually occurs within 2–3 hr with maximal response in 2–4 wk. For the controlled-release tablets, the antihypertensive response occurs within 2 hr with the peak response in 8–10 hr with BP reduction maintained for 24 hr. **t ½, initial:** 1.5–2 hr; **terminal,** 8 hr. Completely metabolized in the liver with 60–65% excreted through the kidneys and 25–30% through the feces. Maximum effect may not be observed for 2–4 weeks.

USES
Essential hypertension, alone or with thiazide diuretics. *Investigational:* Raynaud's phenomenon.

CONTRAINDICATIONS
Lactation.

SPECIAL CONCERNS
Safety and effectiveness have not been determined in children. Use with caution in clients with CHF, especially those taking a beta-adrenergic blocking agent. Bioavailability increases in those over 65 years of age, in impaired hepatic function, and in mild renal impairment.

SIDE EFFECTS
CV: Palpitations, edema, flushing, tachycardia, SOB, hypotension, transient ischemic attack, *stroke*, atrial fibrillation, *ventricular fibrillation, MI,* CHF, angina. **CNS:** Headache, dizziness, fatigue, drowsiness, insomnia, lethargy, nervousness, depression, syncope, amnesia, psychosis, hallucinations, weakness, jitteriness, paresthesia. **GI:** Nausea, abdominal discomfort, diarrhea, vomiting, constipation, dry mouth. **Respiratory:** Dyspnea, cough. **Dermatologic:** Pruritus, urticaria. **Miscellaneous:** Chest pain, rash, pollakiuria, cramps of the legs and feet, nocturia, polyuria, hyperhidrosis, visual disturbances, numbness, throat discomfort, leukopenia, sexual difficulties.

LABORATORY TEST CONSIDERATIONS
↑ LFTs.

DRUG INTERACTIONS
Azole antifungals / ↑ Serum isradipine levels
Beta-blockers / Possible additive or synergistic effects; isradipine may ↓ metabolism of certain beta-blockers
Cimetidine / Possible ↑ serum isradipine levels
Fentanyl / Severe hypotension with a beta-blocker and isradipine
Lovastatin / ↓ Plasma lovastatin levels
Rifampin / ↓ Effect of isradipine

HOW SUPPLIED
Capsule: 2.5 mg, 5 mg; *Tablet, Controlled Release:* 5 mg, 10 mg

DOSAGE
• **CAPSULES (DYNACIRC)**
  Hypertension.
Adults, initial: 2.5 mg twice a day alone or in combination with a thiazide diuretic. If BP is not decreased satisfactorily after 2–4 weeks, the dose may be increased in increments of 5 mg/day at 2 to 4-week intervals up to a maximum of 20 mg/day. Adverse effects increase at doses above 10 mg/day.

• **TABLETS, CONTROLLED-RELEASE (DYNACIRC CR)**
  Hypertension.
Adults: 5 mg once daily alone or with a thiazide diuretic. If needed, dose can be increaed in increments of 5 mg at 2 to 4-week intervals up to a maximum of 20 mg/day. *NOTE:* For clients over 65 years of age, those with impaired hepatic function, and those with mild renal impairmend, the initial dose should be 2.5 mg 2 twice a day for capsules and 5 mg once daily for tablets.

NURSING CONSIDERATIONS

ADMINISTRATION/STORAGE
Store below 30°C (86°F) in a tight container protected from light, moisture, and humidity.

ASSESSMENT
1. Note indications for therapy, disease onset, other therapies trialed and outcome.
2. Monitor VS, EKG, I&O, weight, CXR, and lung sounds.

CLIENT/FAMILY TEACHING
1. Take as directed with or without food. Swallow controlled-release tablets whole; do not bite or divide.
2. Use caution, may cause dizziness and confusion; assess drug effects. Change positions slowly to prevent rapid drop in BP.
3. Report any SOB, swelling of extremities, irregular heart beat, or prolonged dizziness.
4. Avoid alcohol and OTC meds without approval.
5. Report for scheduled lab tests: liver and renal function studies every 3–6 months.

OUTCOMES/EVALUATE
Control of HTN

L

Labetalol hydrochloride

(lah-**BET**-ah-lohl)

CLASSIFICATION(S):
Alpha-beta adrenergic blocking agent

PREGNANCY CATEGORY: C
Rx: Normodyne, Trandate
♣Rx: Apo-Labetalol

SEE ALSO *BETA-ADRENERGIC BLOCKING AGENTS* AND *ANTIHYPERTENSIVE AGENTS*.

ACTION/KINETICS
Decreases BP by blocking both alpha- and beta-adrenergic receptors. Standing BP is lowered more than supine. Significant reflex tachycardia and bradycardia do not occur although AV conduction may be prolonged. **Onset, PO:** 2–4 hr; **IV:** 5 min. **Peak plasma levels, PO:** 1–2 hr. **Peak effects, PO:** 2–4 hr. **Duration, PO:** 8–12 hr. **t ½, PO:** 6–8 hr; **IV:** 5.5 hr. Significant first-pass effect; metabolized in liver. Food increases bioavailability of the drug.

USES
PO: Hypertension, alone or in combination with other drugs (especially thiazide and loop diuretics). **IV:** Severe hypertension. *Investigational:* Pheochromocytoma, clonidine withdrawal hypertension.

CONTRAINDICATIONS
Cardiogenic shock, overt cardiac failure, bronchial asthma, severe bradycardia, greater than first-degree heart block.

SPECIAL CONCERNS
Use with caution during lactation, in impaired renal and hepatic function, in chronic bronchitis and emphysema, in those with a history of heart failure who are well compensated, and in diabetes (may prevent premonitory signs of acute hypoglycemia). Safety and efficacy in children have not been established.

SIDE EFFECTS
See also *Beta-Adrenergic Blocking Agents*.
After PO Use. GI: Diarrhea, cholestasis with or without jaundice. **CNS:** Fatigue, drowsiness, paresthesias, headache, syncope (rare). **GU:** Impotence, priapism, ejaculation failure, difficulty in micturition, Peyronie's disease, acute urinary bladder retention. **Respiratory:** Dyspnea, *bronchospasm*. **Musculoskeletal:** Muscle cramps, asthenia, toxic myopathy. **Dermatologic:** Generalized maculopapular, lichenoid, or urticarial rashes; bullous lichen planus, psoriasis, facial erythema, reversible alopecia. **Ophthalmic:** Abnormal vision, dry eyes. **Miscellaneous:** SLE, positive antinuclear factor, antimitochondrial antibiodies, fever, edema, nasal stuffiness. **After parenteral use. CV:** Ventricular arrhythmias. **CNS:** Numbness, somnolence, yawning. **Renal:** Transient increases in BUN and serum creatinine associated with drops in BP usually in those with prior renal insufficiency. **Miscellaneous:** Pruritus, flushing, wheezing. **After PO or parenteral use. GI:** N&V, dyspepsia, taste distortion, jaundice or hepatic dysfunction (rare). **CNS:** Dizziness, tingling of skin or scalp, vertigo. **Miscellaneous:** Postural hypotension, increased sweating.

LABORATORY TEST CONSIDERATIONS
False + increase in urinary catecholamines or for amphetamine when screening urine for drugs. Transient ↑ serum transaminases, BUN, serum creatinine.

OD OVERDOSE MANAGEMENT
Symptoms: Excessive hypotension and bradycardia. *Treatment:* Induce vomiting or perform gastric lavage. Place clients in a supine position with legs elevated. If required, the following treatment can be used:

- Epinephrine or a beta-2 agonist (aerosol) to treat bronchospasm.
- Atropine or epinephrine to treat bradycardia.
- Digitalis glycoside and a diuretic for cardiac failure; dopamine or dobutamine may also be used.
- Diazepam to treat seizures.
- Norepinephrine (or another vasopressor) to treat hypotension.
- Administration of glucagon (5–10 mg rapidly over 30 sec), followed by continuous infusion of 5 mg/hr, may be effective in treating severe hypotension and bradycardia.

DRUG INTERACTIONS

Beta-adrenergic bronchodilators / ↓ Bronchodilator drug effects; greater dose of bronchodilator may be required

Cimetidine / ↑ Bioavailability of PO labetalol

Glutethimide / ↓ Labetalol effects R/T ↑ liver breakdown

Halothane / ↑ Risk of severe myocardial depression → hypotension

Nitroglycerin / Additive hypotension; labetalol blunts reflex tachycardia due to nitroglycerin without preventing hypotension

Tricyclic antidepressants / ↑ Risk of tremors

HOW SUPPLIED

Injection: 5 mg/mL; *Tablet:* 100 mg, 200 mg, 300 mg

DOSAGE————————

- **TABLETS**

  Hypertension.

  Individualize. Initial: 100 mg twice a day alone or with a diuretic. After 2 or 3 days, using BP as a guide, titrate dosage in increments of 100 mg twice a day, q 2–3 days. **Maintenance:** 200–400 mg twice a day up to 1,200–2,400 mg/day for severe cases.

- **IV**

  Hypertension.

  Individualize. Initial: 20 mg slowly over 2 min; **then,** 40–80 mg q 10 min until desired effect occurs or a total of 300 mg has been given.

- **IV INFUSION**

  Hypertension.

Initial: 2 mg/min; **then,** adjust rate according to response. **Usual dose range:** 50–300 mg.

Transfer from IV to PO therapy.

Initial: 200 mg; **then,** 200–400 mg 6–12 hr later, depending on response. Thereafter, dosage based on response.

NURSING CONSIDERATIONS

ADMINISTRATION/STORAGE

1. When transferring to PO labetalol from other antihypertensive therapy, slowly reduce dosage of current therapy.

2. Full antihypertensive effect is usually seen within the first 1–3 hr after the initial dose or dose increment.

IV 3. To transfer from IV to PO therapy in hospitalized clients, begin when supine BP begins to increase.

4. Not compatible with 5% sodium bicarbonate injection.

5. May give IV undiluted (20 mg over 2 min) or reconstituted with dextrose or saline solutions (infuse at a rate of 2 mg/min). When given by IV infusion, use an infusion control device.

ASSESSMENT

1. Note indications for therapy, other agents trialed and the outcome.

2. Assess effect of labetalol tablets on standing BP before hospital discharge. Obtain standing BP at different times during the day to assess full effects.

3. To reduce chance of orthostatic hypotension, keep supine for 3 hr after receiving parenteral labetalol.

CLIENT/FAMILY TEACHING

1. Take as directed with meals. Do not stop taking abruptly; may cause chest pain.

2. Use caution and change positions slowly; may precipitate sudden drop in BP and cause dizziness. Report any low heart rate, confusion, fever, swelling of extremities, difficulty breathing, night cough, or persistent dizziness. Record heart rate and BP for provider review.

3. May cause increased sensitivity to cold; dress appropriately.

L

4. Avoid alcohol, OTC products (especially cold remedies), high sodium intake, and tobacco.

OUTCOMES/EVALUATE
↓ BP

Lepirudin
(leh-**PEER**-you-din)

CLASSIFICATION(S):
Anticoagulant, thrombin inhibitor
PREGNANCY CATEGORY: B
Rx: Refludan

SEE ALSO ANTICOAGULANTS.

ACTION/KINETICS
Recombinant hirudin from yeast cells; highly specific direct inhibitor of thrombin. One antithrombin unit (ATU) is the amount of lepirudin that neutralizes one unit of World Health Organization preparation 89/588 of thrombin. One molecule of lepirudin binds to one molecule of thrombin, blocking the thrombogenic activity of thrombin. Thus, all thrombin-dependent assays are affected (i.e., activated partial thromboplastin time—aPTT), resulting in an increase in aPTT. **t ½, distribution:** About 10 min; **t ½, elimination:** About 1.3 hr. Systemic clearance is dependent on glomerular filtration rate. About half is excreted in the urine as unchanged drug and other fragments. Thought to be metabolized by release of amino acids via catabolic hydrolysis of the parent drug. The systemic clearance in women is about 25% lower than in men and clearance in the elderly is 20% less than younger clients. Dose must be adjusted based on C_{CR} as elimination half-lives are prolonged up to 2 days.

USES
Anticoagulation in heparin-induced thrombocytopenia (HIT) and associated thromboembolic disease to prevent further complications. *Investigational:* Adjunct to treat unstable angina, acute MI without ST elevation, prevent deep vein thrombosis, and in those undergoing percutaneous coronary intervention.

CONTRAINDICATIONS
Hypersensitivity to hirudins. Lactation.

SPECIAL CONCERNS
Assess risk of therapy in those with an increased risk of bleeding, including recent puncture of large vessels or organ biopsy; anomaly of vessels or organs; recent CVA, stroke, intracerebral surgery or other neuraxial procedures; severe uncontrolled hypertension; bacterial endocarditis; advanced renal impairment; hemorrhagic diathesis; recent major surgery; recent intracranial, GI, intraocular, or pulmonary major bleeding; recent active peptic ulcer. Formation of antihirudin antibodies or serious hepatic injury may increase the anticoagulant effect. Increased risk of allergic reactions in those also receiving thrombolytic therapy (e.g., streptokinase) for acute MI or contrast media for coronary angiography. Intracranial bleeding following concomitant thrombolytic therapy with alteplase or streptokinase may be life-threatening. Safety and efficacy have not been determined in children.

SIDE EFFECTS
Hemorrhagic events: Bleeding from puncture sites and wounds, anemia or isolated drop in hemoglobin, hematoma, hematuria, GI/rectal bleeding, epistaxis, hemothorax, vaginal bleeding, intracranial bleeding, hemoperitoneum, hemoptysis, liver bleeding, lung bleeding, mouth bleeding, retroperitoneal bleeding. **CV:** *Heart failure, pericardial effusion, ventricular fibrillation.* **Allergic reactions:** Cough, *bronchospasms,* stridor, dyspnea, pruritus, urticaria, rash, flushes, chills, *anaphylaxis,* angioedema, *facial/tongue/larynx edema.* **Miscellaneous:** Fever, pneumonia, sepsis, allergic skin reactions, abnormal kidney/liver function, unspecified infections, *multiorgan failure.*

OD **OVERDOSE MANAGEMENT**
Symptoms: Bleeding. *Treatment:* Immediately stop administration. Determine aPTT and other coagulation levels as appropriate. Determine hemoglobin and prepare for blood transfusion. Follow guidelines for treatment of shock. Hemofiltration or hemodialysis may be helpful.

DRUG INTERACTIONS

Coumarin derivatives / ↑ Risk of bleeding

Thrombolytics (streptokinase, TPA) / ↑ Risk of bleeding complications and ↑ effect on aPTT prolongation

HOW SUPPLIED

Powder for Injection: 50 mg

DOSAGE

- **IV**

  Heparin-induced   thrombocytopenia and associated thromboembolic disease.

Adults, initial: 0.4 mg/kg given slowly over 15–20 seconds as a bolus dose followed by 0.15 mg/kg/hr as a continuous IV infusion for 2–10 days or longer if needed. Normally the initial dose is based on body weight; this is valid for clients up to 110 kg; for those over 110 kg, do not increase the initial dosage beyond the 110 kg body weight dose (the maximum bolus dose is 44 mg and the maximal initial infusion dose is 16.5 mg/hr). Adjust dose according to the aPTT ratio (client aPTT at a given time over an aPTT reference value, usually median of the lab normal range for aPTT). The target range for aPTT is 1.5 to 2.5. To avoid initial overdosing, do not start therapy in clients with a baseline aPTT ratio of 2.5 or more.

The bolus and infusion doses must be reduced in known or suspected renal insufficiency (C_{CR} less than 60 mL/min or serum creatinine greater than 1.5 mg/dL).

  Concomitant use with thrombolytics. **Initial IV bolus:** 0.2 mg/kg; **continuous IV infusion:** 0.1 mg/kg/hr.

NURSING CONSIDERATIONS

ADMINISTRATION/STORAGE

[IV] 1. If client is to receive coumarin derivatives for PO anticoagulation after lepirudin, gradually reduce the dose of lepirudin to reach an aPTT ratio just above 1.5 before initiating PO anticoagulation. As soon as an INR of 2 is reached, stop drug.

2. Do not mix with other drugs except water for injection, 0.9% NaCl, or D5W injection.

3. Reconstitution and further dilution are to be done under sterile conditions as follows:

- Use D5W or water for injection for reconstitution

- For further dilution, 0.9% NaCl injection or D5W injection is suitable.

- For rapid, complete reconstitution, inject 1 mL of diluent into the vial and shake gently. A clear, colorless solution is usually obtained in a few seconds, but less than 3 min.

- Do not use solutions that are cloudy or contain particles.

- Use reconstituted solution immediately; it is stable for 24 hr or less at room temperature (i.e., during infusion).

- Warm the product to room temperature before administration.

- Discard any unused solution.

4. For the initial IV bolus, use a 5 mg/mL solution. Prepare as follows:

- Reconstitute one vial (50 mg) with 1 mL of 0.9% NaCl or water for injection.

- To obtain a final concentration of 5 mg/mL, transfer the contents of the vial into a sterile, single-use syringe (10 mL or greater capacity) and dilute the solution to a total volume of 10 mL using water for injection, 0.9% NaCl, or D5W.

5. For continuous IV infusion, use a concentration of 0.2 or 0.4 mg/mL. Prepare as follows:

- Reconstitute two vials (50 mg each) with 1 mL each using either 0.9% NaCl or water for injection.

- To obtain a final concentration of 0.2 or 0.4 mg/mL, transfer the contents of both vials into an infusion bag containing 500 or 250 mL of 0.9% NaCl or D5W.

- The infusion rate (mL/hr) is determined according to body weight).

ASSESSMENT

1. Assess for conditions that preclude therapy. Note allergic reactions with thrombolytic therapy.

2. Monitor LFTs, CBC, bleeding parameters, and renal function studies; reduce dosage with dysfunction.

3. If weight is more than 110 kg, do not increase dosage beyond that weight dose.

4. Monitor carefully at all sites for evidence of excessive bleeding. Have RBCs available for transfusion.

5. Get PTT 4 hr after first dose and at least daily during therapy (more frequently with liver/renal impairment). If PTT ratio >2.5 stop infusion for 2 hr and report.

CLIENT/FAMILY TEACHING
1. Drug is used to anticoagulate those with HIT.
2. Report any evidence of bleeding or oozing from catheter sites, under skin or gums, in urine or stools or adverse effects.
3. Use soft bristled tooth brush, electric razor, night light, and slippers to prevent injury; avoid contact sports or aggressive hugging, juggling or wrestling.

OUTCOMES/EVALUATE
• Inhibition of thromboembolic complications
• PTT ratio 1.5 to 2.5

Lidocaine hydrochloride
(LYE-doh-kayn)

CLASSIFICATION(S):
Antiarrhythmic, Class IB
PREGNANCY CATEGORY: B
Rx: IM: Lidocaine HCl for Cardiac Arrhythmias, LidoPen Auto-Injector. **Direct IV or IV Admixtures:** Lidocaine HCl for Cardiac Arrhythmias, Xylocaine HCl IV for Cardiac Arrhythmias. **IV Infusion:** Lidocaine HCl in 5% Dextrose.
♣Rx: Xylocard

SEE ALSO *ANTIARRHYTHMIC AGENTS.*

ACTION/KINETICS
Shortens the refractory period and suppresses the automaticity of ectopic foci without affecting conduction of impulses through cardiac tissue. Increases the electrical stimulation threshold of the ventricle during diastole. It does not affect BP, CO, or myocardial contractility. **IV, Onset:** 45–90 sec; **duration:** 10–20 min. **IM, Onset:** 5–15 min; **dura-**

tion: 60–90 min. **t ½:** 1–2 hr. **Therapeutic serum levels:** 1.5–6 mcg/mL. **Time to steady-state plasma levels:** 3–4 hr (8–10 hr in clients with AMI). Ninety percent is rapidly metabolized in the liver to active metabolites. Since lidocaine has little effect on conduction at normal antiarrhythmic doses, use in acute situations (instead of procainamide) in instances in which heart block might occur. Is 40–80% protein bound.

USES
IV: Acute ventricular arrhythmias (i.e., following MIs or occurring during surgery). Ineffective against atrial arrhythmias. **IM:** Certain emergency situations (e.g., ECG equipment not available; mobile coronary care unit, under advice of a physician).
Investigational: IV in children who develop ventricular couplets or frequent premature ventricular beats.

CONTRAINDICATIONS
Hypersensitivity to amide-type local anesthetics, Stokes-Adams syndrome, Wolff-Parkinson-White syndrome, severe SA, AV, or intraventricular block (when no pacemaker is present). Use of the IM autoinjector for children.

SPECIAL CONCERNS
Use with caution during labor and delivery, during lactation, and in the presence of liver or severe kidney disease, CHF, marked hypoxia, digitalis toxicity with AV block, severe respiratory depression, or shock. In geriatric clients, the rate and dose for IV infusion should be decreased by one-half and slowly adjusted. Safety and efficacy have not been determined in children.

SIDE EFFECTS
Body as a whole: Malignant hyperthermia characterized by tachycardia, tachypnea, labile BP, metabolic acidosis, temperature elevation. **CV:** Precipitation or aggravation of arrhythmias (following IV use), hypotension, bradycardia *(with possible cardiac arrest), CV collapse.* **CNS:** Dizziness, apprehension, euphoria, lightheadedness, nervousness, drowsiness, confusion, changes in mood, hallucinations, twitching, 'doom anxiety,' *convulsions,* unconsciousness.

Bold Italic = life threatening side effect   ■ = black box warning   ♣ = Available in Canada

Respiratory: Difficulties in breathing or swallowing, ***respiratory depression or arrest.*** **Allergic:** Rash, cutaneous lesions, urticaria, edema, ***anaphylaxis.*** **Other:** Tinnitus, blurred/double vision, vomiting, numbness, sensation of heat or cold, twitching, tremors, soreness at IM injection site, fever, ***venous thrombosis or phlebitis (extending from site of injection),*** extravasation. During anesthesia, CV depression may be the first sign of lidocaine toxicity. During other usage, *convulsions are the first sign of lidocaine toxicity.*

LABORATORY TEST CONSIDERATIONS
↑ CPK following IM use.

OD **OVERDOSE MANAGEMENT**
Symptoms: Dependent on plasma levels. If plasma levels range from 4 to 6 mcg/mL, mild CNS effects are observed. Levels of 6 to 8 mcg/mL may result in significant CNS and CV depression while levels greater than 8 mcg/mL cause hypotension, decreased CO, respiratory depression, obtundation, ***seizures, and coma.*** *Treatment:* Discontinue the drug and begin emergency resuscitative procedures. Seizures can be treated with diazepam, thiopental, or thiamylal. Succinylcholine, IV, may be used if the client is anesthetized. IV fluids, vasopressors, and CPR are used to correct circulatory depression.

DRUG INTERACTIONS
Aminoglycosides / ↑ Neuromuscular blockade
Beta-adrenergic blockers / ↑ Lidocaine levels with possible toxicity
Cimetidine / ↓ Clearance of lidocaine → possible toxicity
Phenytoin / IV phenytoin → excessive cardiac depression
Procainamide / Additive cardiodepressant effects
Succinylcholine / ↑ Succinylcholine action by ↓ plasma protein binding
Tocainide / ↑ Risk of side effects
Tubocurarine / ↑ Neuromuscular blockade

HOW SUPPLIED
IM Injection: 300 mg/3 mL; *Direct IV Injection:* 1%, 2%; *For IV Admixture:* 4%, 10%, 20%; *For IV Infusion:* 0.2%, 0.4%, 0.8%

DOSAGE
• **IV BOLUS**
Antiarrhythmic.
Adults: 50–100 mg at a rate of 25–50 mg/min. Bolus is used to establish rapid therapeutic plasma levels. Repeat if necessary after 5 min interval. Onset of action is 10 sec. **Maximum dose/hr:** 200–300 mg.
• **IV INFUSION**
Antiarrhythmic.
20–50 mcg/kg at a rate of 1–4 mg/min. No more than 200–300 mg/hr should be given. **Pediatric, loading dose:** 1 mg/kg IV or intratracheally q 5–10 min until desired effect reached (maximum total dose: 5 mg/kg).
• **IV CONTINUOUS INFUSION**
Maintain therapeutic plasma levels following loading doses.
Adults: Give at a rate of 1–4 mg/min (20–50 mcg/kg/min). Reduce the dose in clients with heart failure, with liver disease, or who are taking drugs that interact with lidocaine. **Pediatric:** 20–50 mcg/kg/min (usual is 30 mcg/kg/min).
• **IM**
Antiarrhythmic.
Adults: 4.5 mg/kg (approximately 300 mg for a 70-kg adult). Switch to IV lidocaine or oral antiarrhythmics as soon as possible although an additional IM dose may be given after 60–90 min.

NURSING CONSIDERATIONS
ADMINISTRATION/STORAGE
IV 1. *Do not add lidocaine to blood transfusion assembly.*
2. Do not use lidocaine solutions that contain epinephrine to treat arrhythmias. Make certain that vial states, "For Cardiac Arrhythmias." Check prefilled syringes closely to ensure appropriate dose has been obtained. (Lidocaine prefilled syringes come in both milligrams and grams.)
3. Use D5W to prepare solution; this is stable for 24 hr. Administer with an electronic infusion device.
4. Reduce IV bolus dosage in clients over 70 years old, with CHF or liver disease, and if taking cimetidine or pro-

pranolol (i.e., where metabolism of lidocaine is reduced).

ASSESSMENT

1. Note indications for therapy and any hypersensitivity to amide-type local anesthetics.

2. Those with hepatic or renal disease or who weigh less than 45.5 kg will need to be watched closely for adverse side effects; adjust dosage as directed.

3. Document CNS status; report sudden changes in mental status, dizziness, visual disturbances, twitching, and tremors. These symptoms may precede convulsions. Review pulmonary findings; assess for respiratory depression. Monitor liver and renal function studies, electrolytes, VS, and ECG; assess for hypotension and cardiac collapse.

4. View monitor strips for myocardial depression, variations of rhythm, or aggravation of arrhythmia during infusion.

CLIENT/FAMILY TEACHING

1. Drug is used to eradicate ventricular arrhythmias. It is generally administered IV in a continously monitored environment.

2. Report any evidences of dizziness or altered mentation; may be sign of toxicity and progress to seizures and coma.

3. Smoking is not permitted during drug therapy. Refer to smoking cessation for alternative therapy.

OUTCOMES/EVALUATE

• Control of ventricular arrhythmias

• Therapeutic serum drug levels (1.5–6 mcg/mL)

Lisinopril ■ ©

(lie-**SIN**-oh-prill)

CLASSIFICATION(S):
Antihypertensive, ACE inhibitor
PREGNANCY CATEGORY: C
Rx: Prinivil, Zestril
✤**Rx:** Apo-Lisinopril

SEE ALSO *ANGIOTENSIN-CONVERTING ENZYME INHIBITORS.*

ACTION/KINETICS

Both supine and standing BPs are reduced, although the drug is less effective in blacks than in Whites. Although food does not alter the bioavailability of lisinopril, only 25% of a PO dose is absorbed. **Onset:** 1 hr. **Peak serum levels:** 7 hr. **Duration:** 24 hr. Is about 25% bioavailable. **t ½:** 12 hr. 100% of the drug is excreted unchanged in the urine.

USES

(1) Alone or in combination with a diuretic (usually a thiazide) to treat hypertension. (2) Hypertension in children, aged 6–16 years. (3) In combination with digitalis and a diuretic for treating CHF not responding to other therapy. (4) Use within 24 hr of acute MI to improve survival in hemodynamically stable clients (clients should receive the standard treatment, including thrombolytics, aspirin, and beta blockers.

CONTRAINDICATIONS

Use in children less than 6 years of age or in children with a GFR less than 30 mL/min/1.73 m^2.

SPECIAL CONCERNS

■When used during the second and third trimesters of pregnancy, injury and even death can result in the developing fetus. When pregnancy is detected, discontinue as soon as possible.■ Use with caution during lactation. Safety and efficacy have not been established in children. Geriatric clients may manifest higher blood levels. Reduce the dosage in clients with impaired renal function.

SIDE EFFECTS

CV: Hypotension, orthostatic hypotension, angina, tachycardia, palpitations, rhythm disturbances, *stroke*, chest pain, orthostatic effects, peripheral edema, *MI, CVA,* worsening of heart failure, chest sound abnormalities, PVCs, TIAs, decreased blood pressure, atrial fibrillation. **CNS:** Dizziness, headache, fatigue, vertigo, insomnia, depression, sleepiness, paresthesias, malaise, nervousness, confusion, ataxia, impaired memory, tremor, irritability, hypersomnia, peripheral neuropathy, spasm. **GI:** Diarrhea, N&V, dyspepsia, anorexia, constipation, dysgeusia, dry mouth, abdominal pain, flatulence, dry mouth, gastritis, heartburn, GI cramps, weight

---

Bold Italic = life threatening side effect   ■ = black box warning   ✤ = Available in Canada

loss/gain, taste alterations, increased salivation. **Respiratory:** Cough, dyspnea, bronchitis, upper respiratory symptoms, nasal congestion, sinusitis, pharyngeal pain, bronchospasm, asthma, pulmonary edema infiltrates, *pulmonary embolism, pulmonary infarction,* PND, chest discomfort, common cold, pleural effusion, wheezing, painful respiration, epistaxis, laryngitis, pharyngitis, rhinitis, rhinorrhea, orthopnea. **Musculoskeletal:** Asthenia, muscle cramps, pain (neck, hip, leg, knee, arm, joint, shoulder, back, pelvic, flank), myalgia, arthralgia, arthritis, lumbago. **Hepatic:** Hepatitis, hepatocellular/cholestatic jaundice, pancreatitis, hepatomegaly. **Dermatologic:** Rash, pruritus, flushing, increased sweating, urticaria, alopecia, erythema multiforme, photophobia. **GU:** Impotence, oliguria, progressive azotemia, acute renal failure, UTI, anuria, uremia, renal dysfunction, pyelonephritis, dysuria. **Ophthalmic:** Blurred vision, visual loss, diplopia. **Miscellaneous:** *Angioedema (may be fatal if laryngeal edema occurs),* hyperkalemia, neutropenia, anemia, *bone marrow depression,* decreased libido, fever, syncope, vasculitis of the legs, gout, eosinophilia, fluid overload, dehydration, diabetes mellitus, chills, virus infection, edema, *anaphylactoid reaction,* malignant lung neoplasms, hemoptysis, breast pain.

LABORATORY TEST CONSIDERATIONS
↑ Serum potassium, BUN, serum creatinine. ↓ H&H.

OD OVERDOSE MANAGEMENT
Symptoms: Hypotension. *Treatment:* Supportive. To correct hypotension, IV normal saline is treatment of choice. Lisinopril may be removed by hemodialysis.

DRUG INTERACTIONS
Diuretics / Excess ↓ BP
Indomethacin / Possible ↓ lisinopril effect
Potassium-sparing diuretics / Significant ↑ serum potassium

HOW SUPPLIED
Tablet: 2.5 mg, 5 mg, 10 mg, 20 mg, 30 mg, 40 mg

DOSAGE
• **TABLETS**
Essential hypertension, used alone.
Adults, Initial: 10 mg once daily. Adjust dosage depending on response (range: 20–40 mg/day given as a single dose). Doses greater than 80 mg/day do not give a greater effect. **Children over 6 years of age, initial:** 0.07 mg/kg once daily up to 5 mg total). Adjust dose according to BP response; doses above 0.61 mg/kg (or in excess of 40 mg) have not been studied in children.
Essential hypertension in combination with a diuretic.
Initial: 5 mg. The BP-lowering effects of the combination are additive. Reduce dosage in renal impairment as follows: C_{CR}, 10–30 mL/min: Give an initial dose of 5 mg /day for hypertension. C_{CR}, less than 10 mL/min: Give an initial dose of 2.5 mg/day and adjust dose depending on BP response.
CHF.
Initial: 5 mg once daily (2.5 mg/day in clients with hyponatremia) in combination with diuretics and digitalis. **Dosage range:** 5–20 mg/day as a single dose.
Acute MI.
First dose: 5 mg within 24 hr of the onset of symptoms; **then,** 5 mg after 24 hr, 10 mg after 48 hr, and then 10 mg daily. Continue dosing for 6 weeks. In clients with a systolic pressure less than 120 mm Hg when treatment is started or within 3 days after the infarct should be given 2.5 mg. If hypotension occurs (systolic BP less than 100 mm Hg), the dose may be temporarily reduced to 2.5 mg. If prolonged hypotension occurs, withdraw the drug.

NURSING CONSIDERATIONS
⚐ Do not confuse lisinopril with Lioresal (a muscle relaxant). Also, do not confuse Prinivil with Prilosec (a proton pump inhibitor) or Proventil (a sympathomimetic).

ADMINISTRATION/STORAGE
1. To prepare a suspension (200 mL) of a 1 mg/mL concentration, add 10 mL purified water to a polyethylene terephthalate bottle containing ten-20 mg tablets of lisinopril. Shake for at least 1

H = Herbal   IV = Intravenous   ⚐ = sound-alike drug

min. Add 30 mL Bicitra diluent and 160 mL of Ora-Sweet SF to the concentrate in the bottle; shake gently for several seconds to disperse the ingredients. Store the suspension at or below 25°C (77°F) for up to 4 weeks. Shake the suspension before each use.

2. When considering use of lisinopril in a client taking diuretics, discontinue the diuretic, if possible, 2–3 days before beginning lisinopril therapy. If the diuretic cannot be discontinued, the initial dose of lisinopril should be 5 mg; observe closely for at least 2 hr.

3. Maximum antihypertensive effects may not be observed for 2–4 weeks.

4. When starting treatment for CHF, give under medical supervision, especially if SBP is less than 100 mm Hg.

5. With clients whose BP is controlled with lisinopril, 20 mg, plus hydrochlorothiazide 25 mg, given separately should trial Prinzide 12.5 mg or Zestoretic 20–12.5 mg before Prinzide 25 mg or Zestoretic 20–25 mg is used.

6. The maximum recommended daily dose of lisinopril is 80 mg in a single daily dose. Clients usually do not require hydrochlorothiazide in doses exceeding 50 mg/day, especially if combined with other antihypertensives.

7. Use of potassium supplements, potassium-sparing diuretics, or potassium salt substitutes with Prinzide or Zestoretic may lead to increases in serum potassium.

8. Prinzide or Zestoretic is recommended for those with a C_{CR} greater than 30 mL/min.

9. Anticipate reduced dosage with renal insufficiency—initial dose of 10 mg/day if C_{CR} is greater than 30 mL/min, 5 mg/day if C_{CR} is between 10 and 30 mL/min, and 2.5 mg/day in dialysis clients (i.e., C_{CR} less than 10 mL/min).

10. Store tablets from 15–30°C (59–86°F) and protect from moisture.

ASSESSMENT

1. Document indications for therapy, agents trialed and the outcome.

2. Perform physical exam noting cardiopulmonary status, review history for any existing conditions, and labs for any organ dysfunction.

3. Obtain ECG, VS, CXR, and baseline labs. Reduce dose with renal dysfunction.

4. Identify risk factors and those that are modifiable to reduce CHD.

5. Start within 24 hr of AMI in addition to ASA, beta blockers, statins, and thrombolytics to reduce mortality.

CLIENT/FAMILY TEACHING

1. Must be taken as directed at least once a day to control BP.

2. Avoid symptoms of low BP (i.e., rise slowly from sitting or lying position and wait until symptoms subside).

3. Avoid all potassium supplements as well as foods high in potassium, unless otherwise directed.

4. Review drug side effects; report for BP, ECG, and lab studies.

5. Report any new or unusual side effects or any aggravation of existing conditions, as well as sore throat, hoarseness, cough, chest pain, difficulty breathing, or swelling of hands, feet, or face.

6. Do not take nonprescription medications without medical advice as some may affect the action of lisinopril.

OUTCOMES/EVALUATE

• ↓ BP
• Improved survival with acute MI

Losartan potassium ■ⓒ

(loh-**SAR**-tan)

CLASSIFICATION(S):
Antihypertensive, angiotensin II receptor blocker

PREGNANCY CATEGORY: C (first trimester), D (second and third trimesters)

Rx: Cozaar

SEE ALSO *ANGTIOTENSIN II RECEPTOR ANTAGONISTS* AND *ANTIHYPERTENSIVE AGENTS.*

ACTION/KINETICS
Undergoes significant first-pass metabolism (by CYP2C9 and CYP3A4) in the liver, where it is converted to an active carboxylic acid metabolite that is re-

sponsible for most of the angiotensin receptor blockade. About 33% is bioavailable. Rapidly absorbed after PO administration, although food slows absorption. **Peak plasma levels of losartan and metabolite:** 1 hr and 3–4 hr, respectively. When used alone, decease in BP in blacks was less than in nonblacks. **t** $\frac{1}{2}$, **losartan:** 2 hr; **t** $\frac{1}{2}$, **metabolite:** 6–9 hr. **Maximum effects:** 1 week (3 to 6 weeks in some clients). Drug and metabolites are excreted through both the urine (35%) and feces (60%). 98.7% of the drug and 99.8% of the metabolite are bound to plasma proteins.

USES
(1) Antihypertensive, alone or in combination with other antihypertensive drugs. (2) Reduce risk of stroke in clients with hypertension and left ventricular hypertrophy. (3) Nephropathy in type 2 diabetics.

CONTRAINDICATIONS
Use during second and third trimesters of pregnancy due to possible injury and death to developing fetus.

SPECIAL CONCERNS
■Use during the second and third trimester of pregnancy can cause injury and even death to the fetus. When pregnancy is detected, discontinue as soon as possible.■ In severe CHF there is a risk of oliguria and/or progressive azotemia with acute renal failure and/or death (which are rare). In those with unilateral or bilateral renal artery stenosis, there is a risk of increased serum creatinine or BUN. Lower doses are recommended in those with hepatic insufficiency.

SIDE EFFECTS
GI: Diarrhea, dyspepsia, anorexia, constipation, dental pain, dry mouth, flatulence, gastritis, vomiting, taste perversion. **CV:** Angina pectoris, second-degree AV block, vasculitis, *CVA, MI, ventricular tachycardia, ventricular fibrillation,* hypotension, palpitation, sinus bradycardia, tachycardia, orthostatic effects. **CNS:** Dizziness, insomnia, anxiety, anxiety disorder, ataxia, confusion, depression, abnormal dreams, hypesthesia, decreased libido, impaired memory, migraine, nervousness, pares-

thesia, peripheral neuropathy, panic disorder, sleep disorder, somnolence, tremor, vertigo. **Respiratory:** URI, cough, nasal congestion, sinus disorder, sinusitis, dyspnea, bronchitis, pharyngeal discomfort, epistaxis, rhinitis, respiratory congestion. **Musculoskeletal:** Muscle cramps, myalgia, joint swelling, musculoskeletal pain, stiffness, arthralgia, arthritis, fibromyalgia, muscle weakness; pain in the back, legs, arms, hips, knees, shoulders. **Dermatologic:** Alopecia, dermatitis, dry skin, ecchymosis, erythema, flushing, photosensitivity, pruritus, rash, sweating, urticaria. **GU:** Impotence, nocturia, urinary frequency, UTI. **Ophthalmologic:** Blurred vision, burning/stinging in the eye, conjunctivitis, decrease in visual acuity. **Miscellaneous:** Gout, anemia, tinnitus, facial edema, fever, syncope.

LABORATORY TEST CONSIDERATIONS
Minor ↑ BUN, serum creatinine. Occasional ↑ liver enzymes and/or serum bilirubin. Small ↓ H&H.

OD OVERDOSE MANAGEMENT
Symptoms: Hypotension, tachycardia, bradycardia (due to vagal stimulation). *Treatment:* Supportive treatment. Hemodialysis is not indicated.

DRUG INTERACTIONS
Grapefruit juice / ↓ Liver metabolism of losartan to its active form
Indomethacin / ↓ Antihypertensive effect of losartan
Phenobarbital / ↓ Plasma losartan levels (20%)

HOW SUPPLIED
Tablet: 25 mg, 50 mg, 100 mg

DOSAGE
• **TABLETS**
  Hypertension.
Adults: 50 mg once daily with or without food. Total daily doses range from 25 to 100 mg. In those with possible depletion of intravascular volume (e.g., clients treated with a diuretic), use 25 mg once daily. If the antihypertensive effect (measured at trough) is inadequate, a twice-a-day regimen, using the same dose, may be tried; or an increase in dose may give a more satisfactory result. Range of total daily dose: 25–100 mg. If BP is not controlled by losartan

alone, a diuretic (e.g., hydrochlorothiazide) may be added.

Hypertensives with left ventricular hypertrophy.
Initial: 50 mg once daily. Add hydrochlorothiazide, 12.5 mg/day, and/or increase the dose of losartan to 100 mg once daily followed by an increase in hydrochlorothiazide to 25 mg once daily based on BP response.

Nephropathy in type 2 diabetics.
Initial: 50 mg once daily. Increase to 100 mg once daily based on BP response. May be given with insulin and other hypoglycemic drugs.

NURSING CONSIDERATIONS

Ⓒ Do not confuse Cozaar with Zocor (an antihyperlipidemic).

ADMINISTRATION/STORAGE
Store from 15–30°C (59–86°F) and protect from light. Keep container tightly closed.

ASSESSMENT
1. Document indications for therapy, onset, other agents used and outcome.
2. Monitor CBC, microalbumin, renal and LFTs. Correct any volume depletion prior to using to prevent sympathomimetic hypotension. Reduce starting dose with volume depletion or hepatic impairment. Observe for S&S of fluid or electrolyte imbalance.
3. When pregnancy is detected, discontinue as soon as possible.

CLIENT/FAMILY TEACHING
1. Take only as directed with or without food. Do not take with grapefruit juice. Avoid any OTC agents unless directed.
2. Regular exercise, proper low-salt diet, and lifestyle changes (i.e., no smoking, low alcohol, low-fat diet, low stress, adequate rest) may also contribute to enhanced BP control. Avoid salt substitutes containing potassium; may cause high potassium levels with this drug.
3. Do not change positions suddenly, dangle legs before rising, and rest until symptoms subside to prevent low BP.
4. May cause photosensitivity reaction; use precautions.
5. Use effective contraception; report immediately if pregnancy is suspected

because drug use during second and third trimesters is associated with fetal injury and morbidity.

OUTCOMES/EVALUATE
BP control; Cardiac/renal protection

Lovastatin (Mevinolin)   Ⓒ

(**LOW**-vah-**STAT**-in, me-**VIN**-oh-lin)

CLASSIFICATION(S):
Antihyperlipidemic, HMG-CoA reductase inhibitor
PREGNANCY CATEGORY: X
Rx: Altocor, Mevacor
❖**Rx:** Apo-Lovastatin, Gen-Lovastatin, ratio-Lovastatin

SEE ALSO ANTIHYPERLIPIDEMIC AGENTS— HMG-COA REDUCTASE INHIBITORS.

ACTION/KINETICS
Isolated from a strain of *Aspergillus terreus.* Approximately 35% of a dose is absorbed. Extensive first-pass metabolism (by CYP2C9; less than 5% reaches the general circulation. Absorption is decreased by about one-third if the drug is given on an empty stomach rather than with food. **Onset:** Within 2 weeks using multiple doses. **Time to peak plasma levels:** 2–4 hr. **Time to peak effect:** 4–6 weeks using multiple doses. **t ½, elimination:** 1.1–1.7 hr. **Duration:** 4–6 weeks after termination of therapy. Metabolized in the liver (its main site of action) to active metabolites. Over 80% of a PO dose is excreted in the feces, via the bile, and approximately 10% is excreted through the urine. Over 95% is bound to plasma proteins.

USES
Immediate-Release Only: (1) As an adjunct to diet to reduce elevated total and LDL cholesterol in primary hypercholesterolemia (types IIa and IIb) when the response to diet restricted in saturated fat and cholesterol and to other nonpharmacological regimens has been inadequate. (2) As an adjunct to

---

diet to reduce total and LDL cholesterol and apolipoprotein B levels in adolescent boys and girls (who are at least 1 yr postmenarche) and 10–17 years old, with heterozygous familial hypercholesterolemia. Used in those after an adequate trial of diet, the LDL cholesterol remains higher than 189 mg/dL or if LDL cholesterol remains higher than 160 gm/dL *and* there is a positive family history of premature CV disease or 2 or more CV disease risk factors present.

Extended-Release Only: Adjunct to diet to decrease elevated total and LDL cholesterol, apolipoprotein B, and triglycerides and to increase HDL cholesterol in those with primary hypercholesterolemia (heterozygous familial and nonfamilial and mixed dyslipidemia Fredrickson types IIa and IIb) when response to diet restricted in saturated fat and cholesterol and other nonpharmacological measures have been inadequate.

Immediate-Release or Extended-Release: (1) To slow the progression of coronary atherosclerosis in clients with CAD in order to lower total and LDL cholesterol levels to target levels. (2) Primary prevention of coronary heart disease in those without symptomatic CV disease, average to moderately elevated total cholesterol and LDL cholesterol, and below average HDL cholesterol. Used to reduce risk of MI, unstable angina, and coronary revascularization procedures. *Investigational:* Diabetic dyslipidemia, nephrotic hyperlipidemia, familial dysbetalipoproteinemia, and familial combined hyperlipidemia.

ADDITIONAL CONTRAINDICATIONS
Use with mibefradil (Posicor).

SPECIAL CONCERNS
Carefully monitor clients with impaired renal function.

SIDE EFFECTS
See *Antihyperlipidemic Agents—HMG-CoA Reductase Inhibitors.* **CNS:** Headache, dizziness, paresthesia, insomnia. **GI:** Flatus (most common), abdominal pain, cramps, diarrhea, constipation, dyspepsia, N&V, heartburn, dysgeusia, acid regurgitation, dry mouth. **Musculoskeletal:** Myalgia, muscle cramps, arthralgia, leg/shoulder pain, localized pain. **Miscellaneous:** Blurred vision, eye irritation, rash, pruritus, chest pain, alopecia.

LABORATORY TEST CONSIDERATIONS
↑ Risk of elevated serum transaminases in clients with homozygous familial hypercholesterolemia.

ADDITIONAL DRUG INTERACTIONS
Grapefruit juice / ↑ Lovastatin plasma levels R/T ↓ liver metabolism; ↑ risk of myopathy and rhabdomyolysis
Isradipine / ↑ Clearance of lovastatin

HOW SUPPLIED
Tablet, Immediate Release: 10 mg, 20 mg, 40 mg; *Tablet, Extended-Release:* 10 mg, 20 mg, 40 mg, 60 mg

DOSAGE————————————————
• **TABLETS, IMMEDIATE-RELEASE**
Hypercholesterolemia, coronary heart disease, primary prevention of coronary heart disease.
Adults/adolescents, initial: 20 mg once daily with the evening meal. Initiate at 10 mg/day in clients who require smaller reductions. Dose range: 10–80 mg/day in single or two divided doses. Adjust dose at intervals of every 4 weeks, if necessary. If C_{CR} is less than 30 mL/min, use doses greater than 20 mg/day with caution.
Adolescents with heterozygous familial hypercholesterolemia.
Dose range: 10–40 mg/day (maximum). Individualize dose depending on goal of therapy. Start clients with 20 mg/day who require decreases in LDL cholesterol of 20% or more to achieve their goal. For those requiring smaller reductions, start with 10 mg/day. Adjust dose at intervals of 4 weeks or more.
• **TABLETS, EXTENDED-RELEASE**
Hyperlipidemia, coronary heart disease, primary prevention of coronary heart disease.
Initial: 20, 40, or 60 mg once a day at bedtime; range: 10–60 mg/day in single doses. Start with 10 mg once a day for those requiring small reductions in lipid levels. Adjust dose at intervals of 4 weeks or more.

L

NURSING CONSIDERATIONS

€ Do not confuse lovastatin with Lotensin (an ACE inhibitor).

ADMINISTRATION/STORAGE

1. Immediate-release is effective alone or when used together with bile acid sequestrants. Avoid use of extended-release with fibrates or niacin.

2. If lovastatin is used with gemfibrozil, other fibrates, or lipid-lowering doses of niacin (1 g or more), do not exceed a dose of 20 mg/day of lovastatin due to the increased risk of myopathy.

3. Do not exceed a dose of 40 mg/day of lovastatin in clients taking amiodarone or verapamil. Do not exceed a dose of 20 mg/day of lovastatin in clients taking cyclosporine due to the increased risk of myopathy.

4. Store immediate-release tablets between 5–30°C (41–86°F) protected from light in a well-closed, light-resistant container. Store extended-release tablets at controlled room temperature of 20–25°C (68–77°F); avoid excess heat and humidity.

ASSESSMENT

1. Document serum cholesterol profile, other therapies and the outcome.

2. Note hepatic disease and any heavy consumption of alcohol.

3. Determine if pregnant.

4. Request recent eye exam; slight changes have been noted in the lenses of some clients.

5. Assess LFTs q 4–6 weeks for the first 12 mo of therapy. A threefold increase in serum transaminase or new-onset abnormal LFTs is an indication to stop therapy.

6. Assess life-style, including weight, diet (intake of fats, CHOs, and proteins), activity (regular exercise), alcohol consumption, and smoking history. Identify areas that may contribute to increased cholesterol levels.

CLIENT/FAMILY TEACHING

1. Take with meals. Avoid coadministration with grapefruit juice due to increased serum levels of lovastatin. Continue cholesterol-lowering diet and exercise program as prescribed. Cholesterol production by the liver is highest in the evening; drug usually taken with the evening meal.

2. Place client on a standard cholesterol-lowering diet before starting lovastatin and continue during therapy. Adhere to dietary restrictions, daily exercise, and weight loss in the overall management and control of hypercholesterolemia/hyperlipidemia.

3. Practice reliable birth control; drug is pregnancy category X.

4. Report malaise, muscle spasms, or fever. These may be mistaken for the flu, but could be serious side effects of drug therapy.

5. Any RUQ abdominal pain or change in color and consistency of stools should be reported.

6. Periodic LFTs and eye exams are mandatory; report any early visual disturbances.

OUTCOMES/EVALUATE

• ↓ Cholesterol/triglyceride levels
• ↓ Progression of coronary atherosclerosis

Magnesium sulfate

(mag-**NEE**-see-um **SUL**-fayt)

CLASSIFICATION(S):
Anticonvulsant, miscellaneous; saline laxative
PREGNANCY CATEGORY: A

SEE ALSO *ANTICONVULSANTS* AND *LAXATIVES.*

ACTION/KINETICS
Magnesium (Mg) is an essential element for muscle contraction, certain enzyme systems, and nerve transmission. Extracellular fluid levels: 1.5–2.5 mEq/L. Mg depresses the CNS and controls convulsions by blocking release of acetylcholine at the myoneural junction. Also, Mg decreases the sensitivity of the motor end plate to acetylcholine and decreases the excitability of the motor membrane. **Therapeutic anticonvulsant serum levels:** 2.5 or 3–7.5 mEq/L (normal Mg levels: 1.5–2.5 mEq/L). **Onset, IM:** 1 hr; **IV:** immediate. **Duration, IM:** 3–4 hr; **IV:** 30 min. Excreted by the kidneys at a rate proportional to the serum concentration and GFR. Is 30% bound to albumin.

USES
Parenteral. (1) Seizures associated with epilepsy or when abnormally low levels of magneisum may be a contributing factor in convulsions, such as in hypothyroidism or glomerulonephritis. (2) Prevention and treatment of seizures in severe pre-eclampsia or eclampsia without producing deleterious CNS depression in mother or infant. (3) To control hypertension, encephalopathy, and convulsions associated with acute nephritis in children. (4) Replacement therapy in Mg deficiency, especially in acute hypomagnesemia accompanied by signs of tetany. **Oral.** Laxative. *Investigational:* Inhibit premature labor (not a first-line agent). IV use as an adjunct to treat acute exacerbations of moderate to severe asthma in clients who respond poorly to beta agonists. In adults to prevent recurrences of **torsades de pointes** by suppressing early-after depolarization.

CONTRAINDICATIONS
In the presence of heart block or myocardial damage. In toxemia of pregnancy during the 2 hr prior to delivery.

SPECIAL CONCERNS
Use with caution in clients with renal disease because Mg is removed from the body solely by the kidneys. The elderly may require reduced dosage due to impaired renal function. Use with caution during lactation.

SIDE EFFECTS
Magnesium intoxication. **CNS:** Depression. **CV:** Flushing, hypotension, *circulatory collapse, depression of the myocardium.* **Other:** Sweating, hypothermia, muscle paralysis, CNS depression, *respiratory paralysis.* Suppression of knee jerk reflex can be used to determine toxicity. *Respiratory failure may occur if given after knee jerk reflex disappears.* Hypocalcemia with signs of tetany secondary to Mg sulfate when used for eclampsia. *NOTE:* Magneisum toxicity may occur in the newborn especially if the mother has received an IV infusion for more than 24 hr prior to delivery. Elevated Mg levels may persist for up to 7 days in the newborn.

OD **OVERDOSE MANAGEMENT**
Symptoms: Serum levels can predict symptoms of toxicity. Symptoms include *sharp decrease in BP and respiratory paralysis,* changes in ECG (increased PR interval, increased QRS complex, prolonged QT interval), *asystole, heart block.* At serum levels greater than 3 mEq/L there is N&V, weakness, and flushing. Levels greater than 5 mEq/L: ECG changes, including prolonged PR, QRS, and QT intervals. Levels of 7–10 mEq/L: Hypotension, sedation, and loss of DTRs. *Levels greater than*

10 mEq/L: Arrhythmias, muscle paralysis, respiratory arrest, hypotension. Levels greater than 14 mEq/L: Respiratory arrest, asystole, death.
Treatment:
- Use artificial ventilation immediately.
- Have 5–10 mEq of calcium (e.g., 10–20 mL of 10% calcium gluconate) readily available for IV injection to reverse heart block and respiratory depression.
- Hemodialysis and peritoneal dialysis are effective.

DRUG INTERACTIONS
CNS depressants (general anesthetics, sedative-hypnotics, narcotics) / Additive CNS depression
Neuromuscular blocking agents / Possible potentiation of neuromuscular blockade
Streptomycin / ↓ Streptomycin antibiotic activity
Tetracycline / ↓ Tetracycline antibiotic activity
Tobramycin / ↓ Tobramycin antibiotic activity

HOW SUPPLIED
Injection: 4% (0.325 mEq/mL), 8% (0.65 mEq/mL), 12.5% (1 mEq/mL), 50% (4 mEq/mL)

DOSAGE————————————
• IM
Anticonvulsant.
Adults: 1–5 g of a 25–50% solution up to 6 times per day. **Pediatric:** 20–40 mg/kg using the 20% solution (may be repeated if necessary).
Acute nephritis in children.
20–40 mg/kg as needed to control seizures. Dilute the 50% concentration to a 20% solution and give 0.1–0.2 mL/kg of the 20% solution.
• IV
Anticonvulsant.
Adults: 1–4 g using 10–20% solution, not to exceed 1.5 mL/min of the 10% solution.
Seizures associated with eclampsia.
Initial: 10–14 g. To initiate therapy, 4 g Mg sulfate in water for injection or 4–5 g in 250 mL of D5W or 0.9% NaCl may be given IV. Simultaneously, 4–5 g may be given IM into each buttock using undiluted 50% Mg sulfate. Alternatively,

the initial IV dose of 4 g may be given by diluting the 50% solution to a 10% or 20% concentration; the diluted solution (40 mL of a 10% solution or 20 mL of a 20% solution) may be given IV over a period of 3–4 hr. After the initial IV dose, 1–2 g/hr may be given by IV infusion. Subsequent IM doses of 4–5 g may be injected into alternate buttocks q 4 hr, depending on the presence of the patellar reflex, adequate respiratory function, and absences of signs of Mg toxicity. Continue therapy until paroxysms cease.
Hypomagnesemia, mild.
Adults: 1 g as a 50% solution q 6 hr for 4 times (or total of 32.5 mEq/24 hr).
Hypomagnesemia, severe.
Adults: Up to 2 mEq/kg over 4 hr.
• IV INFUSION
Anticonvulsant.
Adults: 4–5 g in 250 mL D5W at a rate not to exceed 3 mL/min.
Hypomagnesemia, severe.
Adults: 5 g (40 mEq) in 1,000 mL D5W or sodium chloride solution by **slow** infusion over period of 3 hr.
Hyperalimentation.
Adults: 8–24 mEq/day; **infants:** 2–10 mEq/day.
• ORAL SOLUTION
Laxative.
Adults: 10–15 g; **pediatric:** 5–10 g.

NURSING CONSIDERATIONS
ADMINISTRATION/STORAGE
1. When used as a laxative, dissolve in a glassful of ice water or other chilled fluid to lessen the disagreeable taste.
2. Dilutions for IM: deep injection of 50% concentrate for adults. Use a 20% solution for children.
[IV] 3. For IV infusion, dilute to a concentration of 20% or less. Generally do not exceed an IV rate of 1.5 mL of a 10% concentration (or its equivalent) per min (150 mg/min), except in severe eclampsia with seizures.
4. Mg sulfate in solution may cause a precipitate when mixed with solutions containing the following: High concentrations of alcohol, alkali carbonates and bicarbonates, alkali hydroxides, arsenates, barium, calcium, clindamycin

phosphate, heavy metals, hydrocortisone sodium succinate, phosphates, polymyxin B sulfate, procaine HCl, salicylates, strontium, and tartrates.

ASSESSMENT

1. Document indications for therapy, onset and characteristics of S&S.
2. Evaluate cardiac status, respirations, and ECG. Monitor I&O.
3. Note any kidney disease. Assess Mg levels (S&S of toxicity begin at 4 mEq/L.) and renal function.
4. With premature labor, continually assess fetal heart rate and intensity and timing of contractions.

INTERVENTIONS

1. Before administering IV check for the following conditions:
- Absent patellar reflexes
- Respirations below 16/min
- Urine output < 100 mL in past 4 hr
- Early signs of hypermagnesemia: flushing, sweating, hypotension, or hypothermia
- Past history of heart block or myocardial damage; prolonged PR and widened QRS intervals
2. Adjust dose of CNS depressants.
3. Digitalis toxicity treated with calcium is extremely dangerous and may result in heart block.
4. With acute MI, administer immediately and continue for 24–48 hr.
5. Do not administer for 2 hr preceding delivery.
6. If mother received continuous IV Mg therapy 24 hr prior to delivery, assess newborn for neurologic and respiratory depression.

CLIENT/FAMILY TEACHING

1. Do not exceed prescribed dose.
2. Ensure well balanced diet, with increased bulk, increased water intake, and regular daily exercise to promote bowel motility.
3. Report adverse side effects or lack of response.

OUTCOMES/EVALUATE

- Control of seizures
- Mg levels (1.8–3 mEq/L)
- Successful evacuation of stool

Methyldopa ©
(meth-ill-**DOH**-pah)

CLASSIFICATION(S):
Antihypertensive, centrally-acting
PREGNANCY CATEGORY: B (PO), C (IV)
♣**Rx:** Apo-Methyldopa, Nu-Medopa

Methyldopate hydrochloride
PREGNANCY CATEGORY: B (PO), C (IV)
Rx: Aldomet Hydrochloride

SEE ALSO *ANTIHYPERTENSIVE AGENTS.*

ACTION/KINETICS

The active metabolite, alpha-methylnorepinephrine, lowers BP by stimulating central inhibitory alpha-adrenergic receptors, false neurotransmission, and/or reduction of plasma renin. Little change in CO. **PO, Onset:** 7–12 hr. **Duration:** 12–24 hr. All effects terminated within 48 hr. Absorption is variable. **IV, Onset:** 4–6 hr. **Duration:** 10–16 hr. Seventy percent of drug excreted in urine. **Full therapeutic effect:** 1–4 days. **t ½:** 1.7 hr. Metabolites excreted in the urine.

USES

PO: Moderate to severe hypertension. Particularly useful for clients with impaired renal function, renal hypertension, resistant cases of hypertension complicated by stroke, CAD, or nitrogen retention. **IV:** Hypertensive crisis. *Investigational:* Hypertension in pregnancy.

CONTRAINDICATIONS

Sensitivity to drug (including sulfites), labile and mild hypertension, pregnancy, active hepatic disease (e.g., acute hepatitis, active cirrhosis), use with MAO inhibitors, or pheochromocytoma. Use if previous methyldopa therapy has been associated with liver disorders.

SPECIAL CONCERNS

Use with caution in clients with a history of liver or kidney disease. A decrease in dose in geriatric clients may prevent syncope.

M

SIDE EFFECTS

CNS: Sedation (transient), weakness, headache, asthenia, dizziness, paresthesias, Parkinson-like symptoms, psychic disturbances, symptoms of CV impairment, choreoathetotic movements, Bell's palsy, decreased mental acuity, verbal memory impairment. **CV:** Bradycardia, orthostatic hypotension, hypersensitivity of carotid sinus, worsening of angina, paradoxical hypertensive response (after IV), myocarditis, CHF, pericarditis, vasculitis. **GI:** N&V, abdominal distention, diarrhea or constipation, flatus, colitis, dry mouth, sore or 'black tongue,' pancreatitis, sialoadenitis, hepatotoxicity, jaundice. **Hematologic:** **Hemolytic anemia,** leukopenia, granulocytopenia, thrombocytopenia, ***bone marrow depression.*** **Endocrine:** Gynecomastia, amenorrhea, galactorrhea, lactation, hyperprolactinemia. **GU:** Impotence, failure to ejaculate, decreased libido. **Dermatologic:** Rash, ***toxic epidermal necrolysis.*** **Hepatic:** Jaundice, hepatitis, liver disorders, abnormal LFTs. **Miscellaneous:** Edema, weight gain, fever, lupus-like symptoms, nasal stuffiness, arthralgia, myalgia, ***septic shock-like syndrome.***

LABORATORY TEST CONSIDERATIONS

Positive Coombs' test. Hepatotoxicity may cause ↑ alkaline phosphatase, AST, ALT, bilirubin, and prothrombin time; also, eosinophilia. Interference with urinary uric acid by phosphotungstate method; serum creatinine by the alkaline picrate method; AST by colorimetric methods.

OD OVERDOSE MANAGEMENT

Symptoms: CNS, GI, and CV, effects including sedation, weakness, lightheadedness, dizziness, coma, bradycardia, acute hypotension, impairment of AV conduction, constipation, diarrhea, distention, flatus, N&V. *Treatment:* Induction of vomiting or gastric lavage if detected early. General supportive treatment with special attention to HR, CO, blood volume, urinary function, electrolyte imbalance, paralytic ileus, and CNS activity. In severe cases, hemodialysis is effective.

DRUG INTERACTIONS

Anesthetics, general / Additive hypotension
Antidepressants, tricyclic / May block methyldopa hypotensive effects
Ferrous gluconate or sulfate / ↓ Bioavailability of methyldopa
Haloperidol / ↑ Haloperidol toxic effects
Levodopa / ↑ Effect of both drugs
Lithium / ↑ Possibility of lithium toxicity
MAO inhibitors / Accumulation of methyldopa metabolites may → excessive sympathetic stimulation
Methotrimeprazine / Additive hypotensive effect
Phenothiazines / Possible ↑ BP
Propranolol / Paradoxical hypertensive crisis
Sympathomimetics / Potentiation of pressor effects → hypertension
Thiazide diuretics / Additive hypotensive effect
Thioxanthenes / Additive hypotensive effect
Tolbutamide / ↑ Hypoglycemia R/T ↓ liver breakdown
Tricyclic antidepressants / ↓ Methyldopa effect
Vasodilator drugs / Additive hypotensive effect
Verapamil / ↑ Methyldopa effect

HOW SUPPLIED

Methyldopa: *Tablet:* 250 mg, 500 mg. **Methyldopate hydrochloride:** *Injection:* 50 mg/mL.

DOSAGE

- **METHYLDOPA TABLETS**
  Hypertension.

Initial: 250 mg 2– 3 times per day for 2 days. Adjust dose q 2 days. If increased, start with evening dose. **Usual maintenance:** 0.5–2.0 g/day in two to four divided doses; **maximum:** 3 g/day. Gradually transfer to and from other antihypertensive agents, with initial dose of methyldopa not exceeding 500 mg. *NOTE:* Do not use combination medication to initiate therapy. **Pediatric, initial:** 10 mg/kg/day in two to four divided doses, adjusting maintenance to a maximum of 65 mg/kg/day (or 3 g/day, whichever is less).

Bold Italic = life threatening side effect   ■ = black box warning   ✦ = Available in Canada

• **METHYLDOPA HCL, IV INFUSION**
Hypertensive crisis.
Adults: 250–500 mg q 6 hr; **maximum:**
1 g q 6 hr for hypertensive crisis. Switch
to PO methyldopa, at same dosage level, when BP is brought under control.
Pediatric: 20–40 mg/kg/day in divided
doses q 6 hr; **maximum:** 65 mg/kg/day
(or 3 g/day, whichever is less).

NURSING CONSIDERATIONS
© Do not confuse Aldomet with Aldoril
(also an antihypertensive).
ADMINISTRATION/STORAGE
1. Tolerance may occur following 2–3
months of therapy. Increasing the dose
or adding a diuretic often restores effect on BP.
[IV] 2. For IV, mix with 100 mL of D5W
or administer in D5W at a concentration
of 10 mg/mL. Infuse over 30–60 min.
ASSESSMENT
1. Document indications for therapy,
onset/characteristics of symptoms, other agents prescribed and outcome.
2. Monitor BP, CBC, renal and LFTs, and
Coombs' test. If blood transfusion required, obtain both direct and indirect
Coombs' tests; if positive, consult he-
matologist.
3. Avoid during pregnancy. Note any
jaundice; contraindicated with active
hepatic disease.
4. Assess for depression and drug tolerance; may occur during the second or
third month of therapy.
CLIENT/FAMILY TEACHING
1. To prevent dizziness and fainting,
rise slowly to a sitting position and dangle legs over the bed edge.
2. Use caution, sedation may occur initially; should disappear once maintenance dose established.
3. In rare cases, may darken or turn
urine blue; not harmful.
4. Withhold and report any of the following symptoms: tiredness, fever, depression, or yellowing of eyes/skin.
5. Continue to follow prescribed diet
and exercise program in the overall
goal of BP control.
6. Do not take any other medications
or remedies unless appoved.
OUTCOMES/EVALUATE
↓ BP

Metolazone   ©
(meh-**TOH**-lah-zohn)

CLASSIFICATION(S):
Diuretic, thiazide
PREGNANCY CATEGORY: B
Rx: Mykrox, Zaroxolyn

SEE ALSO *DIURETICS, THIAZIDE.*
ACTION/KINETICS
Onset: 1 hr. **Peak blood levels, rapid
availability tablets:** 2–4 hr; **t ½, elimination:** About 14 hr. **Peak blood levels, slow availability tablets:** 8 hr. **Duration, rapid or slow availablity tablets:** 24 hr or more. Most excreted
unchanged through the urine.
USES
Slow availability tablets: (1) Edema
accompanying CHF; edema accompanying renal diseases, including nephrotic syndrome and conditions of reduced
renal function. (2) Alone or in combination with other drugs for the treatment
of hypertension.
   Rapid availability tablets: Treatment of newly diagnosed mild to moderate hypertension alone or in combination with other drugs. The rapid
availability tablets are not to be used to
produce diuresis.
   Investigational: Alone or as an adjunct to treat calcium nephrolithiasis,
premanagement of menstrual syndrome, and adjunct treatment of renal
failure.
CONTRAINDICATIONS
Anuria, prehepatic and hepatic coma,
allergy or hypersensitivity to metolazone. Routine use during pregnancy.
Lactation.
SPECIAL CONCERNS
Use with caution in those with severely
impaired renal function and in the elderly. Safety and effectiveness have not
been determined in children.
SIDE EFFECTS
See *Diuretics, Thiazide.* The most commonly reported side effects are diz-

M

ziness, headache, muscle cramps, malaise, lethargy, lassitude, joint pain/swelling, and chest pain. Also, *toxic epidermal necrolysis and Stevens-Johnson syndrome.*

ADDITIONAL DRUG INTERACTIONS

Alcohol / ↑ Hypotensive effect
Barbiturates / ↑ Hypotensive effect
Narcotics / ↑ Hypotensive effect
NSAIDs / ↓ Hypotensive effect of metolazone
Salicylates / ↓ Hypotensive effect of metolazone

HOW SUPPLIED

Tablets: 0.5 mg, 2.5 mg, 5 mg, 10 mg.

DOSAGE

- **SLOW AVAILABILITY TABLETS**

ZAROXOLYN

Edema due to cardiac failure or renal disease.

Adults: 5–20 mg once daily. For those who experience paroxysmal nocturnal dyspnea, a larger dose may be required to ensure prolonged diuresis and saluresis for a 24-hr period.

Mild to moderate essential hypertension.

Adults: 2.5–5 mg once daily.

- **RAPID AVAILABILITY TABLETS**

MYKROX

Mild to moderate essential hypertension.

Adults, initial: 0.5 mg once daily, usually in the morning. If inadequately controlled, the dose may be increased to 1 mg once a day. Increasing the dose higher than 1 mg does not increase the effect.

NURSING CONSIDERATIONS

℃ Do not confuse metolazone with methotrexate (an antineoplastic) or with metoclopramide (a GI stimulant).

ADMINISTRATION/STORAGE

1. Formulations of slow availability tablets should not be interchanged with formulations of rapid availability tablets as they are not therapeutically equivalent.
2. The antihypertensive effect may be observed from 3 to 4 days to 3 to 6 weeks.
3. If BP is not controlled with 1 mg of the rapid availability tablets, add another antihypertensive drug, with a different mechanism of action, to the therapy.
4. Store tablets at room temperature in a tight, light-resistant container.

ASSESSMENT

1. Document indications for therapy, noting onset, duration, and clinical characteristics. Has synergistic effect with furosemide.
2. Monitor BP, ECG, CBC, electrolytes, liver and renal function studies; assess for symptoms of electrolyte imbalance (i.e., ↓ Na/K/Mg/P and hypochloremic alkalosis).

CLIENT/FAMILY TEACHING

1. May take with food. Take exactly as directed; early in the day to prevent nighttime awakening for urination.
2. May cause sudden drop in BP and syncope; use caution and change positions slowly. Avoid alcohol during therapy.
3. Check weight regularly; report increases of more than 3 lb/day or lack of response to extremity swelling.
4. Avoid exposure to sun or bright lights; may cause photosensitivity.
5. May cause potassium depletion; eat a K rich diet (whole grain cereals, legumes, meat, bananas, apricots, orange juice, potatoes, raisins) and keep all F/U appointments for evaluation and lab tests.
6. Report any muscle weakness/cramps, fatigue, nausea, dizziness, or adverse effects.

OUTCOMES/EVALUATE

↓ Edema; ↓ BP

Metoprolol succinate ℃

(me-toe-**PROH**-lohl)

CLASSIFICATION(S):
Beta-adrenergic blocking agent
PREGNANCY CATEGORY: C
Rx: Toprol XL

Metoprolol tartrate

PREGNANCY CATEGORY: B

Rx: Lopressor

♣Rx: Apo-Metoprolol, Apo-Metoprolol (Type L), Betaloc, Betaloc Durules, Gen-Metoprolol, Gen-Metoprolol (Type L), Novo–Metoprol, Nu-Metop, PMS-Metoprolol-B, PMS-Metoprolol-L

SEE ALSO *BETA-ADRENERGIC BLOCKING AGENTS.*

ACTION/KINETICS

Exerts mainly beta-1-adrenergic blocking activity although beta-2 receptors are blocked at high doses. Has no membrane stabilizing or intrinsic sympathomimetic effects. Moderate lipid solubility. **Onset:** 15 min. **Peak plasma levels:** 90 min. **t½:** 3–7 hr. Effect of drug is cumulative. Food increases bioavailability. Exhibits significant first-pass effect. Metabolized in liver and excreted in urine.

USES

Metoprolol Succinate: (1) Alone or with other drugs to treat hypertension. (2) Chronic management of angina pectoris. (3) Treatment of stable, symptomatic (NYHA Class II or III) heart failure of ischemic, hypertensive, or cardiomyopathic origin.

Metoprolol Tartrate: (1) Hypertension (either alone or with other antihypertensive agents, such as thiazide diuretics). (2) Acute MI in hemodynamically stable clients. (3) Angina pectoris. *Investigational:* IV to suppress atrial ectopy in COPD, aggressive behavior, prophylaxis of migraine, ventricular arrhythmias, enhancement of cognitive performance in geriatric clients, essential tremors.

ADDITIONAL CONTRAINDICATIONS

Myocardial infarction in clients with a HR of less than 45 bpm, in second- or third-degree heart block, or if SBP is less than 100 mm Hg. Moderate to severe cardiac failure.

SPECIAL CONCERNS

Safety and effectiveness have not been established in children. Use with caution in impaired hepatic function and during lactation.

LABORATORY TEST CONSIDERATIONS

↑ Serum transaminase, LDH, alkaline phosphatase.

ADDITIONAL DRUG INTERACTIONS

Cimetidine / May ↑ plasma metoprolol levels

Contraceptives, oral / May ↑ metoprolol effects

Diphenhydramine / ↓ Metoprolol clearance → prolonged negative chronotropic and inotropic effects in extensive metabolizers

Hydroxychloroquine / ↑ Bioavailability of metoprolol in homozygous extensive metabolizers

Methimazole / May ↓ metoprolol effects

Phenobarbital / ↓ Metoprolol effect R/T ↑ liver metabolism

Propylthiouracil / May ↓ metoprolol effects

Quinidine / May ↑ metoprolol effects

Rifampin / ↓ Metoprolol effect R/T ↑ liver metabolism

HOW SUPPLIED

Metoprolol succinate: *Tablet, Extended Release:* 25 mg, 50 mg, 100 mg, 200 mg. **Metoprolol tartrate:** *Injection:* 1 mg/mL; *Tablet:* 50 mg, 100 mg

DOSAGE

- **METOPROLOL SUCCINATE EXTENDED RELEASE TABLETS**

  Angina pectoris.

Individualized. Initial: 100 mg/day in a single dose. Dose may be increased slowly, at weekly intervals, until optimum effect is reached or there is a pronounced slowing of HR. Doses above 400 mg/day have not been studied.

  Hypertension.

Initial: 50–100 mg/day in a single dose with or without a diuretic. Dosage may be increased in weekly intervals until maximum effect is reached. Doses above 400 mg/day have not been studied.

  CHF.

Individualize dose. **Initial:** 25 mg once daily for 2 weeks in clients with NYHA Class II heart failure and 12.5 mg once daily in those with more severe heart failure. Double the dose q 2 weeks to the highest dose level tolerated or up to 200 mg.

• **METOPROLOL TARTRATE TABLETS**
Hypertension.
Initial: 100 mg/day in single or divided doses; **then,** dose may be increased weekly to maintenance level of 100–450 mg/day. A diuretic may also be used.
Angina pectoris.
Initial: 100 mg/day in 2 divided doses. Dose may be increased gradually at weekly intervals until optimum response is obtained or a pronounced slowing of HR occurs. Effective dose range: 100–400 mg/day. If treatment is to be discontinued, reduce dose gradually over 1–2 weeks.
Aggressive behavior.
200–300 mg/day.
Essential tremors.
50–300 mg/day.
Prophylaxis of migraine.
50–100 mg twice a day.
Ventricular arrhythmias.
200 mg/day.
• **METOPROLOL TARTRATE INJECTION (IV) AND TABLETS**
Early treatment of MI.
Three IV bolus injections of 5 mg each at approximately 2-min intervals. If clients tolerate the full IV dose, give 50 mg q 6 hr PO beginning 15 min after the last IV dose (or as soon as client's condition allows). This dose is continued for 48 hr followed by **late treatment:** 100 mg twice a day as soon as feasible; continue for 1–3 months (although data suggest treatment should be continued for 1–3 years). In clients who do not tolerate the full IV dose, begin with 25–50 mg q 6 hr PO beginning 15 min after the last IV dose or as soon as client's condition allows.

NURSING CONSIDERATIONS
Ⓒ Do not confuse metoprolol with metoclopramide (GI stimulant), metaproterenol (bronchodilator), or with misoprostol (prostaglandin derivative).

ADMINISTRATION/STORAGE
1. If transient worsening of heart failure occurs, may be treated with increased doses of diuretics. May be necessary to lower the dose of metoprolol or temporarily discontinue.

2. For CHF, do not increase dose until symptoms of worsening have been stabilized. Initial difficulty with titration should not preclude attempts later to use metoprolol.
3. If CHF clients experience symptomatic bradycardia, reduce the dose.
ASSESSMENT
1. Document indications for therapy: CAD, recent MI, and NYHA class.
2. Monitor CXR, CBC, liver/renal function studies, ECG, echocardiogram, EF, and VS.

CLIENT/FAMILY TEACHING
1. Take doses at the same time each day; do not stop suddenly.
2. Take with food.
3. Do not crush or chew the extended release products; swallow tablets whole.
4. Avoid activities that require mental alertness until drug effects realized. Alcohol may intensify the effect.
5. Before taking nonprescription drugs, obtain medical advice as some may affect the action of metoprolol.
6. Continue with diet, regular exercise, and weight loss in the overall plan to control BP.
7. Report any symptoms of fluid overload such as sudden weight gain, SOB, or swelling of extremities. Avoid salt.
8. Dress appropriately; may cause an increased sensitivity to cold. Do not smoke.
9. Keep a log of symptoms, BP and HR readings; report if heart rate <50 or irregular.

OUTCOMES/EVALUATE
• ↓ BP; ↓ anginal attacks
• Prevention of myocardial reinfarction and associated mortality

Mexiletine hydrochloride
(mex-**ILL**-eh-teen)

CLASSIFICATION(S):
Antiarrhythmic, Class IB
PREGNANCY CATEGORY: C
Rx: Mexitil

Bold Italic = life threatening side effect   ■ = black box warning   ✤ = Available in Canada

Rx: Novo-Mexiletine

SEE ALSO *ANTIARRHYTHMIC DRUGS.*

ACTION/KINETICS
Similar to lidocaine but is effective PO. Inhibits the flow of sodium into the cell, thereby reducing the rate of rise of the action potential. The drug decreases the effective refractory period in Purkinje fibers. BP and pulse rate are not affected following use, but there may be a small decrease in CO and an increase in peripheral vascular resistance. Also has both local anesthetic and anticonvulsant effects. **Bioavailability:** About 90%. **Onset:** 30–120 min. **Peak blood levels:** 2–3 hr. **Therapeutic plasma levels:** 0.5–2 mcg/mL. **Plasma t ½:** 10–12 hr. Metabolized in the liver mainly by CYP2D6. Approximately 10% excreted unchanged in the urine; acidification of the urine enhances excretion, whereas alkalinization decreases excretion.

USES
Documented life-threatening ventricular arrhythmias (such as ventricular tachycardia). *Investigational:* Prophylactically to decrease the incidence of ventricular tachycardia and other ventricular arrhythmias in the acute phase of MI. To reduce pain, dysesthesia, and paresthesia associated with diabetic neuropathy.

CONTRAINDICATIONS
Cardiogenic shock, preexisting second- or third-degree AV block (if no pacemaker is present). Use with lesser arrhythmias. Lactation.

SPECIAL CONCERNS
■Clients with asymptomatic, non life-threatening ventricular arrhythmias who had an MI more than 6 days but less than 2 years previously may show an excessive mortality or nonfatal cardiac arrest. Use of mexilitene should be reserved for those with life-threatening ventricular arrhythmias.■ Use with caution in hypotension, severe CHF, or known seizure disorders. Safety and efficacy have not been determined in children.

SIDE EFFECTS
CV: *Worsening of arrhythmias,* palpitations, chest pain, increased ventricular arrhythmias (PVCs), CHF, angina or angina-like pain, hypotension, bradycardia, syncope, *AV block or conduction disturbances,* atrial arrhythmias, hypertension, *cardiogenic shock,* hot flashes, edema, worsening of CHF in those with pre-existing compromised ventricular function. **GI:** High incidence of UGI distress, N&V, heartburn. Also, diarrhea/constipation, changes in appetite, dry mouth, abdominal cramps/pain/discomfort, salivary changes, dysphagia, altered taste, pharyngitis, changes in oral mucous membranes, UGI bleeding, peptic ulcer, esophageal ulceration, dyspepsia, pancreatitis (rare). **CNS:** High incidence of lightheadedness, dizziness, tremor, coordination difficulties, and nervousness. Also, changes in sleep habits, headache, fatigue, weakness, tinnitus, paresthesias, numbness, depression, confusion, difficulty with speech, short-term memory loss, hallucinations, malaise, psychosis, drowsiness, ataxia, *seizures,* loss of consciousness. **Hematologic:** Leukopenia, neutropenia, agranulocytosis, thrombocytopenia. **GU:** Decreased libido, impotence, urinary hesitancy/retention. **Dermatologic:** Rash, dry skin. Rarely, exfoliative dermatitis, and *Stevens-Johnson syndrome.* **Pulmonary:** Dyspnea, laryngeal or pharyngeal changes, pulmonary fibrosis, pulmonary infilatration. **Ophthalmic:** Blurred vision, visual disturbances, nystamus. **Miscellaneous:** Arthralgia, fever, diaphoresis, loss of hair, hiccoughs, syndrome of SLE, myelofibrosis, hypersensitivity reaction.

LABORATORY TEST CONSIDERATIONS
↑ AST. Positive ANA. Abnormal LFTs.

OD OVERDOSE MANAGEMENT
Symptoms: Nausea. CNS symptoms (dizziness, drowsiness, confusion, paresthesias, seizures) usually precede CV symptoms (hypotension, sinus bradycardia, intermittent LBBB, *temporary asystole, AV heart block, ventricular tachyarrhythmias, CV collapse). Massive overdoses cause coma and respiratory arrest. Treatment:* General supportive

treatment. Give atropine to treat hypotension or bradycardia. Give anticonvulsants for seizures. Transvenous cardiac pacing may be helpful. Acidification of the urine may increase rate of excretion.

DRUG INTERACTIONS

Al hydroxide / ↓ Mexiletine absorption
Atropine / ↓ Mexiletine absorption
Caffeine / ↓ Drug clearance (50%)
Cimetidine / ↑ or ↓ Plasma mexiletine levels
Fluvoxamine / ↓ Oral clearance and ↑ in AUC and peak serum levels of mexiletine R/T ↓ liver metabolism by CYP1A2
Mg hydroxide / ↓ Mexiletine absorption
Metoclopramide / ↑ Mexiletine absorption
Narcotics / ↓ Mexiletine absorption
Phenobarbital / ↓ Plasma mexiletine levels
Phenytoin / ↑ Mexiletine clearance → ↓ plasma mexiletine levels
Propafenone / ↓ Metabolic clearance of mexiletine in extensive metabolizers → no differences between extensive and poor metabolizers
Rifampin / ↑ Clearance → ↓ plasma mexiletine levels
Theophylline / ↑ Drug effect R/T ↑ serum levels
Urinary acidifiers / ↑ Rate of mexiletine excretion
Urinary alkalinizers / ↓ Rate of mexiletine excretion

HOW SUPPLIED

Capsule: 150 mg, 200 mg, 250 mg

DOSAGE

• CAPSULES

Antiarrhythmic.

Adults, individualized, initial: 200 mg q 8 hr if rapid control of arrhythmia not required; dosage adjustment may be made in 50- or 100-mg increments q 2–3 days, if required. **Maintenance:** 200–300 mg q 8 hr, depending on response and tolerance of client. If adequate response is not achieved with 300 mg or less q 8 hr, 400 mg q 8 hr may be tried although the incidence of CNS side effects increases. If the drug is effective at doses of 300 mg or less q 8 hr, the same total daily dose may be given in divided doses q 12 hr (e.g., 450 mg q 12 hr). Maximum total daily dose: 1,200 mg.

Rapid control of arrhythmias.
Initial loading dose: 400 mg followed by a 200-mg dose in 8 hr.

Diabetic neuropathy.
Initial: 150 mg/day for 3 days; **then,** 300 mg/day for 3 days. **Maintenance:** 10 mg/kg/day.

NURSING CONSIDERATIONS

ADMINISTRATION/STORAGE

1. If transferring to mexiletine from other class I antiarrhythmics, initiate mexiletine at a dose of 200 mg and then titrate according to the response at the following times: 6–12 hr after the last dose of quinidine sulfate, 3–6 hr after the last dose of procainamide, 6–12 hr after the last dose of disopyramide, or 8–12 hr after the last dose of tocainide.

2. Hospitalize client when transferring to mexiletine if there is a chance that withdrawal of the previous antiarrhythmic may produce life-threatening arrhythmias.

3. When transferring from lidocaine to mexiletine, stop the lidocaine infusion when the first PO dose of mexiletine is given. Maintain the IV line until suppression of the arrhythmia appears satisfactory.

4. Avoid concurrent drugs or diets which may markedly affect urinary pH.

ASSESSMENT

1. Document indications for therapy; list any other agents trialed and the outcome.

2. Note evidence of CHF; assess ECG for AV block.

3. Document pulmonary assessment findings; note SaO_2/PO_2.

4. Monitor ECG, CXR, CBC, electrolytes, renal and LFTs.

5. Reduce dose with severe liver disease and marked right-sided CHF.

6. Assess urinary pH; alkalinity decreases and acidity increases renal drug excretion.

CLIENT/FAMILY TEACHING

1. Take with food or an antacid to ↓ GI upset.

2. Do not stop drug suddenly; maintain acidity level in urine by not changing dietary patterns.

3. Report any bruising, bleeding, fevers, or sore throat or adverse CNS effects such as dizziness, tremor, impaired coordination, N&V.

4. Immediately report any increase in heart palpitations, irregularity, or rate less than 50 bpm.

5. Do not perform tasks that require mental alertness until drug effects are realized.

6. Carry identification that lists drugs currently prescribed. Keep regularly scheduled appointments

OUTCOMES/EVALUATE
- Control of ventricular arrhythmias
- Therapeutic drug levels (0.5–2 mcg/mL)
- ↓ S&S of diabetic neuropathy

Midodrine hydrochloride ■

(**MIH**-doh-dreen)

CLASSIFICATION(S):
Vasopressor
PREGNANCY CATEGORY: C
Rx: ProAmatine
✚Rx: Amatine

ACTION/KINETICS
Midodrine, a prodrug, is converted to an active metabolite—desglymidodrine—that is an alpha-1 agonist. Desglymidodrine produces an increase in vascular tone and elevation of BP by activating alpha-adrenergic receptors of the arteriolar and venous vasculature. No effect on cardiac beta-adrenergic receptors. The active metabolite does not cross the blood-brain barrier; thus, there are no CNS effects. Standing systolic BP is increased by approximately 15–30 mm Hg at 1 hr after a 10-mg dose; duration: 2–3 hr. Rapidly absorbed from the GI tract. Absolute bioavailability of midodrine is 93%. **Peak plasma levels, midodrine:** 30 min; t½: 25 min. **Peak plasma levels, desglymi-**dodrine: 1–2 hr; **t½:** 3–4 hr. The bioavailability of the active metabolite is not affected by food. Desglymidodrine is eliminated in the urine. Neither midodrine nor desglymidodrine are significantly bound to plasma proteins.

USES
Orthostatic hypotension in those whose lives are significantly impaired despite standard clinical care. *Investigational:* Management of stress urinary incontinence.

CONTRAINDICATIONS
Use in severe organic heart disease, acute renal disease, urinary retention, pheochromocytoma, thyrotoxicosis, persistent and excessive supine hypertension.

SPECIAL CONCERNS
■Midodrine can cause marked elevation of supine BP; thus, use only in those whose lives are considerably impaired despite standard clinical care. The basis for use in the treatment of symptomatic orthostatic hypotension is based primarily on a change in a surrogate marker of effectiveness, an increase in systolic BP measured 1 min after standing, a surrogate marker considered likely to correspond to a clinical benefit. Clinical benefits of midodrine, especially improved ability to carry out activities of daily living, have not been verified.■ Use with caution in impaired renal or hepatic function, during lactation, in orthostatic hypotensive clients who are also diabetic, or in those with a history of visual problems or who are also taking fludrocortisone acetate. Safety and efficacy have not been determined in children.

SIDE EFFECTS
CV: Supine hypertension (potentially most serious side effect), sitting hypertension. **CNS:** Paresthesia, pain, headache, feeling of pressure or fullness in the head, confusion, abnormal thinking, nervousness, anxiety. Rarely, dizziness, insomnia, somnolence. **GI:** Dry mouth. Rarely, canker sore, nausea, GI distress, flatulence. **Dermatologic:** Piloerection (goose bumps), pruritus (mainly of the scalp), rash, vasodilation, flushed face. Rarely, erythema multiforme, dry skin.

M

GU: Dysuria, urinary urge/retention/frequency. **Miscellaneous:** Chills, pain. Rarely, visual field defect, skin hyperesthesia, asthenia, backache, pyrosis, leg cramps, canker sore.

OD OVERDOSE MANAGEMENT

Symptoms: Hypertension, piloerection, sensation of coldness, urinary retention. *Treatment*: Emesis and administration of an alpha-adrenergic blocking agent (e.g., phentolamine). Desglymidodrine is dialyzable.

DRUG INTERACTIONS

Alpha-adrenergic agonists (ephedrine, phenylephrine, pseudoephedrine) / ↑ Pressor effects of midodrine

Alpha-adrenergic antagonists (doxazosin, prazosin, terazosin) / Antagonism of the effects of midodrine

Beta-adrenergic blockers / ↑ Risk of bradycardia, AV block, or arrhythmias

Cardiac glycosides / ↑ Risk of bradycardia, AV block, or arrhythmias

Dihydroergotamine / ↑ Pressor effects of midodrine

Fludrocortisone / ↑ Risk of supine hypertension, intraocular pressure and glaucoma

Psychopharmacologic drugs / ↑ Risk of bradycardia, AV block, or arrhythmias

HOW SUPPLIED

Tablet: 2.5 mg, 5 mg, 10 mg

DOSAGE

• **TABLETS**

Orthostatic hypotension.

10 mg 3 times per day given during the daytime hours when the client is upright and pursuing daily activities (e.g., shortly before or upon arising in the morning, midday, and late afternoon–not later than 6:00 p.m.). To control symptoms, dosing may be q 3 hr. Initial dose in impaired renal function: 2.5 mg 3 times per day.

Urinary incontinence.

2.5–5 mg 2–3 times per day.

NURSING CONSIDERATIONS

ASSESSMENT

1. Document onset, duration, and characteristics of symptoms. Note other nonpharmacologic treatments (i.e., support stockings, increased salt in diet, fluid expansion, sleeping with head of bed raised) trialed.

2. Orthostatic hypotension is defined as SBP reductions > 20 mm Hg or DBP of over 10 mm Hg reduction within 3 min of standing; assess carefully on several occasions.

3. Document any acute renal disease, urinary retention, pheochromocytoma, severe organic heart disease, or thyrotoxicosis, as these preclude drug therapy. Assess for liver and renal dysfunction.

CLIENT/FAMILY TEACHING

1. Take during the day while up and around. Do not take after the evening meal or within 4 hr of bedtime.

2. Use OTC products containing phenylephrine (e.g., cold/allergy remedies/diet aids) cautiously; may increase supine BP.

3. May experience supine hypertension; check BP regularly while lying and sitting and keep a record. Stop drug and report blurred vision, pounding in ears, headache, cardiac awareness, increased dizziness/syncope.

OUTCOMES/EVALUATE

Relief of symptomatic orthostatic hypotension: ↓ dizziness, ↓ lightheadedness, ↓ unsteadiness

Milrinone lactate

(**MILL**-rih-nohn)

CLASSIFICATION(S):

Inotropic drug

PREGNANCY CATEGORY: C

Rx: Primacor

ACTION/KINETICS

Selective inhibitor of peak III cyclic AMP phosphodiesterase isozyme in cardiac and vascular muscle, resulting in a direct inotropic effect and a direct arterial vasodilator activity. Also improves diastolic function as manifested by improvements in LV diastolic relaxation. In clients with depressed myocardial function, produces a prompt increase in CO and a decrease in pulmonary wedge pressure and vascular resistance, with-

---

Bold Italic = life threatening side effect   ■ = black box warning   ✤ = Available in Canada

out a significant increase in HR or myocardial oxygen consumption. Causes an inotropic effect in clients who are fully digitalized without causing signs of glycoside toxicity. Also, LV function has improved in clients with ischemic heart disease. **Therapeutic plasma levels:** 150–250 ng/mL. **t½:** 2.3 hr following doses of 12.5–125 mcg/kg to clients with CHF. Metabolized in the liver and excreted primarily through the urine.

USES

Short-term IV treatment of CHF, usually in clients receiving digoxin and diuretics.

CONTRAINDICATIONS

Hypersensitivity to the drug. Use in severe obstructive aortic or pulmonary valvular disease in lieu of surgical relief of the obstruction.

SPECIAL CONCERNS

Use with caution during lactation. Safety and efficacy have not been determined in children.

SIDE EFFECTS

CV: *Ventricular and supraventricular arrhythmias, including ventricular ectopic activity, nonsustained ventricular tachycardia, sustained ventricular tachycardia, and ventricular fibrillation. Infrequently, life-threatening arrhythmias associated with preexisting arrhythmias,* metabolic abnormalities, abnormal digoxin levels, and catheter insertion. Also, hypotension, angina, chest pain. **Miscellaneous:** Mild to moderately severe headaches, hypokalemia, tremor, thrombocytopenia, bronchospasm (rare).

OD OVERDOSE MANAGEMENT

Symptoms: Hypotension. *Treatment:* If hypotension occurs, reduce or temporarily discontinue administration of milrinone until the condition of the client stabilizes. Use general measures to support circulation.

HOW SUPPLIED

Injection: 1 mg/mL; *Injection, premixed:* 200 mcg/mL in D5W

DOSAGE

• **IV INFUSION**

Adults, loading dose: 50 mcg/kg administered slowly over 10 min. **Maintenance, minimum:** 0.59 mg/kg/24 hr (infused at a rate of 0.375 mcg/kg/min); **maintenance, standard:** 0.77 mg/kg/ 24 hr (infused at a rate of 0.5 mcg/kg/ min); **maintenance, maximum:** 1.13 mg/kg/24 hr (infused at a rate of 0.75 mcg/kg/min).

NURSING CONSIDERATIONS

ADMINISTRATION/STORAGE

IV 1. Give IV infusions at rates described in the package insert.

2. Adjust rate depending on the hemodynamic and clinical response.

3. Prepare dilutions using 0.45% or 0.9% NaCl or 5% dextrose injection.

4. Reduce rate in renal impairment (see package insert for chart).

5. Do not give furosemide in IV lines containing milrinone as a precipitate will form.

6. Store at room temperatures of 15–30°C (59–86°F).

ASSESSMENT

1. Document indications, onset and characteristics of symptoms. Identify NYHA class, other medications used and outcome.

2. Monitor CBC, electrolytes, liver/renal function studies. Document ECG, CO, CVP, and PAWP; rule out acute MI.

INTERVENTIONS

1. Monitor I&O, electrolyte levels, and renal function. Potassium loss due to excessive diuresis may cause arrhythmias in digitalized clients; correct hypokalemia.

2. Monitor VS; review parameters for interruption of infusion (e.g., SBP < 80; HR < 50).

3. Observe for increased supraventricular and ventricular arrhythmias on monitor.

OUTCOMES/EVALUATE

• ↑ CO and ↓ PACWP
• Resolution of S&S of CHF
• Therapeutic drug levels (150–250 ng/ mL)

Minoxidil, oral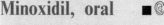
(mih-**NOX**-ih-dil)

CLASSIFICATION(S):
Antihypertensive, peripheral vasodilator

PREGNANCY CATEGORY: C

Rx: Loniten

SEE ALSO *ANTIHYPERTENSIVE AGENTS.*

ACTION/KINETICS
Decreases elevated BP by decreasing peripheral resistance by a direct effect. Causes increase in renin secretion, increase in cardiac rate and output, and salt/water retention. Does not cause orthostatic hypotension. **Onset:** 30 min. **Peak plasma levels:** Reached within 60 min; **plasma t½:** 4.2 hr. **Duration:** 24–48 hr. Ninety percent absorbed from GI tract; excretion: Renal (90% metabolites). The time needed to reach the maximum effect is inversely related to the dose.

USES
Severe hypertension not controllable by the use of a diuretic plus two other antihypertensive drugs. Usually taken with at least two other antihypertensive drugs (a diuretic and a drug to minimize tachycardia such as a beta-adrenergic blocking agent). Can produce severe side effects; reserve for resistant cases of hypertension. Close medical supervision required, including possible hospitalization during initial administration.

CONTRAINDICATIONS
Pheochromocytoma. Within 1 month after a MI. Dissecting aortic aneurysm. Use in milder forms of hypertension.

SPECIAL CONCERNS
■(1) May produce serious side effects. Can cause pericardial effusion, occasionally progressing to tamponade. Can also worsen angina pectoris. Reserve for hypertensive clients who do not respond adequately to maximum therapeutic doses of a diuretic and two other antihypertensive agents. (2) In experimental animals, minoxidil caused several kinds of myocardial lesions and other adverse cardiac effects. (3) Give under close supervision, usually together with a beta-adrenergic blocking agent, to prevent tachycardia and increased myocardial workload. Usually must be given with a diuretic, frequently one acting in the ascending limb of the loop of Henle, to prevent serious fluid accumulation. (4) When first given, hospitalize and monitor clients with malignant hypertension and those already receiving guanethidine to avoid too rapid or large orthostatic decreases in BP.■ Safe use during lactation not established. Use with caution and at reduced dosage in impaired renal function. Geriatric clients may be more sensitive to the hypotensive and hypothermic effects of minoxidil; also, may be necessary to decrease the dose due to age-related decreases in renal function. BP controlled too rapidly may cause syncope, stroke, MI, and ischemia of affected organs. Experience with use in children is limited.

SIDE EFFECTS
CV: Edema, *pericardial effusion that may progress to tamponade* (acute compression of heart caused by fluid or blood in pericardium), CHF, angina pectoris, changes in direction of T waves, increased HR. In children, rebound hypertension following slow withdrawal. **GI:** N&V. **CNS:** Headache, fatigue. **Hypersensitivity:** Rashes, including bullous eruptions and *Stevens-Johnson syndrome.* **Hematologic:** Initially, decrease in hematocrit, hemoglobin, and erythrocyte count but all return to normal. Rarely, thrombocytopenia and leukopenia. **Other:** Hypertrichosis (enhanced hair growth, pigmentation and thickening of fine body hair 3–6 weeks after initiation of therapy), breast tenderness, darkening of skin, temporary edema.

LABORATORY TEST CONSIDERATIONS
Nonspecific changes in ECG. ↑ Alkaline phosphatase, serum creatinine, and BUN.

OD OVERDOSE MANAGEMENT
Symptoms: Excessive hypotension. *Treatment:* Give NSS IV (to maintain BP and urine output). Vasopressors, such

---

as phenylephrine and dopamine, can be used but only in underperfusion of a vital organ.

DRUG INTERACTIONS
Concomitant use with guanethidine may result in severe hypotension.

HOW SUPPLIED
Tablet: 2.5 mg, 10 mg

DOSAGE
- **TABLETS**
  Hypertension.

Adults and children over 12 years, Initial: 5 mg/day. For optimum control, dose can be increased to 10, 20, and then 40 mg in single or divided doses/day. Do not exceed 100 mg/day. **Children under 12 years: Initial,** 0.2 mg/kg/day. Effective dose range: 0.25–1.0 mg/kg/day. Dosage must be titrated to individual response. Do not exceed 50 mg/day. *NOTE:* Clients with renal failure or undergoing dialysis may require smaller doses.

NURSING CONSIDERATIONS

℗ Do not confuse minoxidil with Monopril (an ACE inhibitor).

ADMINISTRATION/STORAGE
1. Give once daily if supine DBP has been reduced less than 30 mm Hg and twice daily (in two equal doses) if it has been reduced more than 30 mm Hg.
2. Wait at least 3 days between dosage adjustments as the full response is not obtained until then. However, if more rapid control is required, may adjust q 6 hr but with careful monitoring.

ASSESSMENT
1. Anticipate BP decreases within 30 min.
2. Note indications for therapy, other agents trialed, and outcome. Be sure diuretic prescribed to relieve fluid accumulation and beta blocker to control tachycardia.
3. Assess cardiopulmonary status; may cause pericardial effusion which may progress to tamponade. Also, may worsen angina pectoris.
4. Monitor VS, CBC, glucose, electrolytes, and renal function studies; adjust dose with dysfunction. Give after dialysis as drug removed by hemodialysis.

CLIENT/FAMILY TEACHING
1. Can be taken with fluids and without regard to meals.
2. Record BP, HR and weight daily; report any S&S of fluid overload (gain of 6 lb/week; swelling of extremities, face, and abdomen; or ↑ SOB).
3. Report any symptoms of chest pain, fainting, dizziness, or ↑ SOB that occurs, especially when lying down.
4. Drug may cause elongation, thickening, and increased pigmentation of body hair; should resolve once discontinued.

OUTCOMES/EVALUATE
↓ BP; control of hypertension

Moricizine hydrochloride
(mor-**IS**-ih-zeen)

CLASSIFICATION(S):
Antiarrhythmic, Class IA
PREGNANCY CATEGORY: B
Rx: Ethmozine

M

SEE ALSO *ANTIARRHYTHMIC DRUGS.*

ACTION/KINETICS
Causes a stabilizing effect on the myocardial membranes as well as local anesthetic activity. Shortens phase II and III repolarization leading to a decreased duration of the action potential and an effective refractory period. Also, there is a decrease in the maximum rate of phase O depolarization and a prolongation of AV conduction in clients with ventricular tachycardia. Whether the client is at rest or is exercising, has minimal effects on cardiac index, stroke index, systemic or pulmonary vascular resistance or ejection fraction, and pulmonary capillary wedge pressure. There is a small increase in resting BP and HR. The time, course, and intensity of antiarrhythmic and electrophysiologic effects are not related to plasma levels of the drug. **Onset:** 2 hr. **Peak plasma levels:** 30–120 min. **t ½:** 1.5–3.5 hr (reduced after multiple dosing). **Duration:** 10–24 hr. Significant first-pass

effect. Metabolized almost completely by the liver with metabolites excreted through both the urine and feces; the drug induces its own metabolism. Food delays the rate of absorption resulting in lower peak plasma levels; however, the total amount absorbed is not changed. Is 95% bound to plasma proteins.

USES
Documented life-threatening ventricular arrhythmias (e.g., sustained VT) where benefits of the drug are determined to outweigh the risks. *Investigational:* Ventricular premature contractions, couplets, and nonsustained VT.

CONTRAINDICATIONS
Preexisting second- or third-degree block, right bundle branch block when associated with bifascicular block (unless the client has a pacemaker), cardiogenic shock. Lactation.

SPECIAL CONCERNS
There is the possibility of increased risk of death when used in clients with non-life-threatening cardiac arrhythmias. Safety and effectiveness in children less than 18 years of age have not been determined. Geriatric clients have a higher rate of side effects. Increased survival rates following use of antiarrhythmic drugs have not been proven in clients with ventricular arrhythmias. Use with caution in clients with sick sinus syndrome due to the possibility of sinus bradycardia, sinus pause, or sinus arrest. Use with caution in clients with CHF.

SIDE EFFECTS
CV: *Proarrhythmias, including new rhythm disturbances or worsening of existing arrhythmias;* ECG abnormalities, including conduction defects, sinus pause, junctional rhythm, AV block; palpitations, ***sustained VT,*** cardiac chest pain, CHF, ***cardiac death,*** hypotension, hypertension, atrial fibrillation, atrial flutter, syncope, bradycardia, ***cardiac arrest, MI, pulmonary embolism,*** vasodilation, thrombophlebitis, ***cerebrovascular events.*** **CNS:** Dizziness (common), anxiety, headache, fatigue, nervousness, paresthesias, sleep disorders, tremor, hypoesthesias, depression, eu-

phoria, somnolence, agitation, confusion, ***seizures,*** hallucinations, loss of memory, vertigo, coma. **GI:** Nausea, dry mouth, abdominal pain, vomiting, diarrhea, dyspepsia, anorexia, ileus, flatulence, dysphagia, bitter taste. **Musculoskeletal:** Asthenia, abnormal gait, akathisia, ataxia, abnormal coordination, dyskinesia, pain. **GU:** Urinary retention, dysuria, urinary incontinence, urinary frequency, impotence, kidney pain, decreased libido. **Respiratory:** Dyspnea, apnea, asthma, hyperventilation, pharyngitis, cough, sinusitis. **Ophthalmologic:** Nystagmus, diplopia, blurred vision, eye pain, periorbital edema. **Dermatologic:** Rash, pruritus, dry skin, urticaria. **Miscellaneous:** Sweating, drug fever, hypothermia, temperature intolerance, swelling of the lips and tongue, speech disorder, tinnitus, jaundice.

LABORATORY TEST CONSIDERATIONS
↑ Bilirubin and liver transaminases.

OD OVERDOSE MANAGEMENT
Symptoms: Vomiting, hypotension, lethargy, worsening of CHF, ***MI, conduction disturbances, arrhythmias (e.g., junctional bradycardia, VT, ventricular fibrillation, asystole), sinus arrest, respiratory failure.*** *Treatment:* In acute overdose, induce vomiting, taking care to prevent aspiration. Hospitalize and closely monitor for cardiac, respiratory, and CNS changes. Provide life support, including an intracardiac pacing catheter, if necessary.

DRUG INTERACTIONS
Cimetidine / ↑ Plasma moricizine levels R/T ↓ excretion
Digoxin / Additive prolongation of the PR interval (but no significant increase in the rate of second- or third-degree AV block)
Propranolol / Additive prolongation of the PR interval
Theophylline / ↓ Plasma theophylline levels R/T ↑ rate of clearance

HOW SUPPLIED
Tablet: 200 mg, 250 mg, 300 mg

DOSAGE————————————————
• **TABLETS**
Antiarrhythmic.

Adults: 600–900 mg/day in equally divided doses q 8 hr. If needed, the dose can be increased in increments of 150 mg/day at 3-day intervals until the desired effect is obtained. In clients with hepatic or renal impairment, the initial dose should be 600 mg or less with close monitoring and dosage adjustment.

NURSING CONSIDERATIONS

ADMINISTRATION/STORAGE

1. When transferring clients from other antiarrhythmics to moricizine, withdraw the previous drug for one to two plasma half-lives before starting moricizine. For example, when transferring from quinidine or disopyramide, moricizine can be started 6–12 hr after the last dose; when transferring from procainamide, moricizine can be initiated 3–6 hr after the last dose; when transferring from mexiletine, propafenone, or tocainide, start 8–12 hr after the last dose; and, when transferring from flecainide, start moricizine 12–24 hr after the last dose.

2. If clients are well controlled on an 8-hr regimen, they might be given the same total daily dose q 12 hr to increase compliance.

ASSESSMENT

1. Document cardiac history, note preexisting conditions and ECG abnormalities.

2. Monitor ECG, electrolytes, CXR, PFTs, liver and renal function studies; correct any electrolyte disturbance and reduce dose with liver or renal dysfunction.

3. Monitor cardiac rhythm closely to observe for drug-induced rhythm disturbances.

4. Antiarrhythmic response may be determined by ECG, exercise testing, or programmed electrical stimulation testing and implantable defibrillators. Assess pacing parameters with pacemakers.

5. Monitor VS and report any persistent temperature elevations.

CLIENT/FAMILY TEACHING

1. Drug is used to terminate life threatening ventricular arrhythmias.

2. Take before meals; food delays rate of absorption.

3. Drug may cause dizziness. Use care when rising from a lying or sitting position. Report any unusual or new side effects.

4. Advise family member or significant other to learn CPR.

OUTCOMES/EVALUATE

Termination of life-threatening ventricular arrhythmias

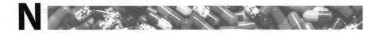

Nadolol ©

(NAY-doh-lohl)

CLASSIFICATION(S):

Beta-adrenergic blocking agent
PREGNANCY CATEGORY: C
Rx: Corgard
✦**Rx:** Apo-Nadol, Novo-Nadolol, ratio-Nadolol

SEE ALSO *BETA-ADRENERGIC BLOCKING AGENTS*.

ACTION/KINETICS

Manifests both beta-1- and beta-2-adrenergic blocking activity. Has no membrane stabilizing or intrinsic sympathomimetic activity. Low lipid solubility. **Peak serum concentration:** 3–4 hr. **t ½:** 20–24 hr (permits once-daily dosage). **Duration:** 17–24 hr. Absorption variable, averaging 30%; steady plasma level achieved after 6–9 days of administration. Excreted unchanged by the kidney.

USES

(1) Hypertension, either alone or with other drugs (e.g., thiazide diuretic). (2)

Long-term management of angina pectoris. *Investigational:* Prophylaxis of migraine, ventricular arrhythmias, aggressive behavior, essential tremor, tremors associated with lithium or parkinsonism, antipsychotic-induced akathisia, rebleeding of esophageal varices, reduce intraocular pressure.

CONTRAINDICATIONS
Use in bronchial asthma or bronchospasm, including severe COPD.

SPECIAL CONCERNS
Dosage has not been established in children.

HOW SUPPLIED
Tablet: 20 mg, 40 mg, 80 mg, 120 mg, 160 mg

DOSAGE
- **TABLETS**
  Hypertension.
  Initial: 40 mg/day; **then,** may be increased in 40 to 80 mg increments until optimum response obtained. **Maintenance:** 40–80 mg/day although up to 240–320 mg/day may be needed.
  Angina.
  Initial: 40 mg/day; **then,** increase dose in 40 to 80 mg increments q 3–7 days until optimum response obtained. **Maintenance:** 40–80 mg/day, although up to 160–240 mg/day may be needed.
  Aggressive behavior.
  40–160 mg/day.
  Antipsychotic-induced akathisia.
  40–80 mg/day.
  Essential tremor.
  120–240 mg/day.
  Lithium-induced tremors.
  20–40 mg/day.
  Tremors associated with parkinsonism.
  80–320 mg/day.
  Prophylaxis of migraine.
  40–80 mg/day.
  Rebleeding of esophageal varices.
  40–160 mg/day.
  Ventricular arrhythmias.
  10–640 mg/day.
  Reduction of intraocular pressure.
  10–20 mg twice a day.
  NOTE: For all uses decrease dose or increase dosage intervals in clients with renal failure.

NURSING CONSIDERATIONS
☙ Do not confuse Corgard with Coreg.
ASSESSMENT
1. Note indications for therapy, medical history, characteristics of S&S, and other agents trialed.
2. Document baseline VS, labs, and ECG.
3. Assess for history of asthma, severe COPD; reduce dose with renal dysfunction.

CLIENT/FAMILY TEACHING
1. Take only as directed; do not stop abruptly.
2. Report any rapid weight gain, increased SOB, or extremity swelling.
3. Do not perform tasks that require mental alertness until drug effects realized; may cause dizziness.
4. May cause increased sensitivity to cold; dress appropriately.
5. Keep log of BP and HR for provider review.

OUTCOMES/EVALUATE
- ↓ BP, ↓ HR
- ↓ Frequency/intensity of angina

Nesiritide
(nih-**SIR**-ih-tide)

CLASSIFICATION(S):
Vasodilator, peripheral
PREGNANCY CATEGORY: C
Rx: Natrecor

ACTION/KINETICS
Nesiritide is a human B-type natriuretic peptide (hBNP) made from *E. coli* using recombinant DNA technology. Human BNP binds to the particulate guanylate cyclase receptor in vascular smooth muscle and endothelial cells, leading to increased intracellular levels of guanosine 3'5'-cyclic monophosphate (cGMP) and smooth muscle cell relaxation. Cyclic GMP serves as a second messenger to dilate veins and arteries. In acutely decompensated CHF, the drug reduces pulmonary capillary wedge pressure and improves dyspnea. **$t\frac{1}{2}$, initial elimination:** About 2 min; **$t\frac{1}{2}$, mean terminal, elimination:** About 18 min.

Bold Italic = life threatening side effect   ■ = black box warning   ✚ = Available in Canada

Human BNP is cleared from the circulation by three mechanisms: (1) Binding to cell surface clearance receptors with subsequent cellular internalization and lysosomal proteolysis; (2) Proteolytic cleavage of the peptide by endopeptidases, such as neutral endopeptidase (present on the vascular lumenal surface); and, (3) renal filtration.

USES

IV treatment of acutely decompensated CHF in those who have dyspnea at rest or with minimal activity.

CONTRAINDICATIONS

Use as primary therapy for those with cardiogenic shock or in those with a systolic BP < 90 mm Hg. Hypersensitivity to any of the product components. Use in those suspected of having, or known to have, low cardiac filling pressures. Use in those for whom vasodilating agents are not appropriate, including valvular stenosis, restrictive or obstructive cardiomyopathy, constrictive pericarditis, pericardial tamponade, or other conditions in which cardiac output is dependent on venous return.

SPECIAL CONCERNS

Use with caution during lactation. Safety and efficacy have not been determined in children.

SIDE EFFECTS

CV: Hypotension (symptomatic, asymptomatic), *ventricular tachycardia,* nonsustained ventricular tachycardia, ventricular extrasystoles, angina pectoris, bradycardia, tachycardia, atrial fibrillation, AV node conduction abnormalities. **CNS:** Headache, insomnia, dizziness, anxiety, confusion, paresthesia, somnolence, tremor. **GI:** N&V. **Dermatologic:** Sweating, pruritus, rash. **Respiratory:** Increased cough, hemoptysis, apnea. **Miscellaneous:** Back pain, abdominal pain, hypersensitivity reactions, catheter pain, fever, injection site reaction, leg cramps, amblyopia, anemia.

LABORATORY TEST CONSIDERATIONS

↑ Creatinine.

DRUG INTERACTIONS

↑ Symptomatic hypotension when used with ACE inhibitors.

HOW SUPPLIED

Powder for injection, lyophilized: 1.58 mg

DOSAGE

• **IV ONLY**

Acutely decompensated CHF.
IV bolus of 2 mcg/kg, followed by a continuous IV infusion of 0.01 mcg/kg/min.

NURSING CONSIDERATIONS

ADMINISTRATION/STORAGE

IV 1. Do not start nesiritide at a dose greater than the recommended dose.
2. Prime the IV tubing with an infusion of 0.25 mL before connecting to the client's vascular access port and prior to giving the bolus or starting the infusion.
3. After preparing the infusion bag, withdraw the bolus volume and give over about 60 seconds through an IV port in the tubing. Immediately following the bolus, infuse nesiritide at a flow rate of 0.1 mL/kg/hr (this will deliver an infusion dose of 0.01 mcg/kg/min).
4. To calculate the appropriate bolus volume and infusion flow rate to deliver 0.01 mcg/kg/min dose, use the following formulas: Bolus volume (mL) = 0.33 x client weight (kg). Infusion flow rate (mL/hr) = 0.1 x client weight (kg).
5. To prepare the infusion, use the following procedure:
• Reconstitute one 1.5 mg vial by adding 5 mL of diluent removed from a prefilled 250 mL plastic IV bag containing the diluent of choice (D5/0.9% NaCl, D5/0.45% NaCl, or D5/0.2% NaCl).
• Do not shake the vial but rock gently so that all surfaces, including the stopper, are in contact with diluent to ensure complete reconstitution. Use only a clear, essentially colorless solution.
• Withdraw the entire contents of the reconstituted vial and add to the 250 mL plastic IV bag. This will yield a solution with a nesiritide concentration of about 6 mcg/mL. Invert the IV bag several times to ensure complete mixing of the solution.
• Use the reconstituted solution within 24 hr, as there are no preservatives in the product. Inspect visually for particulate matter and discoloration prior to use.

6. If hypotension occurs during administration, reduce or discontinue the dose and begin other measures to support BP (e.g., IV fluids, changes in body position). The drug may be restarted at a dose that is reduced by 30% (with no bolus given). Hypotension may be prolonged; thus, before restarting the drug, a period of observation may be needed.

7. Nesiritide is physically and chemically incompatible with injections of heparin, insulin, ethacrynate sodium, bumetamide, enalaprilat, hydralazine, and furosemide. Do not give these drugs as infusions in the same IV catheter as nesiritide.

8. Do not give injectable drugs that contain sodium metabisulfate in the same infusion line; incompatible with nesiritide. Flush the catheter between administration of nesiritide and incompatible drugs.

9. Nesiritide binds to heparin. Thus, **do not** give through a central line heparin-coated catheter.

10. Store at controlled room temperature between 20–25°C (68–77°F) or refrigerated at 2–8°C (36–46°F). Reconstituted vials may be left at controlled room temperature or refrigerated for 24 hr or less. Keep in carton until time of use.

ASSESSMENT

1. Note indications for therapy, other agents trialed, ejection fraction, and NYHA class.

2. For IV use only; avoid infusing through central line heparin-coated catheters.

3. Review list of drugs not compatible for co-administration.

4. Monitor cardiac status, renal function and VS; if SBP < 90 mm Hg reduce dose or stop infusion and report.

5. Administer in a closely monitored environment by trained individuals; monitor heart pressures and assess closely for arrhythmias.

OUTCOMES/EVALUATE

Improved exercise tolerance; ↓ PACWP; ↓ SOB with mild exertion and at rest

Niacin (Nicotinic acid)

(**NYE**-ah-sin, nih-koh-**TIN**-ick **AH**-sid)

CLASSIFICATION(S):
Vitamin B complex
PREGNANCY CATEGORY: C
OTC: Slo-Niacin
Rx: Niacor, Niaspan

Niacinamide

(nye-ah-**SIN**-ah-myd)

PREGNANCY CATEGORY: C

ACTION/KINETICS

Niacin (nicotinic acid) and niacinamide are water-soluble, heat-resistant vitamins prepared synthetically. Niacin (after conversion to the active niacinamide) is a component of the coenzymes nicotinamide-adenine dinucleotide and nicotinamide-adenine dinucleotide phosphate, which are essential for oxidation-reduction reactions involved in lipid metabolism, glycogenolysis, and tissue respiration. Deficiency of niacin results in pellagra, the most common symptoms of which are dermatitis, diarrhea, and dementia. In high doses niacin also produces vasodilation. Niacin, but not nicotinamide, reduces total and LDL cholesterol, triglycerides, and apolipoprotein B-100, and increases HDL cholesterol. Mechanism is unknown but may involve a decrease in esterification of hepatic triglycerides. Rapidly absorbed from the GI tract. **Peak serum levels:** 30–60 min; **t ½:** 20–45 min. About 88% of a PO dose of niacin is eliminated by the kidneys unchanged or as nicotinuric acid.

USES

Niacin. (1) Prophylaxis and treatment of pellagra; niacin deficiency. (2) Adjunct therapy in adults with very high serum triglycerides (Types IV and V hyperlipidemia) who are at risk of pancreatitis and

---

Bold Italic = life threatening side effect   ■ = black box warning   ✢ = Available in Canada

who do not respond adequately to diet. (3) Niaspan: Used in combination with lovastatin as an adjunct to exercise and diet to treat adults with dyslipidemia. **Niacinamide.** Prophylaxis and treatment of pellagra. *Investigational:* Treatment of various dermatologic disorders.

CONTRAINDICATIONS

Severe hypotension, hemorrhage, arterial bleeding, liver dysfunction, active peptic ulcer. Use of the extended-release tablets and capsules in children.

SPECIAL CONCERNS

Extended-release niacin may be hepatotoxic. Use with caution in diabetics, gall bladder disease, in those who consume a large amount of alcohol, and clients with gout.

SIDE EFFECTS

GI: N&V, diarrhea, peptic ulcer activation, abdominal pain, severe hepatic toxicity (including necrosis with high doses). **Dermatologic:** Flushing, warm feeling, skin rash, pruritus, dry skin, itching and tingling feeling, keratosis nigricans. **Other:** Hypotension, headache, macular cystoid edema, amblyopia, rhabdomyolysis (rare). *NOTE:* Megadoses are accompanied by serious toxicity including the symptoms listed in the preceding as well as liver damage, hyperglycemia, hyperuricemia, arrhythmias, tachycardia, and dermatoses.

DRUG INTERACTIONS

Chenodiol / ↓ Effect of chenodiol
HMG-CoA Reductase Inhibitors / ↑ Risk of myopathy and rhabdomyolysis
Probenecid / Niacin may ↓ uricosuric effect of probenecid
Sulfinpyrazone / Niacin ↓ uricosuric effect of sulfinpyrazone
Sympathetic blocking agents / Additive vasodilating effects → postural hypotension

HOW SUPPLIED

Niacin: *Capsule, Extended Release:* 125 mg, 250 mg, 400 mg, 500 mg; *Elixir:* 50 mg/5 mL; *Tablet:* 50 mg, 100 mg, 250 mg, 500 mg; *Tablet, Extended Release:* 250 mg, 500 mg, 750 mg, 1,000 mg. **Niacinamide:** *Tablet:* 100 mg, 500 mg

DOSAGE

Niacin
- **EXTENDED-RELEASE CAPSULES, TABLETS, EXTENDED-RELEASE TABLETS, ELIXIR**
   Pellagra.
Adults: Up to 500 mg/day; **pediatric:** Up to 300 mg/day.
   Antihyperlipidemic.
Adults: 1–2 g of immediate release product 2 or 3 times per day. Initiate therapy at 250 mg as a single dose after the evening meal. Frequency of dosing and total daily dose can be increased every 4–7 days until desired response reached. If adequate response not achieved after 2 months at 1.5–2 g/day, increase at 2–4 week intervals to 3 g/day (i.e., 1 g 3 times per day). Do not exceed 6 g/day. For extended release products, give 500 mg at bedtime for 1–4 weeks; then, 1,000 mg at bedtime during weeks 5–8. If response to 1,000 mg/day is inadequate, increase dose to 1,500 mg/day, up to a maximum of 2,000 mg/day if needed. Do not increase daily dose more than 500 mg in a 4-week period.

Niacinamide
- **TABLETS**
   Pellagra.
Adults: 100–500 mg/day. **Pediatric:** Up to 300 mg/day.

NURSING CONSIDERATIONS

ADMINISTRATION/STORAGE

1. Do not substitute sustained release niacin products for equivalent doses of immediate-release niacin.
2. Niacin, 100 mg/day, plus a statin may increase HDL levels.

ASSESSMENT

1. Note indications for therapy, other agents trialed, and outcome. Monitor glucose, HbA1c, LFTs, and plasma lipid levels.
2. Note any history of CAD, PUD, liver or gallbladder dysfunction.
3. Assess diet, exercise, and any lifestyle changes necessary to decrease coronary risk factors.
4. If and when used with statins monitor LFTs closely as they both utilize the same metabolic pathway.

5. When using the regular strength tablets for hyperlipidemia, start low and go slow to enhance client tolerance. With the extended release tablets, titrate up and advise to take at bedtime with an ASA or small snack to diminish side effects (flushing/hot flashes).

CLIENT/FAMILY TEACHING
1. Take nicotinic acid PO only with cold water (no hot beverages). Can be taken with meals if GI upset occurs.
2. May experience a warm flushing in the face and ears within 2 hr after taking. To prevent/reduce take one aspirin (325 mg) or a small low fat snack 30–60 min prior to dosing. Hot showers, exercise, hot/spicy foods and alcohol may increase these effects.
3. Lie down if feeling weak and dizzy after taking niacin (until this feeling passes) and report if feeling persists.
4. Identify food sources high in niacin (dairy products, meats, tuna, and eggs); assess consumption.
5. With diabetes, do not take niacin unless specifically ordered and then the BS levels must be closely monitored for hyperglycemia; also monitor for ketonuria and glucosuria. Antidiabetic agents may require adjustment.
6. Report any skin color changes or yellowing of the sclera.
7. Clients predisposed to gout may experience flank, joint, or stomach pains; report immediately.
8. If blurred vision or skin lesions occur, remain out of direct sunlight.
9. No unsupervised excessive vitamin ingestion; high doses may impair liver function.
10. Report as scheduled for regular labs and F/U.

OUTCOMES/EVALUATE
• ↓ Triglyceride levels
• Relief of symptoms of pellagra and niacin deficiency

Nicardipine hydrochloride
(nye-**KAR**-dih-peen)

CLASSIFICATION(S):
Calcium channel blocker
PREGNANCY CATEGORY: C
Rx: Cardene, Cardene IV, Cardene SR

SEE ALSO *CALCIUM CHANNEL BLOCKING AGENTS.*

ACTION/KINETICS
Moderately increases CO and HR and significantly decreases peripheral vascular resistance. Slight increase in QT interval and slight to no decrease in myocardial contractility. No effect on QRS complex or PR interval. Nearly 100% absorbed. **Onset of action:** 20 min. **Maximum plasma levels:** 30–120 min. Significant first-pass metabolism. Food (especially fats) will decrease the amount of drug absorbed from the GI tract. Steady-state plasma levels are reached after 2–3 days of therapy. **Therapeutic serum levels:** 0.028–0.050 mcg/mL. **t ½, at steady state:** 8.6 hr. **Maximum BP-lowering effects, immediate release:** 1–2 hr; **maximum BP-lowering effects, sustained release:** 2–6 hr. **Duration:** 8 hr. Metabolized by the liver with excretion through both the urine and feces. More than 95% bound to plasma proteins.

USES
Immediate release: Chronic stable angina (effort-associated angina) alone or in combination with beta-adrenergic blocking agents. **Immediate and sustained release:** Hypertension alone or in combination with other antihypertensive drugs. **IV:** Short-term treatment of hypertension when PO therapy is not desired or possible. *Investigational:* CHF.

CONTRAINDICATIONS
Use in advanced aortic stenosis due to the effect on reducing afterload. During lactation.

SPECIAL CONCERNS
Safety and efficacy in children less than 18 years of age have not been established. Use with caution in clients with CHF, especially in combination with a beta blocker due to the possibility of a negative inotropic effect. Use with caution in clients with impaired liver function, reduced hepatic blood flow, or im-

paired renal function. Initial increase in frequency, duration, or severity of angina.

SIDE EFFECTS

CV: Pedal edema, flushing, increased angina, palpitations, tachycardia, other edema, abnormal ECG, hypotension, postural hypotension, syncope, *MI, AV block,* ventricular extrasystoles, PVD. **CNS:** Dizziness, headache, somnolence, malaise, nervousness, insomnia, abnormal dreams, vertigo, depression, confusion, amnesia, anxiety, weakness, psychoses, hallucinations, paranoia. **GI:** N&V, dyspepsia, dry mouth, constipation, sore throat. **Neuromuscular:** Asthenia, myalgia, paresthesia, hyperkinesia, arthralgia. **Miscellaneous:** Rash, dyspnea, SOB, nocturia, polyuria, allergic reactions, abnormal LFTs, hot flashes, impotence, rhinitis, sinusitis, nasal congestion, chest congestion, tinnitus, equilibrium disturbances, abnormal or blurred vision, infection, atypical chest pain.

OD **OVERDOSE MANAGEMENT**

Symptoms: Marked hypotension, bradycardia, palpitations, flushing, drowsiness, confusion, and slurred speech following PO overdose. Lethal overdose may cause systemic hypotension, bradycardia (following initial tachycardia), and progressive AV block.

Treatment:
• Treatment is supportive. Monitor cardiac and respiratory function.
• If client is seen soon after ingestion, emetics or gastric lavage should be considered, followed by cathartics.
• *Hypotension:* IV calcium, dopamine, isoproterenol, metaraminol, or norepinephrine. Also, provide IV fluids. Place client in Trendelenburg position.
• *Ventricular tachycardia:* IV procainamide or lidocaine; cardioversion may be necessary. Also, provide slow-drip IV fluids.
• *Bradycardia, asystole, AV block:* IV atropine sulfate (0.6–1 mg), calcium gluconate (10% solution), isoproterenol, norepinephrine; also, cardiac pacing may be indicated. Provide slow-drip IV fluids.

DRUG INTERACTIONS

Beta-blockers / Additive or synergistic effects; possible ↓ metabolism of certain beta-blockers
Cimetidine / ↑ Bioavailability of nicardipine → ↑ plasma levels
Cyclosporine / ↑ Plasma levels of cyclosporine possibly leading to renal toxicity
Grapefruit juice / ↑ Bioavailability of nicardipine R/T ↓ liver metabolism of nicardipine in the gut wall
Ranitidine / ↑ Bioavailability of nicardipine
Rifampin / ↓ Nicardipine effects

HOW SUPPLIED

Capsule, Immediate Release: 20 mg, 30 mg; *Capsule, Extended Release:* 30 mg, 45 mg, 60 mg; *Injection:* 2.5 mg/mL

DOSAGE

• **CAPSULES, IMMEDIATE RELEASE**
Angina, Hypertension.
Initial, usual: 20 mg 3 times per day (range: 20–40 mg 3 times per day). Wait 3 days before increasing dose to ensure steady-state plasma levels.

• **CAPSULES, EXTENDED RELEASE**
Hypertension.
Initial: 30 mg twice a day (range: 30–60 mg twice a day).
NOTE: Initial dose in renal impairment: 20 mg 3 times per day. Initial dose in hepatic impairment: 20 mg twice a day.

• **IV**
Hypertension.
Individualize dose. Initial: 5 mg/hr; the infusion rate may be increased to a maximum of 15 mg/hr (by 2.5-mg/hr increments q 15 min). For a more rapid reduction in BP, initiate at 5 mg/hr but increase the rate q 5 min in 2.5-mg/hr increments until a maximum of 15 mg/hr is reached. **Maintenance:** 3 mg/hr. The IV infusion rate to produce an average plasma level similar to a particular PO dose is as follows: 20 mg q 8 hr is equivalent to 0.5 mg/hr; 30 mg q 8 hr is equivalent to 1.2 mg/hr; and 40 mg q 8 hr is equivalent to 2.2 mg/hr.

NURSING CONSIDERATIONS

℮ Do not confuse nicardipine with nifedipine (also a calcium channel

N

blocker). Also, do not confuse Cardene with Cardizem (also a calcium channel blocker).

ADMINISTRATION/STORAGE

1. When used for treating angina, may be administered safely along with sublingual nitroglycerin, prophylactic nitrates, or beta blockers.

2. When used to treat hypertension, may be administered safely along with diuretics or beta blockers.

3. During initial therapy and when dosage is increased, may experience an increase in the frequency, duration, or severity of angina.

4. If transfer to PO antihypertensives other than nicardipine is planned, initiate therapy after discontinuing infusion. If PO nicardipine is used at a dosage regimen of three times daily, give the first dose 1 hr prior to discontinuing infusion.

IV 5. Ampules must be diluted before infusion. Acceptable diluents are D5W, D5/0.45% NaCl, D5W with 40 mEq potassium, 0.45% NaCl, and 0.9% NaCl. Nicardipine is incompatible with 5% $NaHCO_3$ and RL solution.

6. The infusion concentration is 0.1 mg/mL. The diluted product is stable at room temperature for 24 hr.

7. Store ampules at room temperature; freezing does not affect the product. Protect ampules from light and elevated temperatures.

ASSESSMENT

1. Document indications for therapy. List other agents prescribed and the outcome.

2. Note CHF and if beta blockers prescribed, monitor closely.

3. Monitor ECG, liver and renal function studies; note any dysfunction.

4. Monitor VS. When the immediate-release product is used for hypertension, the maximum lowering of BP occurs 1–2 hr after dosing. Evaluate BP at trough (8 hr after dosing). When the sustained-release product is used, maximum lowering of BP occurs 2–6 hr after dosing. Monitor BP frequently during and following IV infusion. Avoid too rapid or excessive decrease in BP and

discontinue infusion if significant hypotension or tachycardia.

CLIENT/FAMILY TEACHING

1. Take at the same time each day.

2. Report any persistent and/or bothersome side effects such as dizziness, flushing, increased chest pain, SOB, weight gain, or swelling of extremities. Avoid activities that require mental alertness until drug effects realized.

3. Maintain proper intake of fluids to avoid constipation. Avoid alcohol; limit caffeine.

4. May experience impotence.

5. Anginal attacks may persist up to 30 min following drug ingestion due to reflex tachycardia; use nitrates as prescribed.

6. Report any change in psychologic state—depression, anxiety, sleep problems, or decreased mental acuity. Particularly important when working with elderly clients since there is a tendency to misdiagnose as senility.

OUTCOMES/EVALUATE

• Control of hypertension

• ↓ Frequency/intensity of anginal attacks

• Therapeutic drug levels (0.028–0.050 mcg/mL)

Nifedipine   ©

(nye-**FED**-ih-peen)

CLASSIFICATION(S):

Calcium channel blocker

PREGNANCY CATEGORY: C

Rx: Adalat, Adalat CC, Afeditab CR, Nifediac CC, Nifedical XL, Procardia, Procardia XL

✦Rx: Adalat XL, Apo-Nifed, Apo-Nifed PA, Novo-Nifedin, Nu-Nifed, Nu-Nifedipine-PA

SEE ALSO *CALCIUM CHANNEL BLOCKING AGENTS*.

ACTION/KINETICS

Variable effects on AV node effective and functional refractory periods. CO is slightly increased while peripheral vascular resistance is significantly decreased. Slight to no increase in HR and slight to no decrease in myocardial con-

---

tractility. **Onset:** 20 min. **Peak plasma levels:** 30 min (up to 4 hr for extended-release). **t ½:** 2–5 hr. 92–95% bound to plasma proteins. **Therapeutic serum levels:** 0.025–0.1 mcg/mL. **Duration:** 4–8 hr (12 hr for extended-release). Low-fat meals may slow the rate but not the extent of absorption. Metabolized in the liver to inactive metabolites with 60–80% excreted in the urine and 15% excreted in the feces.

USES

(1) Vasospastic (Prinzmetal's or variant) angina (except Adalat CC). (2) Chronic stable angina without vasospasm (except Adalat CC), including angina due to increased effort (especially in clients who cannot take beta blockers or nitrates or who remain symptomatic following clinical doses of these drugs). (3) Essential hypertension (sustained-release only). *Investigational:* PO, sublingually, or chewed in hypertensive emergencies. Also prophylaxis of migraine headaches, primary pulmonary hypertension, severe pregnancy-associated hypertension, esophageal diseases, Raynaud's phenomenon, CHF, asthma, premature labor, biliary and renal colic, and cardiomyopathy. To prevent strokes and to decrease the risk of CHF in geriatric hypertensives.

CONTRAINDICATIONS

Hypersensitivity. Lactation.

SPECIAL CONCERNS

Use with caution in impaired hepatic or renal function and in elderly clients. Initial increase in frequency, duration, or severity of angina (may also be seen in clients being withdrawn from beta blockers and who begin taking nifedipine).

SIDE EFFECTS

CV: Peripheral and pulmonary edema, MI, hypotension, palpitations, syncope, CHF (especially if used with a beta blocker), decreased platelet aggregation, arrhythmias, tachycardia. Increased frequency, length, and duration of angina when beginning nifedipine therapy. **GI:** Nausea, diarrhea, constipation, flatulence, abdominal cramps, dysgeusia, vomiting, dry mouth, eructation, gastroesophageal reflux, melena. **CNS:**

Dizziness, lightheadedness, giddiness, nervousness, sleep disturbances, headache, weakness, depression, migraine, psychoses, hallucinations, disturbances in equilibrium, somnolence, insomnia, abnormal dreams, malaise, anxiety. **Dermatologic:** Rash, dermatitis, urticaria, pruritus, photosensitivity, erythema multiforme, ***Stevens-Johnson syndrome.*** **Respiratory:** Dyspnea, cough, wheezing, SOB, respiratory infection; throat, nasal, or chest congestion. **Musculoskeletal:** Muscle cramps or inflammation, joint pain or stiffness, arthritis, ataxia, myoclonic dystonia, hypertonia, asthenia. **Hematologic:** Thrombocytopenia, leukopenia, purpura, anemia. **Other:** Fever, chills, sweating, blurred vision, sexual difficulties, flushing, transient blindness, hyperglycemia, hypokalemia, gingival hyperplasia, allergic hepatitis, hepatitis, tinnitus, gynecomastia, polyuria, nocturia, erythromelalgia, weight gain, epistaxis, facial and periorbital edema, hypoesthesia, gout, abnormal lacrimation, breast pain, dysuria, hematuria.

LABORATORY TEST CONSIDERATIONS

↑ Alkaline phosphatase, CPK, LDH, AST, ALT. Positive Coombs' test.

ADDITIONAL DRUG INTERACTIONS

Anticoagulants, oral / Possibility of ↑ PT
Barbiturates / ↓ Nifedipine effects
Cimetidine / ↑ Bioavailability of nifedipine
Cyclosporine / ↑ Cyclosporine levels and toxicity
Digoxin / ↑ Effect of digoxin by ↓ excretion by kidney
Diltiazem / ↑ Plasma levels of both nifedipine and diltiazem
Grapefruit juice / ↑ Nifedipine plasma levels R/T ↓ metabolism
Itraconazole / ↑ Nifedipine serum levels
Mg sulfate / ↑ Neuromuscular blockade and hypotension
Melatonin / Melatonin may ↓ antihypertensive effect
Nafcillin / Significant ↓ nifedipine plasma levels
Quinidine / Possible ↓ quinidine effect R/T ↓ plasma levels; ↑ risk of hypoten-

sion, bradycardia, AV block, pulmonary edema, and VT

Quinupristin/Dalfopristin / ↑ Nifedipine plasma levels

Ranitidine / ↑ Nifedipine bioavailability

Rifampin ↑ Nifedipine effects

H *St. John's wort* / ↓ Nifedipine plasma levels R/T ↑ metabolism

Tacrolimus / ↑ Tacrolimus levels → ↑ toxicity

Theophylline / Possible ↑ effect of theophylline

Vincristine / ↑ Vincristine levels → ↑ toxicity

HOW SUPPLIED

Capsule: 10 mg, 20 mg; *Tablet, Extended Release:* 30 mg, 60 mg, 90 mg

DOSAGE

• CAPSULES

Individualized. Initial: 10 mg 3 times per day (range: 10–20 mg 3 times per day); **maintenance:** 10–30 mg 3–4 times per day. Clients with coronary artery spasm may respond better to 20–30 mg 3–4 times per day. Doses greater than 120 mg/day are rarely needed while doses greater than 180 mg/day are not recommended.

• EXTENDED-RELEASE TABLETS

Initial: 30 or 60 mg once daily for Nifedical XL or Procardia XL and 30 mg once daily for Adalat CC. Titrate over a 7- to 14-day period. Dosage can be increased as required and as tolerated to a maximum of 120 mg/day for Nifedical XL or Procardia XL and 90 mg/day for Adalat CC.

Investigational: Hypertensive emergencies.

10–20 mg given PO (capsule is punctured several times and then chewed).

NURSING CONSIDERATIONS

℮ Do not confuse nifedipine with nicardipine (also a calcium channel blocker).

ADMINISTRATION/STORAGE

1. Do not exceed a single dose (other than sustained-released) of 30 mg.

2. Before increasing the dose, carefully monitor BP.

3. Use only the sustained-release tablets to treat hypertension.

4. Sublingual nitroglycerin and long-acting nitrates may be used concomitantly with nifedipine.

5. Concomitant therapy with beta-adrenergic blocking agents may be used. In these cases, note any potential drug interactions.

6. Clients withdrawn from beta blockers may manifest symptoms of increased angina which cannot be prevented by nifedipine; in fact, nifedipine may increase the severity of angina in this situation.

7. Clients with angina may be switched to the sustained-release product at the nearest equivalent total daily dose. Use doses greater than 90 mg/day with caution.

8. No rebound effect noted when nifedipine is discontinued. However, if the drug is to be discontinued, decrease dosage gradually with supervision.

9. Protect capsules from light and moisture and store at room temperature in the original container.

10. During initial therapy and when dosage is increased, may experience an increase in the frequency, duration, or severity of angina.

11. Food may decrease the rate but not the extent of absorption; can be taken without regard to meals.

ASSESSMENT

1. Document indications for therapy, other agents trialed/outcome and any sensitivity to CCBs.

2. Note any pulmonary edema, ECG abnormalities, or palpitations. Document K+ levels, BP, and cardiopulmonary assessment findings.

INTERVENTIONS

1. During titration period, note any hypotensive response and increased HR that result from peripheral vasodilation; may precipitate angina.

2. Although beta-blocking drugs may be used concomitantly with chronic stable angina, the combined effects of the drugs cannot be predicted (especially with compromised LV function or cardiac conduction abnormalities). Pronounced hypotension, heart block, and CHF may occur.

Bold Italic = life threatening side effect   ■ = black box warning   ♣ = Available in Canada

3. If therapy with a beta blocker is to be discontinued, gradually decrease dosage to prevent withdrawal syndrome.

CLIENT/FAMILY TEACHING

1. May take with or without food. Sustained-release tablets should not be chewed, crushed, or divided. Grapefruit juice may cause increased serum drug levels.

2. Maintain a fluid intake of 2–3 L/day to avoid constipation. There is no cause for concern if a tablet coating appears in the stool.

3. Do not switch brands, Adalat CC and Procardia XL are not interchangeable as they are not equivalent.

4. Do not use OTC agents unless approved; avoid alcohol and caffeine.

5. Report any symptoms of persistent headache, flushing, nausea, palpitations, weight gain, dizziness, lightheadedness, or lack of response.

6. Keep log of BP reports. Perform weekly weights and note any extremity swelling. This may result from arterial vasodilatation precipitated by nifedipine or the swelling may indicate increasing ventricular dysfunction and should be reported.

7. If also receiving beta-adrenergic blocking agents, report any evidence of hypotension, exacerbation of angina, or evidence of heart failure. Once beta-blocking agents have been discontinued, report increased anginal pain.

OUTCOMES/EVALUATE

- ↓ Frequency and intensity of anginal episodes ↓ BP
- Improved peripheral circulation
- Prevention of strokes and ↓ risk of CHF in geriatric hypertensives

---

Nimodipine

(nye-**MOH**-dih-peen)

CLASSIFICATION(S):
Calcium channel blocker
PREGNANCY CATEGORY: C
Rx: Nimotop
✚**Rx:** Nimotop I.V.

SEE ALSO *CALCIUM CHANNEL BLOCKING AGENTS.*

ACTION/KINETICS

Has a greater effect on cerebral arteries than arteries elsewhere in the body (probably due to its highly lipophilic properties). Mechanism to reduce neurologic deficits following subarachnoid hemorrhage not known. **Peak plasma levels:** 1 hr. **t ½:** 1–2 hr; **t ½, elimination:** 8–9 hr. Undergoes first-pass metabolism in the liver; metabolites excreted through the urine. Over 95% bound to plasma proteins.

USES

Improvement of neurologic deficits due to spasm following subarachnoid hemorrhage (SAH) from ruptured congenital intracranial aneurysms irrespective of the postictus neurological condition. *Investigational:* Migraine headaches and cluster headaches.

CONTRAINDICATIONS

Lactation.

SPECIAL CONCERNS

Safety and efficacy have not been established in children. Use with caution in clients with impaired hepatic function and reduced hepatic blood flow. The half-life may be increased in geriatric clients.

SIDE EFFECTS

CV: Hypotension, peripheral edema, CHF, ECG abnormalities, tachycardia, bradycardia, palpitations, rebound vasospasm, hypertension, hematoma, *DIC, DVT.* **GI:** Nausea, dyspepsia, diarrhea, abdominal discomfort, cramps, *GI hemorrhage,* vomiting. **CNS:** Headache, depression, lightheadedness, dizziness. **Hepatic:** Abnormal LFT, hepatitis, jaundice. **Hematologic:** Thrombocytopenia, anemia, purpura, ecchymosis. **Dermatologic:** Rash, dermatitis, pruritus, urticaria. **Miscellaneous:** Dyspnea, muscle pain or cramps, acne, itching, flushing, diaphoresis, wheezing, hyponatremia.

LABORATORY TEST CONSIDERATIONS

↑ Nonfasting BS, LDH, alkaline phosphatase, ALT. ↓ Platelet count.

ADDITIONAL DRUG INTERACTIONS

Cimetidine / ↑ Nimodipine serum levels
Valproic acid / ↑ AUC of nimodipine

HOW SUPPLIED
Capsule, Liquid-Filled: 30 mg

DOSAGE
• CAPSULES
Adults: 60 mg (two 30 mg capsules) q 4 hr beginning within 96 hr after subarachnoid hemorrhage and continuing for 21 consecutive days. Reduce the dose to 30 mg q 4 hr in clients with hepatic impairment.

NURSING CONSIDERATIONS
ADMINISTRATION/STORAGE
If unable to swallow capsule (e.g., unconscious or at time of surgery), make a hole in both ends of the capsule (soft gelatin) with an 18-gauge needle and withdraw the contents into a syringe. This may be administered into the NG tube and washed down with 30 mL of NSS. Do not administer the contents of the capsule by IV injection or any other parenteral route.

ASSESSMENT
1. Note characteristics of S&S. Initiate therapy within 96 hr of subarachnoid hemorrhage.
2. Obtain baseline labs, determine if pregnant; reduce dose with hepatic dysfunction.
3. Perform baseline neurologic scores and thoroughly document deficits. Monitor BP, I&O, and weights.

CLIENT/FAMILY TEACHING
1. Take the drug on time; sleep must be interrupted to give the medication q 4 hr ATC for 21 days.
2. Report any side effects such as nausea, lightheadedness, irregular heart beat, low BP, dizziness, muscle cramps/pain or swelling of extremities.
3. Avoid activities that require mental alertness until drug effects realized.
4. Report ↑ SOB, the need to take deep breaths on occasion, or wheezing. Keep all F/U visits.

OUTCOMES/EVALUATE
• ↓ Neurologic deficits R/T venospasm after subarachnoid hemorrhage
• Termination of migraine and cluster headaches

Nisoldipine   ©
(NYE-sohl-dih-peen)

CLASSIFICATION(S):
Calcium channel blocker
PREGNANCY CATEGORY: C
Rx: Sular

ACTION/KINETICS
Inhibits the transmembrane influx of calcium into vascular smooth muscle and cardiac muscle, resulting in dilation of arterioles. Has greater potency on vascular smooth muscle than on cardiac muscle. Chronic use results in a sustained decrease in vascular resistance and small increases in stroke index and LV ejection fraction. Weak diuretic effect and no clinically important chronotropic effects. Well absorbed following PO use; however, absolute bioavailability is low due to presystemic metabolism in the gut wall. Foods high in fat result in a significant increase in peak plasma levels. **Maximum plasma levels:** 6–12 hr. **t ½, terminal:** 7–12 hr. Metabolized in the liver and excreted through the urine. Almost completely bound to plasma proteins.

USES
Hypertension alone or in combination with other antihypertensive drugs.

CONTRAINDICATIONS
Use with grapefruit juice as it interferes with metabolism, resulting in a significant increase in plasma levels of the drug. Use in those with known hypersensitivity to dihydropyridine calcium channel blockers. Lactation.

SPECIAL CONCERNS
Geriatric clients may show a two- to threefold higher plasma concentration; use caution in dosing. Use with caution and at lower doses in those with hepatic insufficiency. Use with caution in clients with CHF or compromised ventricular function, especially in combination with a beta blocker.

SIDE EFFECTS
CV: Increased angina and/or MI in clients with CAD. Initially, excessive hypotension, especially in those taking

---

other antihypertensive drugs. Vasodilation, palpitation, atrial fibrillation, **CVA, MI,** CHF, first-degree AV block, hyper/hypotension, JVD, migraine, ventricular extrasystoles, SVT, syncope, systolic ejection murmur, T-wave abnormalities on ECG, venous insufficiency. **Body as a whole:** Peripheral edema, cellulitis, chills, facial edema, fever, flu syndrome, malaise. **GI:** Anorexia, nausea, colitis, diarrhea, dry mouth, dyspepsia, dysphagia, flatulence, gastritis, **GI hemorrhage,** gingival hyperplasia, glossitis, hepatomegaly, increased appetite, melena, mouth ulceration. **CNS:** Headache, dizziness, abnormal dreams/thinking and confusion, amnesia, anxiety, ataxia, cerebral ischemia, decreased libido, depression, hypesthesia, hypertonia, insomnia, nervousness, paresthesia, somnolence, tremor, vertigo. **Musculoskeletal:** Arthralgia, arthritis, leg cramps, myalgia, myasthenia, myositis, tenosynovitis. **Hematologic:** Anemia, ecchymoses, leukopenia, petechiae. **Respiratory:** Pharyngitis, sinusitis, asthma, dyspnea, end-inspiratory wheeze and fine rales, epistaxis, increased cough, laryngitis, pleural effusion, rhinitis. **Dermatologic:** Acne, alopecia, dry skin, exfoliative dermatitis, fungal dermatitis, herpes simplex/zoster, maculopapular rash, pruritus, pustular rash, skin discoloration/ulcer, sweating, urticaria. **GU:** Dysuria, hematuria, impotence, nocturia, urinary frequency, vaginal hemorrhage, vaginitis. **Metabolic:** Gout, hypokalemia, weight gain/loss. **Ophthalmic:** Abnormal vision, amblyopia, blepharitis, conjunctivitis, glaucoma, watery/itchy eyes, keratoconjunctivitis, retinal detachment, temporary unilateral loss of vision, vitreous floater. **Miscellaneous:** Diabetes mellitus, thyroiditis, chest/ear pain, otitis media, tinnitus, taste disturbance.

LABORATORY TEST CONSIDERATIONS
↑ Serum creatine kinase, NPN, BUN, serum creatinine. Abnormal LFTs.

OD OVERDOSE MANAGEMENT
Symptoms: Pronounced hypotension. *Treatment:* Active CV support, including monitoring of CV and respiratory function, elevation of extremities, judicious

use of calcium infusion, pressor agents, and fluids. Dialysis is not likely to be beneficial, although plasmapheresis may be helpful.

DRUG INTERACTIONS
Azole antifungals / ↑ Nisoldipine serum levels; avoid coadministration
Cimetidine / Significant ↑ plasma nisoldipine levels
Ketoconazole / ↑ Plasma nisoldipine levels R/T ↓ liver metabolism
Phenytoin / ↑ Nisoldipine pharmacologic effects
Quinidine / ↑ AUC of nisoldipine but not peak concentration

HOW SUPPLIED
Extended-Release Tablets: 10 mg, 20 mg, 30 mg, 40 mg.

DOSAGE
• **TABLETS, EXTENDED-RELEASE**
  Hypertension.
Dose must be adjusted to the needs of each person. **Initial:** 20 mg once daily; **then,** increase by 10 mg/week or longer intervals to reach adequate BP control. **Usual maintenance:** 20–40 mg once daily. Doses beyond 60 mg once daily are not recommended. **Initial dose, clients over 65 years and those with impaired renal function:** 10 mg once daily.

NURSING CONSIDERATIONS
ℂ Do not confuse nisoldipine with nicardipine or nifedipine.

ADMINISTRATION/STORAGE
1. Closely monitor dosage adjustments in clients over age 65 and those with impaired liver/renal function.
2. Store at controlled room temperature of 20–25°C (68–77°F) protected from light and moisture. Should be dispensed in tight, light-resistant containers.

ASSESSMENT
1. Document indications for therapy, characteristics of symptoms, agents trialed, and outcome.
2. List drugs prescribed to ensure none interact unfavorably. Reduce dosage in the elderly and with liver/renal dysfunction.
3. Obtain baseline VS and ECG; monitor BP closely and note any history/evi-

dence of CHF, CAD, or compromised LV function.

CLIENT/FAMILY TEACHING
1. Swallow tablets whole; do not chew, divide, or crush. Do not take with grapefruit juice or a high-fat meal.
2. Headaches, extremity swelling, and dizziness may occur; use caution and report if persistent.
3. Report as scheduled for BP evaluation during titration period. Maintain BP log and report any new/adverse side effects or loss of BP control.

OUTCOMES/EVALUATE
↓ BP

Nitroglycerin IV
(nye-troh-**GLIH**-sir-in)

CLASSIFICATION(S):
Vasodilator, coronary
PREGNANCY CATEGORY: C
Rx: Nitro-Bid IV, Nitroglycerin in 5% Dextrose

SEE ALSO *ANTIANGINAL DRUGS - NITRATES/NITRITES*.

ACTION/KINETICS
Onset: 1–2 min; **duration:** 3–5 min (dose-dependent).

USES
(1) Hypertension associated with surgery (e.g., associated with ET intubation, skin incision, sternotomy, anesthesia, cardiac bypass, immediate postsurgical period). (2) CHF associated with acute MI. (3) Angina unresponsive to usual doses of organic nitrate or beta-adrenergic blocking agents. (4) Cardiacload reducing agent. (5) Produce controlled hypotension during surgical procedures.

SPECIAL CONCERNS
Dosage has not been established in children.

HOW SUPPLIED
Injection: 5 mg/mL; *Injection Solution:* 25 mg, 50 mg 100 mg, 200 mg

DOSAGE
• **IV INFUSION ONLY**
Initial: 5 mcg/min delivered by precise infusion pump. May be increased by 5 mcg/min q 3–5 min until response is seen. If no response seen at 20 mcg/min, dose can be increased by 10–20 mcg/min until response noted. Monitor titration continuously until client reaches desired level of response.

NURSING CONSIDERATIONS
ADMINISTRATION/STORAGE
IV 1. Dilute with D5W or 0.9% NaCl injection. Not for direct IV use; must first be diluted.
2. Use glass IV bottle only and administration set provided by the manufacturer; is readily adsorbed onto many plastics. Avoid adding unnecessary plastic to IV system.
3. Aspirate medication into a syringe and then inject immediately into a glass bottle (or polyolefin bottle) to minimize contact with plastic.
4. Do not administer with any other medications in the IV system.
5. Do not interrupt IV nitroglycerin for administration of a bolus of any other medication.
6. To provide correct dosage, remove 15 mL of solution from the IV tubing if concentration of solution is changed.
7. Administer solution with infusion device (volumetric) in a closely monitored environment.

ASSESSMENT
1. Document indications/goals of therapy. Assess VS, ECG, and cardiopulmonary assessments.
2. Assess and rate pain, noting location, onset, duration, and any precipitating factors.

INTERVENTIONS
1. Obtain written parameters for BP and pulse; monitor during therapy. Note any evidence of hypotension, nausea, sweating, and/or vomiting. Monitor CVP and/or PA pressure as ordered; document presence of tachycardia or bradycardia:
• Elevate the legs to restore BP.
• Reduce the rate of flow or administer additional IV fluids.
2. Assess for thrombophlebitis at the IV site; remove if reddened.

3. After the initial positive response to therapy, dosage increments will be smaller and made at longer intervals.

4. Sinus tachycardia may occur in client with angina receiving a maintenance dose of nitroglycerin (HR of 80 beats/min or less reduces myocardial demand).

5. Check that topical, PO, or SL doses are adjusted/held if on concomitant IV nitroglycerin.

6. Wean from IV nitroglycerin by gradually decreasing doses to avoid posttherapy or CV distress. Usually initiated when the client is receiving the peak effect from PO or topical vasodilators; monitor for hypertension and angina.

7. Administer nonnarcotic analgesic (usually acetaminophen) because headache is a common side effect of drug therapy.

CLIENT/FAMILY TEACHING

1. Drug is used to lower BP, control chest pain, and/or reduce cardiac work load.

2. Report pain and level so dose may be adjusted to control.

3. Report any headaches so medications to relieve them can be administered.

OUTCOMES/EVALUATE

- Resolution/control of angina
- ↓ BP; ↑ activity tolerance
- ↓ LVEDP (preload) and ↓ systemic vascular resistance (afterload)
- Improvement in S&S of CHF (↑ output, ↓ rales, ↓ CVP)

Nitroglycerin sublingual

CLASSIFICATION(S):
Vasodilator, coronary
PREGNANCY CATEGORY: C
Rx: NitroQuick, Nitrostat, NitroTab

SEE ALSO *ANTIANGINAL DRUGS - NITRATES/NITRITES.*

ACTION/KINETICS
Sublingual. Onset: 1–3 min; **duration:** 30–60 min.

USES
Agent of choice for prophylaxis and treatment of angina pectoris.

SPECIAL CONCERNS
Dosage has not been established in children.

ADDITIONAL DRUG INTERACTIONS
Tadalafil ↑ the hypotensive effect of sublingual nitroglycerin for 24 hr after tadalafil administration.

HOW SUPPLIED
Tablet: 0.3 mg, 0.4 mg, 0.6 mg

DOSAGE
- **SUBLINGUAL TABLETS**

Dissolve 1 tablet under the tongue or in the buccal pouch at first sign of attack; may be repeated in 5 min if necessary (no more than 3 tablets should be taken within 15 min). For prophylaxis, tablets may be taken 5–10 min prior to activities that may precipitate an attack.

NURSING CONSIDERATIONS

ASSESSMENT
Note indications for therapy, characteristics of S&S, and cardiac history/assessments.

CLIENT/FAMILY TEACHING
1. Sit down and place sublingual tablet under the tongue and allow to dissolve; do not swallow until entirely dissolved. May sting when it comes in contact with the mucosa.

2. Take *before* stressful activity, i.e., exercise, sex.

3. Report immediately if pain is not controlled with prescribed dosage (usu. 1 tab q 5 min x 3). Call 911 or for an ambulance as directed by provider if relief not attained.

4. Date sublingual container upon opening. Store in original container at room temperature protected from moisture. Discard unused tablets if 6 months has elapsed since the original container was opened.

5. Encourage family members to learn CPR.

OUTCOMES/EVALUATE
- Angina prophylaxis
- Termination of anginal attack

Nitroglycerin sustained-release capsules

CLASSIFICATION(S):
Vasodilator, coronary
PREGNANCY CATEGORY: C
Rx: Nitroglyn, Nitro-Time

Nitroglycerin sustained-release tablets

PREGNANCY CATEGORY: C
Rx: Nitrong
✦**Rx:** Nitrong SR

SEE ALSO *ANTIANGINAL DRUGS - NITRATES/NITRITES.*

ACTION/KINETICS
Sustained-release. Onset: 20–45 min; **duration:** 3–8 hr.

USES
Prophylaxis and long term treatment of recurrent angina.

SPECIAL CONCERNS
Dosage has not been established in children.

HOW SUPPLIED
Sustained-release capsules: 2.5 mg, 6.5 mg, 9 mg, 13 mg. **Sustained-release tablets:** 2.6 mg, 6.5 mg, 9 mg

DOSAGE————————
• **SUSTAINED-RELEASE CAPSULES, TABLETS**
Initial: 2.5 or 2.6 mg 3 or 4 times per day. Titrate upward to an effective dose until side effects limit dose. Dose may usually be increased by 2.5 or 2.6 mg 2–4 times per day over a period of days or weeks. Doses as high as 26 mg 4 times per day have been reported.

NURSING CONSIDERATIONS

ASSESSMENT
Note indications for therapy, characteristics of S&S, and cardiac history/assessments.

CLIENT/FAMILY TEACHING
1. Drug is used to control/prevent chest pain.

2. Do not chew or crush sustained-release tablets and capsules; not intended for sublingual use.
3. Take smallest effective dose 2–4 times per day with a glass of water. Report if tolerance/lack of response evident.

OUTCOMES/EVALUATE
Angina prophylaxis

Nitroglycerin topical ointment

CLASSIFICATION(S):
Vasodilator, coronary
PREGNANCY CATEGORY: C
Rx: Cellegesic (formerly Anogesic), Nitro-Bid, Nitrol

SEE ALSO *ANTIANGINAL DRUGS - NITRATES/NITRITES.*

ACTION/KINETICS
Onset: 30–60 min; **duration:** 2–12 hr (depending on amount used per unit of surface area).

USES
(1) Prophylaxis and treatment of angina pectoris due to CAD. (2) Pain associated with chronic anal fissures (Cellegesic).

SPECIAL CONCERNS
Dosage has not been established in children.

HOW SUPPLIED
Ointment: 2%
DOSAGE————————
• **TOPICAL OINTMENT (2%)**
1–2 in. (15–30 mg) q 8 hr; up to 4–5 in. (60–75 mg) q 4 hr may be necessary. One inch equals approximately 15 mg nitroglycerin. Determine optimum dosage by starting with $\frac{1}{2}$ in. q 8 hr and increasing by $\frac{1}{2}$ in. with each successive dose until headache occurs; then, decrease to largest dose that does not cause headache. When ending treatment, reduce both the dose and frequency of administration over 4–6 weeks to prevent sudden withdrawal reactions.

NURSING CONSIDERATIONS
ASSESSMENT
Note indications for therapy, characteristics of S&S, and cardiac history/assessments.

CLIENT/FAMILY TEACHING

1. Squeeze ointment carefully onto dose-measuring application papers (packaged with the medicine). Use applicator to spread ointment or fold paper in half and rub back and forth. Clean around tube opening and tightly cap tube after use.

2. Use the paper to spread the ointment onto a nonhairy area of skin. Application to the chest may be psychologically helpful, but may be applied to other nonhairy areas.

3. Rotate sites to prevent irritation. Keep a record of areas used to avoid unnecessary repetitive use of sites.

4. Apply ointment in a thin, even layer covering an area of skin 5–6 in. in diameter; remove last dose. Date and tape the application paper over the area, or cover the area with a piece of plastic wrap-type material. A clear plastic cover causes less leakage of ointment, decreases skin irritation, increases absorption, and prevents clothing stains.

5. Once the dose is established, use the same type of covering to ensure that the same amount of drug is absorbed during each application.

6. To prevent systemic absorption protect skin from contact with ointment. Wash hands thoroughly after application to avoid headache.

7. Remove at bedtime or as directed to prevent tolerance or loss of drug effect. Remember to reapply upon awakening the next morning. Report adverse effects and lack of response.

OUTCOMES/EVALUATE

• Termination/prevention of anginal episodes

• Relief of chronic anal fissure pain

Nitroglycerin transdermal system

CLASSIFICATION(S):
Vasodilator, coronary
PREGNANCY CATEGORY: C

Rx: Deponit 0.2 mg/hr and 0.4 mg/hr; Minitran 0.1 mg/hr, 0.2 mg/hr, 0.4 mg/hr, and 0.6 mg/hr; Nitrek 0.2 mg/hr, 0.4 mg/hr, and 0.6 mg/hr; Nitrodisc 0.2 mg/hr, 0.3 mg/hr, and 0.4 mg/hr; Nitro-Dur 0.1 mg/hr, 0.2 mg/hr, 0.3 mg/hr, 0.4 mg/hr, 0.6 mg/hr, and 0.8 mg/hr; Transderm-Nitro 0.1 mg/hr, 0.2 mg/hr, 0.4 mg/hr, 0.6 mg/hr, and 0.8 mg/hr.

SEE ALSO *ANTIANGINAL DRUGS - NITRATES/NITRITES.*

ACTION/KINETICS
Onset: 30–60 min; **duration:** 8–24 hr. The amount released each hour is indicated in the name.

USES
Prophylaxis of angina pectoris due to CAD. *NOTE:* There is some evidence that nitroglycerin patches stop preterm labor. Also, high-dose nitrate therapy with an ACE inhibitor may cause significant, progressive, and long-term enhancement of exercise tolerance within 2 months of initiation of nitrate therapy.

SPECIAL CONCERNS
Dosage has not been established in children.

HOW SUPPLIED
Film, Extended Release: 0.1 mg/hr, 0.2 mg/hr, 0.3 mg/hr, 0.4 mg/hr, 0.6 mg/hr, 0.8 mg/hr

DOSAGE
• **TOPICAL PATCH**
Initial: 0.2–0.4 mg/hr (initially the smallest available dose in the dosage series) applied each day to skin site free of hair and free of excessive movement (e.g., chest, upper arm). **Maintenance:** Additional systems or strengths may be added depending on the clinical response.

NURSING CONSIDERATIONS
ADMINISTRATION/STORAGE
1. Follow instructions for specific products on package insert.

2. Tolerance is a significant factor affecting efficacy if the system is used continuously for more than 12 hr/day. Thus, a dosage regimen would include a daily period where the patch is on for 12–14 hr and a period of 10–12 hr when the patch is off (i.e., while asleep).

3. Remove patch before defibrillating as patch may explode.

4. The various products differ in the mechanism for the delivery system; the most important factor is the amount of drug released per hour. A wide range of client variability will be noted. Variables in the absorption rate include skin, physical exercise, and elevated ambient temperature.

ASSESSMENT

Note indications for therapy, characteristics of S&S, and cardiac history/assessments.

CLIENT/FAMILY TEACHING

1. Apply as directed at the same time each day. Dry skin completely before applying to a hair free site.

2. Rotate application sites each day to avoid skin irritation. Do not apply to distal extremities or to skin that is irritated, abraded, or scarred. Date patch as a reminder that drug has been administered. Once applied, do not disturb or open patch. Do not stop abruptly.

3. Remove at bedtime or as directed to prevent a diminished response (tolerance) to the drug. Remember to reapply a new system upon awakening the next morning.

4. Report adverse effects or breakthrough pain. Bathing or swimming should not interfere with therapy.

5. When terminating therapy, gradually reduce the dose and frequency of application over 4–6 weeks.

6. Remove patch before defibrillating as patch may explode. Have family/significant other learn CPR.

OUTCOMES/EVALUATE

Control/prevention of anginal episodes

Nitroglycerin translingual spray

CLASSIFICATION(S):
Vasodilator, coronary

PREGNANCY CATEGORY: C

Rx: Nitrolingual, Nitrolingual Pumpspray

SEE ALSO *ANTIANGINAL DRUGS - NITRATES/NITRITES.*

ACTION/KINETICS

Onset: 2 min; **duration:** 30–60 min.

USES

(1) Terminate an acute anginal attack. (2) Prophylactically 10–15 min before beginning activities that can cause an acute anginal attack.

SPECIAL CONCERNS

Dosage has not been established in children.

HOW SUPPLIED

Aerosol Spray: 400 mcg/metered dose

DOSAGE

• **SPRAY**

Termination of acute attack.

One to two metered doses (400–800 mcg) on or under the tongue q 5 min as needed; no more than three metered doses should be administered within a 15-min period.

Prophylaxis.

One to two metered doses (400–800 mcg) 5–10 min before beginning activities that might precipitate an acute attack.

NURSING CONSIDERATIONS

ASSESSMENT

Note indications for therapy, characteristics of S&S, and cardiac history/assessments.

CLIENT/FAMILY TEACHING

1. Do *not* inhale the spray. Spray under or on the tongue 5-10 min before anticipated activity or when pain experienced. Wait 10 sec and then swallow.

2. Seek immediate medical attention if chest pain persists.

3. Have family/significant other learn CPR.

OUTCOMES/EVALUATE

Control/prevention of acute anginal episodes

Nitroprusside sodium ■

(nye-troh-**PRUS**-eyed)

CLASSIFICATION(S):

Antihypertensive, peripheral vasodilator

PREGNANCY CATEGORY: C

Rx: Nitropress

ACTION/KINETICS

Direct action on vascular smooth muscle, leading to peripheral vasodilation of arteries and veins. Acts on excitation-contraction coupling of vascular smooth muscle by interfering with both influx and intracellular activation of calcium. No effect on smooth muscle of the duodenum or uterus and is more active on veins than on arteries. May also improve CHF by decreasing systemic resistance, preload and afterload reduction, and improved CO. **Onset** (drug must be given by IV infusion): 0.5–1 min; **peak effect:** 1–2 min; **t ½:** 2 min; **duration:** Up to 10 min after infusion stopped. Reacts with hemoglobin to produce cyanmethemoglobin and cyanide ion. Caution must be exercised as nitroprusside injection can result in toxic levels of cyanide. However, when used briefly or at low infusion rates, the cyanide produced reacts with thiosulfate to produce thiocyanate, which is excreted in the urine.

USES

(1) Hypertensive crisis to reduce BP immediately. (2) To produce controlled hypotension during anesthesia to reduce bleeding. (3) Acute CHF. *Investigational:* In combination with dopamine for acute MI. Left ventricular failure with coadministration of oxygen, morphine, and a loop diuretic.

CONTRAINDICATIONS

Compensatory hypertension where the primary hemodynamic lesion is aortic coarctation or AV shunting. Use to produce controlled hypotension during surgery in clients with known inadequate cerebral circulation or in moribund clients. Clients with congenital optic atrophy or tobacco amblyopia (both of which are rare). Acute CHF associated with decreased peripheral vascular resistance (e.g., high-output heart failure that may be seen in endotoxic sepsis). Lactation.

SPECIAL CONCERNS

■(1) After reconstitution, nitroprusside is not suitable for direct injection. The reconstituted solution must be further diluted in D5W before infusion. (2) Can cause a precipitous drop in BP. In clients not properly monitored, these decreases can lead to irreversible ischemic injuries or death. Use only when available equipment and personnel allow BP to be monitored continuously. (3) Nitroprusside injection gives rise to important quantities of cyanide except when used briefly or at low (less than 2 mcg/kg/min) infusion rates. This can lead to toxic and potentially lethal levels. The usual dose rate is 0.5–10 mcg/kg/min, but infusion at the maximum rates should never last beyond 10 minutes. If BP has not been adequately controlled after 10 min of infusion at the maximum rate, terminate administration immediately. (4) Monitor acid-base balance and venous oxygen levels; they may indicate cyanide toxicity but these tests provide imperfect guidance.■ Use with caution in hypothyroidism, liver or kidney impairment, during lactation, and in the presence of increased ICP. Geriatric clients may be more sensitive to the hypotensive effects of nitroprusside; also, a decrease in dose may be necessary in these clients due to age-related decreases in renal function.

SIDE EFFECTS

Excessive hypotension. *Large doses may lead to cyanide toxicity.* **Following rapid BP reduction:** Dizziness, nausea, restlessness, headache, sweating, muscle twitching, palpitations, abdominal pain, apprehension, retching, retrosternal discomfort. **Other side effects:** Bradycardia, tachycardia, ECG changes, venous streaking, rash, vomiting or skin rash, methemoglobinemia, decreased platelet aggregation, flushing, ileus, irritation at injection site, hypothyroidism.

N

Symptoms of thiocyanate toxicity: Blurred vision, tinnitus, confusion, hyperreflexia, seizures. **CNS symptoms (transitory):** Restlessness, agitation, increased ICP, and muscle twitching.

OD OVERDOSE MANAGEMENT

Symptoms: Excessive hypotension, cyanide toxicity, thiocyanate toxicity. *Treatment:*

• Measure cyanide levels and blood gases to determine venous hyperoxemia or acidosis.

• To treat cyanide toxicity, discontinue nitroprusside and give sodium nitrite, 4–6 mg/kg (about 0.2 mL/kg) over 2–4 min (to convert hemoglobin into methemoglobin); follow by sodium thiosulfate, 150–200 mg/kg (about 50 mL of the 25% solution). This regimen can be given again, at half the original doses, after 2 hr.

DRUG INTERACTIONS

Concomitant use of other antihypertensives, volatile liquid anesthetics, or certain depressants ↑ nitroprusside response.

HOW SUPPLIED

Powder for injection: 50 mg/vial

DOSAGE————————————

• **IV INFUSION ONLY**

  Hypertensive crisis.

Adults: Average, 3 mcg/kg/min. **Range:** 0.3–10 mcg/kg/min. Smaller dose is required for clients receiving other antihypertensives. **Pediatric:** 1.4 mcg/kg/min adjusted slowly depending on the response.

Monitor BP and use as guide to regulate rate of administration to maintain desired antihypertensive effect. Do not exceed a rate of administration of 10 mcg/kg/min.

NURSING CONSIDERATIONS

ADMINISTRATION/STORAGE

IV 1. Dissolve contents of the vial (50 mg) in 2–3 mL of D5W. Must be further diluted in 250–1,000 mL D5W.

2. If protected from light, reconstituted solution stable for 24 hr. Discard solutions that are any color but light brown.

3. Do not add any other drug or preservative to solution.

4. Protect dilute solutions during administration by wrapping bag and tubing with opaque material such as Aluminum foil or foil-lined bags; change setup every 24 hr. Explain that covering the IV bag protects the medication from light and maintains drug stability. Administer IV solution with an electronic infusion device in a monitored environment.

5. Cyanide toxicity is possible if more than 500 mcg/kg nitroprusside is given faster than 2 mcg/kg/min. To reduce this possibility, sodium thiosulfate can be co-infused with nitroprusside at rates of 5–10 times that of nitroprusside.

6. Protect drug from heat, light, and moisture. Store at 15–30°C (59–86°F).

ASSESSMENT

1. Document indications for therapy, characteristics of S&S, and other therapies trialed.

2. Note any hypothyroidism or B_{12} deficiency. Monitor VS, I&O, ECG, CBC, electrolytes, ABGs, PAWP, renal and LFT's.

INTERVENTIONS

1. Monitor BP closely and titrate infusion. Administer only in a continuously monitored environment.

2. Observe for symptoms of thiocyanate toxicity. Evaluate thiocyanate levels q 48–72 hr; levels should be less than 100 mcg thiocyanate/mL or 3 μmol cyanide/mL. Metabolic acidosis may precede cyanide toxicity.

CLIENT/FAMILY TEACHING

1. Drug is given in a monitored environment to rapidly lower BP and to reduce the workload of the heart.

2. Aluminum foil or foil-lined bags are used to protect solutions from light during administration and to maintain drug stability.

3. Report any adverse side effects or pain at injection site immediately.

OUTCOMES/EVALUATE

• ↓ BP; ↓ Preload/afterload

• Improved S&S of refractory CHF

Bold Italic = life threatening side effect   ■ = black box warning   ✦ = Available in Canada

O

Olmesartan medoxomil ■

(ohl-meh-SAR-tan)

CLASSIFICATION(S):
Antihypertensive agent - angiotensin II receptor antagonist
PREGNANCY CATEGORY: C
Rx: Benicar

SEE ALSO *ANGIOTENSIN II RECEPTOR ANTAGONISTS.*

ACTION/KINETICS
Selectively blocks the binding of angiotensin II to the AT$_1$ receptor in vascular smooth muscle. Angiotensin II is a pressor agent causing vasoconstriction, stimulation of the synthesis of and release of aldosterone, cardiac stimulation, and renal reabsorption of sodium. Rapid and complete converson of olmesartan medoxomil to olmesartan occurs during absorption from the GI tract. Olmesartan itself is not further metabolized. Is about 26% bioavailable. **Peak plasma levels:** 1–2 hr. Food does not affect bioavailability. **Steady-state levels:** Within 3 to 5 days, with no drug accumulation following once daily dosing. **t ½, terminal:** 13 hr. Excreted through the urine (35–50%) and feces (50–65%). Over 99% bound to plasma proteins.

USES
Hypertension, alone or in combination with other antihypertensives.

CONTRAINDICATIONS
Hypersensitivity to the drug or any component of the product. Lactation.

SPECIAL CONCERNS
■Use during the second and third trimester of pregnancy can cause injury and even death to the fetus. When pregnancy is detected, discontinue as soon as possible.■ Safety and efficacy have not been determined in children.

SIDE EFFECTS
CV: Hypotension, especially in volume- and/or salt-depleted clients, tachycardia. **GI:** Diarrhea, abdominal pain, dyspepsia, gastroenteritis, nausea. **CNS:** Headache, vertigo, insomnia. **GU:** Oliguria, progressive azotemia, hematuria, *acute renal failure (rare).* **Musculoskeletal:** Arthralgia, arthritis, myalgia, skeletal pain. **Respiratory:** Bronchitis, pharyngitis, rhinitis, sinusitis, URT. **Body as a whole:** Inflicted injury, flu-like symptoms, fatigue, pain, peripheral edema, rash. **Miscellaneous:** Back/chest pain, facial edema.

LABORATORY TEST CONSIDERATIONS
↑ CPK. Slight ↓ H&H. Hyperglycemia, hypertriglyceridemia, hypercholesterolemia, hyperlipemia, hyperuricemia.

OD **OVERDOSE MANAGEMENT**
Symptoms: Hypotension, tachycardia. *Treatment:* If needed, supportive treatment for symptomatic hypotension.

HOW SUPPLIED
Tablets: 5 mg, 20 mg, 40 mg

DOSAGE
• **Tablets**
Hypertension.
Individualize dosage. **Initial:** 20 mg once daily when used as monotherapy in those not volume-depleted. After 2 weeks of therapy, if further reduction in BP is required, dose may be increased to 40 mg. Doses above 40 mg appear not to have a greater effect. Consider a lower starting dose in those who are volume- and salt-depleted.

NURSING CONSIDERATIONS
ADMINISTRATION/STORAGE
1. Twice-daily dosing has no advantage over once daily dosing.
2. Dosage adjustment is not recommended for the elderly or those with moderate to severe renal or hepatic dysfunction.
3. May be given with or without food.
4. If BP is not controlled with olmesartan alone, a diuretic or other antihypertensive drugs may be added.

O

ASSESSMENT

1. Note disease onset, indications for therapy, characteristics of S&S, other medical problems, and other agents trialed and outcome. List other drugs prescribed to ensure none interact.

2. Monitor BP, hydration status, CBC, electrolytes, liver and renal function studies; note any dysfunction.

CLIENT/FAMILY TEACHING

1. May take with or without food and with other prescribed BP medications.

2. Change positions slowly and avoid dehydration to prevent sudden drop in BP and dizziness.

3. Practice reliable contraception; report if pregnancy suspected as drug may cause fetal death.

4. Continue low fat, low sodium diet, regular exercise, weight loss, smoking and alcohol cessation, and stress reduction in goal of BP control.

5. May experience headaches, coughing, diarrhea, nausea, and joint aches; report if persistent.

6. May alter glucose readings with diabetes.

7. Consume plenty of fluids to ensure adequate hydration.

OUTCOMES/EVALUATE

↓ BP

Papaverine

(pah-**PAV**-er-een)

CLASSIFICATION(S):
Vasodilator, peripheral

PREGNANCY CATEGORY: C

Rx: Pavabid Plateau Caps, Pavagen TD

ACTION/KINETICS

Direct spasmolytic effect on smooth muscle, possibly by inhibiting cyclic nucleotide phosphodiesterase, thus increasing levels of cyclic AMP. This effect is seen in the vascular system, bronchial muscle, and in the GI, biliary, and urinary tracts. Large doses produce CNS sedation and sleepiness. May also directly relax cerebral vessels as it increases cerebral blood flow and decreases cerebral vascular resistance. Depresses cardiac conduction and irritability and prolongs the myocardial refractory period. Localized in fat tissues and liver. Steady plasma concentration maintained when drug is given q 6 hr. **Peak plasma levels:** 1–2 hr. **t ½:** 30–120 min. Sustained-release products may be poorly and erratically absorbed. Metab-

olized in the liver and inactive metabolites excreted in the urine.

USES

Relief of cerebral and peripheral ischemia associated with arterial spasm and myocardial ischemia complicated by arrhythmias.

CONTRAINDICATIONS

Complete AV block.

SPECIAL CONCERNS

Safe use during lactation or for children not established. Use with extreme caution in coronary insufficiency and glaucoma.

SIDE EFFECTS

CV: Flushing of face, hypertension, increase in HR and depth of respiration. Large doses can depress AV and intraventricular conduction, causing serious arrhythmias. Large doses: Depression of atrioventricular and intraventricular conduction leading to serious arrhythmias. **GI:** Nausea, anorexia, abdominal distress, constipation or diarrhea, dry mouth and throat. **CNS:** Headache, drowsiness, sedation, vertigo. **Miscellaneous:** Sweating, malaise, pruritus, skin rashes, chronic hepatitis, hepatic hypersensitivity, jaundice, eosinophilia, altered LFTs.

Bold Italic = life threatening side effect   ■ = black box warning   ✦ = Available in Canada

LABORATORY TEST CONSIDERATIONS
↑ AST, ALT, and bilirubin.

OD OVERDOSE MANAGEMENT

NOTE: Both acute and chronic poisoning may result from use of papaverine. Symptoms are extensions of side effects.

Symptoms (Acute Poisoning): Nystagmus, diplopia, drowsiness, weakness, lassitude, incoordination, coma, cyanosis, *respiratory depression. Treatment (Acute Poisoning):* Delay absorption by giving tap water, milk, or activated charcoal followed by gastric lavage or induction of vomiting and then a cathartic. Maintain BP and take measures to treat respiratory depression and coma. Hemodialysis is effective.

Symptoms (Chronic Poisoning): Ataxia, blurred vision, drowsiness, anxiety, headache, GI upset, depression, urticaria, erythematous macular eruptions, blood dyscrasias, hypotension. *Treatment (Chronic Poisoning):* Discontinue medication. Monitor and treat blood dyscrasias. Provide symptomatic treatment. Treat hypotension by IV fluids, elevation of legs, and a vasopressor with inotropic effects.

DRUG INTERACTIONS
Diazoxide IV / Additive hypotension
Levodopa / ↓ Levodopa effect by blocking dopamine receptors

HOW SUPPLIED
Capsule, Timed Release: 150 mg; *Injection:* 30 mg/mL

DOSAGE
- **CAPSULES, TIMED-RELEASE; INJECTION**

  Ischemia relief.
  150 mg q 12 hr. May be increased to 150 mg q 8 hr or 300 mg q 12 hr in difficult cases.

NURSING CONSIDERATIONS
ASSESSMENT
1. Document indications for therapy, type, onset, and characteristics of symptoms.
2. Determine any cardiac dysfunction; monitor VS, ECG, and LFTs.
3. Document mental status; assess all extremities for color, warmth, and pulses.

CLIENT/FAMILY TEACHING
1. Take with meals or milk to minimize GI upset. Do not crush or chew time release capsules– swallow whole.
2. Do not perform activities that require mental alertness until drug effects are realized; may cause dizziness or drowsiness.
3. Avoid alcohol (may ↑ dizziness).
4. Avoid tobacco products; nicotine causes vasospasm.
5. Report loss of response/worsening of S&S.

OUTCOMES/EVALUATE
↓ Pain symptoms R/T ischemia/vascular spasms

Penbutolol sulfate
(pen-**BYOU**-toe-lohl)

CLASSIFICATION(S):
Beta-adrenergic blocking agent
PREGNANCY CATEGORY: C
Rx: Levatol

SEE ALSO *BETA-ADRENERGIC BLOCKING AGENTS.*

ACTION/KINETICS
Has both beta-1- and beta-2-receptor blocking activity. It has no membrane-stabilizing activity but does possess minimal intrinsic sympathomimetic activity. High lipid solubility. **t ½:** 5 hr. Metabolized in the liver and excreted through the urine. 80–98% protein bound.

USES
Alone or in combination with other antihypertensive drugs for mild to moderate arterial hypertension

CONTRAINDICATIONS
Bronchial asthma or bronchospasms, including severe COPD.

SPECIAL CONCERNS
Dosage has not been established in children. Geriatric clients may manifest increased or decreased sensitivity to the usual adult dose.

HOW SUPPLIED
Tablet: 20 mg

DOSAGE
- **TABLETS**

Hypertension.
Initial: 20 mg/day either alone or with other antihypertensive agents. **Maintenance:** Same as initial dose. Doses greater than 40 mg/day do not result in a greater antihypertensive effect.

NURSING CONSIDERATIONS
ADMINISTRATION/STORAGE
Doses of 10 mg/day are effective but full effects are not evident for 4–6 weeks. The full effect of a 20- to 40-mg dose may not be observed for 2 weeks.
ASSESSMENT
Note other agents trialed and outcome. Assess for asthma or COPD history.
CLIENT/FAMILY TEACHING
1. Avoid activities that require mental alertness until drug effects realized.
2. May cause low BP; to avoid, rise slowly from a sitting or lying position.
3. Take only as prescribed; full effects may not be realized for a month or more.
4. May cause an increased sensitivity to cold; dress appropriately.
5. Avoid alcohol. Do not stop drug suddenly, may exacerbate heart disease.
6. Report any low heart rate, breathing problems/wheezing, depression, confusion, rash, fever, dizziness, cold hands/feet, unusual bruising/bleeding, or sore throat. Keep log of BP for provider review.
OUTCOMES/EVALUATE
↓ BP

Perindopril erbumine ■

(per-**IN**-doh-pril)

CLASSIFICATION(S):
Antihypertensive, ACE inhibitor
PREGNANCY CATEGORY: C (first trimester), D (second and third trimesters)
Rx: Aceon
♣Rx: Coversyl

SEE ALSO ANGIOTENSIN-CONVERTING ENZYME (ACE) INHIBITORS.

ACTION/KINETICS
Converted in the liver to the active perindoprilat. Is about 75% bioavailable. **Time to peak levels:** About 1 hr (2 hr for perindoprilat). **t½, elimination:** 0.8–1 hr (3–10 hr for perindoprilat). Eliminated through the kidney. About 60% of perindopril and 10–20% of perindoprilat are bound to plasma proteins.
USES
Essential hypertension, either alone or combined with other antihypertensive classes, especially thiazide diuretics.
CONTRAINDICATIONS
Use in those with a history of angioedema related to previous ACE inhibitor therapy.
SPECIAL CONCERNS
■When used during the second and third trimesters of pregnancy, ACE inhibitors can cause injury and even death to the developing fetus. When pregnancy is detected, discontinue as soon as possible.■ Safety and efficacy have not been determined in clients with a C_{CR} less than 30 mL/min. There is a higher incidence of angioedema in blacks compared to nonblacks. Use with caution during lactation. Safety and efficacy have not been determined in children.
SIDE EFFECTS
GI: Diarrhea, abdominal pain, N&V, dyspepsia, flatulence, dry mouth, dry mucous membrane, increased appetite, gastroenteritis, *hepatic necrosis/failure.* **CNS:** Headache, dizziness, sleep disorder, paresthesia, depression, migraine, amnesia, vertigo, anxiety, psychosexual disorder. **CV:** Palpitation, abnormal ECG, *CVA, MI,* orthostatic symptoms, hypotension, ventricular extrasystole, vasodilation, syncope, abnormal conduction, heart murmur. **Respiratory:** Cough, sinusitis, URTI, rhinitis, pharyngitis, posterior nasal drip, bronchitis, rhinorrhea, throat disorder, dyspnea, sneezing, epistaxis, hoarseness, pulmonary fibrosis. **Body as a whole:** Asthenia, viral infection, fever, edema, rash, seasonal allergy, malaise, pain, cold/hot sensation, chills, fluid retention, angioedema, *anaphylaxis.* **Muscu-**

Ioskeletal: Back pain, upper extremity pain, lower extremity pain, chest pain, neck pain, myalgia, arthralgia, arthritis. **GU:** UTI, male sexual dysfunction, menstrual disorder, vaginitis, kidney stone, flank pain, urinary frequency, urinary retention. **Dermatologic:** Sweating, skin infection, tinea, pruritus, dry skin, erythema, fever blisters, purpura, hematoma. **Miscellaneous:** Hypertonia, ear infection, injury, tinnitus, facial edema, gout, ecchymosis.

LABORATORY TEST CONSIDERATIONS
↑ Alkaline phosphatase, uric acid, cholesterol, AST, ALT, creatinine, glucose. ↓ Potassium. Hematuria, proteinuria.

DRUG INTERACTIONS
Concomitant use of diuretics may cause an excessive ↓ BP.

HOW SUPPLIED
Tablets: 2 mg, 4 mg, 8 mg

DOSAGE————————————

• **TABLETS**
Uncomplicated essential hypertension.
Adults, initial: 4 mg once daily (may also be given in 2 divided doses). May increase dose until BP, when measured just before the next dose, is controlled. **Usual maintenance:** 4–8 mg, up to a maximum of 16 mg/day. For elderly clients, initially give 4 mg/day in 1 or 2 divided doses. Dose may then be titrated gradually upward; give doses greater than 8 mg/day cautiously.
Use with a diuretic for essential hypertension.
If possible, discontinue the diuretic 2–3 days before beginning perindopril therapy. If BP is not controlled with perindopril, resume the diuretic. When using both drugs, use an initial dose of 2–4 mg of perindopril daily in 1 or 2 divided doses. Carefully supervise until BP has stabilized.
In clients with a C_{CR} less than 30 mL/min, give an initial dose of 2 mg/day. Daily dose should not exceed 8 mg.

NURSING CONSIDERATIONS
ASSESSMENT
1. Note indications for therapy, other medical conditions, previous agents trialed, and outcome.

2. Monitor electrolytes, U/A, microalbumin, CBC, renal and LFTs; reduce dose with renal dysfunction.

CLIENT/FAMILY TEACHING
1. Take as directed at the same time(s) each day. Do not perform activities that require mental alertness until drug effects known.
2. May experience cough, headaches, palpitations, sinusitis and dizziness; report if persistent.
3. Continue lifestyle changes useful in controlling BP; i.e., regular exercise, weight loss, low fat/salt diet, smoking cessation, reduced alcohol intake, and stress reduction.
4. Monitor BP at different times during the day and keep a log for provider review.
5. Practice reliable contraception. Report any unusual side effects and avoid all OTC agents esp. cold/cough remedies without provider approval.

OUTCOMES/EVALUATE
Control of HTN; ↓ BP

Phenylephrine hydrochloride
(fen-ill-**EF**-rin)

P

CLASSIFICATION(S):
Sympathomimetic
PREGNANCY CATEGORY: C
OTC: Nasal Solution: Afrin Children's Pump Mist, Little Colds for Infants & Children, Little Noses Gentle Formula (Infants & Children), Neo-Synephrine 4-Hour Extra Strength, Neo-Synephrine 4-Hour Mild Formula, Neo-Synephrine 4-Hour Regular Strength, Rhinall, Vicks Sinex Ultra Fine Mist, 4-Way Fast Acting. **Ophthalmic Solution:** AK-Nefrin, Prefrin Liquifilm, Relief. **Oral Tablet:** AH-chew D.
Rx: Ophthalmic Solution: AK-Dilate, Mydfrin 2.5%, Neo-Synephrine, Neo-Synephrine Viscous, Phenoptic. **Parenteral:** Neo-Synephrine.

SEE ALSO *SYMPATHOMIMETIC DRUGS.*

ACTION/KINETICS

Stimulates alpha-adrenergic receptors, producing pronounced vasoconstriction and hence an increase in both SBP and DBP; reflex bradycardia results from increased vagal activity. Also acts on alpha receptors producing vasoconstriction in the skin, mucous membranes, and the mucosa as well as mydriasis by contracting the dilator muscle of the pupil. Resembles epinephrine, but it has more prolonged action and few cardiac effects. **IV, Onset:** immediate; **duration:** 15–20 min. **IM, SC: Onset,** 10–15 min; **duration:** 0.5–2 hr for IM and 50–60 min for SC. **Nasal decongestion (topical), Onset:** 15–20 min; **duration:** 30 min–4 hr. **Ophthalmic, time to peak effect for mydriasis:** 15–60 min for 2.5% solution and 10–90 min for 10% solution. **Duration:** 0.5–1.5 hr for 0.12%, 3 hr for 2.5%, and 5–7 hr with 10% (when used for mydriasis). Excreted in urine.

USES

Parenteral: (1) Vascular failure in shock, shock-like states, drug-induced hypotension or hypersensitivity. (2) To maintain BP during spinal and inhalation anesthesia; to prolong spinal anesthesia. As a vasoconstrictor in regional analgesia. (3) Paroxysmal SVT. **Oral:** (1) Temporary relief of nasal congestion due to the common cold, hay fever, or other upper respiratory allergies. (2) Nasal congestion associated with sinusitis. (3) Promote nasal or sinus drainage. **Nasal:** Nasal congestion due to allergies, sinusitis, common cold, hay fever, or other upper respiratory allergies. **Ophthalmologic, 0.12%:** Temporary relief of redness of the eye associated with colds, hay fever, wind, dust, sun, smog, smoke, contact lens. **2.5% and 10%:** (1) Decongestant and vasoconstrictor. (2) Treatment of uveitis with posterior synechiae. (3) Open-angle glaucoma. (4) Refraction without cycloplegia, ophthalmoscopic examination, funduscopy, prior to surgery.

CONTRAINDICATIONS

Severe hypertension, VT.

SPECIAL CONCERNS

Use with extreme caution in geriatric clients, severe arteriosclerosis, bradycardia, partial heart block, myocardial disease, hyperthyroidism and during pregnancy and lactation. Systemic absorption with nasal or ophthalmic use. Use of the 2.5% or 10% ophthalmic solutions in children may cause hypertension and irregular heart beat. In geriatric clients, chronic use of the 2.5% or 10% ophthalmic solutions may cause rebound miosis and a decreased mydriatic effect.

SIDE EFFECTS

CV: Reflex bradycardia, arrhythmias (rare). **CNS:** Headache, excitability, restlessness. **Ophthalmologic:** Rebound miosis and decreased mydriatic response in geriatric clients, blurred vision.

OD OVERDOSE MANAGEMENT
Symptoms: Ventricular extrasystoles, short paroxysms of ventricular tachycardia, sensation of fullness in the head, tingling of extremities. *Treatment:* Administer an alpha-adrenergic blocking agent (e.g., phentolamine).

ADDITIONAL DRUG INTERACTIONS

Anesthetics, halogenated hydrocarbon / May sensitize myocardium → serious arrhythmias
Bretylium / ↑ Effect of phenylephrine → possible arrhythmias
Guanethidine / Possible ↑ pressor effect of phenylephrine → severe hypertension
Oxytocic drugs / Possible severe persistent hypertension
Tricyclic antidepressants / Possible ↑ or ↓ sensitivity to IV phenylephrine

HOW SUPPLIED

Nasal. *Solution/Spray:* 0.125%, 0.25%, 0.5%, 1%; **Oral:** *Tablet, chewable:* 10 mg. **Ophthalmic.** *Solution:* 0.12%, 2.5%, 10%. **Parenteral.** *Injection:* 10 mg/mL

DOSAGE

- **IM, IV, SC**
  Vasopressor, mild to moderate hypotension.
  Adults: 2–5 mg (range: 1–10 mg), not to exceed an initial dose of 5 mg IM or SC repeated no more often than q 10–15 min; or, 0.2 mg (range: 0.1–0.5

mg), not to exceed an initial dose of 0.5 mg IV repeated no more often than q 10–15 min. **Pediatric:** 0.1 mg/kg (3 mg/m^2) IM or SC repeated in 1–2 hr if needed.

Vasopressor, severe hypotension and shock.

Adults: 10 mg by continuous IV infusion using 250–500 mL D5W or 0.9% NaCl injection given at a rate of 0.1–0.18 mg/min initially; **then,** give at a rate of 0.04–0.06 mg/min.

Prophylaxis of hypotension during spinal anesthesia.

Adults: 2–3 mg IM or SC 3–4 min before anesthetic given; subsequent doses should not exceed the previous dose by more than 0.1–0.2 mg. No more than 0.5 mg should be given in a single dose. **Pediatric:** 0.044–0.088 mg/kg IM or SC.

Hypotensive emergencies during spinal anesthesia.

Adults, initial: 0.2 mg IV; dose can be increased by no more than 0.2 mg for each subsequent dose not to exceed 0.5 mg/dose.

Prolongation of spinal anesthesia.

2–5 mg added to the anesthetic solution increases the duration of action up to 50% without increasing side effects or complications.

Vasoconstrictor for regional anesthesia.

Add 1 mg to every 20 mL of local anesthetic solution. If more than 2 mg phenylephrine is used, pressor reactions can be expected.

Paroxysmal SVT.

Initial: 0.5 mg (maximum) given by rapid IV injection (over 20–30 seconds). Subsequent doses are determined by BP and should not exceed the previous dose by more than 0.1–0.2 mg and should never be more than 1 mg.

• **NASAL SOLUTION, NASAL SPRAY**
Adults and children over 12 years of age: 2–3 gtt of the 0.25% or 0.5% solution into each nostril q 3–4 hr as needed. In resistant cases, the 1% solution can be used but no more often than q 4 hr. **Children, 6–12 years of age:** 2–3 gtt of the 0.25% solution not more often than q 4 hr. **Children, 2–less than**

6 years of age: 1 dropperful of the 0.25% oral drops PO q 4 hr, not to exceed 6 doses in a 24-hr period. Or, 2–3 gtt of these 0.125% nasal solution into each nostril, not more than q 4 hr.

• **TABLETS, CHEWABLE**
Nasal congestion.

Adults: 1–2 tablets (10–20 mg) q 4 hr. **Children, 6–less than 12 years of age:** 1 tablet (10 mg) q 4 hr.

• **OPHTHALMIC SOLUTION, 0.12%**
Minor eye irritations.

1–2 gtt of the 0.12% solution in the eye(s) up to 4 times per day as needed.

• **OPHTHALMIC SOLUTION, 2.5%, 10%**
Vasoconstriction, pupillary dilation.

1 gtt of the 2.5% or 10% solution on the upper limbus a few minutes following 1 gtt of topical anesthetic (prevents stinging and dilution of solution by lacrimation). An additional drop may be needed after 1 hr.

Uveitis.

1 gtt of the 2.5% or 10% solution with atropine. To free recently formed posterior synechiae, 1 gtt of the 2.5% or 10% solution to the upper surface of the cornea. Continue treatment the following day, if needed. In the interim, apply hot compresses for 5–10 min 3 times per day using 1 gtt of 1% or 2% atropine sulfate before and after each series of compresses.

Glaucoma.

1 gtt of 10% solution on the upper surface of the cornea as needed. Both the 2.5% and 10% solutions may be used with miotics in clients with open-angle glaucoma.

Surgery.

2.5% or 10% solution 30–60 min before surgery for wide dilation of the pupil.

Refraction.

Adults: 1 gtt of a cycloplegic (homatropine HBr, atropine sulfate, cyclopentolate, tropicamide HCl, or a combination of homatropine and cocaine HCl) in each eye followed in 5 min with 1 gtt of 2.5% phenylephrine solution and in 10 min with another drop of cycloplegic. The eyes are ready for refraction in 50–60 min. **Children:** 1 gtt of atropine sulfate, 1%, in each eye followed in

P

10–15 min with 1 gtt of phenylephrine solution, 2.5%, and in 5–10 min with a second drop of atropine sulfate, 1%. The eyes are ready for refraction in 1–2 hr.

Ophthalmoscopic examination.
1 gtt of 2.5% solution in each eye. The eyes are ready for examination in 15–30 min and the effect lasts for 1–3 hr.

NURSING CONSIDERATIONS
ADMINISTRATION/STORAGE
1. Store drug in a brown bottle and away from light.
2. Instill a drop of local anesthetic before administering the 10% ophthalmic solution.
IV 3. For IV administration, dilute each 1 mg with 9 mL of sterile water and administer over 1 min. Further dilution of 10 mg in 500 mL of dextrose, Ringer's, or saline solution may be titrated to client response.
4. Monitor infusion site closely to avoid extravasation. If evident, administer SC phentolamine locally to prevent tissue necrosis.
5. Prolonged exposure to air or strong light may result in oxidation and discoloration. Do not use solution if it changes color, becomes cloudy, or contains a precipitate.

ASSESSMENT
1. Document indications for therapy, type, onset, and characteristics of symptoms; note goals of therapy.
2. During IV administration monitor cardiac rhythm and BP continuously until stabilized, noting any evidence of bradycardia or arrhythmias.

CLIENT/FAMILY TEACHING
1. Review frequency, method of administration, and care of containers.
2. Ophthalmic instillations and nasal decongestants may produce systemic sympathomimetic effects; chronic excessive use may cause rebound congestion.
3. Wear sunglasses in bright light. Report if symptoms of photosensitivity and blurred vision persist after 12 hr. Blurred vision should decrease with repeated use.

4. With ophthalmic solution, report if there is no relief of symptoms within 5 days. Remove contact lens as some solutions may stain.
5. When using for nasal decongestion, blow nose before administering; report if no relief of symptoms within 3 days. Rebound nasal congestion may occur with longer therapy.

OUTCOMES/EVALUATE
- ↑ BP
- Termination of paroxysmal SVT
- Relief of nasal congestion
- ↓ Conjunctivitis/allergic S&S
- Dilatation of pupils

Potassium Salts
CLASSIFICATION(S):
Electrolyte

Potassium acetate, parenteral
PREGNANCY CATEGORY: C

Potassium gluconate and Potassium chloride
Rx: Oral Solution and Powder for Oral Solution: Kolyum

Potassium gluconate and Potassium citrate
Rx: Oral Solution: Twin-K

Potassium acetate, Potassium bicarbonate, and Potassium citrate (Trikates)
Rx: Oral Solution: Tri-K

Potassium bicarbonate
Rx: Oral Solution: K + Care ET

Potassium bicarbonate and Citric acid
Rx: Effervescent Tablets: K+ Care ET

Potassium bicarbonate and Potassium chloride
Rx: Effervescent Tablets: Klorvess, Klor-Con/EF, K-Lyte/Cl, K-Lyte/Cl 50
❧**Rx: Effervescent Granules:** Neo-K. **Effervescent Tablets:** Potassium-Sandoz

Potassium bicarbonate and Potassium citrate
Rx: Effervescent Tablets: K-Lyte, Effer-K, Effervescent Potassium

Potassium chloride
Rx: Extended-Release Capsules: K-Lease, K-Norm, Micro-K 10 Extencaps., Micro-K Extencaps. **Extended-Release Tablets:** K+ 10, Kaon-Cl, Kaon-Cl-10, K-Dur 10 and 20, Klor-Con 8 and 10, Klor-Con M10, M15, and M20, Klotrix, K-Tab, Slow-K, Ten-K. **Injection:** Potassium Chloride for Injection Concentrate. **Oral Solution:** Cena-K 10% and 20%, Kaochlor 10%, Kaochlor S-F 10%, Kaon-Cl 20% Liquid, Kay Ciel, Klorvess 10% Liquid, Potasalan, Rum-K. **Powder for Oral Solution:** Gen-K, K+ Care, Kay Ciel, K-Lor, Klor-Con Powder, Klor-Con/25 Powder, K-Lyte/Cl Powder, Micro-K LS.
❧**Rx: Extended-Release Tablets:** Apo-K, K-Long, K-Lyte/Cl, Slow-K. **Oral Solution:** K-10, Kaochlor-10 and -20, KCl 5%.

Potassium chloride, Potassium bicarbonate, and Potassium citrate
Rx: Effervescent Granules: Klorvess Effervescent Granules

Potassium gluconate
Rx: Elixir: Kaon, Kaylixir, K-G Elixir

GENERAL STATEMENT
Potassium is the major cation of the body's intracellular fluid. It is essential for the maintenance of important physiologic processes, including cardiac, smooth, and skeletal muscle function, acid-base balance, gastric secretions, renal function, protein and carbohydrate metabolism. Symptoms of hypokalemia include weakness, cardiac arrhythmias, fatigue, ileus, hyporeflexia or areflexia, tetany, polydipsia, and, in severe cases, flaccid paralysis and inability to concentrate urine. Loss of potassium is usually accompanied by a loss of chloride resulting in hypochloremic metabolic alkalosis.

The usual adult daily requirement of potassium is 40–80 mg. In adults, the normal extracellular concentration of potassium ranges from 3.5 to 5 mEq/L with the intracellular levels being 150–160 mEq/L. Extracellular concentrations of up to 5.6 mEq/L are normal in children.

Both hypokalemia and hyperkalemia, if uncorrected, can be fatal; thus, potassium must always be administered cautiously.

ACTION/KINETICS
Potassium is readily and rapidly absorbed from the GI tract. Though a number of salts can be used to supply the potassium cation, potassium chloride is the agent of choice since hypochloremia frequently accompanies potassium deficiency. Dietary measures can often prevent and even correct potassium deficiencies. Potassium-rich foods include most meats (beef, chicken, ham, turkey, veal), fish, beans, broc-

P

coli, brussels sprouts, lentils, spinach, potatoes, milk, bananas, dates, prunes, raisins, avocados, watermelon, cantaloupe, apricots, and molasses.

From 80 to 90% of potassium intake is excreted by the kidney and is partially reabsorbed from the glomerular filtrate.

USES

PO: (1) Treat hypokalemia due to digitalis intoxication, diabetic acidosis, diarrhea and vomiting, familial periodic paralysis, certain cases of uremia, hyperadrenalism, starvation and debilitation, and corticosteroid or diuretic therapy. (2) Hypokalemia with or without metabolic acidosis and following surgical conditions accompanied by nitrogen loss, vomiting and diarrhea, suction drainage, and increased urinary excretion of potassium. (3) Prophylaxis of potassium depletion when dietary intake is not adequate in the following conditions: Clients on digitalis and diuretics for CHF, hepatic cirrhosis with ascites, excess aldosterone with normal renal function, significant cardiac arrhythmias, potassium-losing nephropathy, and certain states accompanied by diarrhea. *Investigational:* Mild hypertension.

NOTE: Use potassium chloride when hypokalemia is associated with alkalosis; potassium bicarbonate, citrate, acetate, or gluconate should be used when hypokalemia is associated with acidosis.

IV: (1) Prophylaxis and treatment of moderate to severe potassium loss when PO therapy is not feasible. (2) Potassium acetate is used as an additive for preparing specific IV formulas when client needs cannot be met by usual nutrient or electrolyte preparations. (3) Potassium acetate is also used in the following conditions: Marked loss of GI secretions due to vomiting, diarrhea, GI intubation, or fistulas; prolonged parenteral use of potassium-free fluids (e.g., dextrose or NSS); diabetic acidosis, especially during treatment with insulin and dextrose infusions; prolonged diuresis; metabolic alkalosis; hyperadrenocorticism; primary aldosteronism; overdose of adrenocortical steroids, testosterone, or corticotropin; attacks of hereditary or familial periodic paralysis; during the healing phase of burns or scalds; and cardiac arrhythmias, especially due to digitalis glycosides.

CONTRAINDICATIONS

Severe renal function impairment with azotemia or oliguria, postoperatively before urine flow has been reestablished. Crush syndrome, Addison's disease, hyperkalemia from any cause, anuria, heat cramps, acute dehydration, severe hemolytic reactions, adynamia episodica hereditaria, clients receiving potassium-sparing diuretics or aldosterone-inhibiting drugs. Solid dosage forms in clients in whom there is a reason for delay or arrest in passage of tablets through the GI tract.

SPECIAL CONCERNS

Safety during lactation and in children has not been established. Geriatric clients are at greater risk of developing hyperkalemia due to age-related changes in renal function. Administer with caution in the presence of cardiac and renal disease. Potassium loss is often accompanied by an obligatory loss of chloride resulting in hypochloremic metabolic alkalosis; thus, the underlying cause of the potassium loss should be treated.

SIDE EFFECTS

Hypokalemia. CNS: Dizziness, mental confusion. **CV:** Arrhythmias; weak, irregular pulse; hypotension, *heart block,* ECG abnormalities, *cardiac arrest.* **GI:** Abdominal distention, anorexia, N&V, **Neuromuscular:** Weakness, paresthesia of extremities, flaccid paralysis, areflexia, muscle or *respiratory paralysis,* weakness and heaviness of legs. **Other:** Malaise.

Hyperkalemia. CV: Bradycardia, then tachycardia, *cardiac arrest.* **GI:** N&V, diarrhea, abdominal cramps, GI bleeding or obstruction. Ulceration or perforation of the small bowel from enteric-coated potassium chloride tablets. **GU:** Oliguria, anuria. **Neuromuscular:** Weakness, tingling, paralysis. **Other:** Skin rashes, hyperkalemia.

Effects due to solution or IV technique used. Fever, infection at injection site, venous thrombosis, phlebitis

---

Bold Italic = life threatening side effect   ■ = black box warning   ✦ = Available in Canada

extending from injection site, extravasation, venospasm, hypervolemia, hyperkalemia.

OD **OVERDOSE MANAGEMENT**
Symptoms: Mild (5.5–6.5 mEq/L) to moderate (6.5–8 mEq/L) hyperkalemia (may be asymptomatic except for ECG changes). ECG changes include progression in height and peak of T waves, lowering of the R wave, decreased amplitude and eventually disappearance of P waves, prolonged PR interval and QRS complex, shortening of the QT interval, *ventricular fibrillation, death. Muscle weakness that may progress to flaccid quadriplegia and respiratory failure,* although dangerous cardiac arrhythmias usually occur before onset of complete paralysis. *Treatment (plasma potassium levels greater than 6.5 mEq/L):* All measures must be monitored by ECG. Measures consist of actions taken to shift potassium ions from plasma into cells by:

• **Sodium bicarbonate:** IV infusion of 50–100 mEq over period of 5 min. May be repeated after 10–15 minutes if ECG abnormalities persist.

• **Glucose and insulin:** IV infusion of 3 g glucose to 1 unit regular insulin to shift potassium into cells.

• **Calcium gluconate—or other calcium salt** (only for clients not on digitalis or other cardiotonic glycosides): IV infusion of 0.5–1 g (5–10 mL of a 10% solution) over period of 2 min. Dosage may be repeated after 1–2 min if ECG remains abnormal. When ECG is approximately normal, the excess potassium should be removed from the body by administration of polystyrene sulfonate, hemodialysis, or peritoneal dialysis (clients with renal insufficiency), or other means.

• **Sodium polystyrene sulfonate, hemodialysis, peritoneal dialysis:** To remove potassium from the body.

DRUG INTERACTIONS
ACE inhibitors / May cause potassium retention → hyperkalemia
Digitalis glycosides / Cardiac arrhythmias

Potassium-sparing diuretics / Severe hyperkalemia with possibility of cardiac arrhythmias or arrest

HOW SUPPLIED
Potassium acetate, parenteral: *Injection:* 2 mEq/mL, 4 mEq/mL. **Potassium acetate, potassium bicarbonate, and potassium citrate:** *Liquid:* 45 mEq/15 mL. **Potassium bicarbonate:** *Tablet, effervescent:* 25 mEq, 650 mg. **Potassium bicarbonate and potassium citrate:** *Tablet, effervescent:* 25 mEq. **Potassium bicarbonate and potassium chloride:** *Granule for reconstitution:* 20 mEq; *Tablet, effervescent:* 25 mEq, 50 mEq. **Potassium chloride:** *Capsule, extended release:* 8 mEq, 10 mEq; *Injection:* 1.5 mEq/mL, 2 mEq/mL, 10 mEq/50 mL, 10 mEq/100 mL, 20 mEq/50 mL, 20 mEq/100 mL, 30 mEq/100 mL, 40 mEq/100 mL, 100 mEq/L, 200 mEq/L; *Liquid:* 20 mEq/15 mL, 30 mEq/15 mL, 40 mEq/15 mL; *Powder for reconstitution:* 20 mEq, 25 mEq, 200 mEq; *Tablet:* 180 mg; *Tablet, extended release:* 8 mEq, 10 mEq, 20 mEq.
Potassium gluconate: *Elixir:* 20 mEq/15 mL; *Tablet:* 486 mg, 500 mg, 550 mg, 595 mg, 610 mg, 620 mg; *Tablet, extended release:* 595 mg.
Potassium gluconate and potassium citrate: *Liquid:* 20 mEq/15 mL.

DOSAGE
Highly individualized. Oral administration is preferred because the slow absorption from the GI tract prevents sudden, large increases in plasma potassium levels. Dosage is usually expressed as mEq/L of potassium. The bicarbonate, chloride, citrate, and gluconate salts are usually administered PO. The chloride, acetate, and phosphate may be administered by **slow IV** infusion.

• **IV INFUSION**
Serum K less than 2.0 mEq/L.
400 mEq/day at a rate not to exceed 40 mEq/hr. Use a maximum concentration of 80 mEq/L.
Serum K more than 2.5 mEq/L.
200 mEq/day at a rate not to exceed 20 mEq/hr. Use a maximum concentration of 40 mEq/L.
Pediatric: Up to 3 mEq potassium/kg (or 40 mEq/m^2) daily. Adjust the volume

P

administered depending on the body size.

• **EFFERVESCENT GRANULES, EFFERVESCENT TABLETS, ELIXIR, EXTENDED-RELEASE CAPSULES, EXTENDED RELEASE GRANULES, EXTENDED-RELEASE TABLETS, ORAL SOLUTION, POWDER FOR ORAL SOLUTION, TABLETS**

Prophylaxis of hypokalemia.
16–24 mEq/day.

Potassium depletion.
40–100 mEq/day.

NOTE: Usual dietary intake of potassium is 40–250 mEq/day.

For clients with accompanying metabolic acidosis, use an alkalizing potassium salt (potassium bicarbonate, potassium citrate, potassium acetate, or potassium gluconate).

NURSING CONSIDERATIONS

℘ Do not confuse K-Phos Neutral with Neutra-Phos-K.

ADMINISTRATION/STORAGE

1. Give PO doses 2–4 times per day. Correct hypokalemia slowly over a period of 3–7 days to minimize risk of hyperkalemia.

2. With esophageal compression, administer dilute liquid solutions of potassium rather than tablets.

IV 3. Do not administer potassium IV undiluted. Usual method is to administer by slow IV infusion in dextrose solution at a concentration of 40–80 mEq/L and at a rate not to exceed 10–20 mEq/hr.

4. Avoid "layering" by inverting container during addition of potassium solution and properly agitating the prepared IV solution. Squeezing the plastic container will not prevent KCL from settling to the bottom. Never add potassium to an IV bottle that is hanging.

5. Check site of administration frequently for pain and redness because drug is extremely irritating.

6. In critical clients, KCl may be given slow IV in a solution of saline (unless contraindicated) since dextrose may lower serum potassium levels by producing an intracellular shift.

7. Administer all concentrated potassium infusions and riders with an infusion control device.

8. Have sodium polystyrene sulfonate (Kayexalate) available for oral or rectal administration in the event of hyperkalemia.

ASSESSMENT

1. Note indications for therapy; document electrolytes and ECG. List all drugs and OTC agents consumed.

2. Note any impaired renal function. Assess for adequate urinary flow before administering potassium. Impaired function can lead to hyperkalemia.

INTERVENTIONS

1. Withhold and report if abdominal pain, distention, or GI bleeding occurs.

2. Complaints of weakness, fatigue, or the presence of cardiac arrhythmias may be symptoms of hypokalemia indicating a low *intracellular* potassium level, although the level may appear to be within normal limits.

3. Monitor I&O. Withhold drug and report oliguria, anuria, or azoturia.

4. Observe for S&S of adrenal insufficiency or extensive tissue breakdown.

5. Report complaints of weakness or heaviness of the legs, the presence of a gray pallor, cold skin, listlessness, mental confusion, flaccid paralysis, hypotension, or cardiac arrhythmias (S&S of hyperkalemia).

6. Monitor serum potassium levels during parenteral therapy; normal level is 3.5–5.0 mEq/L.

CLIENT/FAMILY TEACHING

1. Dilute or dissolve PO liquids, effervescent tablets, or soluble powders in 3–8 oz of cold water, fruit or vegetable juice, or other suitable liquid and drink slowly. Chill to improve taste. Take all products with plenty of water.

2. If GI upset occurs, products can be taken after meals or with food with a full glass of water.

3. Swallow enteric-coated tablets and extended-release capsules and tablets; do not chew or dissolve in the mouth.

4. Do not use salt substitutes concomitantly with potassium preparations.

5. If receiving potassium-sparing diuretics, such as spironolactone or triam-

terene, do not take potassium supplements or eat foods high in potassium.
6. Identify high-potassium sources in the diet: Spinach, collards, brussel sprouts, beet greens, tomato juice, celery. Once parenteral potassium is discontinued, ingest potassium-rich foods such as citrus juices, bananas, apricots, raisins, and nuts. The daily adult requirement is usually 40–80 mg. A dietitian may assist with meal planning.
7. Avoid self-prescribed enemas, and large amounts of licorice.
8. Report any adverse side effects and keep all visits for lab and exams.

OUTCOMES/EVALUATE
Correction of potassium deficiency; potassium levels within desired range

Pravastatin sodium
(prah-vah-**STAH**-tin)

CLASSIFICATION(S):
Antihyperlipidemic, HMG-CoA reductase inhibitor
PREGNANCY CATEGORY: X
Rx: Pravachol
✦Rx: Apo-Pravastatin, Lin-Pravastatin, Nu-Pravastatin

SEE ALSO ANTIHYPERLIPIDEMIC - HMG-COA REDUCTASE INHIBITORS

ACTION/KINETICS
Rapidly absorbed from the GI tract; absolute bioavailability is 17%. **Peak plasma levels:** 1–1.5 hr. Significant first-pass extraction and metabolism in the liver, which is the site of action of the drug; thus, plasma levels may not correlate well with lipid-lowering effectiveness. **t ½, elimination:** 77 hr (including metabolites). Metabolized in the liver; excreted in the urine (about 20%) and feces (70%). Potential accumulation of drug with renal or hepatic insufficiency. *NOTE:* A product (Pravigard PAC) is now available that contains pravastatin sodium, 40 mg, and aspirin, 81 mg, to be used with diet to reduce the occurrence of heart attacks, strokes, and death in those with heart disease. About 50% bound to plasma proteins.

USES
(1) Adjunct to diet to reduce elevated total cholesterol, LDL cholesterol, apolipoprotein B, and triglyceride levels and to increase HDL cholesterol in patients with primary hypercholesterolemia and mixed dyslipidemia (Fredrickson Type IIa and IIb). (2) Adjunct therapy to diet for the treatment of patients with elevated serum triglyceride levels (Fredrickson Type IV). (3) Treatment of patients with primary dysbetalipoproteinemia (Fredrickson Type III) who do not respond adequately to diet. (4) Adjunct to diet and lifestyle modification to treat heterozygous familial hypercholesterolemia in children and adolescents 8 years of age and older if after an adequate trial of diet the following are present: LDL-C remains 190 mg/dL or greater or LDL-C remains 160 mg/dL and there is a positive family history of premature CV disease or 2 or more other cardiovascular disease factors are present. (5) Primary prevention of coronary events. Indicated to reduce the risk of myocardial infarction; reduce the risk of undergoing myocardial revascularization procedures; reduce the risk of stroke and stroke/transient ischemic attack; and slow the progression of coronary atherosclerosis in hypercholesterolemic patients without clinically evident coronary heart disease. (6) Secondary prevention of cardiovascular events. Indicated to reduce the risk of total mortality by reducing coronary death; reduce the risk of myocardial infarction; reduce the risk of undergoing myocardial revascularization procedures; reduce the risk of stroke and stroke/transient ischemic attack; and slow the progression of coronary atherosclerosis in patients with clinically evident coronary heart disease.

CONTRAINDICATIONS
Active liver disease or unexplained, persistent elevations of serum transaminases. Pregnancy and lactation.

SPECIAL CONCERNS
Use with caution in clients with a history of liver disease or renal insufficiency.

SIDE EFFECTS

Musculoskeletal: Rhabdomyolysis with renal dysfunction secondary to myoglobinuria, myalgia, myopathy, arthralgias, localized pain, muscle cramps, leg cramps, bursitis, tenosynovitis, myasthenia, tendinous contracture, myositis. **CNS:** CNS vascular lesions characterized by *perivascular hemorrhage,* edema, and mononuclear cell infiltration of perivascular spaces; headache, dizziness, psychic disturbances. Dizziness, vertigo, memory loss, anxiety, insomnia, somnolence, abnormal dreams, emotional lability, incoordination, hyperkinesia, torticollis, psychic disturbances. **GI:** N&V, diarrhea, abdominal pain, cramps, constipation, flatulence, heartburn, anorexia, gastroenteritis, dry mouth, rectal hemorrhage, esophagitis, eructation, glossitis, mouth ulceration, increased appetite, stomatitis, cheilitis, duodenal ulcer, dysphagia, enteritis, melena, gum hemorrhage, stomach ulcer, tenesmus, ulcerative stomach. **CV:** Palpitation, vasodilation, syncope, migraine, postural hypotension, phlebitis, arrhythmia. **Hepatic:** Hepatitis (including chronic active hepatitis), fatty change in liver, cirrhosis, *fulminant hepatic necrosis, hepatoma,* pancreatitis, cholestatic jaundice, biliary pain. **GU:** Gynecomastia, erectile dysfunction, loss of libido, cystitis, hematuria, impotence, dysuria, kidney calculus, nocturia, epididymitis, fibrocystic breast, albuminuria, breast enlargement, nephritis, urinary frequency, incontinence, retention and urgency, abnormal ejaculation, vaginal or uterine hemorrhage, menorrhagia, UTI. **Ophthalmic:** Progression of cataracts, lens opacities, ophthalmoplegia. **Hypersensitivity reaction:** Vasculitis, purpura, polymyalgia rheumatica, *angioedema,* lupus erythematosus–like syndrome, thrombocytopenia, *hemolytic anemia,* leukopenia, positive ANA, arthritis, arthralgia, urticaria, asthenia, ESR increase, fever, chills, photosensitivity, malaise, dyspnea, *toxic epidermal necrolysis, Stevens-Johnson syndrome.* **Dermatologic:** Alopecia, pruritus, rash, skin nodules, discoloration of skin, dryness of skin and mucous membranes, changes in hair and nails, contact dermatitis, sweating, acne, urticaria, eczema, seborrhea, skin ulcer. **Neurologic:** Dysfunction of certain cranial nerves resulting in alteration of taste, impairment of extraocular movement, and facial paresis; paresthesia, peripheral neuropathy, tremor, vertigo, memory loss, peripheral nerve palsy. **Respiratory:** Common cold, rhinitis, cough. **Hematologic:** Anemia, transient asymptomatic eosinophilia, thrombocytopenia, leukopenia, ecchymosis, lymphadenopathy, petechiae. **Miscellaneous:** Cardiac chest pain, fatigue, influenza.

LABORATORY TEST CONSIDERATIONS

↑ CPK, AST, ALT, alkaline phosphatase, bilirubin. Abnormalities in thyroid function tests.

ADDITIONAL DRUG INTERACTIONS

Bile acid sequestrants / ↓ Bioavailability of pravastatin

Clofibrate / ↑ Risk of myopathy

HOW SUPPLIED

Tablet: 10 mg, 20 mg, 40 mg, 80 mg

DOSAGE

- **TABLETS**

Adults, initial: 40 mg once daily (at any time of the day) with or without food. A dose of 80 mg/day can be used if the 40 mg dose does not achieve desired results. Use a starting dose of 10 mg/day at bedtime in renal/hepatic dysfunction, in those taking concomitant immunosuppressants, and in the elderly (maximum maintenance dose for these clients is 20 mg/day). **Children, 8–13 years of age (inclusive):** 20 mg once daily. Doses greater than 20 mg have not been studied in this population. **Adolescents, 14–18 years of age, initial:** 40 mg once daily. Doses greater than 40 mg have not been studied in this population.

NURSING CONSIDERATIONS

℘ Do not confuse Pravachol with Prevacid (proton pump inhibitor) or propranolol (a beta-adrenergic blocking agent).

ADMINISTRATION/STORAGE

1. In clients taking immunosuppressants (e.g., cyclosporine), begin pravastatin therapy at 10 mg/day at bedtime

and titrate to higher doses with caution. Usual maximum dose is 20 mg/day.

2. Place on a standard cholesterol-lowering diet for 3–6 months before beginning pravastatin and continue during therapy.

3. Drug may be taken without regard to meals.

4. When given with a bile-acid binding resin (e.g., cholestyramine, colestipol), give pravastatin either 1 hr or more before or 4 or more hr after the resin.

5. The maximum effect is seen within 4 weeks during which time periodic lipid determinations should be undertaken.

ASSESSMENT

1. Determine that secondary causes for hypercholesterolemia are ruled out. Secondary causes include hypothyroidism, poorly controlled diabetes mellitus, dysproteinemias, obstructive liver disease, nephrotic syndrome, alcoholism, and other drug therapy.

2. Determine if pregnant.

3. Assess for liver disease if alcohol is abused or before initiating therapy, before increasing the dose, or as clinically indicated.

4. Document all CAD risk factors. Initiate therapy during hospitalization for MI/angioplasty procedure.

5. Monitor cholesterol profile, CBC, liver and renal function studies.

INTERVENTIONS

1. Obtain LFTs prior to pravastatin therapy and 6 weeks after starting therapy; if WNL may monitor at 6-month intervals.

2. Pravastatin should be discontinued if markedly elevated CPK levels occur or myopathy is diagnosed.

3. Pravastatin should be discontinued temporarily in clients experiencing an acute or serious condition (e.g., sepsis, hypotension, major surgery, trauma, uncontrolled epilepsy, or severe metabolic, endocrine, or electrolyte disorders) predisposing to the development of renal failure secondary to rhabdomyolysis.

CLIENT/FAMILY TEACHING

1. Take as directed at bedtime.

2. Review the prescribed dietary recommendations (restricted cholesterol and saturated fats); continue diet during drug therapy.

3. Continue a regular exercise program and strive to attain recommended weight loss.

4. Report unexplained muscle pain, tenderness, or weakness, especially if accompanied by malaise or fever.

5. Practice reliable barrier contraception; report if pregnancy is suspected as drug therapy is hazardous to a developing fetus.

6. Report severe GI upset, unusual bruising/bleeding, vision changes, dark urine or light colored stools.

7. Avoid prolonged or excessive exposure to direct or artificial sunlight.

OUTCOMES/EVALUATE

↓ Serum cholesterol and LDL levels; MI prophylaxis in those with atherosclerosis and hypercholesterolemia

Prazosin hydrochloride

(**PRAY**-zoh-sin)

CLASSIFICATION(S):

Antihypertensive, alpha-1-adrenergic blocking drug

PREGNANCY CATEGORY: C

Rx: Minipress

❧Rx: Apo-Prazo, Novo-Prazin, Nu-Prazo

SEE ALSO *ALPHA-1-ADRENERGIC BLOCKING AGENTS* AND *ANTIHYPERTENSIVE AGENTS.*

ACTION/KINETICS

Produces selective blockade of postsynaptic alpha-1-adrenergic receptors. Dilates arterioles and veins, thereby decreasing total peripheral resistance and decreasing DBP more than SBP. CO, HR, and renal blood flow are not affected. Can be used to initiate antihypertensive therapy; most effective when used with other agents (e.g., diuretics, beta-adrenergic blocking agents). **Onset:** 2 hr. Absorption not affected by food. **Maximum effect:** 2–3 hr; **duration:** 6–12 hr.

t ½: 2–3 hr. Full therapeutic effect: 4–6 weeks. Metabolized extensively; excreted primarily in feces.

USES
Mild to moderate hypertension alone or in combination with other antihypertensive drugs. *Investigational:* CHF refractory to other treatment. Raynaud's disease, BPH.

SPECIAL CONCERNS
Safe use in children has not been established. Use with caution during lactation. Geriatric clients may be more sensitive to the hypotensive and hypothermic effects; may be necessary to decrease the dose due to age-related decreases in renal function.

SIDE EFFECTS
First-dose effect: Marked hypotension and syncope 30–90 min after administration of initial dose (usually 2 or more mg), increase of dosage, or addition of other antihypertensive agent. **CNS:** Dizziness, drowsiness, headache, fatigue, paresthesias, depression, vertigo, nervousness, hallucinations. **CV:** Palpitations, syncope, tachycardia, orthostatic hypotension, aggravation of angina. **GI:** N&V, diarrhea or constipation, dry mouth, abdominal pain, pancreatitis. **GU:** Urinary frequency/incontinence, impotence, priapism. **Respiratory:** Dyspnea, nasal congestion, epistaxis. **Dermatologic:** Pruritus, rash, sweating, alopecia, lichen planus. **Miscellaneous:** Asthenia, edema, symptoms of lupus erythematosus, blurred vision, tinnitus, arthralgia, myalgia, reddening of sclera, eye pain, conjunctivitis, edema, fever.

LABORATORY TEST CONSIDERATIONS
↑ Urinary metabolites of norepinephrine, VMA.

OD OVERDOSE MANAGEMENT
Symptoms: Hypotension, *shock.* *Treatment:* Keep client supine to restore BP and HR. If shock is manifested, use volume expanders and vasopressors; maintain renal function.

DRUG INTERACTIONS
Antihypertensives (other) / ↑ Antihypertensive effect
Beta-adrenergic blocking agents / Enhanced acute postural hypotension after first dose of prazosin
Clonidine / ↓ Antihypertensive effect
Diuretics / ↑ Antihypertensive effect
Indomethacin / ↓ Effect of prazosin
Nifedipine / ↑ Hypotensive effect
Propranolol / Especially pronounced additive hypotensive effect
Verapamil / ↑ Hypotensive effect; ↑ sensitivity to prazosin-induced postural hypotension

HOW SUPPLIED
Capsule: 1 mg, 2 mg, 5 mg

DOSAGE
- **CAPSULES**
  Hypertension.
  Individualized: Initial, 1 mg 2–3 times per day; **maintenance:** if necessary, increase gradually to 6–15 mg/day in two to three divided doses. Do not exceed 20 mg/day, although some clients have benefited from doses of 40 mg daily. If used with diuretics or other antihypertensives, reduce dose to 1–2 mg 3 times per day. **Pediatric, less than 7 years of age, initial:** 0.25 mg 2–3 times per day adjusted according to response. **Pediatric, 7–12 years of age, initial:** 0.5 mg 2–3 times per day adjusted according to response.

NURSING CONSIDERATIONS
ADMINISTRATION/STORAGE
Reduce the dose to 1 or 2 mg 3 times per day if a diuretic or other antihypertensive agent is added to the regimen and then retitrate client.

ASSESSMENT
Note indications for therapy, other agents trialed and outcome. Assess cardiopulmonary status and renal function.

CLIENT/FAMILY TEACHING
1. Take the first dose at bedtime. Also, take the first dose of each increment at bedtime to reduce the incidence of syncope.
2. Do not drive or operate machinery for 24 hr after the first dose; may cause dizziness and drowsiness.
3. Food may delay absorption and minimize side effects of the drug.
4. Avoid rapid changes in body position that may precipitate weakness, dizziness, and syncope. Lie down or sit down and put head below knees to avoid fainting if a rapid heartbeat is felt.

---

5. Avoid dangerous situations that may lead to fainting.

6. Report any bothersome side effects because reduction in dosage may be indicated. Use sips of water and sugarless gum or candies for dry mouth effects.

7. Do not stop medication unless directed.

8. Avoid cold, cough, and allergy medications. The sympathomimetic component of such medications will interfere with the action of prazosin.

9. Comply with prescribed drug regimen; full drug effect may not be evident for 4–6 weeks.

OUTCOMES/EVALUATE

↓ BP; ↓ symptoms of refractory CHF

Procainamide hydrochloride ■

(proh-**KAYN**-ah-myd)

CLASSIFICATION(S):
Antiarrhythmic, Class IA
PREGNANCY CATEGORY: C
Rx: Procanbid
✤**Rx:** Apo-Procainamide, Procan SR

SEE ALSO *ANTIARRHYTHMIC DRUGS.*

ACTION/KINETICS

Produces a direct cardiac effect to prolong the refractory period of the atria and to a lesser extent the bundle of His-Purkinje system and ventricles. Large doses may cause AV block. Some anticholinergic and local anesthetic effects. **Onset, PO:** 30 min; **IV:** 1–5 min. **Time to peak effect, PO:** 90–120 min; **IM:** 15–60 min; **IV,** immediate. **Duration:** 3 hr. **t ½:** 2.5–4.7 hr. **Therapeutic serum level:** 4–8 mcg/mL. **Protein binding:** 15%. From 40 to 70% excreted unchanged. Metabolized in the liver (16–21% by slow acetylators and 24–33% by fast acetylators) to the active N-acetylprocainamide (NAPA); has antiarrhythmic properties with a longer half-life than procainamide.

USES

Documented ventricular arrhythmias (e.g., sustained ventricular tachycardia) that may be life threatening in clients where benefits of treatment clearly outweigh risks. *NOTE:* Antiarrhythmic drugs have not been shown to improve survival in clients with ventricular arrhythmias. *Investigational:* Atrial fibrillation/flutter.

CONTRAINDICATIONS

Hypersensitivity to drug, complete AV heart block, lupus erythematosus, torsades de pointes, asymptomatic ventricular premature depolarizations. Lactation.

SPECIAL CONCERNS

■(1) Prolonged use of procainamide often leads to development of a positive antinuclear antibody (ANA) test, with or without symptoms of lupus erythematosus-like syndrome. If a positive ANA titer develops, assess the benefit/risk ratio related to continued procainamide therapy. (2) Use should be reserved for those with life-threatening ventricular arrhythmias. (3) Agranulocytosis, bone marrow depression, neutropenia, hypoplastic anemia, and thrombocytopenia have been reported. Most cases occurred after recommended dosage. Fatalities have occurred (usually with agranulocytosis). Because most of these events occur during the first 12 weeks of therapy, it is recommended that CBC, including WBC, differential, and platelet counts be performed weekly for the first 3 months of therapy and periodically thereafter. Perform CBC promptly if the client develops any signs of infection (e.g., fever, chills, sore throat, stomatitis), bruising, or bleeding. If any of these hematologic disorders occur, discontinue therapy. Blood counts usually return to normal within 1 month after discontinuation. Use caution in those with pre-existing bone marrow failure or cytopenia of any type.■ There is an increased risk of death in those with non-life-threatening arrhythmias. Although used in children, safety and efficacy have not been established. Use with extreme caution in clients for whom a sudden drop in BP could be

P

detrimental, in CHF, acute ischemic heart disease, or cardiomyopathy. Also, use with caution in clients with liver or kidney dysfunction, preexisting bone marrow failure or cytopenia of any type, development of first-degree heart block while on procainamide, myasthenia gravis, and those with bronchial asthma or other respiratory disorders. May cause more hypotension in geriatric clients; also, in this population, the dose may have to be decreased due to age-related decreases in renal function.

SIDE EFFECTS

Body as a whole: Lupus erythematosus–like syndrome especially in those on maintenance therapy and who are slow acetylators. Symptoms include arthralgia, pleural or abdominal pain, arthritis, pleural effusion, pericarditis, fever, chills, myalgia, skin lesions, hematologic changes. **CV:** Following IV use: Hypotension, ***ventricular asystole or fibrillation, partial or complete heart block.*** Rarely, second-degree heart block after PO use. **GI:** N&V, diarrhea, anorexia, bitter taste, abdominal pain. **Hematologic:** Thrombocytopenia, ***agranulocytosis,*** neutropenia, hypoplastic anemia. Rarely, ***hemolytic anemia.*** **Dermatologic:** Urticaria, pruritus, angioneurotic edema, flushing, maculopapular rash. **CNS:** Depression, dizziness, weakness, giddiness, psychoses with hallucinations. **Other:** Granulomatous hepatitis, weakness, fever, chills.

LABORATORY TEST CONSIDERATIONS

May affect LFTs. False + ↑ in serum alkaline phosphatase. Positive ANA test. High levels of lidocaine and meprobamate may inhibit fluorescence of procainamide and NAPA.

OD **OVERDOSE MANAGEMENT**

Symptoms: Plasma levels of 10–15 mcg/mL are associated with toxic symptoms. Progressive widening of the QRS complex, prolonged QT or PR intervals, lowering of R and T waves, increased AV block, increased ventricular extrasystoles, ***ventricular tachycardia or fibrillation.*** IV overdose may result in hypotension, CNS depression, tremor, respiratory depression.
Treatment:

• Induce emesis or perform gastric lavage followed by administration of activated charcoal.
• To treat hypotension, give IV fluids and/or a vasopressor (dopamine, phenylephrine, or norepinephrine).
• Infusion of ⅙ molar sodium lactate IV reduces the cardiotoxic effects.
• Hemodialysis (but not peritoneal dialysis) is effective in reducing serum levels.
• Renal clearance can be enhanced by acidification of the urine and with high flow rates.
• A ventricular pacing electrode can be inserted as a precaution in the event AV block develops.

DRUG INTERACTIONS

Acetazolamide / ↑ Procainamide effect R/T ↓ kidney excretion
Amiodarone / ↑ Procainamide levels
Antiarrhythmics (e.g., lidocaine, disopyramide, quinidine) / Additive effects on the heart; quinidine may also ↑ procainamide and metabolite levels
Anticholinergic agents, atropine / Additive antivagal effects on AV conduction
Antihypertensive agents / Additive hypotensive effect
Cholinergic agents / Anticholinergic activity of procainamide antagonizes effect of cholinergic drugs
Cimetidine / ↑ Procainamide effect R/T ↓ renal clearance
Disopyramide / ↑ Risk of enhanced prolongation of conduction or depression of contractility and hypotension
Ethanol / Effect of procainamide may be altered, but because the main metabolite is active as an antiarrhythmic, specific outcome not clear
H *Henbane leaf* / ↑ Anticholinergic effects
Kanamycin / ↑ Kanamycin-induced muscle relaxation
Lidocaine / Additive cardiodepressant effects
Mg salts / ↑ Mg-induced muscle relaxation
Neomycin / ↑ Neomycin-induced muscle relaxation
Ofloxacin / See *Quinolones;* also, possible ↑ procainamide levels

---

Bold Italic = life threatening side effect   ■ = black box warning   ✚ = Available in Canada

Propranolol / ↑ Serum procainamide levels

Quinidine / ↑ Risk of enhanced prolongation of conduction or depression of contractility and hypotension

Quinolones / ↑ Risk of life-threatening cardiac arrhythmias, including torsades de pointes

Ranitidine / ↑ Procainamide effect R/T ↓ renal clearance

Sodium bicarbonate / ↑ Procainamide effect R/T ↓ kidney excretion

Succinylcholine / ↑ Succinylcholine-induced muscle relaxation

Thioridazine / Possible synergistic or additive prolongation of the QTc interval and ↑ risk for life-threatening cardiac arrhythmias, including torsades de pointes

Trimethoprim / ↑ Procainamide effect R/T ↑ serum levels

Ziprasidone / Possible synergistic or additive prolongation of the QTc interval and ↑ risk for life-threatening cardiac arrhythmias, including torsades de pointes

HOW SUPPLIED

Capsule: 250 mg, 375 mg, 500 mg; *Injection:* 500 mg/mL; *Tablet, Immediate Release:* 250 mg, 375 mg, 500 mg; *Tablet, Extended Release:* 250 mg, 500 mg, 750 mg, 1000 mg

DOSAGE

• **CAPSULES, EXTENDED-, IMMEDIATE-RELEASE TABLETS**

Adults, initial: Up to 50 mg/kg/day in divided doses q 3 hr. **Usual, 40–50 kg:** 250 mg q 3 hr or 500 mg q 6 hr of immediate release; 500 mg q 6 hr of sustained-release; or, 1 g q 12 hr of Procanbid; **60–70 kg:** 375 mg q 3 hr or 750 mg q 6 hr of immediate release; 750 mg q 6 hr of sustained-release; or, 1.5 g q 12 hr of Procanbid; **80–90 kg:** 500 mg q 3 hr or 1 g q 6 hr of immediate release; 1 g q 6 hr of sustained-release; or, 2 g q 12 hr of Procanbid; **over 100 kg:** 625 mg q 3 hr or 1.25 g q 6 hr of immediate release; 1.25 g q 6 hr of sustained-release; or, 2.5 g q 12 hr of Procanbid.

• **IM**

Ventricular arrhythmias.

Adults, initial: 50 mg/kg/day divided into fractional doses of $\frac{1}{8}$–$\frac{1}{4}$ given q

3–6 hr until PO therapy is possible. If more than 3 injections are given, assess client factors as age, renal function, clinical response, and blood procainamide and n-acetylprocainamide levels in adjusting further doses.

Arrhythmias associated with surgery or anesthesia.

Adults: 100–500 mg.

• **IV**

Initial loading infusion: Slowly inject into a vein or tubing at a rate not to exceed 50 mg/min; doses of 100 mg may be given q 5 min until arrhythmia is suppressed or until 500 mg has been given. Wait at least 10 min to allow for more distribution into tissues before resuming. Alternatively, a loading infusion containing 20 mg/mL (1 g diluted to 50 mL with D5W) may be given at a constant rate of 1 mL/min for 25–30 min to deliver 500–600 mg. Maximum dosage either by repeated bolus injections or loading infusion is 1 g. **Maintenance infusion:** 2–6 mg/min.

NURSING CONSIDERATIONS

ADMINISTRATION/STORAGE

1. Extended-release tablets are not recommended for use in children or for initiating treatment.

2. IM therapy may be used as an alternative to PO in clients with less threatening arrhythmias but who are nauseated or vomiting, who cannot take anything PO (e.g., preoperatively), or who have malabsorptive problems.

3. If more than three IM injections are required, assess the age, renal function, and blood levels of procainamide and NAPA; adjust dosage accordingly.

IV 4. Reserve IV use for emergency situations.

5. For IV initial therapy, dilute the drug with D5W; give a maximum of 1 g slowly to minimize side effects by one of the following methods:

• Direct injection into a vein or into tubing of an established infusion line at a rate not to exceed 50 mg/min. Dilute either the 100- or 500-mg/mL vials prior to injection to facilitate control of the dosage rate. Doses of 100 mg may be given q 5 min until arrhythmia is suppressed or until 500 mg has been given (then wait 10 or more min before resuming administration).

• Loading infusion containing 20 mg/mL (1 g diluted with 50 mL of D5W) given at a constant rate of 1 mL/min for 25–30 min to deliver 500–600 mg.

6. For IV maintenance infusion, dose is usually 2–6 mg/min. Administer with electronic infusion device.

7. Discard solutions that are darker than light amber or otherwise colored. Solutions that have turned slightly yellow on standing may be used. Consult pharmacist if unsure.

ASSESSMENT

1. Document indications for therapy, type, onset, and characteristics of symptoms. List other agents prescribed and the outcome.

2. Assess cardiopulmonary status and note findings. Note any sensitivity to tartrazine, pregnancy, or heart block.

3. Monitor VS, ECG, CBC, electrolytes, ANA titers, liver and renal function studies.

INTERVENTIONS

1. Place in a supine position during IV infusion and monitor BP. Discontinue if SBP falls 15 mm Hg or more during administration or if increased SA or AV block is noted.

2. Reduce dose with liver or renal dysfunction, or if client <120 lb.

3. Assess for symptoms of SLE, manifested by polyarthralgia, arthritis, pleuritic pain, fever, myalgia, and skin lesions. ANA titer may become positive in 60% of those taking this drug without lupus— like S&S; may progress to SLE if drug is not dicontinued.

CLIENT/FAMILY TEACHING

1. Take with a full glass of water to lessen GI symptoms. Take either 1 hr before or 2 hr after meals.

2. If GI symptoms are severe and persistent may take with meals or with a snack to ensure adherence.

3. Sustained-release preparations should be swallowed whole. They should not be crushed, broken, or chewed. The wax matrix of sustained-release tablets may be evident in the stool and is considered normal.

4. Report any sore throat, fever, rash, chills, bruising, diarrhea or increased palpitations. With long term use may note loss of effectiveness.

5. Do not take any OTC drugs, do not stop suddenly. Report any adverse side effects, i.e., irregular pulse, anxiety, sudden fatigue.

OUTCOMES/EVALUATE

• Termination of arrhythmias with restoration of stable cardiac rhythm

• Therapeutic drug levels (4–8 mcg/mL)

Propafenone hydrochloride ■

(proh-pah-**FEN**-ohn)

CLASSIFICATION(S):
Antiarrhythmic, Class IC

PREGNANCY CATEGORY: C

Rx: Rythmol, Rythmol SR

✤**Rx:** Apo-Propafenone

ACTION/KINETICS

Manifests local anesthetic effects and a direct stabilizing action on the myocardium. Reduces upstroke velocity (Phase O) of the monophasic action potential, reduces the fast inward current carried by sodium ions in the Purkinje fibers, increases diastolic excitability threshold, and prolongs the effective refractory period. Also, spontaneous activity is decreased. Slows AV conduction and causes first-degree heart block. Has slight beta-adrenergic blocking activity. Almost completely absorbed after PO administration. **Peak plasma levels:** 3.5 hr. **Therapeutic plasma levels:** 0.5–3 mcg/mL. Significant first-pass effect. Most metabolize rapidly (**t**½: 2–10 hr) to two active metabolites: 5-hydroxypropafenone and N-depropylpropafenone. However, approximately 10% (as well as those taking quinidine) metabolize the drug more slowly (**t**½: 10–32 hr). Because the 5-hydroxy metabolite is not formed in slow metabolizers and because steady-state levels are reached after 4–5 days in all clients, the recommended dosing regimen is the same for all clients.

USES

Immediate-Release. (1) Prolong the time to recurrence of paroxysmal atrial fibrillation/flutter associated with disabling symptoms in clients without structural heart disease. (2) To prolong the time to recurrence of paroxysmal supraventricular tachycardia associated with disabling symptoms in clients without structural heart disease. (3) Treatment of ventricular arrhythmias, such as sustained ventricular tachycardia, that are life-threatening. **Extended-Release.** Prolong the time to recurrence of symptomatic atrial fibrillation in clients without structural heart disease. *NOTE:* Antiarrhythmic drugs have not been shown to improve survival in clients with ventricular arrhythmias. *Investigational:* Arrhythmias associated with Wolff-Parkinson-White syndrome.

CONTRAINDICATIONS

Uncontrolled CHF, cardiogenic shock, sick sinus node syndrome or AV block in the absence of an artificial pacemaker, bradycardia, marked hypotension, bronchospastic disorders, electrolyte disorders, hypersensitivity to the drug. MI more than 6 days but less than 2 years previously. Use to control ventricular rate during atrial fibrillation. Use with lesser ventricular arrhythmias, even if clients are symptomatic. Lactation.

SPECIAL CONCERNS

■The National Heart, Lung, and Blood Institute's Cardiac Arrhythmia Suppression Trial (CAST) reported that clients with asymptomatic non-life-threatening ventricular arrhythmias who had an MI more than 6 days but less than 2 years previously, an increased rate of death or reversed cardiac arrest rate was seen in clients treated with encainide or flecainide (Class 1C antiarrhythmics) compared with that seen in those receiving a placebo. The applicability of the CAST results to other populations (e.g., those without recent MI) or other antiarrhythmic drugs is uncertain, but at present, it is prudent to consider any 1C antiarrhythmic to have a signifcant risk in clients with structural heart disease. Given the lack of any evidence that these drugs improve survival, antiarrhythmic drugs should generally be avoided in those with non-life-threatening ventricular arrhythmias, even if the clients are experiencing unpleasant, but not life-threatening symptoms or signs.■ May cause new or worsened arrhythmias or CHF. Use with caution during labor and delivery. Safety and effectiveness have not been determined in children. Use with caution in clients with impaired hepatic or renal function. Geriatric clients may require lower dosage. Monitor clients taking propafenone and an inhibitor of CYP1A2, CYP2D6, or CYP3A4 metabolizing enzymes; dosage adjustment may be necessary.

SIDE EFFECTS

CV: *New or worsened arrhythmias.* First-degree AV block, intraventricular conduction delay, palpitations, PVCs, proarrhythmia, bradycardia, atrial fibrillation, angina, syncope, CHF, *ventricular tachycardia, second-degree AV block,* increased QRS duration, chest pain, hypotension, bundle branch block. Less commonly, atrial flutter, AV dissociation, flushing, hot flashes, sick sinus syndrome, sinus pause or arrest, SVT, prolongation of the PR and QRS interval, *cardiac arrest.* **CNS:** Dizziness, headache, anxiety, drowsiness, fatigue, loss of balance, ataxia, insomnia. Less commonly, abnormal speech/dreams/ vision, confusion, depression, memory loss, *apnea,* psychosis/mania, vertigo, *seizures, coma,* numbness, paresthesias. **GI:** Unusual taste, constipation, nausea and/or vomiting, dry mouth, anorexia, flatulence, abdominal pain, cramps, diarrhea, dyspepsia. Less commonly, gastroenteritis and liver abnormalities (cholestasis, hepatitis, elevated enzymes). **Hematologic:** *Agranulocytosis,* increased bleeding time, anemia, granulocytopenia, bruising, leukopenia, purpura, thrombocytopenia. **Miscellaneous:** Blurred vision, dyspnea, weakness, rash, edema, tremors, diaphoresis, joint pain, possible decrease in spermatogenesis. Less commonly, tinnitus, un-

P

usual smell sensation, alopecia, eye irritation, hyponatremia, inappropriate ADH secretion, impotence, increased glucose, kidney failure, lupus erythematosus, muscle cramps or weakness, nephrotic syndrome, pain, pruritus, exacerbation of myasthenia gravis.

LABORATORY TEST CONSIDERATIONS
↑ ANA titers, alkaline phosphatase, AST, ALT.

OD OVERDOSE MANAGEMENT
Symptoms: Bradycardia, hypotension, IA and intraventricular conduction disturbances, somnolence. ***Rarely, high-grade ventricular arrhythmias and seizures.*** *Treatment:* To control BP and cardiac rhythm, defibrillation and infusion of dopamine or isoproterenol. If seizures occur, diazepam, IV, can be given. External cardiac massage and mechanical respiratory assistance may be required.

DRUG INTERACTIONS
Drugs that inhibit CYP2D6, CYP1A2, and CYP3A4 may lead to increased plasma levels of propafenone; monitor such situations carefully.
Beta-adrenergic blockers / ↑ Levels of beta blockers metabolized by the liver
Cimetidine / ↓ Propafenone plasma levels → ↑ effects
Cyclosporine / ↑ Cyclosporine blood trough levels; ↓ renal function
Desipramine / ↑ Desipramine levels
Digoxin / ↑ Plasma digoxin levels → ↓ digoxin dose
Local anesthetics / May ↑ risk of CNS side effects
Mexiletine / ↓ Metabolic clearance of mexiletine in extensive metabolizers → no differences between extensive and poor metabolizers
Quinidine / ↑ Propafenone serum levels in rapid metabolizers → possible ↑ effect
Rifamycins / ↓ Propafenone effect R/T ↑ clearance
Ritonavir / Large ↑ in serum propafenone levels; do not use together
SSRIs / Certain SSRIs may inhibit the metabolism (by CYP2D6) of propafenone
Theophylline / ↑ Theophylline levels → possible toxicity
Warfarin / May ↑ warfarin plasma levels; ↓ warfarin dose

HOW SUPPLIED
Capsules, Extended-Release: 225 mg, 325 mg, 425 mg; *Tablets, Immediate Release:* 150 mg, 225 mg, 300 mg

DOSAGE———————————
• **CAPSULES, EXTENDED-RELEASE**
Sympatomatic atrial fibrillation without structural heart disease.
Individualize dosage based on response and tolerance. **Initial:** 225 mg q 12 hr; increase in 5 day or more intervals to 325 mg q 12 hr. Increase to 425 mg q 12 hr if needed.
• **TABLETS, IMMEDIATE-RELEASE**
Titrate on basis of response and tolerance. **Adults, initial:** 150 mg q 8 hr; dose may be increased at a minimum of q 3–4 days to 225 mg q 8 hr and, if necessary, to 300 mg q 8 hr. The safety and efficacy of doses exceeding 900 mg/day have not been established.

NURSING CONSIDERATIONS
ADMINISTRATION/STORAGE
1. Always initiate therapy in a hospital setting.
2. Consider dose reduction in those in whom significant widening of the QRS complex or second- or third-degree AV block occurs. Consider dose reduction in those with hepatic impairment.
3. Increase the dose of the immediate-release tablets more gradually during the initial treatment phase in the elderly or in those with marked previous myocardial damage.
4. There is no evidence that the use of propafenone affects the survival or incidence of sudden death with recent MI or SVT.

ASSESSMENT
1. Note indications for therapy noting ECG and baseline arrhythmias; note any cardiac problems and list drugs prescribed.
2. Monitor CBC, electrolytes, liver and renal function studies. Determine any renal or hepatic disease.
3. Report any significant widening of the QRS complex or any evidence of second- or third-degree AV block. May induce new or more severe arrhyth-

---

Bold Italic = life threatening side effect   ■ = black box warning   ✦ = Available in Canada

mias; titrate dose based on client response and tolerance.

4. Increase dose more gradually in elderly clients as well as those with previous myocardial damage.

5. Evaluate hematologic studies for anemia, agranulocytosis, leukopenia, thrombocytopenia, or altered prothrombin and coagulation times.

CLIENT/FAMILY TEACHING

1. Drink adequate quantities of fluid (2–3 L/day) and add bulk to the diet to avoid constipation.

2. The sustained-release capsules can be taken with or without food. Do not crush or further divide the contents of the capsule.

3. May experience dizziness or unusual taste in the mouth; report if interferes with walking, eating, or nutritional status.

4. Report any increased chest pain, SOB, blurred vision, palpitations, unusual bruising/bleeding, or S&S of liver failure such as yellow eyes, dark-yellow urine, or yellow skin.

5. Report any urinary tract problems, decreased urinary output, or adverse side effects.

6. Record BP and pulse readings for provider review.

OUTCOMES/EVALUATE

• Termination of life-threatening VT; restoration of stable rhythm

• Therapeutic drug levels (0.5–3 mcg/mL)

Propranolol hydrochloride ©

(proh-**PRAN**-oh-lohl)

CLASSIFICATION(S):

Beta-adrenergic blocking agent
PREGNANCY CATEGORY: C
Rx: Inderal, Inderal LA, InnoPran XL, Propranolol Intensol
✽**Rx:** Apo-Propranolol, Nu-Propranolol

SEE ALSO *BETA-ADRENERGIC BLOCKING AGENTS.*

ACTION/KINETICS

Manifests both beta-1- and beta-2-adrenergic blocking activity. Antiarrhythmic action is due to both beta-adrenergic receptor blockade and a direct membrane-stabilizing action on the cardiac cell. Has no intrinsic sympathomimetic activity and has high lipid solubility. **Onset, PO:** 30 min; **IV:** immediate. **Maximum effect:** 1–1.5 hr. **Duration:** 3–5 hr. **t ½:** 2–3 hr (8–11 hr for long-acting). **Therapeutic serum level, antiarrhythmic:** 0.05–0.1 mcg/mL. Completely metabolized by liver and excreted in urine. Although food increases bioavailability, absorption may be decreased.

USES

(1) Hypertension, alone or in combination with other antihypertensive agents. (2) Angina pectoris when caused by coronary atherosclerosis. (3) Hypertrophic subaortic stenosis (especially to treat exercise or other stress-induced angina, palpitations, and syncope). (4) MI. (5) Adjunctive treatment of pheochromocytoma after primary therapy with an alpha-adrenergic blocker. (6) Prophylaxis of migraine. (7) Essential tremor (familial or hereditary). (8) Cardiac arrhythmias, including supraventricular, ventricular, tachyarrhythmias of digitalis intoxication and resistant tachyarrhythmias due to excessive catecholamines during anesthesia. *Investigational:* Schizophrenia, tremors due to parkinsonism, aggressive behavior, antipsychotic-induced akathisia, rebleeding due to esophageal varices, situational anxiety, acute panic attacks, gastric bleeding in portal hypertension, vaginal contraceptive, anxiety, alcohol withdrawal syndrome, winter depression.

CONTRAINDICATIONS

Bronchial asthma, bronchospasms including severe COPD.

SPECIAL CONCERNS

It is dangerous to use propranolol for pheochromocytoma unless an alpha-adrenergic blocking agent is already in use.

ADDITIONAL SIDE EFFECTS

Psoriasis-like eruptions, skin necrosis, SLE (rare).

P

H = Herbal   IV = Intravenous   © = sound-alike drug

LABORATORY TEST CONSIDERATIONS

↑ Blood urea, serum transaminase, alkaline phosphatase, LDH. Interference with glaucoma screening test.

ADDITIONAL DRUG INTERACTIONS

Gabapentin / Possible paroxysmal dystonic movements in the hands

Haloperidol / Severe hypotension

Hydralazine / ↑ Effect of both agents

Methimazole / May ↑ propranolol effects

Phenobarbital / ↓ Propranolol effect R/T ↑ liver breakdown

Propylthiouracil / May ↑ Propranolol effects

Rifampin / ↓ Propranolol effect R/T ↑ liver breakdown

Rizatriptan / ↑ AUC and peak rizatriptan levels R/T ↓ rizatriptan metabolism

Smoking / ↓ Serum levels and ↑ clearance of propranolol

HOW SUPPLIED

Capsule, sustained release: 60 mg, 80 mg, 120 mg, 160 mg; *Injection:* 1 mg/mL; *Oral Solution:* 4 mg/mL, 8 mg/mL; *Oral Solution Concentrate:* 80 mg/mL; *Tablet:* 10 mg, 20 mg, 40 mg, 60 mg, 80 mg, 90 mg

DOSAGE

• **SUSTAINED-RELEASE CAPSULES, ORAL SOLUTION, ORAL SOLUTION CONCENTRATE, TABLETS**

Hypertension.

Initial: 40 mg twice a day or 80 mg of sustained-release/day; **then,** increase dose to maintenance level of 120–240 mg/day given in two to three divided doses or 120–160 mg of sustained-release medication once daily. Do not exceed 640 mg/day. **Pediatric, initial:** 0.5 mg/kg twice a day; dose may be increased at 3- to 5-day intervals to a maximum of 1 mg/kg twice a day Calculate the dosage range by weight and not by body surface area.

Angina.

Initial: 80–320 mg 2–4 times per day; or, 80 mg of sustained-release once daily; **then,** increase dose gradually to maintenance level of 160 mg/day of sustained-release capsule. Do not exceed 320 mg/day.

Arrhythmias.

10–30 mg 3–4 times per day given after meals and at bedtime.

Hypertrophic subaortic stenosis.

20–40 mg 3–4 times per day before meals and at bedtime or 80–160 mg of sustained-release medication given once daily.

MI prophylaxis.

180–240 mg/day given in three to four divided doses. Do not exceed 240 mg/day.

Pheochromocytoma, preoperatively.

60 mg/day for 3 days before surgery, given concomitantly with an alpha-adrenergic blocking agent.

Pheochromocytoma, inoperable tumors.

30 mg/day in divided doses.

Migraine.

Initial: 80 mg sustained-release medication given once daily; **then,** increase dose gradually to maintenance of 160–240 mg/day in divided doses. If a satisfactory response has not been observed after 4–6 weeks, discontinue the drug and withdraw gradually.

Essential tremor.

Initial: 40 mg twice a day; **then,** 120 mg/day up to a maximum of 320 mg/day.

Aggressive behavior.

80–300 mg/day.

Antipsychotic-induced akathisia.

20–80 mg/day.

Tremors associated with Parkinson's disease.

160 mg/day.

Rebleeding from esophageal varices.

20–180 mg twice a day

Schizophrenia.

300–5,000 mg/day.

Acute panic symptoms.

40–320 mg/day.

Anxiety.

80–320 mg/day.

Intermittent explosive disorder.

50–1,600 mg/day.

Nonvariceal gastric bleeding in portal hypertension.

24–480 mg/day.

• **IV**

Life-threatening arrhythmias or those occurring under anesthesia.

1–3 mg not to exceed 1 mg/min; a second dose may be given after 2 min, with subsequent doses q 4 hr. Begin PO therapy as soon as possible. Although use in pediatrics is not recommended, investigational doses of 0.01–0.1 mg/kg/dose, up to a maximum of 1 mg/dose (by slow push), have been used for arrhythmias.

NURSING CONSIDERATIONS

ⓔ Do not confuse propranolol with Pravachol (antihyperlipidemic). Also, do not confuse Inderal with Inderide (an antihypertensive) or with Isordil (a coronary vasodilator).

ADMINISTRATION/STORAGE

1. Do not administer for a minimum of 2 weeks after MAO drug use.

IV 2. Reserve IV use for life-threatening arrhythmias or those occurring during anesthesia.

3. If signs of serious myocardial depression occur, slowly infuse isoproterenol (Isuprel) IV.

4. For IV use, dilute 1 mg in 10 mL of D5W and administer IV over at least 1 min. May be further reconstituted in 50 mL of dextrose or saline solution and infused IVPB over 10–15 min.

5. After IV administration, have emergency drugs and equipment available to combat hypotension or circulatory collapse.

ASSESSMENT

1. Document indications for therapy, characteristics of symptoms, other agents trialed, and outcome.

2. Note ECG, VS, and cardiopulmonary assessment. Assess for pulmonary disease, bronchospasms, or depression.

3. Report rash, fever, and/or purpura; S&S of hypersensitivity reaction.

4. Monitor VS, I&O. Observe for S&S of CHF (e.g., SOB, rales, edema, and weight gain).

CLIENT/FAMILY TEACHING

1. May cause drowsiness; assess drug response before performing activities that require mental alertness.

2. Sustained-release products are usually taken at bedtime. It is recommended that InnoPran XL be taken about 10 p.m. on an empty stomach or with food.

3. Do not smoke; smoking decreases serum levels and interferes with drug clearance.

4. May mask symptoms of hypoglycemia; monitor FS carefully.

5. Keep log of BP and pulse for provider review; report significant changes.

6. Do not stop abruptly; may precipitate hypertension, myocardial ischemia, or cardiac arrhythmias.

7. Dress appropriately; may cause increased sensitivity to cold.

8. Avoid alcohol and any OTC agents containing alpha-adrenergic stimulants or sympathomimetics.

9. Report any persistent side effects, e.g., skin rashes, abnormal bleeding, unusual crying, or feelings of depression.

OUTCOMES/EVALUATE

- ↓ BP, ↓ HR
- ↓ Angina; prophylaxis of myocardial reinfarction
- Migraine prophylaxis
- Control of tachyarrhythmias
- Therapeutic drug levels as an antiarrhythmic (0.05–0.1 mcg/mL)

Protamine sulfate
(**PROH**-tah-meen)

P

CLASSIFICATION(S):
Heparin antagonist
PREGNANCY CATEGORY: C

ACTION/KINETICS

A strong basic polypeptide that complexes with strongly acidic heparin to form an inactive stable salt. The complex has no anticoagulant activity. Heparin is neutralized within 5 min after IV protamine. **Duration:** 2 hr (but depends on body temperature). The t ½ of protamine is shorter than heparin; thus, repeated doses may be required. Upon metabolism, the complex may liberate heparin (heparin rebound).

USES

Only for treatment of heparin overdose.

CONTRAINDICATIONS
Previous intolerance to protamine. Use to treat spontaneous hemorrhage, post-partum hemorrhage, menorrhagia, or uterine bleeding. Administration of over 50 mg over a short period.

SPECIAL CONCERNS
Use with caution during lactation. Safety and efficacy have not been determined in children. Rapid administration may cause severe hypotension and anaphylaxis.

SIDE EFFECTS
CV: Sudden fall in BP, bradycardia, transitory flushing, warm feeling, *acute pulmonary hypertension, circulatory collapse (possibly irreversible) with myocardial failure* and decreased CO. Pulmonary edema in clients on cardiopulmonary bypass undergoing CV surgery. **Anaphylaxis:** Severe respiratory distress, capillary leak, and noncardiogenic pulmonary edema. **GI:** N&V. **CNS:** Lassitude. **Other:** Dyspnea, back pain in conscious clients undergoing cardiac catheterization, hypersensitivity reactions.

OD OVERDOSE MANAGEMENT
Symptoms: Bleeding. Rapid administration may cause dyspnea, bradycardia, flushing, warm feeling, severe hypotension, hypertension. In assessing overdose, there may be the possibility of multiple drug overdoses leading to drug interactions and unusual pharmacokinetics. *Treatment:* Replace blood loss with blood transfusions or fresh frozen plasma. Fluids, epinephrine, dobutamine, or dopamine to treat hypotension.

HOW SUPPLIED
Injection: 10 mg/mL

DOSAGE
• **SLOW IV**

Give no more than 50 mg of protamine sulfate in any 10-min period. One mg of protamine sulfate can neutralize about 90 USP units of heparin derived from lung tissue or about 115 USP units of heparin derived from intestinal mucosa. *NOTE:* The dose of protamine sulfate depends on the amount of time that has elapsed since IV heparin administration. For example, if 30 min has elapsed, one-half the usual dose of protamine sulfate may be sufficient because heparin is cleared rapidly from the circulation.

NURSING CONSIDERATIONS

ADMINISTRATION/STORAGE
IV 1. Incompatible with several penicillins and with cephalosporins.
2. To minimize side effects, give slowly over 10 min. May also be diluted in 50 mL of D5W or saline solution and administered at a rate of 50 mg over 10–15 min. Do not store diluted solutions.
3. Refrigerate at 2–8°C (36–46°F).

ASSESSMENT
1. Determine amount, time of overdose, and source to ensure appropriate antidote dosing.
2. Request type and crossmatch; assess need for fresh frozen plasma or whole blood.
3. Coagulation studies should be performed 5–15 min after protamine has been administered; repeat in 2–8 hr to assess for heparin rebound (increased bleeding, lowered BP, and/or shock).
4. Monitor VS, I&O; assess for sudden fall in BP, bradycardia, dyspnea, transitory flushing, or sensations of warmth.

OUTCOMES/EVALUATE
Stable H&H; control of heparin-induced hemorrhage

Q

Quinapril hydrochloride ■ ©
(**KWIN**-ah-prill)

CLASSIFICATION(S):
Antihypertensive, ACE inhibitor
PREGNANCY CATEGORY: D
Rx: Accupril

SEE ALSO ANGIOTENSIN-
CONVERTING ENZYME INHIBITORS.

ACTION/KINETICS
Onset: 1 hr. **Time to peak serum levels:** 1 hr. **Peak effect:** 2–4 hr. Bioavailability is about 60%. Metabolized to quinaprilat, the active metabolite. **t ½, quinaprilat:** 2–3 hr. **Duration:** 24 hr. Significantly bound to plasma proteins. Food reduces absorption. Metabolized with approximately 60% excreted through the urine and 40% excreted in the feces. Also appears to improve endothelial function, an early marker of coronary atherosclerosis. About 97% is bound to plasma proteins.

USES
(1) Alone or in combination with a thiazide diuretic for the treatment of hypertension. (2) Adjunct with a diuretic or digitalis to treat CHF in those not responding adequately to diuretics or digitalis.

SPECIAL CONCERNS
■When used during the second and third trimesters of pregnancy, injury and even death can result in the developing fetus. When pregnancy is detected, discontinue as soon as possible.■ Use with caution during lactation. Safety and effectiveness have not been determined in children. Geriatric clients may be more sensitive to the effects of quinapril and manifest higher peak quinaprilat blood levels.

SIDE EFFECTS
CV: Vasodilation, tachycardia, *heart failure,* palpitations, chest pain, hypo-tension, *MI, CVA, hypertensive crisis,* angina pectoris, orthostatic hypotension, *cardiac rhythm disturbances, cardiogenic shock.* **GI:** Dry mouth or throat, constipation, diarrhea, N&V, abdominal pain, hepatitis, pancreatitis, *GI hemorrhage.* **CNS:** Somnolence, vertigo, insomnia, sleep disturbances, paresthesias, nervousness, depression, headache, dizziness, fatigue. **Hematologic:** *Agranulocytosis,* bone marrow depression, thrombocytopenia. **Dermatologic:** *Angioedema of the lips, tongue, glottis, and larynx;* sweating, pruritus, exfoliative dermatitis, photosensitivity, dermatopolymyositis, flushing, rash. **Body as a whole:** Malaise, edema, back pain. **GU:** Oliguria and/or progressive azotemia and rarely *acute renal failure and/or death in severe heart failure.* Impotence. Worsening renal failure. **Respiratory:** Pharyngitis, cough, asthma, bronchospasm, dyspnea. **Musculoskeletal:** Myalgia, arthralgia. **Miscellaneous:** Oligohydramnios in fetuses exposed to the drug in utero. Syncope, hyperkalemia, amblyopia, viral infection.

OD OVERDOSE MANAGEMENT
Symptoms: Commonly, hypotension. *Treatment:* IV infusion of normal saline to restore blood pressure.

DRUG INTERACTIONS
Potassium-containing salt substitutes / ↑ Risk of hyperkalemia
Potassium-sparing diuretics / ↑ Risk of hyperkalemia
Potassium supplements / ↑ Risk of hyperkalemia
Tetracyclines / ↓ Absorption R/T high Mg^+ content of quinapril tablets

HOW SUPPLIED
Tablet: 5 mg, 10 mg, 20 mg, 40 mg

DOSAGE
• **TABLETS**
Hypertension, client not on diuretics.
Initial: 10 or 20 mg once daily; **then,** adjust dosage based on BP response at peak (2–6 hr) and trough (predose)

Q

blood levels. The dose should be adjusted at 2-week intervals. **Maintenance:** 20, 40, or 80 mg daily as a single dose or in two equally divided doses; usual dose is 10–40 mg/day. With impaired renal function, the initial dose should be 10 mg if the C_{CR} is greater than 60 mL/min, 5 mg if the C_{CR} is between 30 and 60 mL/min, and 2.5 mg if the C_{CR} is between 10 and 30 mL/min. If the initial dose is well tolerated, the drug may be given the following day as a twice a day regimen.

Hypertension, client on diuretics.
Initial: 5 mg with careful supervision for several hr until BP stabilizes.

CHF.
Initial: 5 mg twice a day. If this dose is well tolerated, titrate clients at weekly intervals until an effective dose, usually 20–40 mg daily in two equally divided doses, is attained. Undesirable hypotension, orthostasis, or azotemia may prevent this dosage level from being reached.

NURSING CONSIDERATIONS

❡ Do not confuse Accupril with Accutane (antiacne drug) or with Aciphex (proton pump inhibitor).

ADMINISTRATION/STORAGE
1. If taking a diuretic, discontinue the diuretic 2–3 days prior to beginning quinapril. If the BP is not controlled, reinstitute the diuretic. If the diuretic cannot be discontinued, the initial dose should be 5 mg.
2. If the antihypertensive effect decreases at the end of the dosing interval with once-daily therapy, consider either twice-daily administration or increasing the dose.
3. If the initial dose is well tolerated for treating CHF, quinapril may be given as a twice a day regimen. In the absence of excessive hypotension or significant renal function deterioration, the dose may be increased at weekly intervals, based on clinical and hemodynamic responses.
4. The antihypertensive effect may not be observed for 1–2 weeks.

ASSESSMENT
1. Note indications for therapy, all medical conditions, and other agents trialed.
2. Observe infants exposed to quinapril in utero for the development of hypotension, oliguria, and hyperkalemia.
3. If angioedema occurs, stop drug, assess airway, and observe until swelling resolved. Antihistamines may help relieve symptoms.
4. Monitor VS, I&O, weights, electrolytes, CBC, microalbumin, and renal function studies. Agranulocytosis and bone marrow depression seen more often with renal impairment, especially if collagen vascular disease (e.g., SLE, scleroderma) present.
5. Clients with unilateral or bilateral renal artery stenosis may manifest increased BUN and serum creatinine if given quinapril. Assess renal function closely especially during the first few weeks of therapy; reduce dose with renal dysfunction. Monitor renal function and serum K^+ during therapy.

CLIENT/FAMILY TEACHING
1. Take as directed; take 1–2 hr before food or antacids as they will reduce absorption. Avoid foods high in potassium or potassium supplements. Consume adequate fluids to prevent dehydration; hot weather and exercise may increase loss.
2. Avoid activities that require mental alertness until drug effects realized as the drug may cause dizziness or drowsiness. Change positions slowly to prevent sudden low BP.
3. Report any unusual bruising/bleeding, fever, sore throat, cough, or persistent side effects.
4. Any increased SOB, palpitations, swelling, or persistent nonproductive cough should be evaluated as well as rash and altered taste perception.
5. Keep a log of BP and HR readings at different times for provider review.
6. Practice reliable contraception; report if pregnancy suspected.
7. Some OTC drugs may affect the action of quinapril; obtain medical advice before taking OTC drugs.

OUTCOMES/EVALUATE
↓ BP

Bold Italic = life threatening side effect   ■ = black box warning   ✤ = Available in Canada

Quinidine gluconate ®

(**KWIN**-ih-deen)

CLASSIFICATION(S):
Antiarrhythmic, Class IA
PREGNANCY CATEGORY: C
Rx: Quinidine Gluconate Injection

Quinidine sulfate

PREGNANCY CATEGORY: C
Rx: Quinidex Extentabs
✤**Rx:** Apo-Quinidine

SEE ALSO *ANTIARRHYTHMIC AGENTS.*

ACTION/KINETICS
Reduces the excitability of the heart and depresses conduction velocity and contractility. Prolongs the refractory period and increases conduction time. It also decreases CO and possesses anticholinergic, antimalarial, antipyretic, and oxytocic properties. **PO: Onset:** 0.5–3 hr. **Maximum effects, after IM:** 30–90 min. **t½:** 6–7 hr. **Time to peak levels, PO:** 3–5 hr for gluconate salt and 1–1.5 hr for sulfate salt. **IM:** 1 hr. **Therapeutic serum levels:** 2–6 mcg/mL. **Duration:** 6–8 hr for tablets/capsules and 12 hr for extended-release tablets. Metabolized by liver. Urine pH affects rate of urinary excretion (10–50% excreted unchanged). From 60–80% bound to plasma proteins.

USES
(1) Premature atrial, AV junctional, and ventricular contractions. (2) Treatment and control of atrial flutter, established atrial fibrillation, paroxysmal atrial tachycardia, paroxysmal AV junctional rhythm, paroxysmal and chronic atrial fibrillation, paroxysmal ventricular tachycardia not associated with complete heart block. (3) Maintenance therapy after electrical conversion of atrial flutter or fibrillation. The parenteral route is indicated when PO therapy is not feasible or immediate effects are required. *Investigational:* Gluconate salt for life-threatening *Plasmodium falciparum* malaria.

CONTRAINDICATIONS
Hypersensitivity to drug or other cinchona drugs. Myasthenia gravis, history of thrombocytopenic purpura associated with quinidine use, digitalis intoxication evidenced by arrhythmias or AV conduction disorders. Also, complete heart block, left bundle branch block, or other intraventricular conduction defects manifested by marked QRS widening or bizarre complexes. Complete AV block with an AV nodal or idioventricular pacemaker, aberrant ectopic impulses and abnormal rhythms due to escape mechanisms. History of drug-induced torsades de pointes or long QT syndrome.

SPECIAL CONCERNS
Safety in children and during lactation has not been established. Use with extreme caution in clients in whom a sudden change in BP might be detrimental or in those suffering from extensive myocardial damage, subacute endocarditis, bradycardia, coronary occlusion, disturbances in impulse conduction, chronic valvular disease, considerable cardiac enlargement, frank CHF, and renal or hepatic disease. Use with caution in acute infections, hyperthyroidism, muscular weakness, respiratory distress, and bronchial asthma. The dose in geriatric clients may have to be reduced due to age-related changes in renal function.

SIDE EFFECTS
CV: Widening of QRS complex, hypotension, *cardiac asystole,* ectopic ventricular beats, *ventricular tachycardia/ flutter or fibrillation, torsades de pointes,* paradoxical tachycardia, *arterial embolism,* ventricular extrasystoles (one or more every 6 beats), prolonged QT interval, *complete AV block.* **GI:** N&V, abdominal pain, anorexia, diarrhea, urge to defecate as well as urinate, esophagitis (rare). **CNS:** Syncope, headache, confusion, excitement, vertigo, apprehension, delirium, dementia, ataxia, depression. **Dermatologic:** Rash, urticaria, exfoliative dermatitis, photosensitivity, flushing with intense pruri-

Q

tus, eczema, psoriasis, pigmentation abnormalities. **Allergic:** Acute asthma, angioneurotic edema, *respiratory arrest,* dyspnea, fever, *vascular collapse,* purpura, vasculitis, hepatic dysfunction (including granulomatous hepatitis), *hepatic toxicity.* **Hematologic:** Hypoprothrombinemia, *acute hemolytic anemia,* thrombocytopenic purpura, *agranulocytosis,* thrombocytopenia, leukocytosis, neutropenia, shift to left in WBC differential. **Ophthalmologic:** Blurred vision, mydriasis, alterations in color perception, decreased field of vision, double vision, photophobia, optic neuritis, night blindness, scotomata. **Other:** Liver toxicity including hepatitis, lupus nephritis, tinnitus, decreased hearing acuity, arthritis, myalgia, increase in serum skeletal muscle CPK, lupus erythematosus.

LABORATORY TEST CONSIDERATIONS
False + or ↑ PSP, 17-ketosteroids, PT.

OD OVERDOSE MANAGEMENT
Symptoms: **CNS:** Lethargy, confusion, *coma, seizures, respiratory depression or arrest,* headache, paresthesia, vertigo. CNS symptoms may be seen after onset of CV toxicity. **GI:** Vomiting, diarrhea, abdominal pain, hypokalemia, nausea. **CV:** Sinus tachycardia, *ventricular tachycardia or fibrillation, torsades de pointes, depressed automaticity and conduction* (including bundle branch block, sinus bradycardia, SA block, prolongation of QRS and QTc, sinus arrest, AV block, ST depression, T inversion), syncope, *heart failure.* Hypotension due to decreased conduction and CO and vasodilation. **Miscellaneous:** Cinchonism, visual and auditory disturbances, hypokalemia, tinnitus, acidosis.
Treatment:
• Perform gastric lavage, induce vomiting, and administer activated charcoal if ingestion is recent.
• Monitor ECG, blood gases, serum electrolytes, and BP.
• Institute cardiac pacing, if necessary.
• Acidify the urine.
• Use artificial respiration and other supportive measures.

• Infusions of ⅙ molar sodium lactate IV may decrease the cardiotoxic effects.
• Treat hypotension with metaraminol or norepinephrine after fluid volume replacement.
• Use phenytoin or lidocaine to treat tachydysrhythmias.
• Hemodialysis is effective but not often required.

DRUG INTERACTIONS
Acetazolamide, Antacids / ↑ Quinidine effect R/T ↓ renal excretion
Amiodarone / ↑ Quinidine levels with possible fatal cardiac dysrhythmias
Anticholinergic agents, Atropine / Additive effect on blockade of vagus nerve action
Anticoagulants, oral / Additive hypoprothrombinemia with possible hemorrhage
Barbiturates / ↓ Quinidine effect R/T ↑ liver breakdown
 Belladonna leaf/root / Increased anticholinergic effect
Cholinergic agents / Quinidine antagonizes effect of cholinergic drugs
Cimetidine / ↑ Quinidine effect R/T ↓ liver breakdown
Digoxin / ↑ Symptoms of digoxin toxicity
Disopyramide / Either ↑ disopyramide levels or ↓ quinidine levels
Guanethidine / Additive hypotensive effect
Grapefruit juice / ↓ Quinidine absorption and inhibition of quinidine metabolism; effects on the QTc interval delayed and reduced
H *Henbane leaf* / ↑ Anticholinergic effects
Itraconazole / ↑ Risk of tinnitus and ↓ hearing
H *Lily-of-the-valley* / ↑ Effect and side effects of quinidine
Methyldopa / Additive hypotensive effect
Metoprolol / ↑ Metoprolol effect in fast metabolizers
Neuromuscular blocking agents / ↑ Respiratory depression
Nifedipine / ↓ Quinidine effect
H *Pheasant's eye herb* / ↑ Effect and side effects of quinidine

Phenobarbital, Phenytoin / ↓ Quinidine effect R/T ↑ rate of liver metabolism
Potassium / ↑ Quinidine effect
Procainamide / ↑ Procainamide effects with possible toxicity
Propafenone / ↑ Serum propafenone levels in rapid metabolizers
Propranolol / ↑ Propranolol effect in fast metabolizers
Rifampin / ↓ Quinidine effect R/T ↑ liver breakdown
 H *Scopolia root* / ↑ Quinidine effect
Skeletal muscle relaxants / ↑ Skeletal muscle relaxation
Sodium bicarbonate / ↑ Quinidine effect R/T ↓ renal excretion
H *Squill* / ↑ Effect and side effects of quinidine
Sucralfate / ↓ Serum quinidine levels → ↓ effect
Thiazide diuretics / ↑ Quinidine effect R/T ↓ renal excretion
Tricyclic antidepressants / ↑ TCA effect R/T ↓ clearance
Verapamil / ↓ Verapamil clearance → ↑ hypotension, bradycardia, AV block, VT, and pulmonary edema

HOW SUPPLIED

Quinidine gluconate: *Injection:* 80 mg/mL; *Tablet, Extended Release:* 324 mg.
Quinidine sulfate: *Tablet:* 200 mg, 300 mg; *Tablet, Extended Release:* 300 mg

DOSAGE————————

• **QUINIDINE SULFATE TABLETS**
Premature atrial and ventricular contractions.
Adults: 200–300 mg 3–4 times per day.
Paroxysmal SVTs.
Adults: 400–600 mg q 2–3 hr until the paroxysm is terminated.
Conversion of atrial flutter.
Adults: 200 mg q 2–3 hr for five to eight doses; daily doses can be increased until rhythm is restored or toxic effects occur.
Conversion of atrial flutter, maintenance therapy.
Adults: 200–300 mg 3–4 times per day. Large doses or more frequent administration may be required in some clients.
• **QUINIDINE GLUCONATE AND QUINIDINE SULFATE EXTENDED-RELEASE TABLETS**
All uses.

Adults: 300–600 mg q 8–12 hr.
• **QUINIDINE GLUCONATE INJECTION (IM OR IV)**
Acute tachycardia.
Adults, initial: 600 mg IM; **then,** 400 mg IM repeated as often as q 2 hr.
Arrhythmias.
Adults: 330 mg IM or less IV (as much as 500–750 mg may be required).
P. falciparum malaria.
Two regimens may be used. (1) *Loading dose:* 15 mg/kg in 250 mL NSS given over 4 hr; **then,** 24 hr after beginning the loading dose, institute 7.5 mg/kg infused over 4 hr and given q 8 hr for 7 days or until PO therapy can be started. (2) **Loading dose:** 10 mg/kg in 250 mL NSS infused over 1–2 hr followed immediately by 0.02 mg/kg/min for up to 72 hr or until parasitemia decreases to less than 1% or PO therapy can be started.

NURSING CONSIDERATIONS

ⓒ Do not confuse quinidine with quinine (an antimalarial) or with clonidine (an antihypertensive).

ADMINISTRATION/STORAGE

1. A preliminary test dose may be given. **Adults:** 200 mg quinidine sulfate or quinidine gluconate administered PO or IM. **Children:** Test dose of 2 mg/kg of quinidine sulfate.
2. The extended-release forms are not interchangeable.
IV 3. Prepare IV solution by diluting 10 mL of quinidine gluconate injection (800 mg) with 50 mL of D5W; give at a rate of 1 mL/min.
4. Use only colorless clear solution for injection. Light may cause quinidine to crystallize, which turns solution brownish.

ASSESSMENT

1. Note any allergic reactions to antiarrhythmic drugs or tartrazine, which is found in some formulations. Perform a test dose; observe for hypersensitivity reactions and check for intolerance.
2. Document indications for therapy, onset, and symptom characteristics.
3. Obtain CXR; monitor electrolytes, CBC, liver and renal function studies.

H = Herbal   IV = Intravenous   ⓒ = sound-alike drug

4. Assess VS and ECG; note heart and lung findings.

INTERVENTIONS

1. Report any increased AV block, prolonged PR or QT intervals, cardiac irritability, or rhythm suppression during IV administration and stop drug therapy.
2. Monitor I&O, VS; observe for ↓ BP. Drug induces urinary alkalization.
3. Report any neurologic deficits/sensory impairment (i.e., numbness, confusion, psychosis, depression, or involuntary movements).
4. Report any persistent diarrhea. Among the elderly, there is a higher risk of toxicity, reduced CO, and unpredictable effects from drug.
5. Clients with long-standing atrial fibrillation or CHF with atrial fibrillation run a risk of embolization from mural thrombi when converting to sinus rhythm. Ensure antiocoagulated to prevent thromboembolism.
6. Monitor LFTs, PT/INR to ensure no adverse drug side effects.

CLIENT/FAMILY TEACHING

1. Take with food to minimize GI effects.
2. Avoid activities that require mental alertness until drug effects realized; may cause dizziness or blurred vision.
3. Add fruit and grain to diet. A high intake of fruits and vegetables (alkaline-ash foods) may prolong drug half-life. However, avoid grapefruit juice if taking quinidine sulfate extended-release tablets. Intake of salt may increase the plasma levels of quinidine.
4. Report any of the following symptoms:
- Severe skin rash, hives, or itching
- Severe headache
- Unexplained fever
- Ringing in the ears, buzzing, or hearing loss
- Unusual bruising or bleeding
- Blurred vision
- Irregular heart beat, palpitations, or faintness
- Continued diarrhea
5. Wear dark glasses if light sensitive.
6. Report for labs, ECG, PFTs, and eye exams.

OUTCOMES/EVALUATE

- Restoration of stable rhythm
- Therapeutic drug levels (2–6 mcg/mL)

R

Ramipril ■ⓒ

(RAM-ih-prill)

CLASSIFICATION(S):
Antihypertensive, ACE inhibitor
PREGNANCY CATEGORY: D
Rx: Altace

SEE ALSO ANGIOTENSIN-CONVERTING ENZYME INHIBITORS.

ACTION/KINETICS

Onset: 1–2 hr. From 50–60% bioavailable. **Time to peak serum levels:** 1 hr (1–2 hr for ramiprilat, the active metabolite). **Peak effect:** 3–6 hr. Ramiprilat has approximately six times the ACE inhibitory activity than ramipril. **t½:** 1–2 hr (9–18 hr for ramiprilat); prolonged in impaired renal function. **Duration:** 24 hr. Metabolized in the liver with 60% excreted through the urine and 40% in the feces. Food decreases the rate, but not the extent, of absorption of ramipril. About 73% of ramipril and 56% of ramiprilat bound to plasma proteins.

USES

(1) Alone or in combination with other antihypertensive agents (especially thiazide diuretics) for the treatment of hypertension. (2) Treatment of CHF following MI to decrease risk of CV death and decrease the risk of failure-related hospitalization and progression to severe or resistant heart failure. (3) Reduce risk of stroke, MI, and death from

---

Bold Italic = life threatening side effect   ■ = black box warning   ✚ = Available in Canada

CV causes in clients over 55 years with a history of CAD, stroke, peripheral vascular disease, or with diabetes and one other risk factor (e.g., elevated cholesterol, cigarette smoking). Can be used in addition to other therapy, including antihypertensive, antiplatelet, or lipid-lowering therapy.

CONTRAINDICATIONS
Lactation.

SPECIAL CONCERNS
■When used during the second and third trimesters of pregnancy, injury and even death can result in the developing fetus. When pregnancy is detected, discontinue as soon as possible.■ Geriatric clients may manifest higher peak blood levels of ramiprilat. May cause hyperkalemia, especially when used with salt substitutes.

SIDE EFFECTS
CV: Hypotension, chest pain, palpitations, angina pectoris, orthostatic hypotension, *MI, CVA, arrhythmias.* **GI:** N&V, abdominal pain, diarrhea, dysgeusia, anorexia, constipation, dry mouth, dyspepsia, enzyme changes suggesting pancreatitis, dysphagia, gastroenteritis, increased salivation. **CNS:** Headache, dizziness, fatigue, insomnia, sleep disturbances, somnolence, depression, nervousness, malaise, vertigo, anxiety, amnesia, *convulsions,* tremor. **Respiratory:** Cough, dyspnea, URI, asthma, *bronchospasm.* **Hematologic:** Leukopenia, anemia, eosinophilia. Rarely, decreases in hemoglobin or hematocrit. **Dermatologic:** Diaphoresis, photosensitivity, pruritus, rash, dermatitis, purpura, alopecia, erythema multiforme, urticaria. **Body as a whole:** Paresthesias, angioedema, asthenia, syncope, fever, muscle cramps, myalgia, arthralgia, arthritis, neuralgia, neuropathy, influenza, edema. **Miscellaneous:** Impotence, tinnitus, hearing loss, vision disturbances, epistaxis, weight gain, proteinuria, angioneurotic edema, edema, flu syndrome.

LABORATORY TEST CONSIDERATIONS
↓ H&H.

HOW SUPPLIED
Capsule: 1.25 mg, 2.5 mg, 5 mg, 10 mg

DOSAGE
• **CAPSULES**
Hypertension.
Initial: 2.5 mg once daily in clients not taking a diuretic; **maintenance:** 2.5–20 mg/day as a single dose or two equally divided doses.
CHF following MI.
Initial: 2.5 mg twice a day. Clients intolerant of this dose may be started on 1.25 mg twice a day. The target maintenance dose is 5 mg twice a day.
Reduce risk of MI, stroke, death in clients 55 and over with risk factors.
Initial: 2.5 mg/day for 1 week followed by 5 mg/day for the next 3 weeks. **Maintenance:** 10 mg/day. If the client is hypertensive or post-MI, the dose can be divided. *NOTE:* In clients with a C_{CR} of 40 mL/min/m^2 or less, doses of 25% of those normally used should cause full therapeutic levels of ramiprilat. For use in hypertension, start with 1.25 mg once daily; dose may be titrated upward until BP is controlled or to a maximum of 5 mg/day. For use in heart-failure post MI, start with 1.25 mg once daily. Dose may be increased to 1.25 mg twice a day, up to a maximum of 2.5 mg twice a day, depending on response and tolerability.

NURSING CONSIDERATIONS
℗ Do not confuse Altace with Artane (cholinergic blocking agent).

ADMINISTRATION/STORAGE
1. If the antihypertensive effect decreases at the end of the dosing interval with once-daily dosing, consider either twice-daily administration or an increase in dose.
2. If taking a diuretic, discontinue the diuretic 2–3 days prior to beginning ramipril. If BP is not controlled, reinstitute the diuretic. If the diuretic cannot be discontinued, consider an initial dose of ramipril of 1.25 mg.

ASSESSMENT
Note indications for therapy, other agents trialed and the outcome. Monitor BP, K^+, microalbumin, CBC, liver and renal fuction to ensure no abnormality.

R

CLIENT/FAMILY TEACHING

1. For ease of swallowing, may mix contents of the capsule with water, apple juice, or apple sauce.
2. Use caution; drug may cause drowsiness or dizziness and low BP effects with sudden changes in position.
3. Report any persistent, dry, nonproductive cough, increased SOB, edema, significant weight gain, or unusual bruising/bleeding.
4. Do not take any OTC agents, including potassium/potassium-based salt supplements without approval.
5. Record BP at different times of day/night for provider review.

OUTCOMES/EVALUATE

- ↓ BP
- ↓ Mortality with AMI/DM

Reteplase recombinant

(**REE**-teh-place)

CLASSIFICATION(S):

Thrombolytic, tissue plasminogen activator
PREGNANCY CATEGORY: C
Rx: Retavase

ACTION/KINETICS

Plasminogen activator that catalyzes the cleavage of endogenous plasminogen to generate plasmin. Plasmin, in turn, degrades the matrix of the thrombus, causing a thrombolytic effect. **t ½:** 13 to 16 min. Cleared primarily by the liver and kidney.

USES

Acute MI in adults for improvement of ventricular function, reduction of the incidence of CHF, and reduction of mortality. *Investigational:* Clearance of occluded venous catheters, thrombolytic treatment of acute and chronic DVT, treatment of massive pulmonary embolism with a double bolus, with heparin and percutaneous transluminal angioplasty to treat thrombosed polytetrafluoroethylene hemodialysis arteriovenous grafts.

CONTRAINDICATIONS

Active internal bleeding; history of CVA; recent intracranial or intraspinal surgery or trauma; intracranial neoplasm, arteriovenous malformation, or aneurysm; known bleeding diathesis; severe uncontrolled hypertension.

SPECIAL CONCERNS

Use with caution during lactation. Safety and efficacy have not been determined in children.

SIDE EFFECTS

Bleeding disorders: From internal bleeding sites, including intracranial, retroperitoneal, GI, GU, or respiratory. *Hemorrhage may occur.* From superficial bleeding sites, including venous cutdowns, arterial punctures, sites of recent surgery. **CV: *Cholesterol embolism,*** coronary thrombolysis resulting in arrhythmias associated with perfusion (no different from those seen in the ordinary course of acute MI), cardiogenic shock, sinus bradycardia, accelerated idioventricular rhythm, ventricular premature depolarizations, SVT, ventricular tachycardia, *ventricular fibrillation,* AV block, pulmonary edema, *heart failure, cardiac arrest, recurrent ischemia, myocardial rupture, cardiac tamponade, venous thrombosis or embolism, electromechanical dissociation, mitral regurgitation, pericardial effusion, pericarditis.* **Hypersensitivity:** Serious allergic reactions. *NOTE:* Many of the CV side effects listed are frequent sequelae of MI and may or may not be attributable to reteplase recombinant.

LABORATORY TEST CONSIDERATIONS

↓ Plasminogen, fibrinogen. Degradation of fibrinogen in blood samples removed for analysis.

DRUG INTERACTIONS

Use with abciximab, aspirin, dipyridamole, heparin, or vitamin K antagonists may increase the risk of bleeding.

HOW SUPPLIED

Powder for Injection, lyophilized: 10.4 international units (18.1 mg)

DOSAGE—————————

- **IV ONLY**
  Acute MI.
  Adults: 10 + 10 unit double-bolus injection. Each bolus is given over 2 min,

---

with the second bolus given 30 min after initiation of the first bolus injection.

NURSING CONSIDERATIONS
ADMINISTRATION/STORAGE
IV 1. Initiate treatment as soon as possible after symptom onset.

2. Have available antiarrhythmic therapy for bradycardia and/or ventricular irritability.

3. Give each bolus by an IV line in which no other medication is being simultaneously infused/injected. Do not add any other medication to the reteplase solution. If drug is to be given through an IV line containing heparin, flush normal saline or D5W through the line prior to and following reteplase injection.

4. Reconstitution is performed using the diluent, syringe, needle, and dispensing pin provided with the drug as follows:

• Remove the flip-cap from one vial of sterile water (preservative free), and, with the syringe provided, withdraw 10 mL of the sterile water.

• Open the package containing the dispensing pin. Remove the needle from the syringe and discard. Remove the protective cap from the spike end of the dispensing pin and connect the syringe to the dispensing pin. Remove the protective flip-cap from one vial of reteplase.

• Remove the protective cap from the spike end of the dispensing pin, and insert the spike into the vial of reteplase. Transfer the 10 mL of sterile water through the dispensing pin into the vial.

• With the dispensing pin and syringe still attached to the vial, gently swirl the vial to dissolve the reteplase. *Do not shake.*

• Withdraw the 10 mL of reconstituted reteplase back into the syringe (a small amount will remain due to overfill).

• Detach the syringe from the dispensing pin, and attach the sterile 20-gauge needle provided. The solution is ready to administer.

5. Since reteplase contains no antibacterial preservatives, reconstitute just prior to use. When reconstituted as directed, the solution may be used within 4 hr when stored at 2–30°C (36–86°F).

6. Keep the kit sealed until use and store at 2–25°C (36–77°F).

ASSESSMENT
1. Document indications for therapy, noting onset, pain level, and characteristics of chest pain.

2. List drugs currently prescribed to ensure none interact unfavorably.

3. Note evidence of CVA, internal bleeding, trauma, neurosurgery, or bleeding disorders.

4. Obtain CBC, type and cross, coagulation times, cardiac panel, and liver and renal function studies.

5. Note cardiopulmonary assessments and ECG.

INTERVENTIONS
1. During administration, continuously monitor cardiac rhythm. Have medications available for management of arrhythmias. Record VS every 15 min during infusion and for 2 hr following.

2. Administer first dose over 2 min and the second dose 30 min later if no serious bleeding is observed. In the event of any uncontrolled bleeding, terminate the heparin infusion and withhold the second dose.

3. Observe all puncture sites and areas for evidence of bleeding. Arterial sticks require 30 min of manual pressure followed by application of a pressure dressing.

4. Assess for reperfusion reactions such as:

• Arrhythmias usually of short duration, which may include bradycardia or ventricular tachycardia

• Reduction of chest pain

• Return of elevated ST segment and smaller Q waves

5. Maintain bedrest and observe for S&S of abnormal bleeding (hematuria, hematemesis, melena, CVA, cardiac tamponade).

CLIENT/FAMILY TEACHING
1. Review goals of therapy and inherent risks of drug therapy during acute coronary artery occlusion.

R

2. To be effective, therapy should be instituted as soon as possible after symptom onset.

3. Encourage family members to learn CPR.

OUTCOMES/EVALUATE
Improved ventricular function; ↓ incidence of CHF, and ↓ mortality with AMI

Rosuvastatin calcium
(roe-SUE-vuh-stah-tin)

CLASSIFICATION(S):
Antihyperlipidemic, HMG-CoA reductase inhibitor
PREGNANCY CATEGORY: X
Rx: Crestor

SEE ALSO ANTIHYPERLIPIDEMIC AGENTS, HMG-COA REDUCTASE INHIBITORS.

ACTION/KINETICS
Reduces total cholesterol, LDL-C, ApoB, and nonHDL-C in clients with homozygous and heterozygous familial hypercholesterolemia, nonfamilial forms of hypercholesterolemia, and mixed dyslipidemia. Also, reduces triglycerides and increases HDL-C. **Peak plasma levels:** 3–5 hr. Absolute bioavailability is about 20%. About 10% metabolized by CYP2C9 to N-desmethyl rosuvastatin which has some activity. Excreted primarily (90%) in the feces. **t ½, elimination:** About 19 hr. Severe renal or hepatic insufficiency significantly increase plasma levels. About 95% bound to plasma proteins.

USES
(1) As an adjunct to diet in heterozygous familial and nonfamilial hypercholesterolemia. (2) Adjunct to diet in mixed dyslipidemia (Fredrickson Type IIa and IIb). (3) Adjunct to diet in elevated serum triglyceride levels (Fredrickson type IV). (4) Reduce LDL-C, total-C, and Apo-B in homozygous familial hypercholesterolemia (as an adjunct to other lipid-lowering treatments).

CONTRAINDICATIONS
Pregnancy and lactation. Use in clients with active liver disease or with unexplained persistent elevations of serum transaminases.

SPECIAL CONCERNS
Use with caution in clients who consume substantial amounts of alcohol and/or have a history of liver disease. Use with caution in those 65 years and older, in hypothyroidism, and renal insufficiency (all predispose clients to myopathy). Cases (rare) of rhabomyolysis with acute renal failure secondary to myoglobinuria have been reported.

SIDE EFFECTS
The most frequent side effects are myalgia, constipation, asthenia, abdominal pain, and nausea. **Musculoskeletal:** Rhabdomyolysis with acute renal failure, myalgia, muscle aches, muscle weakness, arthritis, arthralgia, pathological fracture, myasthenia, myositis. **CNS:** Headache, dizziness, insomnia, hypertonia, paresthesia, depression, anxiety, vertigo, neuralgia. **GI:** Diarrhea, dyspepsia, abdominal pain, nausea, constipation, gastroenteritis, vomiting, flatulence, periodontal abscess, gastritis, hepatitis, pancreatitis. **Respiratory:** Pharyngitis, rhinitis, sinusitis, bronchitis, increased cough, dyspnea, pneumonia, asthma. **Body as a whole:** Asthenia, flu syndrome, accidental injury, infection, pain, peripheral edema, syncope. **CV:** Hypertension, angina pectoris, vasodilation, palpitation, arrhythmia. **Hypersensitivity:** Facial edema, thrombocytopenia, leukopenia, vesiculobullous rash, urticaria, angioedema. **Miscellaneous:** Back pain, chest pain, pelvic pain, neck pain, UTI, diabetes mellitus, anemia, ecchymosis, rash, pruritus, kidney damage/failure, organ failure, photosensitivity reaction.

LABORATORY TEST CONSIDERATIONS
↑ Serum transaminases (up to 3 or more times ULN), creatine kinase, bilirubin, glutamyl transpeptidase. Proteinuria, microscopic hematuria, hyperglycemia. Thyroid function abnormalities.

DRUG INTERACTIONS

Antacids, Al/Mg combination / ↓ Rosuvastastin plasma levels; give antacid 2 hr after rosuvastatin

Cyclosporine / Significant ↑ of rosuvastastin C$_{max}$ and AUC → ↑ risk of myopathy

Gemfibrozil / Significant ↑ of rosuvastatin C$_{max}$ and AUC → ↑ risk of myopathy

Oral contraceptives / ↑ Plasma levels of ethinyl estradiol and norgestrel

Warfarin / Significant ↑ INR

HOW SUPPLIED

Tablet: 5 mg, 10 mg, 20 mg, 40 mg

DOSAGE————————————

• **TABLETS**

Heterozygous familial and nonfamilial hypercholesterolemia, Mixed dyslipidemia (Fredrickson Type IIa and IIb).

Individualize therapy. **Initial:** 10 mg once daily (use 5 mg once daily for those requiring less aggressive LDL-C reductions or who have predisposing factors for myopathy). For clients with marked hypercholesterolemia (LDL-C greater than 190 mg/dL) and aggressive lipid targets, consider a 20-mg starting dose. Reserve the 40-mg dose for those who have not achieved goal LDL-C at 20 mg.

Homozygous familial hypercholesterolemia.

Initial: 20 mg once daily. **Maximum recommended dose:** 40 mg daily. Use as an adjunct to other lipid-lowering treatments.

NOTE: For clients with severe renal impairment (C$_{CR}$ less than 30 mL/min/1.73 m^2 not on hemodialysis), use an initial dose of 5 mg once daily; dosage should not exceed 10 mg once daily.

NURSING CONSIDERATIONS

ADMINISTRATION/STORAGE

1. Temporarily withhold rosuvastatin in clients with an acute, serious condition suggestive of myopathy or predisposing to the development of renal failure secondary to rhabdomyolysis (e.g., sepsis, hypotension, major surgery, trauma, uncontrolled seizures and severe metabolic, endocrine, and electrolyte disorders).

2. Before beginning rosuvastatin therapy, try to control hypercholesterolemia with appropriate diet and exercise, weight reduction in obese clients, and treatment of underlying medical problems. Continue cholesterol-lowering diet during drug treatment.

3. In clients taking cyclosporine, limit the rosuvastatin dose to 5 mg once daily.

4. The effect of rosuvastatin on LDL-C and total cholesterol may be enhanced if used with a bile acid binding resin such as gemfibrozil. If gemfibrozil is used with rosuvastatin, limit the dose of rosuvastatin to 10 mg once daily.

5. Consider a dose reduction in clients on 40 mg rosuvastatin therapy with unexplained persistent proteinuria during routine urinalysis.

6. Store at controlled room temperature protected from moisture.

ASSESSMENT

1. Note indications for therapy: plaque stability or elevated TG/LDL cholesterol in CAD.

2. Monitor CBC, cholesterol profile, liver, CPK, and renal function studies. Schedule LFTs at the beginning of therapy and semiannually for the first year of therapy. Special attention should be paid to elevated serum transaminase levels.

3. List all medications prescribed to ensure none interact unfavorably. Identify/list risk factors.

4. Assess level of adherence to weight reduction, exercise, and cholesterol-lowering diet and BP or BS control. Note any alcohol abuse.

CLIENT/FAMILY TEACHING

1. Take once daily with or without food as directed. Do not use antacid for 2 hr after consuming drug.

2. Report any S&S of infections, unexplained muscle pain, tenderness/weakness (especially if accompanied by fever or malaise), surgery, trauma, or metabolic disorders.

3. Review importance of following a low-cholesterol diet, regular exercise, low alcohol consumption, and not smoking in the overall plan to reduce

R

serum cholesterol levels and inhibit progression of CAD.

4. Not for use during pregnancy; use barrier contraception.

5. Report as scheduled for labs and F/U to assess drug response.

OUTCOMES/EVALUATE
↓ Total cholesterol and triglycerides
↑ HDL

Simvastatin ©

(**sim**-vah-**STAH**-tin)

CLASSIFICATION(S):
Antihyperlipidemic, HMG-CoA reductase inhibitor
PREGNANCY CATEGORY: X
Rx: Zocor

SEE ALSO *ANTIHYPERLIPIDEMIC AGENTS, HMG–COA REDUCTASE INHIBITORS.*

ACTION/KINETICS
Does not reduce basal plasma cortisol or testosterone levels or impair renal reserve. **Peak therapeutic response:** 4–6 weeks. Approximately 85% absorbed; significant first-pass effect with less than 5% of a PO dose reaching the general circulation. **t ½:** 3 hr. Metabolites excreted in the feces (60%) and urine (13%). Increased levels seen in those with hepatic and severe renal insufficiency. About 95% bound to plasma proteins.

USES
(1) Adjunct to diet to reduce elevated total and LDL cholesterol, apoprotein B, and triglyceride levels in hypercholesterolemia and mixed dyslipidemia (types IIa and IIb) when the response to diet and other approaches has been inadequate. (2) To increase HDL cholesterol in primary hypercholesterolemia and mixed dyslipidemias. (3) Treatment of isolated hypertriglyceridemia (Frederickson IV) and hyperlipoproteinemia (type III). (4) In coronary heart disease and hypercholesterolemia to reduce risk of total mortality by reducing coronary death; to reduce the risk of non-

fatal MI; to reduce the risk for undergoing myocardial revascularization procedures; to reduce the risk of stroke or TIAs. (5) As an adjunct to diet to reduce total and LDL cholesterol and Apo-B levels in adolescent boys and girls who are at least 1 year postmenarche, 10–17 years of age, with heterozygous familial hypercholesterolemia. Given if after an adequate trial of diet therapy, LDL cholesterol remains 190 mg/dL or greater or LDL cholesterol remains 160 mg/dL or greater and there is a positive family history of premature CV disease or 2 or more other CV disease risk factors are present in the adolescent client. *Investigational:* Heterozygous familial hypercholesterolemia, familial combined hyperlipidemia, diabetic dyslipidemia in NIDD, hyperlipidemia secondary to the nephrotic syndrome, and homozygous familial hypercholesterolemia in clients with defective LDL receptors. *NOTE:* Simvastatin reduces risks of fatal and nonfatal heart attacks and strokes, as well as reduces the need for bypass surgery and angioplasty.

CONTRAINDICATIONS
Use if pregnant, planning to become pregnant, or while breastfeeding.

SPECIAL CONCERNS
Use with caution in clients who have a history of liver disease/consume large quantities of alcohol or with drugs that affect steroid levels or activity. Higher plasma levels may be observed in clients with hepatic and severe renal insufficiency. Safety and efficacy have not been determined in children less than 18 years of age.

SIDE EFFECTS

Musculoskeletal: Rhabdomyolysis with renal dysfunction secondary to myoglobinuria, myopathy, arthralgias. **GI:** N&V, diarrhea, abdominal pain, constipation, flatulence, dyspepsia, pancreatitis, anorexia, stomatitis. **Hepatic:** Hepatitis (including chronic active hepatitis), cholestatic jaundice, cirrhosis, fatty change in liver, *fulminant hepatic necrosis, hepatoma.* **Neurologic:** Dysfunction of certain cranial nerves resulting in alteration of taste, impairment of extraocular movement, and facial paresis. Paresthesia, peripheral neuropathy, peripheral nerve palsy. **CNS:** Headache, tremor, vertigo, memory loss, anxiety, insomnia, depression. **Hypersensitivity reactions:** Although rare, the following symptoms have been noted: *Angioedema, anaphylaxis,* lupus erythematous–like syndrome, vasculitis, purpura, thrombocytopenia, leukopenia, *hemolytic anemia,* polymyalgia rheumatica, positive ANA, ESR increase, arthritis, arthralgia, asthenia, urticaria, photosensitivity, chills, fever, flushing, malaise, dyspnea, *toxic epidermal necrolysis, erythema multiforme (including Stevens-Johnson syndrome).* **GU:** Gynecomastia, loss of libido, erectile dysfunction. **Ophthalmologic:** Lens opacities, ophthalmoplegia. **Hematologic:** Transient asymptomatic eosinophilia, anemia, thrombocytopenia, leukopenia. **Miscellaneous:** URI, asthenia, alopecia, edema.

LABORATORY TEST CONSIDERATIONS

↑ CPK, AST, ALT.

ADDITIONAL DRUG INTERACTIONS

Amiodarone / Possibility of myopathy, muscle weakness, and rhabdomyolysis; if used together, do not give client more than 20 mg/day of simvastatin
Bosentan / ↓ Simvastatin levels R/T ↑ metabolism
Carbamazepine / ↓ Simvastatin AUC, peak levels, and shortended t½ R/T ↑ metabolism by CYP3A4
Clarithromycin / ↑ Risk of severe myopathy and rhabdomyolysis
Diltiazem ↑ Risk of myopathy R/T ↑ simvastatin plasma levels

Erythromycin / ↑ Risk of severe myopathy and rhabdomyolysis
Grapefruit juice / Chronic use of grapefruit juice ↑ simvastatin plasma levels due to ↓ liver metabolism
Nefazodone / ↑ Risk of myopathy
Protease inhibitors (e.g., nelfinavir, ritonavir) / ↑ Simvastatin plasma levels → ↑ risk of myopathy
H   *St. John's wort* / ↓ Simvastatin plasma levels → ↓ efficacy
Verapamil / ↑ Risk of myopathy
Warfarin / ↑ INR

HOW SUPPLIED

Tablet: 5 mg, 10 mg, 20 mg, 40 mg, 80 mg

DOSAGE

- **TABLETS**

  Hyperlipidemia, Coronary heart disease.

Adults, initially: 20 mg once daily in the evening; **maintenance:** 5–80 mg/day as a single dose in the evening. Consider a starting dose of 5 mg/day for clients on immunosuppressants (e.g., cyclosporine), those with LDL less than 190 mg/dL, or in those with severe renal insufficiency. Consider a starting dose of 10 mg/day for clients with LDL greater than 190 mg/dL. Consider a starting dose of 40 mg as an alternative for those who require a reduction of more than 45% in their LDL cholesterol (most often those with CAD). For geriatric clients, the starting dose should be 5 mg/day with maximum LDL reductions seen with 20 mg or less daily. Do not exceed 10 mg/day if used in combination with fibrates or niacin.

  Homozygous familial hypercholesterolemia.

Adults: 40 mg/day in the evening or 80 mg/day in 3 divided doses of 20 mg, 20 mg, and an evening dose of 40 mg. Use as an adjunct to other lipid-lowering treatments.

  Adolescents 10–17 years of age with heterozygous familial hypercholesterolemia.

Initial: 10 mg once a day in the evening. **Dose range:** 10–40 mg/day (maximum). Individualize dose. Adjust at intervals of 4 weeks or more.

S

H = Herbal   IV = Intravenous   © = sound-alike drug

NURSING CONSIDERATIONS

℮ Do not confuse Zocor (trade name for simvastatin) with Cozaar (an antihypertensive) or with Zoloft (an antidepressant).

ADMINISTRATION/STORAGE

1. Place client on a standard cholesterol-lowering diet for 3–6 months before starting simvastatin. Continue the diet during drug therapy.
2. May give without regard to meals.
3. Dosage may be adjusted at intervals of at least 4 weeks.
4. In clients taking cyclosporine together with simvastatin, begin therapy with 5 mg/day of simvastatin; do not exceed 10 mg/day.
5. In clients taking amiodarone or verapamil together with simvastatin, the dose of simvastatin should not exceed 20 mg/day.
6. Simvastatin is effective alone or together with bile acid sequestrants. Avoid use of simvastatin with gemfibrozil, other fibrates, or lipid-lowering doses (1 g/day or more) of niacin unless the benefit of further alteration in lipid levels is likely to outweigh the increased risk of the drug combination. However, if simvastatin is used together with fibrates or niacin, do not exceed 10 mg/day of simvastatin.

ASSESSMENT

1. Note indications for therapy: plaque stability or elevated TG/LDL cholesterol in CAD.
2. Monitor CBC, cholesterol profile, liver, CPK, and renal function studies. Schedule LFTs at the beginning of therapy and semiannually for the first year of therapy. A LFT should be done before the dose is increased to 80 mg, three months after the change, and twice a year thereafter. Special attention should be paid to elevated serum transaminase levels.
3. List all medications prescribed to ensure none interact unfavorably. Anticipate reduced dose with certain drug combinations. Identify/list risk factors.
4. Assess level of adherence to weight reduction, exercise, and cholesterol-lowering diet, and BP or BS control. Note any alcohol abuse.

CLIENT/FAMILY TEACHING

1. Take once or twice daily as directed. More preferable in evening.
2. A low-cholesterol diet must be followed during drug therapy. Consult dietitian for assistance in meal planning and food preparation. Do not take with grapefruit juice. May enjoy grapefruit juice at other times during the day.
3. Report any S&S of infections, unexplained muscle pain, tenderness/weakness (especially if accompanied by fever or malaise), surgery, trauma, or metabolic disorders. Report as scheduled for lab tests, eye exam, and F/U.
4. Review importance of regular exercise, low alcohol consumption, smoking abstinence, and following a low-cholesterol diet in the overall plan to reduce serum cholesterol levels and inhibit progression of CAD.
5. Not for use during pregnancy; use barrier contraception.
6. May experience sun sensitivity; take precautions to avoid sun or use sun protection.

OUTCOMES/EVALUATE

↓ Serum triglycerides and LDL cholesterol levels; cardiovascular risk reduction

Sotalol hydrochloride ■
(**SOH**-tah-lol)

CLASSIFICATION(S):
Beta-adrenergic blocking agent
PREGNANCY CATEGORY: B
Rx: Betapace, Betapace AF, Sotalol HCl AF
✦Rx: Apo-Sotalol, Gen-Sotalol, Lin-Sotalol, Novo-Sotalol, Nu-Sotalol, PMS-Sotalol, ratio-Sotalol, Rhoxal-sotalol, Sotacor

SEE ALSO *BETA-ADRENERGIC BLOCKING AGENTS.*

ACTION/KINETICS
Blocks both beta-1- and beta-2-adrenergic receptors; has no membrane-stabi-

lizing activity or intrinsic sympathomimetic activity. Has both Group II and Group III antiarrhythmic properties (dose dependent). Significantly increases the refractory period of the atria, His-Purkinje fibers, and ventricles. Also prolongs the QTc and JT intervals. **t ½:** 12 hr. Not metabolized; excreted unchanged in the urine.

USES
(1) Treatment of documented ventricular arrhythmias such as life-threatening sustained VT. (2) Betapace AF is used for maintenance of normal sinus rhythm in those with symptomatic atrial fibrillation/atrial flutter who are in sinus rhythm; since Betapace AF can cause life-threatening ventricular arrhythmias, reserve use for those who are highly symptomatic. *Do not substitute Betapace for Betapace AF.*

CONTRAINDICATIONS
Use in asymptomatic PVCs or supraventricular arrhythmias due to the proarrhythmic effects of sotalol. Congenital or acquired long QT syndromes. Use in clients with hypokalemia or hypomagnesemia until the imbalance is corrected, as these conditions aggravate the degree of QT prolongation and increase the risk for torsades de pointes.

SPECIAL CONCERNS
■(1) To minimize the risk of induced arrhythmia, those initiated or reinitiated on Betapace or Betapace AF should be placed for a minimum of 3 days (on their maintenance dose) in a facility that can provide cardiac resuscitation, continuous electrocardiographic monitoring, and calculations of creatinine clearance. Consult the package insert for detailed instructions regarding dose selection and special cautions for those with renal impairment. (2) Do not substitute Betapace for Betapace AF because of significant differences in labeling (e.g., patient package insert, dosing administration, and safety information).■ Clients with sustained ventricular tachycardia and a history of CHF appear to be at the highest risk for serious proarrhythmia. Dose, presence of sustained ventricular tachycardia, females, excessive prolongation of the QTc interval, and history of cardiomegaly or CHF are risk factors for torsades de pointes. Use with caution in clients with chronic bronchitis or emphysema and in asthma if an IV agent is required. Use with extreme caution in clients with SSS associated with symptomatic arrhythmias due to the increased risk of sinus bradycardia, sinus pauses, or sinus arrest. Reduce dosage in impaired renal function. Safety and efficacy in children have not been established. Do *not* interchange Betapace and Betapace AF due to significant differences in dosage and safety, although clients can be transferred to Betapace AF from Betapace.

ADDITIONAL SIDE EFFECTS
CV: *New or worsened ventricular arrhythmias, including sustained VT or ventricular fibrillation that might be fatal. Torsades de pointes.*

HOW SUPPLIED
Betapace Tablets: 80 mg, 120 mg, 160 mg, 240 mg; **Betapace AF Tablets**: 80 mg, 120 mg,160 mg; **Sotalol HCl:** 80 mg, 120 mg, 160 mg, 240 mg

DOSAGE

- **BETAPACE TABLETS**
  Ventricular arrhythmias.

Adults, initial: 80 mg twice a day. The dose may be increased to 240 or 320 mg/day after appropriate evaluation. **Usual:** 160–320 mg/day given in two or three divided doses. Clients with life-threatening refractory ventricular arrhythmias may require doses ranging from 480 to 640 mg/day (due to potential proarrhythmias; use these doses only if the potential benefit outweighs the increased risk of side effects). Use the following doses in clients with impaired renal function: 80 mg twice a day if C_{CR} is greater than 60 mL/min, 80 mg once daily if the C_{CR} is between 30 and 59 mL/min, and 80 mg every 36–48 hr if the CCR is between 10 and 29 mL/min. Individualize dose if the C_{CR} is < 10 mL/min.

- **BETAPACE AF TABLETS**
  Maintenance of normal sinus rhythm in those with symptomatic atrial fibrillation/atrial flutter who are in sinus rhythm.

S

Dose individualized according to calculated creatinine clearance. **Initial:** 80 mg. **Maintenance:** 80 mg twice a day if C_{CR} is greater than 60 mL/min and 80 mg once daily if the C_{CR} is between 40 and 60 mL/min. Do not use in clients with a C_{CR} less than 40 mL/min. Can be titrated upward to 120 mg during initial hospitalization or after discharge on 80 mg in the event of recurrence, by re-hospitalization and repeating the same steps used during initiation of therapy. An increase in dose to 160 mg twice a day or daily can be considered if the 120 mg dose does not reduce the frequency of early relapse of AFIB/AF and is tolerated without excessive QT interval prolongation. Doses higher than 160 mg twice a day are associated with an increased incidence of torsade de pointes.

NURSING CONSIDERATIONS
ADMINISTRATION/STORAGE
1. Adjust dosage gradually, allowing 2–3 days between increments in dosage. This allows steady-state plasma levels to be reached and QT intervals to be monitored.
2. Undertake dosage initiation and increases in a hospital with facilities for cardiac rhythm monitoring. Dosage must be individualized only after appropriate clinical assessment.
3. Proarrhythmias can occur during initiation of therapy and with each dosage increment.
4. In clients with impaired renal function, alter the dosing interval as follows: if C_{CR} is 30–60 mL/min, the dosing interval is 24 hr; if C_{CR} is 10–30 mL/min, the dosing interval should be 36–48 hr. If C_{CR} is less than 10 mL/min, dose must be individualized. Undertake dosage adjustments in clients with impaired renal function only after five to six doses at the intervals described.
5. Before initiating sotalol, withdraw previous antiarrhythmic therapy with careful monitoring for a minimum of 2–3 plasma half-lives if condition permits.

6. Do not initiate sotalol after amiodarone is discontinued until the QT interval is normalized.
Initiation and Maintenance of Betapace AF Therapy
1. Determine the QT interval prior to initiation of therapy using an average of 5 beats. If the baseline QT is greater than 450 msec (JT equal to or greater than 330 msec if QRS over 100 msec), do not use Betapace AF.
2. Calculate the creatinine clearance.
3. Initiate the correct dose of Betapace AF, depending on the creatinine clearance (see *Dosage*).
4. Begin continuous ECG monitoring with QT interval measurements 2–4 hr after each dose.
5. If the 80 mg dose is tolerated and the QT interval remains less than 500 msec after at least 3 days (after 5 or 6 doses if client is receiving once daily dosing), the client can be discharged. Alternatively, during hospitalization, the dose can be increased to 120 mg twice a day if the 80 mg dose does not reduce the frequency and relapses of AFIB/AFL. Once again, the client is followed for 3 days on this dose (or 5 or 6 doses if receiving once daily dosing).
6. If the 120 mg dose twice a day or daily does not reduce the frequency of early relapses of AFIB/AFL and is tolerated without excessive QT interval prolongation (520 msec or longer), Betapace AF can be increased to 160 mg twice a day or daily, provided appropriate monitoring is undertaken.
7. Re-evaluate renal function and QT regularly if medically warranted. If QT is 520 msec or greater (JT 430 msec or greater if QRS is over 100 msec), reduce the dose of Betapace AF and monitor QT carefully until QT returns to less than 520 msec.
8. If the QT interval is 520 msec or greater while on the lowest maintenance dose (80 mg), discontinue the drug.
9. If renal function decreases, reduce the daily dose in half and administer the drug once daily.

10. If a dose is missed, the next dose should not be doubled. The next dose should be taken at the usual time.

11. Before starting Betapace AF, withdraw previous antiarrhythmic therapy, with careful monitoring, for a minimum of 2 or 3 plasma half-lives if the clinical condition permits.

12. Do not initiate Betapace AF after amiodarone until the QT interval is normalized.

ASSESSMENT

1. Perform a thorough nursing history; note any cardiomegaly or CHF.

2. Obtain ECG and document QT interval; note symptoms associated with arrhythmia.

3. Client should be in a closely monitored environment with VS and ECG monitored during initiation and adjustment of sotalol. Monitor VS, I&O, electrolytes, Mg^+ level, renal and LFTs.

CLIENT/FAMILY TEACHING

1. Take on an empty stomach as food decreases absorption.

2. Take exactly as directed and do not stop abruptly; drug controls symptoms but does not cure condition.

3. Avoid activities that require mental alertness until drug effects realized; may cause dizziness/drowsiness.

4. Report increased chest pain/SOB, night cough, swelling of feet and ankles, increased fatigue, low heart rate, or unsteady gait.

5. Continue dietary and exercise guidelines as prescribed and healthy lifestyle changes. Avoid alcohol and OTC agents.

OUTCOMES/EVALUATE

Control/conversion of life-threatening arrhythmias to stable cardiac rhythm

Spironolactone

(speer-oh-no-**LAK**-tohn)

CLASSIFICATION(S):

Diuretic, potassium-sparing

PREGNANCY CATEGORY: D

Rx: Aldactone

✦Rx: Novo-Spiroton

SEE ALSO *DIURETICS, THIAZIDES.*

ACTION/KINETICS

Mild diuretic that acts on the distal tubule to inhibit sodium exchange for potassium, resulting in increased secretion of sodium and water and conservation of potassium. An aldosterone antagonist. Manifests a slight antihypertensive effect. Interferes with synthesis of testosterone and may increase formation of estradiol from testosterone, thus leading to endocrine abnormalities. **Onset:** Urine output increases over 1–2 days. **Peak:** 2–3 days. **Duration:** 2–3 days, and declines thereafter. Metabolized to an active metabolite (canrenone). **t ½:** 13–24 hr for canrenone. Canrenone is excreted through the urine (primary) and the bile. Almost completely bound to plasma protein.

USES

(1) Primary hyperaldosteronism, including diagnosis, short-term preoperative treatment, long-term maintenance therapy for those who are poor surgical risks and those with bilateral micronodular or macronodular adrenal hyperplasia. (2) Edema when other approaches are inadequate or ineffective (e.g., CHF, cirrhosis of the liver, nephrotic syndrome). (3) Essential hypertension (usually in combination with other drugs). (4) Prophylaxis of hypokalemia in clients taking digitalis. *Investigational:* Hirsutism, treat symptoms of PMS, with testolactone to treat familial male precocious puberty (short-term treatment), acne vulgaris. In severe heart failure with recommended therapies to reduce mortality.

CONTRAINDICATIONS

Acute renal insufficiency, progressive renal failure, hyperkalemia, and anuria. Clients receiving potassium supplements, amiloride, or triamterene.

SPECIAL CONCERNS

Use during pregnancy only if benefits clearly outweigh risks. Use with caution in impaired renal function. Geriatric clients may be more sensitive to the usual adult dose.

SIDE EFFECTS

Electrolyte: Hyperkalemia, hyponatremia (characterized by lethargy, dry mouth, thirst, tiredness). **GI:** Diarrhea,

S

cramps, ulcers, gastritis, gastric bleeding, vomiting. **CNS:** Drowsiness, ataxia, lethargy, mental confusion, headache. **Endocrine:** Gynecomastia, menstrual irregularities, impotence, bleeding in postmenopausal women, deepening of voice, hirsutism. **Dermatologic:** Maculopapular or erythematous cutaneous eruptions, urticaria. **Miscellaneous:** Drug fever, breast carcinoma, gynecomastia, hyperchloremic metabolic acidosis in hepatic cirrhosis (decompensated), *agranulocytosis.* NOTE: Spironolactone has been shown to be tumorigenic in chronic rodent studies.

DRUG INTERACTIONS

ACE inhibitors / Significant hyperkalemia
Anesthetics, general / Additive hypotension
Anticoagulants, oral / Inhibited by spironolactone
Antihypertensives / ↑ Hypotensive effect of both agents; ↓ dosage, especially of ganglionic blockers, by one-half
Captopril / ↑ Risk of significant hyperkalemia
Digoxin / ↑ Half-life of digoxin → ↓ clearance. Spironolactone may ↓ inotropic effect of digoxin.
Diuretics, others / Often given together due to potassium-sparing effect of spironolactone. Possible severe hyponatremia; monitor closely
Lithium / ↑ Risk of lithium toxicity R/T ↓ renal clearance
Norepinephrine / ↓ NE effect
Potassium salts / Hyperkalemia R/T spironolactone conserving potassium excessively. Rarely used together
Salicylates / Large doses may ↓ spironolactone effects
Triamterene / Possible hazardous hyperkalemia

HOW SUPPLIED

Tablet: 25 mg, 50 mg, 100 mg

DOSAGE————————

• **TABLETS**

Edema.
Adults, initial: 100 mg/day (range: 25–200 mg/day) in two to four divided doses for at least 5 days; **maintenance:** 75–400 mg/day in two to four divided doses. **Pediatric:** 3.3 mg/kg/day as a single dose or as two to four divided doses.

Antihypertensive.
Adults, initial: 50–100 mg/day as a single dose or as two to four divided doses—give for at least 2 weeks; **maintenance:** adjust to individual response.
Pediatric: 1–2 mg/kg in a single dose or in two to four divided doses.

Hypokalemia.
Adults: 25–100 mg/day as a single dose or two to four divided doses.

Diagnosis of primary hyperaldosteronism.
Adults: 400 mg/day for either 4 days (short-test) or 3–4 weeks (long-test).

Hyperaldosteronism, prior to surgery.
Adults: 100–400 mg/day in two to four doses prior to surgery.

Hyperaldosteronism, chronic-therapy.
Use lowest possible dose.

Hirsutism.
50–200 mg/day.

Symptoms of PMS.
25 mg 4 times per day beginning on day 14 of the menstrual cycle.

Familial male precocious puberty, short-term.
Spironolactone, 2 mg/kg/day, and testolactone, 20–40 mg/kg/day, for at least 6 months.

Acne vulgaris.
100 mg/day.

Reduce mortality in severe CHF.
25–50 mg/day with other therapies (e.g., ACE inhibitor, loop diuretic).

NURSING CONSIDERATIONS

ADMINISTRATION/STORAGE

1. When used as the sole drug to treat edema, maintain the initial dose for at least 5 days. After that, adjustments may be made. If the dosage is not effective, a second diuretic may be added, especially one that acts in the proximal tubules.

2. When administered to small children, tablets may be crushed and given as a suspension in cherry syrup.

3. Food may increase the absorption of spironolactone.

4. Protect the drug from light.

Bold Italic = life threatening side effect   ■ = black box warning   ✦ = Available in Canada

ASSESSMENT

1. Document indications for therapy, other agents prescribed, and outcome.
2. Monitor ABGs, ECG, CBC, blood sugar, uric acid, serum electrolytes, and liver and renal function studies. With cardiac disease, be alert for irregularities R/T hypokalemia. Record VS, I&O, and weights.
3. If client develops dysuria, urinary frequency, or renal spasm, obtain a urinalysis and urine culture.
4. Assess for drug tolerance characterized by edema and reduced urine output.

CLIENT/FAMILY TEACHING

1. Take as directed with a snack or meals to minimize GI upset. Report if nausea, bloating, anorexia, vomiting, or diarrhea persist.
2. Avoid foods or salt substitutes high in potassium; drug is potassium-sparing. Record BP and weight twice a week for provider review. Report any evidence of increased swelling of extremities or weight gain/loss of more than 5 lb (2.2 kg) weekly.
3. Do not drive/operate dangerous machinery until drug effects realized; may cause drowsiness or unsteady gait.
4. Drug may cause breast swelling and diminished sex drive by reducing testosterone levels.
5. Report if deep, rapid respirations, headaches, or mental slowing occurs; may indicate hyperchloremic metabolic acidosis.
6. Drug is metabolized in the liver. Report jaundice, tremors, or mental confusion; may develop hepatic encephalopathy with liver disease.

OUTCOMES/EVALUATE

- Enhanced diuresis with ↓ edema
- ↓ BP
- Antagonism of high levels of aldosterone
- Prevention of hypokalemia
- Reduced mortality in CAD with CHF

Streptokinase

(strep-toe-**KYE**-nayz)

CLASSIFICATION(S):

Thrombolytic enzyme

PREGNANCY CATEGORY: C

Rx: Streptase

ACTION/KINETICS

Most clients have a natural resistance to streptokinase that must be overcome with the loading dose before the drug becomes effective. Streptokinase acts with plasminogen to produce an "activator complex," which enhances the conversion of plasminogen to plasmin. Plasmin then breaks down fibrinogen, fibrin clots, and other plasma proteins, promoting the dissolution (lysis) of the insoluble fibrin trapped in intravascular emboli and thrombi. Also, inhibitors of streptokinase, such as alpha-2-macroglobulin, are rapidly inactivated by streptokinase. **Onset:** rapid; **duration:** 12 hr. **t ½, activator complex:** 23 min.

USES

(1) DVT. (2) Arterial thrombosis and embolism. (3) Acute evolving transmural MI. (4) Pulmonary embolism. (5) Clearing of occluded arteriovenous and IV cannulae. *Investigational:* Chronic arterial occlusions, retinal vessel thrombosis, hemolytic-uremic syndrome, renal artery thrombosis, renal cortical necrosis.

CONTRAINDICATIONS

Any condition presenting a risk of hemorrhage, such as recent surgery or biopsies, delivery within 10 days, ulcerative disease. Arterial emboli originating from the left side of the heart. Also, hepatic or renal insufficiency, tuberculosis, recent cerebral embolism, thrombosis, hemorrhage, SBE, rheumatic valvular disease, thrombocytopenia. Streptokinase resistance in excess of 1 million international units. Use to restore patency to IV catheters.

SPECIAL CONCERNS

The use of streptokinase in septic thrombophlebitis may be hazardous. History of significant allergic response. Safety in children has not been established. Geriatric clients have an increased risk of bleeding during therapy. Serious reactions, including hypotension, hypersensitivity, apnea, and bleeding have been associated with using streptokinase for restoring catheter patency.

SIDE EFFECTS
CV: Superficial bleeding, ***severe and internal bleeding, involving GI, GU, retroperitoneal, or intracerebral sites.*** **Allergic:** Nausea, headache, breathing difficulties, ***fever, shivering in acute MI, bronchospasm, angioneurotic edema,*** urticaria, flushing, musculoskeletal pain, vasculitis, interstitial nephritis, periorbital swelling, delayed hypersensitivity reactions (e.g., vasculitis, interstitial nephritis). **Other:** Fever, respiratory depression, back pain, possible development of Guillain-Barre syndrome, development of antistreptokinase antibody (i.e., streptokinase may be ineffective if administered between 5 days and 6 months following prior use of streptokinase or following streptococcal infections).

LABORATORY TEST CONSIDERATIONS
↓ Fibrinogen, plasminogen. ↑ Thrombin time, PT, and activated PTT.

DRUG INTERACTIONS
Anticoagulants and drugs that alter platelet function (e.g., aspirin, NSAIDs, aspirin, dipyridamole, GP IIb/IIIa inhibitors) ↑ the risk of serious bleeding when given with streptokinese.

HOW SUPPLIED
Powder for injection: 250,000 international units, 750,000 international units, 1.5 million international units

DOSAGE
- **IV INFUSION**
  DVT, Pulmonary embolism, Arterial thrombosis or embolism.
Loading dose: 250,000 international units over 30 min (use the 1,500,000 international units vial diluted to 90 mL); **maintenance:** 100,000 international units/hr for 24–72 hr for arterial thrombosis or embolism, 72 hr for deep vein thrombosis, and 24 hr (72 hr if deep vein thrombosis is suspected) for pulmonary embolism.
  Acute evolving transmural MI.
1,500,000 international units within 60 min (use the 1,500,000 international units vial diluted to a total of 45 mL).
  Arteriovenous cannula occlusion.

Before using, try to clear cannula using heparinized saline solution (syringe technique). If adequate flow does not occur, slowly instill 250,000 international units in 2-mL IV solution into each occluded limb of cannula and clamp off; **then,** after 2 hr aspirate cannula limbs, flush with saline, and reconnect cannula.
- **INTRACORONARY INFUSION**
  Acute evolving transmural MI.
20,000 international units by bolus; **then,** 2,000 international units/min for 60 min (total dose of 140,000 international units). Use the 250,000 international units vial diluted to 125 mL.

NURSING CONSIDERATIONS
ADMINISTRATION/STORAGE
IV 1. NaCl injection USP or D5W is the preferred diluent for IV use.
2. For AV cannulae, dilute 250,000 units with 2 mL of NaCl injection or D5W.
3. Reconstitute gently, as directed, without shaking vial.
4. Use within 24 hr of reconstitution.
5. Use an electronic infusion device to administer streptokinase and do not add any other medications to the line. Note any redness and/or pain at the site of infusion; may need to further dilute to prevent phlebitis.
6. Have emergency drugs and equipment available. Have corticosteroids and aminocaproic acid available for excessive bleeding.
7. Do not add other medication to streptokinase.

ASSESSMENT
1. Document indications for therapy, type, onset, and characteristics of symptoms.
2. Note any history of tuberculosis, SBE, ulcerative disease, recent surgery, or streptococcal infection.
3. Assess for bleeding tendency, heart disease, and/or allergic drug reactions.
4. Identify other drugs taking such as aspirin or NSAIDs that could increase bleeding times.
5. Clients with high allergy potential or high streptokinase antibody titer may benefit by skin testing prior to starting therapy. Drug may not be effective if

---

administered within 5 days to 6 months of a strep infection or previous use.
6. Obtain baseline lab studies; ensure that bleeding studies, type and cross-match, and streptokinase resistance have been completed before initiation of therapy.

INTERVENTIONS

1. Observe in a continously monitored environment; document rhythm strips and VS.
2. Check access sites for evidence of bleeding. Test stool, urine, and emesis for occult blood.
3. During IV therapy, arterial sticks require 30 min of manual pressure followed by application of a pressure dressing. To prevent bruising, avoid unnecessary handling of client.
4. If IM injections necessary, apply pressure after withdrawing the needle to prevent hematoma and bleeding from the puncture site. Observe injection sites and postoperative wounds for bleeding during therapy
5. If excessive bleeding develops from an invasive procedure, discontinue therapy and call for packed RBCs and plasma expanders *other than dextran.*
6. To prevent new thrombus formation, or rethrombosis, IV heparin and oral anticoagulants are used when therapy is concluded.

7. Note allergic reactions, ranging from anaphylaxis to moderate and mild reactions. These usually can be controlled with antihistamines and corticosteroids.
8. Fever reaction may be treated with acetaminophen.
9. Following recanalization of an occluded coronary artery, clients may develop reperfusion reactions; these may include:

* Reperfusion arrhythmias (accelerated idioventricular rhythm, sinus bradycardia) usually of short duration.
* Reduction of chest pain
* Return of elevated ST segment to near baseline levels

CLIENT/FAMILY TEACHING

1. Review inherent benefits and risks of drug therapy.
2. To be effective, the therapy should be instituted within 4–6 hr of onset of symptoms of acute MI.
3. Report any symptoms or side effects immediately.
4. Encourage family members or significant other to learn CPR.

OUTCOMES/EVALUATE

* Lysis of emboli/thrombi with restoration of normal blood flow
* ↓ Myocardial infarct size; improved ventricular function
* Catheter patency in previously occluded AV or IV cannulae

Telmisartan ■

(tell-mih-**SAR**-tan)

CLASSIFICATION(S):

Antihypertensive, angiotensin II receptor blocker

PREGNANCY CATEGORY: C (first trimester), D (second and third trimesters)

Rx: Micardis

SEE ALSO *ANGIOTENSIN II RECEPTOR ANTAGONISTS AND ANTIHYPERTENSIVES.*

ACTION/KINETICS

Control of BP in blacks is less than in whites. Is from 42–58% bioavailable (depending on dose). **Time to maximum levels:** 30–60 min. **t ½, terminal:** About 24 hr. Excreted mainly in the feces by way of the bile. Over 99.5% bound to plasma protein.

USES

Hypertension alone or in combination with other antihypertensives.

SPECIAL CONCERNS

■Use during the second and third trimester of pregnancy can cause injury and even death to the fetus. When pregnancy is detected, discontinue as soon as possible.■ Use with caution in impaired hepatic function or in biliary obstructive disorders. Clients on dialysis may develop orthostatic hypotension.

SIDE EFFECTS

GI: Diarrhea, dyspepsia, heartburn, N&V, abdominal pain. **CNS:** Dizziness, headache, fatigue, anxiety, nervousness. **Musculoskeletal:** Pain, including back/neck pain; myalgia. **Respiratory:** URI, sinusitis, cough, pharyngitis, influenza. **Miscellaneous:** Chest pain, UTI, peripheral edema, hypertension.

LABORATORY TEST CONSIDERATIONS

↑ Creatinine (in small number of clients). ↓ Hemoglobin.

OD OVERDOSE MANAGEMENT

Symptoms: Hypotension, dizziness, tachycardia or bradycardia. *Treatment:* Supportive for hypotension.

DRUG INTERACTIONS

↑ Digoxin peak plasma and trough levels.

HOW SUPPLIED

Tablets: 20 mg, 40 mg, 80 mg

DOSAGE

- **TABLETS**
  Antihypertensive.

Individualize dose. **Adults, initial:** 40 mg/day. **Maintenance:** 20–80 mg/day. If additional BP reduction is desired beyond that achieved with 80 mg/day, add a diuretic.

NURSING CONSIDERATIONS

ADMINISTRATION/STORAGE

1. May be taken with or without food.
2. Correct depletion of intravascular volume or begin therapy under close supervision.

ASSESSMENT

1. Note onset and duration of disease, other agents trialed and the outcome.
2. Symptomatic hypotension may occur in clients who are volume- or salt-depleted. Correct prior to using telmisartan, use a lower starting dose and monitor closely.

3. With renal dialysis may develop orthostatic hypotension; monitor BP closely.
4. Monitor ECG, H&H, renal, LFTs and VS. With hepatic or renal dysfunction, use cautiously.

CLIENT/FAMILY TEACHING

1. Take as directed at the same time daily with or without food.
2. Do not remove tablets from blisters until just before administration.
3. Regular exercise, low-salt diet, and life-style changes (i.e., no smoking, low alcohol, low-fat diet, low stress, adequate rest) contribute to enhanced BP control.
4. Use effective contraception; report pregnancy as drug use during second and third trimesters is associated with fetal injury and morbidity.

OUTCOMES/EVALUATE

↓ BP

Tenecteplase

(teh-**NECK**-teh-plays)

CLASSIFICATION(S):
Thrombolytic, tissue plasminogen activator
PREGNANCY CATEGORY: C
Rx: TNKase

ACTION/KINETICS

A tissue plasminogen activator produced by recombinant DNA. It binds to fibrin and converts plasminogen to plasmin. In the presence of fibrin, tenecteplase conversion of plasminogen to plasmin is increased relative to conversion in the absence of fibrin. Following the drug there are decreases in circulating fibrinogen. **t½, initial disposition:** 20–24 min; **terminal disposition:** 90–130 min. Metabolized in the liver.

USES

Reduce mortality due to acute myocardial infarction.

CONTRAINDICATIONS

Active internal bleeding, history of CVA, within 2 months of intracranial or intraspinal surgery or trauma, intracranial neoplasm, arteriovenous malformation

---

or aneurysm, known bleeding diathesis, severe uncontrolled hypertension. IM use.

SPECIAL CONCERNS

There is the possibility of cholesterol embolization and arrhythmias associated with reperfusion. Use with caution in the elderly, weighing the benefits versus risks, including bleeding. Use with caution during lactation. Safety and efficacy have not been determined in children.

SIDE EFFECTS

Bleeding. Most common side effect. Major bleeding includes hematoma, GI tract, urinary tract, puncture site (including cardiac catheterization site), retroperitoneal, respiratory tract. Minor bleeding includes hematoma, urinary tract, puncture site (including cardiac catheterization site), pharyngeal, GI tract, and epistaxis. **CV:** Cardiogenic shock, arrrhythmias, AV block, *heart failure, cardiac arrest,* recurrent myocardial ischemia, *myocardial reinfarction/rupture, cardiac tamponade,* pericarditis, pericardial effusion, mitral regurgitation, thrombosis, embolism, electromechanical dissociation. **Miscellaneous:** Pulmonary edema, N&V, hypotension, fever, *serious allergic or anaphylactic reactions.*

LABORATORY TEST CONSIDERATIONS

Results of coagulation tests or measures of fibrinolytic activity may be unreliable; specific precautions must be taken to prevent in vitro artifacts. Degradation of fibrinogen in blood samples removed for analysis is possible.

DRUG INTERACTIONS

Heparin, vitamin K antagonists, aspirin, dipyridamole, and GP IIb/IIIa inhibitors may increase the risk of bleeding if given prior to, during, or after tenecteplase therapy.

HOW SUPPLIED

Powder for injection, lyophilized: 50 mg

DOSAGE————————————
• **IV**

AMI.

Dose is based on client weight, but not to exceed 50 mg. Given as a single bolus dose over 5 sec. **Less than 60 kg:** 30 mg (6 mL); **60 kg–less than 70 kg:**

35 mg (7 mL); **70 kg– less than 80 kg:** 40 mg (8 mL); **80 kg– less than 90 kg:** 45 mg (9 mL); **90 kg and over:** 50 mg (10 mL).

NURSING CONSIDERATIONS

ADMINISTRATION/STORAGE

IV 1. Initiate treatment as soon as possible after the onset of symptoms of MI.

2. Reconstitute and administer as follows:

• Aseptically withdraw 10 mL sterile water for injection from that supplied. Use the red hub cannula syringe filling device. Do not discard the shield assembly. Do *not* use bacteriostatic water for injection.

• Inject the entire contents of the syringe (10 mL) into the tenecteplase vial. Direct the stream into the powder. Slight foaming may occur; any large bubbles will dissipate if allowed to stand undisturbed for several minutes.

• Swirl contents gently until completely dissolved. Do not shake. The reconstituted product is colorless to pale yellow and is transparent with a concentration of 5 mg/mL and pH of about 7.3.

• Determine the appropriate dose of tenecteplase and withdraw the correct volume (in mL) from the reconstituted vial with the syringe. Discard any unused portion.

• With the correct dose in the syringe, stand the shield vertically on a flat surface with the green side down and passively recap the red hub cannula.

• Remove the entire shield assembly, including the red hub cannula by twisting counter clockwise. The shield assembly also contains the clear-ended blunt plastic cannula; retain for split septum IV access.

• Administer as a single IV bolus over 5 sec.

3. Tenecteplase contains no preservatives; thus, reconstitute immediately before use.

4. If given in an IV line with dextrose, precipitation may occur. Flush dextrose-containing lines with a saline-containing solution prior to and following single bolus administration of tenecteplase.

---

5. Store lyophilized tenecteplase at controlled temperatures not to exceed 30°C (86°F) or under refrigeration at 2–8°C (36–46°F).

6. If reconstituted drug is not used immediately, refrigerate the tenecteplase vial at 2–8°C (36–46°F) and use within 8 hr.

ASSESSMENT

1. Note indications for therapy identifying symptom onset and site of infarct.

2. Do not use with active internal bleeding, history of CVA, recent: intracranial bleed, spinal surgery, trauma or neoplasm; AV malformation, aneurysm, or uncontrolled HTN.

3. Obtain baseline cardiac enzymes, weight, CBC, bleeding times, type and crossmatch. Monitor for S&S active bleeding, stop heparin infusion and report.

4. Assess for reperfusion arrhythmias after therapy which may include accelerated idioventricular rhythm, sinus bradycardia of short duration, and return of elevated ST segment to near baseline.

CLIENT/FAMILY TEACHING

1. Review inherent benefits and risks of drug therapy. Maintain bed rest during therapy.

2. To be effective, the therapy should be instituted as soon as possible after symptom onset of AMI.

3. Report any adverse side effects i.e. sudden severe headache or active bleeding immediately.

4. Encourage family members or significant other to learn CPR.

OUTCOMES/EVALUATE

↓ Mortality with AMI; resolution on MI

Terazosin ©

(ter-**AY**-zoh-sin)

CLASSIFICATION(S):

Antihypertensive, alpha-1-adrenergic blocking drug

PREGNANCY CATEGORY: C

Rx: Hytrin

♣Rx: Apo-Terazosin, Novo-Terazosin, Nu-Terazosin, PMS-Tarazosin, ratio-Terazosin

ACTION/KINETICS

Blocks postsynaptic alpha-1-adrenergic receptors, leading to a dilation of both arterioles and veins, and ultimately, a reduction in BP. Both standing and supine BPs are lowered with no reflex tachycardia. Also relaxes smooth muscle of the prostate and bladder neck. Usefulness in BPH is due to alpha-1 receptor blockade, which relaxes the smooth muscle of the prostate and bladder neck and relieves pressure on the urethra. Bioavailability is not affected by food. **Onset:** 15 min. **Peak plasma levels:** 1–2 hr. t $\frac{1}{2}$: 9–12 hr. **Duration:** 24 hr. Excreted unchanged and as inactive metabolites in both the urine and feces.

USES

(1) Hypertension, alone or in combination with diuretics or beta-adrenergic blocking agents. (2) Symptoms of benign prostatic hyperplasia.

SPECIAL CONCERNS

Use with caution during lactation. Safety and efficacy have not been determined in children. Geriatric clients may be more sensitive to the hypotensive and hypothermic effects of terazosin.

SIDE EFFECTS

First-dose effect: Marked postural hypotension and syncope. **CV:** Palpitations, tachycardia, postural hypotension, syncope, *arrhythmias,* chest pain, vasodilation, atrial fibrillation. **CNS:** Dizziness, headache, somnolence, drowsiness, nervousness, paresthesia, depression, anxiety, insomnia, vertigo. **Respiratory:** Nasal congestion, dyspnea, sinusitis, epistaxis, bronchitis, *bronchospasm,* cold or flu symptoms, increased cough, pharyngitis, rhinitis. **GI:** Nausea, constipation, diarrhea, dyspepsia, dry mouth, vomiting, flatulence, abdominal discomfort or pain. **Musculoskeletal:** Asthenia, arthritis, arthralgia, myalgia, joint disorders, back pain, pain in extremities, neck and shoulder pain, muscle cramps. **Miscellaneous:** Peripheral edema, weight gain, blurred vision, impotence, chest pain, fever, gout, pruri-

---

Bold Italic = life threatening side effect   ■ = black box warning   ♣ = Available in Canada

tus, rash, sweating, urinary frequency, UTI, tinnitus, conjunctivitis, abnormal vision, edema, facial edema, thrombocytopenia, priapism.

LABORATORY TEST CONSIDERATIONS
↓ H&H, WBCs, albumin.

OD OVERDOSE MANAGEMENT
Symptoms: Hypotension, drowsiness, shock. *Treatment:* Restore BP and HR. Client should be kept supine; vasopressors may be indicated. Volume expanders can be used to treat shock.

DRUG INTERACTIONS
When used with finasteride → ↑ finasteride plasma levels.

HOW SUPPLIED
Capsule: 1 mg, 2 mg, 5 mg, 10 mg

DOSAGE

- **CAPSULES**
  Hypertension.
  Individualized, initial: 1 mg at bedtime (this dose is not to be exceeded); **then,** increase dose slowly to obtain desired response. **Range:** 1–5 mg/day; doses as high as 20 mg may be required in some clients. Doses greater than 20 mg daily do not provide further BP control.
  Benign prostatic hyperplasia.
  Initial: 1 mg/day; dose should be increased to 2 mg, 5 mg, and then 10 mg once daily to improve symptoms and/or urinary flow rates. Doses greater than 20 mg daily have not been studied.

NURSING CONSIDERATIONS

ⓒ Do not confuse terazosin with temazepam (a sedative-hypnotic).

ADMINISTRATION/STORAGE
1. The initial dosing regimen must be carefully observed to minimize severe hypotension.
2. Monitor BP 2–3 hr after dosing and at end of dosing interval to ensure BP control maintained.
3. Consider an increase in dose or twice a day dosing if BP control is not maintained at 24-hr interval.
4. To prevent dizziness or fainting due to a drop in BP, take the initial dose at bedtime; the daily dose can be given in the morning.
5. If terazosin must be discontinued for more than a few days, reinstitute the initial dosing regimen if restarted.

6. Due to additive effects, use caution when combined with other antihypertensive agents.
7. When treating BPH, a minimum of 4–6 weeks of 10 mg/day may be needed to determine if a beneficial effect has occurred.

ASSESSMENT
1. Document onset, duration, and characteristics of symptoms.
2. Assess prostate gland, PSA level, and BPH score.
3. A gradual increase in dose until symptom control, i.e., 1 mg/day for 7 days, then 2 mg/day for 7 days, then 3 mg/day for 7 days, then 4 mg/day for 7 days, and then 5 mg /day, may assist to diminish adverse effects and enhance compliance, especially in the elderly.

CLIENT/FAMILY TEACHING
1. Take initial dose at bedtime to minimize side effects. Do not stop abruptly or titration must restart. Use caution when performing activities that require mental alertness until drug effects realized.
2. Do not drive or undertake hazardous tasks for 12 hr after the first dose and after increasing dose or reinstituting therapy.
3. Avoid symptoms of dizziness (drop in BP) by rising slowly from a sitting or lying position and waiting until symptoms subside.
4. Record weight twice a week; report persistent side effects or excessive weight gain or ankle edema.
5. Report if nighttime urinary frequency increases. Keep F/U visits for DRE and labs.

OUTCOMES/EVALUATE
- Improvement in BPH symptoms
- ↓ BP

Ticlopidine hydrochloride ■ ⓒ
(tie-**KLOH**-pih-deen)

CLASSIFICATION(S):
Antiplatelet drug

PREGNANCY CATEGORY: B
Rx: Ticlid
♣Rx: Apo-Ticlopidine, Gen-Ticlopidine, Nu-Ticlopidine, PMS-Ticlopidine, Rhoxal-ticlopidine

ACTION/KINETICS
Irreversibly inhibits ADP-induced platelet-fibrinogen binding and subsequent platelet-platelet interactions. This results in inhibition of both platelet aggregation and release of platelet granule constituents as well as prolongation of bleeding time. **Peak plasma levels:** 2 hr. **Maximum platelet inhibition:** 8–11 days after 250 mg twice a day. **Steady-state plasma levels:** 14–21 days. **t ½, elimination:** 4–5 days. After discontinuing therapy, bleeding time and other platelet function tests return to normal within 14 days. Rapidly absorbed; bioavailability is increased by food. Extensively metabolized by the liver with approximately 60% excreted through the kidneys; 23% is excreted in the feces (with one-third excreted unchanged). Clearance of the drug decreases with age. 98% bound to plasma proteins.

USES
(1) With aspirin to decrease the incidence of subacute stent thrombosis in clients undergoing successful coronary stent implantation. (2) Reduce the risk of fatal or nonfatal thrombotic stroke in clients who have manifested precursors of stroke or who have had a completed thrombotic stroke. Due to the risk of neutropenia or agranulocytosis, reserve for clients who are intolerant to aspirin therapy or who have failed aspirin therapy. *Investigational:* Chronic arterial occlusion, coronary artery bypass grafts, intermittent claudication, open heart surgery, primary glomerulonephritis, subarachnoid hemorrhage, sickle cell disease, uremic clients with AV shunts or fistulas.

CONTRAINDICATIONS
Use in the presence of neutropenia and thrombocytopenia, hemostatic disorder, or active pathologic bleeding such as bleeding peptic ulcer or intracranial bleeding. Severe liver impairment. Lactation.

SPECIAL CONCERNS
■(1) Can cause life-threatening hematological side effects, including neutropenia/agranulocytosis and thrombotic thrombocytopenic purpura. (2) Severe hematological side effects may occur within a few days of starting therapy. The incidence of thrombotic thrombocytopenic purpura peaks after about 3–4 weeks of therapy and neutropenia peaks at about 4–6 weeks with both declining thereafter. Only a few cases have been seen after more than 3 months of therapy. (3) Hematological side effects cannot be reliably predicted by any demographic or clinical characteristics. During the first 3 months of therapy, hematologically and clinically monitor those receiving ticlopidine for evidence of neutropenia or thrombotic thrombocytopenic purpura (TTP). Immediately discontinue if there is any evidence of neutropenia or TTP.■ Use with caution in clients with ulcers (i.e., where there is a propensity for bleeding). Consider reduced dosage in impaired renal function. Geriatric clients may be more sensitive to the effects of the drug. Safety and effectiveness have not been established in children less than 18 years of age.

SIDE EFFECTS
Hematologic: *Neutropenia, agranulocytosis, thrombotic thrombocytopenia purpura,* thrombocytopenia, pancytopenia, immune thrombocytopenia, *hemolytic anemia with reticulocytosis.* **GI:** Diarrhea, N&V, GI pain, dyspepsia, flatulence, anorexia, GI fullness, peptic ulcer. **Hepatic:** Hepatitis, cholestatic jaundice, hepatocellular jaundice, *hepatic necrosis.* **Bleeding complications:** Ecchymosis, hematuria, epistaxis, conjunctival hemorrhage, *GI bleeding,* perioperative bleeding, posttraumatic bleeding, *intracerebral bleeding (rare).* **Dermatologic:** Maculopapular or urticarial rash, pruritus, urticaria. Rarely, erythema multiforme, exfoliative dermatitis, *Stevens-Johnson syndrome.* **CNS:** Dizziness, headache. **Neuromuscular:** Asthenia, SLE, peripheral neurop-

athy, arthropathy, myositis. **Miscellaneous:** Tinnitus, pain, allergic pneumonitis, vasculitis, nephrotic syndrome, renal failure, angioedema, hyponatremia, serum sickness.

LABORATORY TEST CONSIDERATIONS
↑ Alkaline phosphatase, ALT, AST, serum cholesterol, and triglycerides. Abnormal LFTs.

DRUG INTERACTIONS
Antacids / ↓ Ticlopidine plasma levels
Aspirin / ↑ Effect of aspirin on collagen-induced platelet aggregation
Carbamazepine / ↑ Carbamazepine plasma levels → toxicity
Cimetidine / ↓ Ticlopidine clearance R/T ↓ liver metabolism
Digoxin / Slight ↓ in digoxin plasma levels
H *Evening primrose oil* / Potential for ↑ antiplatelet effect
H *Feverfew* / Potential for ↑ antiplatelet effect
H *Garlic* / Potential for ↑ antiplatelet effect
H *Ginger* / Potential for ↑ antiplatelet effect
H *Ginkgo biloba* / Potential for ↑ antiplatelet effect
H *Ginseng* / Potential for ↑ antiplatelet effect
H *Grapeseed extract* / Potential for ↑ antiplatelet effect
Phenytoin / ↑ Phenytoin plasma levels → somnolence and lethargy
Theophylline / ↑ Theophylline plasma levels R/T ↓ clearance

HOW SUPPLIED
Tablet: 250 mg

DOSAGE

• **TABLETS**
Reduce risk of thrombotic stroke, Adjunct with aspirin to reduce subacute stent thrombosis.
250 mg twice a day.

NURSING CONSIDERATIONS
℃ Do not confuse Ticlid with Tequin (a fluoroquinolone antibiotic).
ADMINISTRATION/STORAGE
1. To increase bioavailability and decrease GI discomfort, take with food or just after eating.
2. If switched from an anticoagulant or fibrinolytic drug to ticlopidine, discon-

tinue the former drug before initiation of ticlopidine therapy.
3. IV methylprednisolone (20 mg) may normalize prolonged bleeding times, usually within 2 hr.

ASSESSMENT
1. Note indications for therapy; assess for liver disease, bleeding disorders, or ulcer disease. Ascertain aspirin intolerance.
2. See increased use of clopidogrel due to less side effect profile and once daily dosing advantage.
3. Determine baseline hematologic profile (e.g., CBC, PT, PTT, INR), liver and renal function studies. Monitor CBC biweekly to screen for possibly fatal thrombotic thrombocytopenic purpura (↓ platelets and ↓ WBCs).

CLIENT/FAMILY TEACHING
1. Take with food or after meals to minimize GI upset.
2. It may take longer than usual to stop bleeding; report unusual bleeding as severe hematological side effects may occur.
3. Brush teeth with a soft-bristle tooth brush, use an electric razor for shaving, wear shoes when ambulating, use caution and avoid injury, as bleeding times may be prolonged.
4. During the first 3 months of therapy, low white blood count can occur, resulting in an increased risk of infection. Come for scheduled blood tests and report any symptoms of infection (e.g., fever, chills, sore throat).
5. Any severe or persistent diarrhea, SC bleeding, skin rashes, or evidence of cholestasis (e.g., yellow skin or sclera, dark urine, light-colored stools) should be reported.

OUTCOMES/EVALUATE
Prevention of a complete or recurrent cerebral thrombotic event

Timolol maleate ℃
(TIE-moh-lohl)

CLASSIFICATION(S):
Beta-adrenergic blocking agent

H = Herbal   IV = Intravenous   ℃ = sound-alike drug

PREGNANCY CATEGORY: C

Rx: Betimol, Blocadren, Istalol, Timoptic, Timoptic-XE

✤**Rx:** Apo-Timol, Apo-Timop, Gen-Timolol, Novo-Timol, Nu-Timolol, PMS-Timolol, ratio-Timolol, Rhoxal-timolol

SEE ALSO *BETA-ADRENERGIC BLOCKING AGENTS.*

ACTION/KINETICS

Exerts both beta-1- and beta-2-adrenergic blocking activity. Has minimal sympathomimetic effects, direct myocardial depressant effects, or local anesthetic action. Does not cause pupillary constriction or night blindness. The mechanism of the protective effect in MI is not known. **Peak plasma levels:** 1–2 hr. **t ½:** 4 hr. Metabolized in the liver. Metabolites and unchanged drug excreted through the kidney. Also reduces both elevated and normal IOP, whether or not glaucoma is present; thought to act by reducing aqueous humor formation and/or by slightly increasing outflow of aqueous humor. Does not affect pupil size or visual acuity. For use in eye: **Onset:** 30 min. **Maximum effect:** 1–2 hr. **Duration:** 24 hr.

USES

Tablets: (1) Hypertension (alone or in combination with other antihypertensives such as thiazide diuretics). (2) Reduce CV mortality and risk of reinfarction in clinically stable MI survivors. (3) Prophylaxis of migraine. *Investigational:* Ventricular arrhythmias and tachycardias, essential tremors.

Ophthalmic solution (Betimol, Timoptic): Lower IOP in chronic open-angle glaucoma, selected cases of secondary glaucoma, ocular hypertension, aphakic (no lens) clients with glaucoma.

Gel-Forming Solution (Timoptic-XE): Reduce elevated IOP in open-angle glaucoma or ocular hypertension.

CONTRAINDICATIONS

Hypersensitivity to drug. Bronchial asthma or bronchospasm including severe COPD.

SPECIAL CONCERNS

Use ophthalmic preparation with caution in clients for whom systemic beta-adrenergic blocking agents are contraindicated. Safe use in children not established.

SIDE EFFECTS

Systemic following use of tablets: See *Beta-Adrenergic Blocking Agents.* **Following use of ophthalmic product:** Few. Occasionally, ocular irritation, local hypersensitivity reactions, slight decrease in resting HR.

DRUG INTERACTIONS

When used ophthalmically, possible potentiation with systemically administered beta-adrenergic blocking agents.

HOW SUPPLIED

Ophthalmic gel forming solution: 0.25%, 0.5%; *Ophthalmic solution:* 0.25%, 0.5%; *Tablet:* 5 mg, 10 mg, 20 mg

DOSAGE

• **TABLETS**

Hypertension.

Initial: 10 mg twice a day alone or with a diuretic; **maintenance:** 20–40 mg/day (up to 60 mg/day in two doses may be required), depending on BP and HR. If dosage increase is necessary, wait 7 days.

MI prophylaxis in clients who have survived the acute phase.

10 mg twice a day.

Migraine prophylaxis.

Initially: 10 mg twice a day. **Maintenance:** 20 mg/day given as a single dose; total daily dose may be increased to 30 mg in divided doses or decreased to 10 mg, depending on the response and client tolerance. If a satisfactory response for migraine prophylaxis is not obtained within 6–8 weeks using the maximum daily dose, discontinue the drug.

Essential tremor.

10 mg/day.

• **OPHTHALMIC SOLUTION (BETIMOL OR TIMOPTIC, EACH 0.25% OR 0.5%)**

Glaucoma,

1 gtt of 0.25–0.50% solution in each eye twice a day. If the decrease in intraocular pressure is maintained, reduce dose to 1 gtt once a day.

• **ISATOL OPHTHALMIC**

Glaucoma.

Initial: 1 gtt per affected eye once daily in the morning.

Bold Italic = life threatening side effect   ■ = black box warning   ✤ = Available in Canada

- **OPHTHALMIC GEL-FORMING SOLUTION (TIMOPTIC-XE 0.25% OR 0.5%)**
  Glaucoma.
  1 gtt once daily.

NURSING CONSIDERATIONS

 Do not confuse timolol with atenolol, each of which is a beta-adrenergic blocking drug.

ADMINISTRATION/STORAGE

1. When transferring from another antiglaucoma agent, continue old medication on day 1 of timolol therapy (1 gtt of 0.25% solution). Then, discontinue former therapy. Initiate with 0.25% solution. Increase to 0.50% solution if response is insufficient. Further dosage increases are ineffective.

2. When transferring from several antiglaucoma agents, individualize the dose. If one of the agents is a beta-adrenergic blocking agent, discontinue it before starting timolol. Dosage adjustments should involve one drug at a time at 1-week intervals. Continue the antiglaucoma drugs with the addition of timolol, 1 gtt of 0.25% solution twice a day (if response is inadequate, 1 gtt of 0.5% solution may be used twice a day). The following day, discontinue one of the other antiglaucoma agents while continuing the remaining agents or discontinue based on client response.

3. Before using the gel, invert the closed container and shake once before each use.

4. Administer other ophthalmics at least 10 min before the gel.

5. The ocular hypotensive effect has been maintained when switching clients from timolol solution given twice a day to the gel once daily.

ASSESSMENT

1. Document indications for therapy, onset, and characteristic S&S.

2. Monitor VS, IOPs, renal, and LFTs.

CLIENT/FAMILY TEACHING

1. Review procedure for ophthalmic administration.

- Apply finger lightly to lacrimal sac for 1 min following administration.

- Regular intraocular measurements by an ophthalmologist are required be-

cause ocular hypertension may recur without any overt S&S.

2. When tablets used for long-term prophylaxis against MI, do not interrupt therapy; abrupt withdrawal may precipitate reinfarction.

3. Do not perform tasks such as driving or operating machinery until drug effects are realized; may cause dizziness.

4. Report any evidence of rash, dizziness, heart palpitations, SOB, edema, or depression. May cause increased sensitivity to cold; dress appropriate.

5. With diabetes, drug may mask S&S of hypoglycemia. Keep log of FS and BP for provider review.

6. Continue lifestyle modifications (i.e., weight reduction, regular exercise, reduced intake of sodium and alcohol, and no smoking) in the overall goal of BP control.

OUTCOMES/EVALUATE

- ↓ BP
- Myocardial reinfarction prophylaxis
- Migraine prophylaxis
- ↓ Intraocular pressures

Tinzaparin sodium ■

(tin-**ZAH**-pah-rin)

CLASSIFICATION(S):
Anticoagulant, low molecular weight heparin
PREGNANCY CATEGORY: B
Rx: Innohep

SEE ALSO *HEPARIN, LOW MOLECULAR WEIGHT*

ACTION/KINETICS

Maximum plasma levels: 0.25–0.87 international units/mL within 4 to 5 hr after a single SC dose of 4,500 international units. Metabolized in the liver. **t ½:** 3–4 hr. Excreted mainly in the urine. Clearance is reduced in impaired renal function.

USES

Treat acute symptomatic deep vein thrombosis (DVT) with or without pulmonary embolism when given with warfarin sodium. *Investigational:* Prophylaxis of DVT (which may lead to pulmonary embolism) in clients undergoing moderate risk surgery, orthopedic surgery, hip fracture surgery, or neurosurgery at risk for thromboembolic complications.

ADDITIONAL CONTRAINDICATIONS

Use in those with a history of heparin-induced thrombocytopenia (HIT). Sensitivity to heparin, sulfites, benzyl alcohol, or pork products. Mixing with other injections or infusions.

SPECIAL CONCERNS

■(1) When spinal/epidural anesthesia or spinal puncture is used, those anticoagulated or scheduled to be anticoagulated with low molecular weight heparins or heparinoids to prevent thromboembolic complications are at risk of developing a spinal or epidural hematoma that can result in long-term or permanent paralysis. Risk is increased using indwelling epidural catheters for giving analgesics or by the concurrent use of drugs affecting hemostasis, such as NSAIDs, platelet inhibitors, or other anticoagulants. Risk also appears to increase by traumatic or repeated spinal or epidural puncture. (2) Frequently monitor for signs and symptoms of neurological impairment. If observed, immediate treatment is required. (3) The physician should consider potential benefits vs risk before neuraxial intervention in clients anticoagulated or to be anticoagulated for thromboprophylaxis.■ Use with caution in pregnancy and only if clearly needed since benzyl alcohol in the product may cross the placenta and cause a fatal 'gasping syndrome' in premature neonates. Use with caution during lactation. Safety and efficacy have not been determined in children.

SIDE EFFECTS

CV: Bleeding, *hemorrhage,* hypo/hypertension, tachycardia, angina pectoris, deep leg thrombophlebitis, peripheral ischemia, hemoptysis, ocular hemorrhage, rectal bleeding. **Hematologic:** Thrombocytopenia, anemia, agranulocytosis, pancytopenia. **GI:** N&V, abdominal pain, diarrhea, constipation, flatulence, GI disorder, dyspepsia, cholestatic hepatitis. **CNS:** Headache, dizziness, insomnia, confusion. **GU:** Priapism, UTI, hematuria, urinary retention, dysuria. **Respiratory:** *Pulmonary embolism,* dyspnea, epistaxis, pneumonia, respiratory disorder. **Dermatologic:** Rash, erythematous rash, pruritus, bullous eruption, skin disorder, epidermal necrolysis, ischemic necrosis, urticaria. **At injection site:** Mild local irritation, pain, hematoma, ecchymosis, necrosis, abscess. **Hypersensitivity:** *Anaphylaxis,* angioedema. **Body as a whole:** Fever, impaired healing, infection. **Miscellaneous:** Back/chest pain, pain, rash, neonatal hypotonia.

ADDITIONAL DRUG INTERACTIONS

Anticoagulants, oral / ↑ Risk of bleeding
Dextran / ↑ Risk of bleeding
Thrombolytics / ↑ Risk of bleeding

HOW SUPPLIED

Injection: 20,000 anti-Factor Xa units/mL

DOSAGE

- **SC ONLY**
  Deep vein thrombosis.
  175 anti-Factor IX units/kg once daily for 6 days or until client is adequately anticoagulated with warfarin (INR at least 2.0 for two consecutive days). Initiate warfarin when appropriate (usually 1–3 days after tinzaparin initiation).

NURSING CONSIDERATIONS

ADMINISTRATION/STORAGE

1. Do not give IM or IV.
2. Do not mix with other injections or infusions.
3. To assure withdrawal of the correct volume, use an appropriately calibrated syringe.
4. Inspect visually before administration to ensure there is no particulate matter or discoloration of the vial contents.
5. Position clients either supine or sitting and give by deep SC injection. Alternate injections between left and right anterolateral and left and right posterolateral abdominal wall. Vary the injection site daily. Introduce the entire length of the needle into a skin fold held between the thumb and forefinger; hold the skin fold throughout the

injection. To minimize bruising, do not rub the injection site after completing the injection.

6. Dosage adjustments are not required for the elderly and those with renal impairment.

7. Store between 15–30°C (59–86°F).

ASSESSMENT

1. Assess for any active major bleeding, HIT, or any hypersensitivity to heparin sulfite, benzyl alcohol or pork products.

2. Use cautiously with history of recent GI ulcerations, diabetic retinopathy, hemorrhage, uncontrolled HTN, or bleeding diathesis.

3. Confirm PE by segmental lung scan defect and/or DVT by US. Start SC tinzaparin treatment x 6 days; add coumadin on day 2 and titrate to an INR of 2–3.

4. Weigh client; calculate dose for client weight (kg x 0.00875 mL/Kg = volume in mL to be administered SC).

5. Monitor PT, INR, platelet count, CBC, renal function and FOB.

CLIENT/FAMILY TEACHING

1. Review indications for therapy, self administration techniques, and importance of site rotation.

2. To administer, lie down or sit and give by deep SC injection only. Alternate sites between the left and right anterolateral and left and right posterolateral abdominal wall. Vary the injection site daily.

3. Insert the whole length of the needle into a skin fold held between the thumb and forefinger. Hold the skin fold throughout the injection.

4. To minimize bruising do not rub site after administering and avoid OTC agents such as NSAIDS or aspirin.

5. Use caution to prevent injury; avoid contact sports, excessive jostling and use soft bristle tooth bush, and use electric razor to prevent bleeding.

6. Report any unusual bruising, bleeding, chest pain, acute SOB, itching, rash, or swelling. Keep F/U to evaluate blood tests and response.

OUTCOMES/EVALUATE

- Anticoagulation and prevention of complications R/T clot formation
- Resolution of DVT

Tirofiban hydrochloride
(**ty**-roh-**FYE**-ban)

CLASSIFICATION(S):
Antiplatelet drug
PREGNANCY CATEGORY: B
Rx: Aggrastat

ACTION/KINETICS

Non–peptide antagonist of the platelet glycoprotein (GP) IIb/IIIa receptor, which is the major platelet surface receptor involved in platelet aggregation. Activation of the receptor leads to binding of fibrinogen and von Willebrand's factor to platelets, and thus aggregation. Tirofiban is a reversible antagonist of fibrinogen binding to the GP IIb/IIIa receptor, thus inhibiting platelet aggregation. **t ½:** About 2 hr. Cleared from the plasma mainly unchanged by renal excretion (65%) and feces (25%). Plasma clearance is lower in clients over 65 years of age and is significantly decreased in those with a C_{CR} less than 30 mL/min.

USES

In combination with heparin for acute coronary syndrome (ACS), including those being treated medically and those undergoing PTCA or atherectomy.

CONTRAINDICATIONS

Active internal bleeding or history of diathesis within the previous 30 days; history of intracranial hemorrhage, intracranial neoplasm, AV malformation, or aneurysm; history of thrombocytopenia following prior use of tirofiban; history of stroke within 30 days or any history of hemorrhagic stroke; major surgical procedure or severe physical trauma within the last month; history, findings, or symptoms suggestive of aortic dissection; severe hypertension (systolic BP greater than 180 mm Hg or diastolic BP greater than 110 mm Hg); concomitant use of another parenteral GP IIb/IIIa inhibitor; acute pericarditis.

T

SPECIAL CONCERNS

Use with caution in clients with a platelet count less than 150,000/mm^3 in hemorrhagic retinopathy or with other drugs that affect hemostasis (e.g., warfarin). Safety and efficacy in children less than 18 years of age have not been established. Safety when used in combination with thrombolytic drugs has not been determined.

SIDE EFFECTS

Most common is bleeding, including intracranial bleeding, retroperitoneal bleeding, major GI and GU bleeding. Female and elderly clients have a higher incidence of bleeding than male or younger clients.

Miscellaneous: Nausea, fever, headache, bradycardia, coronary artery dissection, dizziness, edema or swelling, leg/pelvic pain, vasovagal reaction, sweating.

LABORATORY TEST CONSIDERATIONS

↓ H&H, platelets. ↑ Urine and FOB.

OD OVERDOSE MANAGEMENT

Symptoms: Bleeding, including minor mucocutaneous bleeding events and minor bleeding at the site of cardiac catheterization. *Treatment:* Assess clinical condition. Adjust or cease infusion, as appropriate. Can be removed by hemodialysis.

DRUG INTERACTIONS

Aspirin / ↑ Bleeding
H *Evening primrose oil* / Potential for ↑ antiplatelet effect
H *Feverfew* / Potential for ↑ antiplatelet effect
H *Garlic* / Potential for ↑ antiplatelet effect
H *Ginger* / Potential for ↑ antiplatelet effect
H *Ginkgo biloba* / Potential for ↑ antiplatelet effect
H *Ginseng* / Potential for ↑ antiplatelet effect
H *Grapeseed extract* / Potential for ↑ antiplatelet effect
Heparin / ↑ Bleeding
Levothyroxine / ↑ Tirofiban clearance
Omeprazole / ↑ Tirofiban clearance

HOW SUPPLIED

Injection: 50 mcg/mL; *Injection, Concentrate:* 250 mcg/mL

DOSAGE

- **IV**
  Acute coronary syndrome.
  Initial: 0.4 mcg/kg/min for 30 min; **then,** 0.1 mcg/kg/min. Use half the usual rate in those with severe renal impairment. Consult package insert for the guide to dosage adjustment by weight of the client.

NURSING CONSIDERATIONS

ADMINISTRATION/STORAGE

IV 1. May be given in the same IV line as heparin, dopamine, lidocaine, potassium chloride, and famotidine. Do not give in the same IV line as diazepam.
2. Tirofiban injection (250 mcg/mL) must be diluted to the same strength as tirofiban injection premixed (50 mcg/mL). One of three methods can be used to achieve a final concentration of 50 mcg/mL (mix well prior to use):
- Withdraw and discard 100 mL from a 500 mL bag of either sterile 0.9% NaCl or D5W; replace this volume with 100 mL of tirofiban injection (i.e., from two 50 mL vials).
- Withdraw and discard 50 mL from a 250 mL bag of either sterile 0.9% NaCl or D5W and replace this volume with 50 mL of tirofiban injection (i.e., from two-25 mL vials or one-50 mL vial).
- Add the contents of a 25 mL vial to a 100 mL bag of sterile 0.9% NaCl or D5W.
3. Tirofiban injection premix comes in 500 mL *Intravia* containers with 0.9% NaCl and tirofiban, 50 mcg/mL. To open the *Intravia* container, remove the dust cover. The plastic may be opaque due to moisture absorption during sterilization; the opacity will decrease gradually. Check for leaks by firmly squeezing the inner bag. Lack of sterility may be suspected if leaks are found; discard the solution. Do not use unless the solution is clear and the seal is intact.
4. Do not add other drugs or remove tirofiban from the bag without a syringe.
5. Do not use plastic containers in series connections as an air embolism can result by drawing air from the first container if it is empty.

Bold Italic = life threatening side effect   ■ = black box warning   ♣ = Available in Canada

6. Store at 25°C (77°F); do not freeze and protect from light.

7. Discard any unused solution 24 hr after start of the infusion.

ASSESSMENT

1. Note indications for therapy, onset, and characteristics of symptoms.

2. Determine any history of intracranial hemorrhage or neoplasm, AV malformation, or aneurysm.

3. Monitor VS, H&H, platelets, PTT initially and 6 hr after loading infusions of tirofiban and heparin and daily; monitor renal function studies and reduce dosage with dysfunction (C_{CR} < 30 mL/min).

CLIENT/FAMILY TEACHING

1. Drug is used IV with heparin to reduce death and symptoms associated with heart vessel blockage.

2. May experience bleeding so all sites will be carefully assessed and blood work evaluated frequently.

3. May experience dizziness; use caution. Stop smoking now.

4. Encourage family to learn CPR.

OUTCOMES/EVALUATE

Inhibition of platelet aggregation with ↓ refractory ischemia, MI, and death

Tocainide ■
hydrochloride
(toe-**KAY**-nyd)

CLASSIFICATION(S):
Antiarrhythmic, Class IB
PREGNANCY CATEGORY: C
Rx: Tonocard

SEE ALSO *ANTIARRHYTHMIC AGENTS.*

ACTION/KINETICS

Similar to lidocaine. Decreases the excitability of cells in the myocardium by decreasing sodium and potassium conductance. Increases pulmonary and aortic arterial pressure and slightly increases peripheral resistance. Effective in both digitalized and nondigitalized clients. **Peak plasma levels:** 0.5–2 hr. **$t\frac{1}{2}$:** 11–15 hr. **Therapeutic serum levels:** 4–10 mcg/mL. **Duration:** 8 hr. From 28 to 55% is excreted unchanged in the urine. Alkalinization decreases the excretion of the drug although acidification does not produce any changes in excretion. About 10% bound to plasma proteins.

USES

Life-threatening ventricular arrhythmias, including ventricular tachycardia. Has not been shown to improve survival in clients with ventricular arrhythmias. *Investigational:* Myotonic dystrophy, trigeminal neuralgia.

CONTRAINDICATIONS

Allergy to amide-type local anesthetics, second- or third-degree AV block in the absence of artificial ventricular pacemaker. Lactation.

SPECIAL CONCERNS

■(1) Agranulocytosis, bone marrow depression, leukopenia, neutropenia, aplastic/hypoplastic anemia, thrombocytopenia and sequelae, such as septicemia and shock, have occurred in those receiving tocainide (most within the recommended dosage range). Fatalities have occurred. Since most of these events have occurred during the first 12 weeks of therapy, perform CBCs, including WBC, differential, and platelet counts at weekly intervals for the first 3 months of therapy, and frequently thereafter. (2) Perform CBCs promptly if the client develops any signs of infection (e.g., fever, chills, sore throat, stomatitis), bruising, or bleeding. If any of these disorders are noted, discontinue tocainide and begin appropriate treatment if necessary. Blood counts usually return to normal within 1 month of discontinuing the drug. Use with caution in those with preexisting bone marrow failure or cytopenia of any type. (3) Pulmonary fibrosis, interstitial pneumonitis, fibrosing alveolitis, pulmonary edema, and pneumonia have occured. Many of these events occured in those who were seriously ill and fatalities have resulted. The experiences are usually characterized by bilateral infiltrates on x-ray and are frequently associated with dyspnea and cough; fever may be present. Instruct clients to report promptly any pulmonary symptoms (e.g., exertional dyspnea, cough, wheezing). Chest x-rays are advisable. If these pulmonary disorders develop, discontinue tocainide.■ Increased risk of death when used in those with non-life-threatening cardiac arrhythmias. Safety and efficacy have not been established in children. Use with caution in clients with impaired renal or hepatic function (dose may have to be decreased). Geriatric clients may have an increased risk of dizziness and hypotension; the dose may have to be reduced in these clients due to age-related impaired renal function.

SIDE EFFECTS

CV: *Increased arrhythmias,* increased ventricular rate (when given for atrial flutter or fibrillation), CHF, tachycardia, hypotension, **conduction disturbances,** bradycardia, chest pain, LV failure, palpitations. **CNS:** Dizziness, vertigo, headache, tremors, confusion, disorientation, hallucinations, ataxia, paresthesias, numbness, nervousness, altered mood, anxiety, incoordination, walking disturbances. **GI:** N&V, anorexia, diarrhea. **Respiratory:** *Pulmonary fibrosis, fibrosing alveolitis,* interstitial pneumonitis, *pulmonary edema,* pneumonia. **Hematologic:** Leukopenia, *agranulocytosis,* hypoplastic anemia, *aplastic anemia,* bone marrow depression, neutropenia, *thrombocytopenia and sequelae as septicemia and septic shock.* **Musculoskeletal:** Arthritis, arthralgia, myalgia. **Dermatologic:** Rash, skin lesion, diaphoresis. **Other:** Blurred vision, visual disturbances, nystagmus, tinnitus, hearing loss, lupus-like syndrome.

LABORATORY TEST CONSIDERATIONS

Abnormal LFTs (esp. in early therapy). ↑ ANA.

OD OVERDOSE MANAGEMENT

Symptoms: Initially are CNS symptoms including tremor (see above). GI symptoms may follow (see above). *Treatment:* Gastric lavage and activated charcoal may be useful. In the event of respiratory depression or arrest or seizures, maintain airway and provide artificial ventilation. An IV anticonvulsant (e.g., diazepam, thiopental, thiamylal, pentobarbital, secobarbital) may be required if seizures are persistent.

DRUG INTERACTIONS

Cimetidine / ↓ Tocainide bioavailability
Metoprolol / Additive effects on wedge pressure and cardiac index
Rifampin / ↓ Tocainide bioavailability

HOW SUPPLIED

Tablet: 400 mg, 600 mg

DOSAGE

• **TABLETS**
   Antiarrhythmic.
Adults, individualized, initial: 400 mg q 8 hr, up to a maximum of 2,400 mg/day; **maintenance:** 1,200–1,800 mg/day in divided doses. Total daily dose of 1,200 mg may be adequate in clients with liver or kidney disease.
   Myotonic dystrophy.
800–1,200 mg/day.
   Trigeminal neuralgia.
20 mg/kg/day in three divided doses.

NURSING CONSIDERATIONS

ASSESSMENT

1. Document indications for therapy, type, onset, and characteristics of symptoms. List other agents trialed.
2. Monitor ECG, CBC (weekly x 3 months), electrolytes, liver and renal function studies; correct potassium deficits. Document cardiac and pulmonary assessment findings.

CLIENT/FAMILY TEACHING

1. Take in the morning with food to minimize GI upset. Check and record pulse, note if irregular.
2. Do not drive or operate machinery until drug effects are realized; may cause drowsiness or dizziness.
3. Report any abnormal bruising, bleeding, fever, sore throat, or chills (S&S of blood dyscrasia).
4. Avoid alcohol during therapy.
5. Pulmonary symptoms such as wheezing, coughing, or SOB should be reported immediately; may indicate pulmonary fibrosis.

OUTCOMES/EVALUATE

• Control of lethal ventricular arrhythmias
• ↓ Muscle spasm and pain
• Therapeutic drug levels (4–10 mcg/mL)

Bold Italic = life threatening side effect   ■ = black box warning   ♣ = Available in Canada

Torsemide ■ ©
(TOR-seh-myd)

CLASSIFICATION(S):
Diuretic, loop
PREGNANCY CATEGORY: B
Rx: Demadex

SEE ALSO *DIURETICS, LOOP.*

ACTION/KINETICS
Onset, IV: Within 10 min; **PO:** Within 60 min. **Peak effect, IV:** Within 60 min; **PO:** 60–120 min. **Duration:** 6–8 hr. **t ½:** 210 min. Metabolized by the liver and excreted through the urine. Food delays the time to peak effect by about 30 min, but the overall bioavailability and the diuretic activity are not affected.

USES
(1) Congestive heart failure. (2) Acute or chronic renal failure. (3) Hepatic cirrhosis. (4) Hypertension.

CONTRAINDICATIONS
Lactation.

SPECIAL CONCERNS
■Loop diuretics are potent drugs; excess amounts can lead to a profound diuresis with water and electrolyte depletion. Careful medical supervision is required and dosage must be individualized.■ Clients sensitive to sulfonamides may show allergic reactions to torsemide. Safety and efficacy in children have not been determined.

SIDE EFFECTS
CNS: Headache, dizziness, asthenia, insomnia, nervousness, syncope. **GI:** Diarrhea, constipation, nausea, dyspepsia, edema, *GI hemorrhage,* rectal bleeding. **CV:** ECG abnormality, chest pain, atrial fibrillation, hypotension, *ventricular tachycardia,* shunt thrombosis. **Respiratory:** Rhinitis, increase in cough. **Musculoskeletal:** Arthralgia, myalgia. **Miscellaneous:** Sore throat, excessive urination, rash.

LABORATORY TEST CONSIDERATIONS
Hyperglycemia, hyperuricemia, hypokalemia, hypovolemia.

HOW SUPPLIED
Injection: 10 mg/mL; *Tablet:* 5 mg, 10 mg, 20 mg, 100 mg

DOSAGE
• **TABLETS, IV**
Congestive heart failure.
Adults, initial: 10 or 20 mg once daily.
Chronic renal failure.
Adults, initial: 20 mg once daily.
Hepatic cirrhosis.
Adults, initial: 5 or 10 mg once daily given with an aldosterone antagonist or a potassium-sparing diuretic.
Hypertension.
Adults, initial: 5 mg once daily. If this dose does not lead to an adequate decrease in BP within 4–6 weeks, the dose may be increased to 10 mg once daily. If the 10 mg dose is not adequate, an additional antihypertensive agent is added to the treatment regimen.

NURSING CONSIDERATIONS
© Do not confuse torsemide with furosemide (also a loop diuretic).

ADMINISTRATION/STORAGE
1. If the response is inadequate for the initial dose used for CHF, chronic renal failure, or hepatic cirrhosis, the dose can be doubled until the desired diuretic response is obtained. Doses greater than 200 mg for CHF or chronic renal failure and greater than 40 mg for hepatic cirrhosis have not been adequately studied.
2. May be given without regard for meals.
3. It is not necessary to adjust the dose for geriatric clients.
IV 4. Give the IV dose slowly over a period of 2 min or as a continuous infusion.
5. Oral and IV doses are therapeutically equivalent; may switch to and from the IV form with no change in dose.

ASSESSMENT
1. Document indications for therapy, onset and characteristics of symptoms. List agents trialed and the outcome.
2. Document pulmonary, renal, and CV assessments. Note any sensitivity to sulfonamides.
3. Monitor VS, weight, I&O, blood sugar, uric acid, BUN, creatinine, and potassium; drug may increase blood sugar and uric acid levels.

T

CLIENT/FAMILY TEACHING

1. Take only as directed. May take with food to decrease GI upset.
2. With hypertension, keep a BP log for provider review.
3. Report immediately any chest pain, increased SOB, or sudden weight gain with edema.
4. Drug may cause dizziness, lightheadedness, and fatigue; use caution. Rise slowly from a sitting or lying position to minimize low BP effects.
5. May experience blurred vision, yellowing of vision, or sensitivity to sunlight. Report any unusual, persistent symptoms or lack of response.

OUTCOMES/EVALUATE

- ↓ Edema; ↑ diuresis; ↓ BP
- Reduction of interdialysis weight gain and promotion of Na, Cl, and water excretion

Trandolapril ■

(tran-**DOHL**-ah-pril)

CLASSIFICATION(S):
Antihypertensive, ACE inhibitor
PREGNANCY CATEGORY: C (first trimester); D (second and third trimesters)
Rx: Mavik

SEE ALSO ANGIOTENSIN CONVERTING ENZYME (ACE) INHIBITORS.

ACTION/KINETICS

Rapidly absorbed; food slows rate, but not amount absorbed. Metabolized in liver to active trandolaprilat. **Onset:** 2–4 hr. Bioavailability is about 10% (70% of trandolaprilat, the active metabolite). Food slows absorption. **Peak plasma levels, trandolapril:** 30–60 min; **trandolaprilat:** 4–10 hr. **t ½, trandolapril:** About 5 hr; **t ½, trandoprilat:** About 10 hr. **Peak effect:** 4–8 hr. **Duration:** 24 hr. About ⅓ trandolaprilat is excreted in urine and ⅔ in feces. About 80% is bound to plasma proteins.

USES

(1) Hypertension, alone or in combination with other antihypertensives such as hydrochlorothiazide. (2) For stable clients who have left-ventricular systolic dysfunction or who are symptomatic from CHF within the first few days after an acute MI.

CONTRAINDICATIONS

In those with a history of angioedema with ACE inhibitors.

SPECIAL CONCERNS

■When used during the second and third trimesters of pregnancy, injury and even death can result in the developing fetus. When pregnancy is detected, discontinue as soon as possible.■ Safety and efficacy have not been determined in children.

SIDE EFFECTS

See also *ACE Inhibitors.* **Hypersensitivity: *Angioedema.* CNS:** Dizziness, headache, fatigue, insomnia, paresthesias, drowsiness, vertigo, anxiety. **GI:** Diarrhea, dyspepsia, gastritis, abdominal pain, vomiting, constipation, pancreatitis. **CV:** Hypotension, bradycardia, chest pain, *cardiogenic shock*, intermittent claudication, stroke. **Respiratory:** Cough, dyspnea, URTI, epistaxis, throat inflammation. **Hepatic: *Hepatic failure,*** including cholestatic jaundice, *fulminant hepatic necrosis, death.* **Dermatologic:** Photosensitivity, pruritus, rash. **GU:** UTI, impotence, decreased libido. **Miscellaneous:** Neutropenia, syncope, myalgia, asthenia, muscle cramps, hypocalcemia, intermittent claudication, edema, extremity pain, gout.

LABORATORY TEST CONSIDERATIONS

Hyperkalemia, hypocalcemia. ↑ Serum uric acid, BUN, creatinine.

DRUG INTERACTIONS

Diuretics / Excessive hypotensive effects
Diuretics, potassium-sparing: ↑ Risk of hyperkalemia
Lithium / ↑ Risk of lithium toxicity

HOW SUPPLIED

Tablet: 1 mg, 2 mg, 4 mg.

DOSAGE

- **TABLETS**
  Hypertension.
  Initial: 1 mg once daily in nonblack clients (2 mg once daily in black clients) for those not receiving a diuretic. Adjust dosage according to response; usually, adjustments are made at intervals of 1 week. **Maintenance, usual:** 4 mg once

---

T

daily (twice daily dosing may be needed in some). If BP is still not adequately controlled, diuretic may be added.

Heart failure post–MI/Left ventricular dysfunction post–MI.

Initial: 1 mg/day. Then, increase the dose, as tolerated, to a target dose of 4 mg/day. If 4 mg is not tolerated, continue with the highest tolerated dose. If C_{CR} is less than 30 mL/min or if there is hepatic cirrhosis, initial dose is 0.5 mg daily. Titrate dose to optimal response.

NURSING CONSIDERATIONS
ADMINISTRATION/STORAGE
1. If client is on a diuretic, discontinue 2 to 3 days prior to beginning therapy with trandolapril to reduce likelihood of hypotension. If diuretic can not be discontinued, use an initial trandolapril dose of 0.5 mg. Titrate subsequent dosage.
2. Store tablets from 20–25°C (68–77°F).

ASSESSMENT
1. Note indications for therapy, disease onset, other agents trialed and outcome.
2. Monitor BP, cardiac status, CBC, electrolytes, liver and renal function studies; reduce dosage with impairment.

CLIENT/FAMILY TEACHING
1. Take only as directed.
2. May experience cough, dizziness, and diarrhea; report if persistent.
3. Practice reliable contraception; stop drug and report if pregnancy suspected.
4. Continue lifestyle changes i.e., regular exercise, smoking/alcohol cessation, low fat, low salt diet in overall goal of BP control.

OUTCOMES/EVALUATE
• ↓ BP
• Control of heart failure/ventricular dysfunction after MI

Treprostinil sodium
(treh-**PROSS**-tih-nill)

CLASSIFICATION(S):
Antiplatelet drug

PREGNANCY CATEGORY: B
Rx: Remodulin

ACTION/KINETICS
Causes direct dilation of pulmonary and systemic arterial vascular beds and inhibition of platelet aggregation. Also causes a dose-related negative inotropic and lusitropic effect. Rapidly and completely absorbed after SC infusion. Steady state levels occurred in about 10 hr. Metabolized in the liver and excreted in the urine and feces. **t ½, terminal:** 2–4 hr.

USES
Reduce symptoms associated with exercise in pulmonary arterial hypertension with NYHA Class II through IV symptoms.

CONTRAINDICATIONS
Known hypersensitivity.

SPECIAL CONCERNS
Use with caution in renal or hepatic impairment, during lactation, and in the elderly. Safety and efficacy have been been determined in children.

SIDE EFFECTS
At site of injection: Infusion site pain and reaction, bleeding/bruising, erythema, induration, rash, problems with the infusion system. **GI:** Nausea, diarrhea. **CNS:** Headache, dizziness. **CV:** Vasodilation, hypotension. **Miscellaneous:** Rash, jaw pain, edema, pruritus.

OD OVERDOSE MANAGEMENT
Symptoms: Extensions of pharmacological effects, including flushing, headache, hypotension, N&V, diarrhea. *Treatment:* Symptoms are usually self-limiting and are treated with reducing or withholding the drug.

DRUG INTERACTIONS
Anticoagulants / ↑ Risk of bleeding especially in clients maintained on anticoagulants
Antihypertensive drugs / Significant BP reduction
Diuretics / Significant BP reduction
Vasodilators / Significant BP reduction

HOW SUPPLIED
Injection: 1 mg/mL, 2.5 mg/mL, 5 mg/mL, 10 mg/mL

DOSAGE

- **Continuous SC infusion**
  Pulmonary arterial hypertension.
Initial: 1.25 ng/kg/min. If this dose can not be tolerated, reduce to 0.625 ng/kg/min. Increase the infusion rate in increments of no more than 1.25 ng/kg/min per week for the first 4 weeks and then no more than 2.5 ng/kg/min per week for the remaining duration of infusion, depending on the response. Doses above 40 ng/kg/hr have not been studied sufficiently. In clients with mild or moderate hepatic insufficiency, decrease the initial dose to 0.625 ng/kg/min and increase cautiously.

NURSING CONSIDERATIONS

ADMINISTRATION/STORAGE

IV 1. To be given without further dilution of the product.

2. Use the following formula to calculate infusion rates: Infusion rate (mL/hr) = Dose (ng/kg/min) x weight (kg) x (0.00006/treprostinil dosage strength concentration [mg/mL]).

3. A single reservoir syringe can be given up to 72 hr at 37°C (99°F). Do not use a single vial for more than 14 days after initial introduction into the vial.

4. Given by continuous SC infusion via a self-inserted SC catheter using an infusion pump designed for SC drug delivery.

5. To avoid interruptions in drug delivery, the client must have available a backup infusion pump and SC infusion sets.

6. To prevent worsening symptoms, avoid abrupt withdrawal or sudden large increases in dosage of the drug.

7. Unopened vials are stable until the date indicated if stored from 15–25°C (59–77°F).

ASSESSMENT

1. Note NYHA stage and symptom characteristics. List other agents trialed and the outcome. Identify if transplant candidate.

2. Document cardiopulmonary assessment findings and catherization results. Monitor renal and LFTs, use cautiously with dysfunction.

CLIENT/FAMILY TEACHING

1. Drug is administered as a continuous infusion through a SC catheter with an infusion pump for an extended period of time.

2. Review proper administration techniques, catheter insertion, site care, drug loading and pump maintenance/alarms/care. Refer to home infusion agency for management/support.

3. Report any adverse drug effects i.e., headache, N&V, anxiety/restlessness and infusion site pain so dose can be adjusted to control these effects yet improve present functioning level/exercise tolerance.

4. Keep close contact and all F/U visits to assess status and heart disease progression. May eventually require conversion to IV therapy.

OUTCOMES/EVALUATE

↑ Exercise tolerance ↑ CO

Triamterene   ©

(try-**AM**-ter-een)

CLASSIFICATION(S):
Diuretic, potassium-sparing
PREGNANCY CATEGORY: B
Rx: Dyrenium

SEE ALSO *DIURETICS*.

ACTION/KINETICS

Acts directly on the distal tubule to promote the excretion of sodium—which is exchanged for potassium or hydrogen ions—bicarbonate, chloride, and fluid. It increases urinary pH and is a weak folic acid antagonist. **Onset:** 2–4 hr. **Peak effect:** 6–8 hr. **Duration:** 7–9 hr. **t ½:** 3 hr. From one-half to two-thirds of the drug is bound to plasma protein. Metabolized to hydroxytriamterene sulfate, which is also active. About 20% is excreted unchanged through the urine.

USES

(1) Edema due to CHF. (2) Hepatic cirrhosis. (3) Nephrotic syndrome. (4) Steroid therapy. (5) Secondary hyperaldosteronism. (6) Idiopathic edema. May be used alone or with other diuretics. *Investigational:* Prophylaxis and treatment

---

of hypokalemia, adjunct in the treatment of hypertension.

CONTRAINDICATIONS
Hypersensitivity to drug, severe or progressive renal insufficiency, severe hepatic disease, anuria, hyperkalemia, hyperuricemia, gout, history of nephrolithiasis. Lactation.

SPECIAL CONCERNS
Safety and efficacy have not been determined in children.

SIDE EFFECTS
Electrolyte: Hyperkalemia, electrolyte imbalance. **GI:** Nausea, vomiting (may also be indicative of electrolyte imbalance), diarrhea, dry mouth. **CNS:** Dizziness, drowsiness, fatigue, weakness, headache. **Hematologic:** Megaloblastic anemia, thrombocytopenia. **Renal:** Azotemia, interstitial nephritis. **Miscellaneous:** *Anaphylaxis,* photosensitivity, hypokalemia, jaundice, muscle cramps, rash.

OD OVERDOSE MANAGEMENT
Symptoms: Electrolyte imbalance, especially hyperkalemia. Also, nausea, vomiting, other GI disturbances, weakness, hypotension, reversible acute renal failure. *Treatment:* Immediately induce vomiting or perform gastric lavage. Evaluate electrolyte levels and fluid balance and treat if necessary. Dialysis may be beneficial.

DRUG INTERACTIONS
Amantadine / ↑ Amantadine toxic effects R/T ↓ renal excretion
Angiotensin-converting enzyme inhibitors / Significant hyperkalemia
Antihypertensives / Potentiated by triamterene
Captopril / ↑ Risk of significant hyperkalemia
Cimetidine / ↑ Bioavailability and ↓ clearance of triamterene
Digitalis / Inhibited by triamterene
Indomethacin / ↑ Risk of nephrotoxicity and acute renal failure
Lithium / ↑ Chance of toxicity R/T ↓ renal clearance
Potassium salts / Additive hyperkalemia
Spironolactone / Additive hyperkalemia

HOW SUPPLIED
Capsule: 50 mg, 100 mg

DOSAGE
• **CAPSULES.**
Diuretic.
Adults, initial: 100 mg twice a day after meals; **maximum daily dose:** 300 mg.

NURSING CONSIDERATIONS
ℰ Do not confuse Triamterene with Trimipramine

ADMINISTRATION/STORAGE
1. Minimize nausea by giving the drug after meals.
2. Dosage is usually reduced by one-half when another diuretic is added to the regimen.

ASSESSMENT
1. Document indications for therapy and other agents trialed; list agents prescribed to ensure none interact.
2. Assess for alcoholism; megaloblastic anemia may occur because triamterene is a weak antagonist of folic acid.
3. Monitor BP, weight, ECG, CBC, BS, uric acid, electrolytes, I&O, and renal function.

CLIENT/FAMILY TEACHING
1. Take in the a.m. with food to minimize GI upset/nausea. Take care, drug may cause dizziness.
2. Report any sore throat, rash, fever (S&S of blood dyscrasia), or lack of effectiveness.
3. Persistent headaches, drowsiness, vomiting, restlessness, mental wandering, lethargy, and foul breath may be signs of uremia; report.
4. Avoid alcohol and OTC agents. Also avoid potassium supplements, salt substitutes that contain potassium, and foods high in potassium; drug is potassium-sparing.
5. Urine may appear pale fluorescent blue.
6. Avoid direct sunlight for prolonged periods; may cause a photosensitivity reaction. Use sunscreens, sunglasses, hat, long sleeves, and pants when exposed.

OUTCOMES/EVALUATE
↓ Edema; ↑ diuresis; ↓ BP

—*COMBINATION DRUG*—

Triamterene and Hydrochlorothiazide

(try-**AM**-teh-reen, hy-droh-**kloh**-roh-**THIGH**-ah-zyd)

CLASSIFICATION(S):

Antihypertensive, combination drug
PREGNANCY CATEGORY: C
Rx: Dyazide, Maxzide, Maxide-25 MG
✚**Rx:** Apo-Triazide, Novo-Triamzide, Nu-Triazide

SEE ALSO *HYDROCHLOROTHIAZIDE* **AND** *TRIAMTERENE*.

CONTENT

Capsules. *Diuretic:* Hydrochlorothiazide, 25 or 50 mg. *Diuretic:* Triamterene, 50 or 100 mg. **Tablets.** *Diuretic:* Hydrochlorothiazide, 25 or 50 mg. *Diuretic:* Triamterene, 37.5 or 75 mg. (In Canada the tablets contain 25 mg of hydrochlorothiazide and 50 mg triamterene).

USES

Hypertension or edema in clients who manifest hypokalemia on hydrochlorothiazide alone. In clients requiring a diuretic and in whom hypokalemia cannot be risked (i.e., clients with cardiac arrhythmias or those taking digitalis). Usually not the first line of therapy, except for clients in whom hypokalemia should be avoided.

CONTRAINDICATIONS

Clients receiving other potassium-sparing drugs such as amiloride and spironolactone. Use in anuria, acute or chronic renal insufficiency, significant renal impairment, preexisting elevated serum potassium.

SPECIAL CONCERNS

Use with caution during lactation. Geriatric clients may be more sensitive to the hypotensive and electrolyte effects of this combination; also, age-related decreases in renal function may require a decrease in dosage.

LABORATORY TEST CONSIDERATIONS

Triamterene may impart blue fluorescence to urine, interfering with fluorometric assays (e.g., lactic dehydrogenase, quinidine). ↑ BUN, creatinine. ↑ Serum uric acid in clients predisposed to gouty arthritis.

HOW SUPPLIED

See Content

DOSAGE

• **CAPSULES**
Hypertension or edema.
Adults: Triamterene/hydrochlorothiazide: 37.5 mg/25 mg—1–2 capsules given once daily with monitoring of serum potassium and clinical effect. Triamterene/hydrochlorothiazide: 50 mg/25 mg—1–2 capsules twice a day after meals. Some clients may be controlled using 1 capsule every day or every other day. No more than 4 capsules should be taken daily.

• **TABLETS**
Hypertension or edema.
Adults: Triamterene/hydrochlorothiazide: 37.5 mg/25 mg—1–2 tablets/day (determined by individual titration with the components). Or, triamterene/hydrochlorothiazide: 75 mg/50 mg—1 tablet daily.

NURSING CONSIDERATIONS

ADMINISTRATION/STORAGE

Monitor clients who are transferred from less bioavailable formulations of triamterene and hydrochlorothiazide for serum potassium levels following the transfer.

ASSESSMENT

1. Document indications for therapy and other agents trialed; list agents prescribed to ensure none interact.
2. Assess for alcoholism; megaloblastic anemia may occur because triamterene is a weak antagonist of folic acid.
3. Monitor BP, weight, ECG, CBC, BS, uric acid, electrolytes, I&O, and renal function.

CLIENT/FAMILY TEACHING

1. Drug is used to lower BP and reduce swelling of extremities. Take in the A.M. with food to minimize GI upset/nausea. Use care, drug may cause dizziness. Report as scheduled for F/U.

Bold Italic = life threatening side effect   ■ = black box warning   ✚ = Available in Canada

T

2. Report any adverse effects including sore throat, rash, or fever (S&S of blood dyscrasia) or lack of effectiveness.

3. Persistent headaches, drowsiness, vomiting, restlessness, mental wandering, lethargy, and foul breath may be signs of uremia; report.

4. Avoid alcohol and OTC agents. Also avoid potassium supplements, salt substitutes that contain potassium, and foods high in potassium; drug is potassium-sparing.

5. Urine may appear pale fluorescent blue.

6. Avoid direct sunlight for prolonged periods; may cause a photosensitivity reaction. Use sunscreens, sunglasses, hat, and long sleeves and pants when exposed.

OUTCOMES/EVALUATE
• Control of hypertension
• Resolution of edema

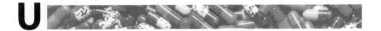

Urokinase
(your-oh-**KYE**-nayz)

CLASSIFICATION(S):
Thrombolytic enzyme
PREGNANCY CATEGORY: B
Rx: Abbokinase

ACTION/KINETICS
Urokinase converts plasminogen to plasmin; plasmin then breaks down fibrin clots, fibrinogen, and other plasma proteins. A decrease in plasma fibrinogen and plasminogen and increased circulating FDP may persist for 12–24 hr. **Onset:** rapid; **duration:** 12 hr. **t ½:** < 20 min, although effect on coagulation disappears after a few hours.

USES
(1) Lysis of acute, massive pulmonary thromboemboli. (2) Adults for the lysis of pulmonary emboli accompanied by unstable hemodynamics (e.g., failure to maintain BP without supportive measures). *Investigational:* Lyse clots in AV cannulae.

CONTRAINDICATIONS
Active internal bleeding, history of CVA, within 2 months of intracranial or intraspinal surgery or trauma, recent cardiopulmonary resuscitation, intracranial neoplasm, arteriovenous malformation or aneurysm, known bleeding diathesis, severe uncontrolled arterial hypertension. Any condition presenting a risk of hemorrhage, such as recent surgery or biopsies, delivery within 10 days, pregnancy, ulcerative disease. Also hepatic or renal insufficiency, tuberculosis, recent cerebral embolism, thrombosis, hemorrhage, SBE, rheumatic valvular disease, thrombocytopenia.

SPECIAL CONCERNS
Use in septic thrombophlebitis may be hazardous. Produced from cultures of human source materials; thus, there is the potential to transmit infectious agents, although procedures are used to reduce such risk. Use with caution during lactation. Safe use in children has not been established.

SIDE EFFECTS
CV: Superficial bleeding, *severe internal bleeding, MI, stroke, cardiac arrest,* cerebral and distal vascular embolization, cholesterol emboli, pulmonary edema, reperfusion ventricular arrhythmias, decreased hematocrit, transient hypotension or hypertension, tachycardia. **Allergic:** Rarely, skin rashes, *anaphylaxis, bronchospasm,* orolingual edema, urticaria, pruritus. **Infusion reaction:** Hypoxia, cyanosis, dyspnea, tachycardia, hypotension, hypertension, acidosis, fever and/or chills/rigor, back pain, N&V. **Other:** Thrombocytopenia, diaphoresis, chest pain, substernal pain.

U

DRUG INTERACTIONS

Anticoagulants and drugs that alter platelet function (e.g., aspirin, NSAIDs, dipyridamole, GP IIb/IIIa inhibitors) ↑ the risk of serious bleeding when given with urokinase.

HOW SUPPLIED

Powder for injection, lyophilized: 250,000 international units

DOSAGE————————————

- **IV INFUSION ONLY**
  Pulmonary embolism.

Loading dose: 4,400 interrnational units/kg mixed with either 0.9% NaCl or D5W given at a rate of 90 mL/hr over 10 min; **maintenance:** 4,400 international units/kg/hr given at a rate of 15 mL/hr for 12 hr. At the end of therapy, treat with continuous IV heparin to prevent thrombosis recurrence. Do not begin anticoagulation until aPTT has decreased to less than twice the normal control value (about 3–4 hr after completing infusion). If heparin is used, do not give a loading dose of heparin. Follow with oral anticoagulants.

NURSING CONSIDERATIONS

ADMINISTRATION/STORAGE

IV 1. Reconstitute only with sterile water for injection without preservatives. Do not use bacteriostatic water.

2. To reconstitute, roll and tilt the vial but do not shake. Reconstitute immediately before using.

3. Dilute reconstituted urokinase before IV administration in 0.9% NSS or D5W.

4. At the end of therapy for pulmonary embolism, ensure that the total dose is given by using the following flush procedure: Give a solution of 0.9% NaCl or D5W via the pump approximately equal to the volume of the tubing in the infusion set. Flush the admixture from the entire length of the infusion set at a rate of 15 mL/hr.

5. Discard any unused portion.

6. Type and cross and have blood for transfusion available. Aminocaproic acid may be employed with severe bleeding or hemorrhage.

7. Store the powder for injection at 2–8°C (36–46°F).

ASSESSMENT

1. Note indications for therapy, type, onset, and symptom characteristics.

2. Monitor ECG, CBC, PT, PTT, liver and renal function studies.

3. Assess for conditions that may preclude drug therapy (recent surgery, cerebral embolism, thrombosis, hermorrhage, SBE, thrombocytopenia, pregnancy, TB).

4. Have additional IV access and Heparin drip ready for therapy.

INTERVENTIONS

1. Check access sites for evidence of bleeding. Test stools, urine, and emesis for occult blood.

2. During IV therapy, arterial sticks require 30 min of manual pressure followed by application of a pressure dressing. To prevent bruising, avoid unnecessary handling of client.

3. If IM injections necessary, apply pressure after withdrawing the needle to prevent hematoma and bleeding from the puncture site. Observe injection sites and postoperative wounds for bleeding during therapy

4. Use FFP or cryoprecipitate for bleeding.

CLIENT/FAMILY TEACHING

1. Review benefits and risks of drug therapy. Drug is used to break up clots with pulmonary embolism from coronary arteries that are obstructed or to unblock venous catheters.

2. For best results, the therapy should be instituted within 4–6 hr of onset of S&S of MI and within one week of other thrombic event.

3. Report any spontaneous bleeding or adverse side effects immediately.

4. Encourage family members or significant other to learn CPR.

OUTCOMES/EVALUATE

- Lysis of thrombi with restoration of blood flow and prevention of tissue infarction

U

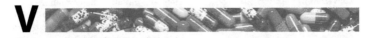

Valsartan ■
(val-**SAR**-tan)

CLASSIFICATION(S):
Antihypertensive, angiotensin II receptor blocker
PREGNANCY CATEGORY: C (1st trimester), D (2nd and 3rd trimesters)
Rx: Diovan

SEE ALSO *ANGIOTENSIN II RECEPTOR ANTAGONISTS* AND *ANTIHYPERTENSIVE AGENTS.*

ACTION/KINETICS
Reduces both BP and left ventricular hypertrophy. About 25% bioavailable. Food decreases absorption. **Peak plasma levels:** 2–4 hr. **t ½:** 6 hr. Eliminated mostly unchanged in feces (83%) and urine (about 13%). 95% bound to plasma proteins.

USES
(1) Alone or in combination to treat hypertension. (2) Heart failure (NYHA class II to IV) in those intolerant to ACE inhibitors. *Investigational:* Life-saving treatment for heart attack clients.

SPECIAL CONCERNS
■Use during the second and third trimester of pregnancy can cause injury and even death to the fetus. When pregnancy is detected, discontinue as soon as possible.■ Use with caution in severe hepatic or renal impaired function. May increase the death rate in clients also taking beta blockers and ACE inhibitors for CHF.

SIDE EFFECTS
CNS: Headache, dizziness, fatigue, anxiety, insomnia, paresthesia, somnolence. **GI:** Abdominal pain, diarrhea, nausea, constipation, dry mouth, dyspepsia, flatulence. **Respiratory:** URI, cough, rhinitis, sinusitis, pharyngitis, dyspnea. **Body as a whole:** Viral infection, edema, asthenia, allergic reaction. **Musculoskeletal:** Arthralgia, back pain, muscle cramps, myalgia. **Dermatologic:** Pruritus, rash. **Miscellaneous:** Palpitations, vertigo, neutropenia, impotence.

LABORATORY TEST CONSIDERATIONS
↓ H&H. ↑ Serum potassium, liver enzymes, serum bilirubin.

HOW SUPPLIED
Tablets: 40 mg, 80 mg, 160 mg, 320 mg

DOSAGE
- **TABLETS**
  Hypertension.
Adults, initial: 80 or 160 mg once daily as monotherapy in clients who are not volume depleted. A higher dose may be used in those requiring greater reductions. **Dose range:** 80–320 mg once daily. If additional antihypertensive effect is needed, dose may be increased to 160 mg or 320 mg once daily or diuretic may be added (has greater effect when valsartan dose increases beyond 80 mg).
  Heart failure.
Adults, initial: 40 mg twice a day. Increase dose to 80 and 160 mg twice a day as tolerated. Consider dose reduction of concomitant diuretics. Concomitant use with both an ACE inhibitor and beta-blocker is not recommended.

NURSING CONSIDERATIONS

ADMINISTRATION/STORAGE
1. Give on an empty stomach.
2. Antihypertensive effect is usually seen within 2 weeks with maximum reduction after 4 weeks.
3. Store between 15–30°C (59–86°F) in a tight container protected from moisture.

ASSESSMENT
1. Note disease onset, indications for therapy, characteristics of S&S, other problems, and other agents trialed and outcome. List other drugs prescribed to ensure none interact.
2. Monitor CBC, electrolytes, liver and renal function studies; note dysfunction.

V

CLIENT/FAMILY TEACHING

1. May take with or without food (works better without) and with other prescribed BP medications.

2. Change positions slowly and avoid dehydration to prevent sudden drop in BP and dizziness.

3. Practice reliable contraception; report if pregnancy suspected as drug may cause fetal death. Do not take if client becomes pregnant.

4. Continue low fat, low sodium diet, regular exercise, weight loss, smoking and alcohol cessation, and stress reduction in goal of BP control.

5. May experience headaches, coughing, diarrhea, nausea, and joint aches; report if persistent.

6. Before taking OTC drugs, obtain medical advice as some may affect the action of valsartan.

OUTCOMES/EVALUATE

↓ BP

Verapamil ©

(ver-**AP**-ah-mil)

CLASSIFICATION(S):

Calcium channel blocker

PREGNANCY CATEGORY: C

Rx: Calan, Calan SR, Covera-HS, Isoptin SR, Verelan, Verelan PM

✦**Rx:** Apo-Verap, Chronovera, Gen-Verapamil, Gen-Verapamil SR, Isoptin, Isoptin I.V., Isoptin SR, Novo-Veramil, Novo-Veramil SR, Nu-Verap

SEE ALSO *CALCIUM CHANNEL BLOCKING AGENTS.*

ACTION/KINETICS

Slows AV conduction and prolongs effective refractory period. IV doses may slightly increase LV filling pressure. Moderately decreases myocardial contractility and peripheral vascular resistance. Worsening of heart failure may result if verapamil is given to clients with moderate to severe cardiac dysfunction. **Onset, PO:** 30 min; **IV:** 3–5 min. **Time to peak plasma levels (PO):** 1–2 hr (5–7 hr for extended-release). **t ½, PO:** 4.5–12 hr with repetitive dos-

ing; **IV, initial:** 4 min; **final:** 2–5 hr. **Therapeutic serum levels:** 0.08–0.3 mcg/mL. **Duration, PO:** 8–10 hr (24 hr for extended-release); **IV:** 10–20 min for hemodynamic effect and 2 hr for antiarrhythmic effect. Metabolized to norverapamil, which possesses 20% of the activity of verapamil. *NOTE:* Covera HS is designed to deliver verapamil in concert with the 24-hr circadian variations in BP. Verelan PM allows for bedtime dosing and incorporates a 4- to 5-hr delay in drug delivery so there are maximum plasma levels in the morning.

USES

PO, Immediate-Release: (1) Angina pectoris due to coronary artery spasm (Prinzmetal's variant), chronic stable angina including angina due to increased effort, unstable angina (preinfarction, crescendo). (2) With digitalis to control rapid ventricular rate at rest and during stress in chronic atrial flutter or atrial fibrillation. (3) Prophylaxis of repetitive paroxysmal supraventricular tachycardia. (4) Essential hypertension. **PO, Extended-Release:** (1) Essential hypertension (Covera-HS only). (2) Angina (Covera-HS only). **IV:** (1) Paroxysmal supraventricular tachyarrhythmias. (2) Atrial flutter or fibrillation. *Investigational:* Manic depression (alternate therapy), exercise-induced asthma, recumbent nocturnal leg cramps, hypertrophic, cluster headaches.

CONTRAINDICATIONS

Severe hypotension, second- or third-degree AV block, cardiogenic shock, severe CHF, sick sinus syndrome (unless client has artificial pacemaker), severe LV dysfunction. Cardiogenic shock and severe CHF unless secondary to SVT that can be treated with verapamil. Lactation. Use of verapamil, IV, with beta-adrenergic blocking agents (as both depress myocardial contractility and AV conduction). Ventricular tachycardia.

SPECIAL CONCERNS

Infants less than 6 months of age may not respond to verapamil. Use with caution in hypertrophic cardiomyopathy, impaired hepatic and renal function, and in the elderly.

SIDE EFFECTS

CV: CHF, bradycardia, **AV block, asystole,** premature ventricular contractions and tachycardia (after IV use), peripheral and pulmonary edema, hypotension, syncope, palpitations, AV dissociation, **MI, CVA. GI:** Nausea, constipation, abdominal discomfort or cramps, dyspepsia, diarrhea, dry mouth. **CNS:** Dizziness, headache, sleep disturbances, depression, amnesia, paranoia, psychoses, hallucinations, jitteriness, confusion, drowsiness, vertigo. IV verapamil may increase intracranial pressure in clients with supratentorial tumors at the time of induction of anesthesia. **Dermatologic:** Rash, dermatitis, alopecia, urticaria, pruritus, erythema multiforme, **Stevens-Johnson syndrome. Respiratory:** Nasal or chest congestion, dyspnea, SOB, wheezing. **Musculoskeletal:** Paresthesia, asthenia, muscle cramps or inflammation, decreased neuromuscular transmission in Duchenne's muscular dystrophy. **Other:** Blurred vision, equilibrium disturbances, sexual difficulties, spotty menstruation, sweating, rotary nystagmus, flushing, gingival hyperplasia, polyuria, nocturia, gynecomastia, claudication, hyperkeratosis, purpura, petechiae, bruising, hematomas, tachyphylaxis.

LABORATORY TEST CONSIDERATIONS

↑ Alkaline phosphatase, transaminase.

OD OVERDOSE MANAGEMENT

Symptoms: Extension of side effects. *Treatment:* Beta-adrenergics, IV calcium, vasopressors, pacing, and resuscitation.

ADDITIONAL DRUG INTERACTIONS

Amiodarone / Possible cardiotoxicity with ↓ CO; monitor closely
Antihypertensive agents / Additive hypotensive effects
Antineoplastics / ↓ Verapamil absorption by several antineoplastics
Atorvastatin / ↑ Atorvastatin plasma levels
Barbiturates / ↓ Verapamil bioavailability
Buspirone / ↑ Buspirone effects
Calcium salts / ↓ Verapamil effect; can reverse clinical and toxic effects of verapamil

Carbamazepine / ↑ Carbamazepine effect R/T ↓ liver breakdown
Cimetidine / ↑ Verapamil bioavailability
Clarithromycin / Possible severe hypotension and bradycardia
Cyclosporine / ↑ Cyclosporine plasma levels → possible renal toxicity
Digoxin / ↑ Risk of digoxin toxicity R/T ↑ plasma levels
Disopyramide / Additive depressant effects on myocardial contractility and AV conduction
Dofetilide ↑ Dofetilide plasma levels → ↑ risk of ventricular arrhythmias
Ethanol / Prolonged and ↑ ethanol effects
Etomidate / Anesthetic effect may be ↑ with prolonged respiratory depression and apnea
Grapefruit juice / ↑ Verapamil plasma levels R/T ↓ liver metabolism
Imipramine / ↑ Imipramine serum levels
Lithium / ↓ Lithium levels; lithium toxicity also observed
Muscle relaxants, nondepolarizing / ↑ Neuromuscular blockade R/T verapamil effect on calcium channels
Prazosin / Acute hypotensive effect
Quinidine / Possibility of bradycardia, hypotension, AV block, VT, and pulmonary edema
Ranitidine / ↑ Verapamil bioavailability
Rifampin / ↓ Verapamil effect
Sirolimus / ↑ Sirolimus plasma levels
Sulfinpyrazone / ↑ Verapamil clearance
Tacrolimus / ↑ Tacrolimus plasma levels → ↑ toxicity
Theophylline / ↑ Theophylline effect
Vitamin D / ↓ Verapamil effect
Warfarin / Possible ↑ effect of either drug R/T ↓ plasma protein binding
   NOTE: Since verapamil is significantly bound to plasma proteins, interaction with other drugs bound to plasma proteins may occur.

HOW SUPPLIED

Capsule, Extended-Release: 100 mg, 120 mg, 180 mg, 200 mg, 240 mg, 300 mg; *Capsule, Sustained-Release:* 120 mg, 180 mg, 240 mg, 360 mg; *Injection:* 2.5 mg/mL; *Tablet:* 40 mg, 80 mg, 120 mg; *Tablet, Extended-Release:* 120 mg, 180 mg,

---

240 mg; *Tablet, Sustained-Release:* 120 mg, 180 mg, 240 mg

DOSAGE

- **TABLETS, IMMEDIATE-RELEASE**
  Angina at rest and chronic stable angina.

Individualized. Adults, initial: 80–120 mg 3 times per day (40 mg 3 times per day if client is sensitive to verapamil); **then,** increase dose to total of 240–480 mg/day.

Arrhythmias.

Dosage range in digitalized clients with chronic atrial fibrillation: 240–320 mg/day in divided doses 3 –4 times per day.

Prophylaxis of paroxysmal supraventricular tachycardia.

240–480 mg/day in divided doses 3–4 times per day in nondigitalized clients. Maximum effects: During first 48 hr.

Essential hypertension.

Initial, when used alone: 80 mg 3 times per day. Doses up to 360–480 mg daily may be used. Effects are seen in the first week of therapy. In the elderly or in people of small stature, initial dose should be 40 mg 3 times per day.

Prophylaxis of migraine headache.

40–80 mg 3–4 times per day.

- **EXTENDED- AND SUSTAINED-RELEASE CAPSULES AND TABLETS**
  Essential hypertension.

Covera-HS, initial: 180 mg at bedtime. If an adequate response is not reached, the dose can be increased as follows: 240 mg each evening, 360 mg each evening, or 480 mg each evening. **Verelan PM:** 200 mg/day at bedtime. If an adequate response is not reached, the dose can be increased as follows: 300 mg each evening or 400 mg each evening. **Calan SR or Isoptin SR, initial:** 180 mg in the a.m. with food. If an adequate response is not reached, the dose may be increased as follows: 240 mg each morning, 180 mg each morning plus 180 mg each evening (or 240 mg each morning plus 120 mg each evening), or 240 mg q 12 hr. **Verelan, initial:** 120 mg once daily in the morning. If an adequate response is not reached, the dose may be increased as follows: 180 mg in the morning, 240 mg in the morning (usual dose), 360 mg in the morning, or 480 mg in the morning

- **IV, SLOW**
  Supraventricular tachyarrhythmias.

Adults, initial: 5–10 mg (0.075–0.15 mg/kg) as an IV bolus given over 2 min (over 3 min in older clients); **then,** 10 mg (0.15 mg/kg) 30 min later if response is not adequate. **Infants, up to 1 year:** 0.1–0.2 mg/kg (0.75–2 mg) given as an IV bolus over 2 min; **1–15 years:** 0.1–0.3 mg/kg (2–5 mg, not to exceed 5 mg total dose) over 2 min. If response to initial dose is inadequate, it may be repeated after 30 min, but not more than a total of 10 mg should be given to clients from 1 to 15 years of age.

NURSING CONSIDERATIONS

℮ Do not confuse Isoptin with Intropin.

ADMINISTRATION/STORAGE

1. The SR tablets (120 mg) may be useful for small stature and elderly clients who require less medication.

2. Take the SR tablets with food.

3. Verelan pellet filled capsules may be carefully opened and the contents sprinkled on a spoonful of applesauce. Swallow the applesauce immediately without chewing and follow with a glass of cool water to ensure complete swallowing of the pellets. Subdividing the contents of a capsule is not recommended.

IV 4. Before administration, inspect ampules for particulate matter or discoloration.

5. Administer IV dosage under continuous ECG monitoring with resuscitation equipment readily available.

6. Give as a slow IV bolus (5–10 mg) over 2 min (3 min to elderly clients) to minimize toxic effects.

7. Store ampules at 15–30°C (59–86°F) and protect from light.

8. Do not give verapamil in an infusion line containing 0.45% NaCl with $NaHCO_3$ because a crystalline precipitate will form.

9. Do not give verapamil by IV push in the same line used for nafcillin infusion because a milky white precipitate will form.

Bold Italic = life threatening side effect   ■ = black box warning   ✤ = Available in Canada

10. Do not mix with albumin, amphotericin B, hydralazine, trimethoprim/sulfamethoxazole, or diluted with sodium lactate in PVC bags.

11. Verapamil will precipitate in any solution with a pH greater than 6.

12. Always individualize dose in the elderly because the pharmacologic effects are more pronounced and more prolonged.

ASSESSMENT

1. Document indications for therapy, onset and characteristics of S&S. List agents trialed and outcome.

2. Review list of prescribed medications to ensure none interact.

3. Monitor VS, ECG, CBC, liver and renal function studies; reduce dose with hepatic or renal impairment, compromised cardiac function, and in those prescribed beta blockers.

INTERVENTIONS

1. Monitor VS; assess for bradycardia and hypotension, symptoms that may indicate overdosage. Verapamil may lower BP to dangerously low levels if BP already low.

2. *Do not* administer concurrently with IV beta-adrenergic blocking agents.

3. Unless treating verapamil overdosage, withhold any medication that may elevate calcium levels.

4. Clients receiving concurrent digoxin therapy should be assessed for symptoms of toxicity and have digoxin levels checked periodically.

5. If disopyramide is to be used, do not administer for at least 48 hr before to 24 hr after verapamil dose.

6. Administer extended-release tablets with food to minimize fluctuations in serum levels.

CLIENT/FAMILY TEACHING

1. Take SR capsule in the a.m. with food; do not cut, crush, or chew; swallow capsules whole.

2. Drug may cause dizziness and sudden drop in BP; use caution until drug effects realized.

3. Keep a log of BP and pulse for provider review. Report any unusual bruising/bleeding or adverse effects.

4. Avoid alcohol, CNS depressants, and any OTC agents without approval.

5. Continue lifestyle modifications (low-fat and low-salt diet, decreased caloric and alcohol consumption, weight loss, no smoking, and regular exercise) in the overall goal of BP control.

6. Increase bulk and fiber in diet to prevent constipation. With higher doses constipation occurs more frequently. Report if bothersome or pronounced, as psyllium may be prescribed or, if severe, drug therapy may be changed.

OUTCOMES/EVALUATE

• ↓ Frequency/severity of anginal attacks
• Control of BP
• Restoration of stable rhythm
• Therapeutic drug levels (0.08–0.3 mcg/mL)

Warfarin sodium

(**WAR**-far-in)

CLASSIFICATION(S):
Anticoagulant, coumarin derivative
PREGNANCY CATEGORY: X
Rx: Coumadin, Jantoven

♣**Rx:** Apo-Warfarin, Gen-Warfarin, Taro-Warfarin

ACTION/KINETICS
Interferes with synthesis of vitamin K–dependent clotting factors resulting in depletion of clotting factors II, VII, IX, and X. Has no direct effect on an established thrombus although therapy may prevent further extension of a formed clot as well as secondary thromboembolic problems. Well absorbed from the

GI tract although food affects the rate (but not the extent) of absorption. Suitable for parenteral administration. **Peak activity:** 3–4 days; **duration:** 2–5 days. **t ½:** 20–60 hours. Highly bound to plasma proteins. Metabolized in the liver and inactive metabolites are excreted through the urine and feces.

USES

(1) Prophylaxis and/or treatment of venous thrombosis and its extension, and pulmonary embolism. (2) Prophylaxis and/or treatment of the thromboembolic complications associated with atrial fibrillation and/or cardiac valve replacement. (3) Reduction of the risk of death, recurrent myocardial infarction, and thromboembolic events such as stroke or systemic embolization after myocardial infarction.

CONTRAINDICATIONS

Lactation. Hemorrhagic tendencies, blood dyscrasias, CNS surgery, ophthalmic or traumatic surgery, inadequate lab facility, threatened abortion, eclampsia, preeclampsia, major regional lumbar block anesthesia, malignant HTN, pregnancy and unsupervised senile, alcoholic or psychotic patients. Bleeding of GI, GU or respiratory tract, aneurysms, pericarditis and pericardial effusion, bacterial endocarditis, cerebrovascular hemorrhage, spinal puncture, procedures with potential for uncontrollable bleeding.

SPECIAL CONCERNS

Geriatric clients may be more sensitive. Anticoagulant use in the following clients leads to increased risk: Trauma, infection, renal insufficiency, sprue, vitamin K deficiency, severe to moderate hypertension, polycythemia vera, severe allergic disorders, vasculitis, indwelling catheters, severe diabetes, anaphylactic disorders, surgery or trauma resulting in large exposed raw surfaces. Use with caution in impaired hepatic and renal function. Safety and efficacy have not been determined in children less than 18 years of age. Careful monitoring and dosage regulation are required during dentistry and surgery.

SIDE EFFECTS

CV: *Hemorrhage* is the main side effect and may occur from any tissue or organ. Symptoms of hemorrhage include headache, paralysis; pain in the joints, abdomen, or chest; difficulty in breathing or swallowing; SOB, unexplained swelling or shock. **GI:** N&V, diarrhea, sore mouth, mouth ulcers, anorexia, abdominal cramping, paralytic ileus, intestinal obstruction (due to intramural or submucosal hemorrhage). **Hepatic:** Hepatotoxicity, cholestatic jaundice. **Dermatologic:** Dermatitis, exfoliative dermatitis, urticaria, alopecia, necrosis or gangrene of the skin and other tissues (due to protein C deficiency). **Miscellaneous:** Pyrexia, red-orange urine, priapism, leukopenia, systemic cholesterol microembolization ("purple toes" syndrome), hypersensitivity reactions, compressive neuropathy secondary to hemorrhage adjacent to a nerve (rare).

LABORATORY TEST CONSIDERATIONS

False ↓ levels of serum theophylline determined by Schack and Waxler UV method (warfarin and dicumarol).

OD OVERDOSE MANAGEMENT

Symptoms: Early symptoms include melena, petechiae, microscopic hematuria, oozing from superficial injuries (e.g., nicks from shaving, excessive bruising, bleeding from gums after teeth brushing), excessive menstrual bleeding. *Treatment:* Discontinue therapy. Administer parenteral phytonadione (e.g., 5–25 mg parenterally). In emergency situations, 200–250 mL fresh frozen plasma or commercial factor IX complex. Fresh whole blood may be needed in clients unresponsive to phytonadione.

DRUG INTERACTIONS

Warfarin is responsible for more adverse drug interactions than any other group. Clients on anticoagulant therapy must be monitored carefully each time a drug is added or withdrawn. Monitoring usually involves determination of PT or INR. In general, a lengthened PT or INR means potentiation of the anticoagulant. Since potentiation may mean hemorrhages, a lengthened PT or INR warrants **reduction of the dosage of**

---

the anticoagulant. However, the anticoagulant dosage must again be increased when the second drug is discontinued. A shortened PT or INR means inhibition of the anticoagulant and may require an increase in dosage.

Acetaminophen / ↑ Anticoagulant effect

Alcohol, ethyl / Chronic use ↓ warfarin effect

Aminoglutethimide / ↓ Warfarin effect R/T ↑ liver breakdown

Aminoglycoside antibiotics / ↑ Warfarin effect R/T interference with vitamin K

Amiodarone / ↑ Warfarin effect R/T ↓ liver breakdown

Androgens / ↑ Warfarin effect

Ascorbic acid / ↓ Warfarin effect by unknown mechanism

H *Avocado* / Possible ↓ warfarin effect (↓ INR)

Barbiturates / ↓ Warfarin effect R/T ↑ liver breakdown

Beta-adrenergic blockers / ↑ Warfarin effect

Bosentan / Possible ↓ INR

H *Bromelain* / ↑ Tendency for bleeding

Capecitabine / ↑ Risk of bleeding and altered coagulation

Carbamazepine / ↓ Warfarin effect R/T ↑ liver breakdown

Celecoxib / ↑ PT & INR

Cephalosporins / ↑ Warfarin effect R/T effects on platelet function

Chloral hydrate / ↑ Warfarin effect R/T ↓ plasma protein binding

Chloramphenicol / ↑ Warfarin effect R/T ↓ liver breakdown

Cholestyramine / ↓ Anticoagulant effect R/T binding and ↓ absorption from GI tract

Cimetidine / ↑ Anticoagulant effect R/T ↓ liver breakdown

H *Cinchona bark* / ↑ Anticoagulant effect

Clarithromycin / ↑ Warfarin effect R/T ↓ liver metabolism

Clofibrate / ↑ Anticoagulant effect

Contraceptives, oral / ↓ Anticoagulant effect R/T ↑ activity of certain clotting factors (VII and X); rarely, the opposite effect of ↑ risk of thromboembolism

Contrast media containing iodine / ↑ Warfarin effect by ↑ PT

Corticosteroids / ↑ Warfarin effect; also ↑ risk of GI bleeding R/T steroids ulcerogenic effect

Cyclophosphamide / ↑ Anticoagulant effect

H *Danshen* / Possible ↑ warfarin effects

Dextrothyroxine / ↑ Warfarin effect

Dicloxacillin / ↓ Warfarin effect

Diflunisal / ↑ Anticoagulant effect and ↑ risk of bleeding R/T effect on platelet function and GI irritation

Disulfiram / ↑ Warfarin effect

H *Dong quai* / Potential for ↑ anticoagulant effects

Erythromycin / ↑ Warfarin effect R/T ↓ liver metabolism

Estrogens / ↓ Anticoagulant response by ↑ activity of certain clotting factors; rarely, the opposite effect of ↑ risk of thromboembolism

Etretinate / ↓ Warfarin effect R/T ↑ liver breakdown

H *Evening primrose oil* / Potential to ↓ platelet aggregation

H *Feverfew* / Potential to ↓ platelet aggregation

Fluconazole / ↑ Warfarin effect

H *Garlic* / Potential to ↓ platelet aggregation

Gatifloxacin / ↑ INR values

Gemfibrozil / ↑ Warfarin effect

H *Ginger* / Potential to ↓ platelet aggregation

H *Ginkgo biloba* / Potential to ↓ platelet aggregation

H *Ginseng, panax* / Potential to ↓ platelet aggregation

Glucagon / ↑ Warfarin effect

Glutethimide / ↓ Warfarin effect R/T ↑ liver breakdown

H *Grapeseed extract* / Potential to ↓ platelet aggregation

Griseofulvin / ↓ Warfarin effect

Hydantoins / ↑ Warfarin effect; also, ↑ hydantoin serum levels

Hypoglycemics, oral / ↑ Warfarin effect R/T ↓ plasma protein binding; also, ↑ effect of sulfonylureas

Ifosfamide / ↑ Warfarin effect R/T ↓ liver breakdown and displacement from protein binding sites

W

Indomethacin / ↑ Warfarin effect R/T effect on platelet function; also, indomethacin is ulcerogenic → GI hemorrhage

Isoniazid / ↑ Warfarin effect

Itraconazole / Anticoagulant effect is enhanced

Ketoconazole / ↑ Warfarin effect

Loop diuretics / ↑ Warfarin effect by displacement from protein binding sites

Lovastatin / ↑ Warfarin effect R/T ↓ liver breakdown

Metronidazole / ↑ Warfarin effect R/T ↓ liver breakdown

Miconazole / ↑ Bleeding or bruising

Mineral oil / ↑ Hypoprothrombinemia by ↓ absorption of vitamin K from GI tract; also mineral oil may ↓ absorption of warfarin from GI tract

Moricizine / ↑ Warfarin effect

Nafcillin / ↓ Warfarin effect

Nalidixic acid / ↑ Warfarin effect R/T displacement from protein binding sites

Nevirapine / Possible ↓ anticoagulant effect

NSAIDs / ↑ Warfarin effect; ↑ risk of bleeding R/T effects on platelet function and GI irritation

Omeprazole / ↑ Warfarin effect R/T ↓ liver breakdown

Orlistat / Possible ↑ INR

Oxandrolone / Large ↑ in INR; dose of warfarin may have to be greatly ↓

Penicillins / ↑ Warfarin effect → ↑ risk of bleeding R/T effects on platelet function

Propafenone / ↑ Warfarin effect R/T ↓ liver breakdown

Propoxyphene / ↑ Warfarin effect

Quinidine, quinine / ↑ Warfarin effect R/T ↓ liver breakdown

Quinolones / ↑ Warfarin effect

Rifampin / ↓ Anticoagulant effect R/T ↑ liver breakdown

Ritonavir / Possible ↓ anticoagulant effect

Rofecoxib / Significant ↑ INR

H *St. John's wort* / Possible ↓ warfarin plasma levels R/T ↑ metabolism

Salicylates / ↑ Warfarin effect and ↑ risk of bleeding R/T effect on platelet function and GI irritation

Spironolactone / ↓ Warfarin effect R/T hemoconcentration of clotting factors due to diuresis

Streptokinase / ↑ Warfarin effect

Sucralfate / ↓ Warfarin effect

Sulfamethoxazole and Trimethoprim / ↑ Warfarin effect R/T ↓ liver breakdown

Sulfinpyrazone / ↑ Anticoagulant effect R/T ↓ liver breakdown and inhibition of platelet aggregation

Sulfonamides / ↑ Sulfonamide effects

Sulindac / ↑ Warfarin effect

Tamoxifen / ↑ Warfarin effect

Tetracyclines / ↑ Warfarin effect R/T interference with vitamin K

Thiazide diuretics / ↓ Warfarin effect R/T hemoconcentration of clotting factors due to diuresis

Thioamines / ↑ Warfarin effect

Thiopurines / ↓ Warfarin effect R/T ↑ synthesis or activation of prothrombin

Thyroid hormones / ↑ Anticoagulant effect with ↑ risk of bleeding

Tolterodine / Prolonged INR values

Trazodone / ↓ Warfarin effect

Trastuzumab / Increased risk of bleeding

Troglitazone / Possible ↑ warfarin effect R/T ↓ liver breakdown or displacement from plasma proteins

Urokinase / ↑ Warfarin effect

Vitamin A / Possible ↑ anticoagulant effect if using large doses of Vitamin A

Vitamin C / Slightly prolonged PT

Vitamin E / ↑ Warfarin effect R/T interference with vitamin K

Vitamin K / ↓ Warfarin effect

HOW SUPPLIED

Powder for injection, lyophilized: 5 mg; *Tablet:* 1 mg, 2 mg, 2.5 mg, 3 mg, 4 mg, 5 mg, 6 mg, 7.5 mg, 10 mg

DOSAGE

• **TABLETS, IV**

Adults: ≥ 18 years: Adjust dose based on PT/INR. Give IV as alternate to PO. Initial: 2-5mg qd. Usual: 2-10mg qd. Venous Thromboembolism (including pulmonary embolism): INR 2-3. Atrial Fibrillation: INR 2-3. Post-MI: Initiate 2-4 weeks post-infarct and maintain INR 2.5-3.5. Mechanical/Bioprosthetic Heart Valve: INR 2-3 for 12 weeks after valve insertion, then INR 2.5-3.5 long term.

Bold Italic = life threatening side effect   ■ = black box warning   ♣ = Available in Canada

NURSING CONSIDERATIONS

ADMINISTRATION/STORAGE

1. Frequent monitoring of PT/INR is recommended during the first week of therapy, or during adjustment periods, and monthly thereafter.

2. Do not change brands; there may be differences in bioavailability.

3. To transfer from heparin therapy, give heparin and warfarin together from the first day (as there is a delayed onset of oral anticoagulant effects). Alternatively, warfarin may be started on the third to sixth day of heparin therapy.

4. Levels of anticoagulation that are recommended for specific indications by the American College of Chest Physicians and the National Heart, Lung, and Blood Institute should be followed.

5. Protect from light; store at controlled room temperature. Dispense in a tight, light-resistant container.

IV 6. Give IV as slow bolus over 1–2 min into peripheral vein.

7. Reconstitute for IV use by adding 2.7 mL sterile water for injection. Inspect for particulate matter and discoloration.

8. After reconstitution, injection is stable for 4 hr at room temperature. There is no preservative; take care to assure sterility of prepared solution.

9. Do not use the vial for multiple use; discard unused solution.

ASSESSMENT

1. Note indications for therapy, timeframe (i.e., DVT (initial) 6 months; recurrent/multiple and heart valve replacement — lifetime), and desired PT/INR range.

2. List drugs currently prescribed to ensure that none interacts unfavorably by increasing or decreasing PT as a result of competition for protein binding at receptor sites.

3. Note any bleeding tendencies. Review PMH for conditions that may preclude therapy: PUD, chronic GI tract ulcerations, alcoholic, severe renal or liver dysfunction, endocardial infections.

4. Determine if pregnant. May cause fetal malformations and neonatal hemorrhage.

5. Monitor ECG, CBC, PT/PTT, INR, renal and LFTs.

6. Some clients may be managed/discharged early on low molecular weight heparin injections and coumadin until desired INR obtained. Adjust oral anticoagulant weekly, especially if receiving one of the many drugs known to interact or compete.

7. Have available vitamin K, FFP, or factor IX concentrate for warfarin overdoses.

INTERVENTIONS

1. Request written parameters noting the desired range for PT or INR, once anticoagulated (orally). It usually takes 36–48 hr for drug to reach steady state; therefore allow time to equilibrate. The INR is the PT ratio (test/control) obtained from human brain thromboplastin and is universally considered most accurate to calculate dosage.

2. Drug inhibits production of factors II, VII, IX, and X; onset in response is delayed because of degradation of clotting factors that have already been synthesized.

3. Question about bleeding (gums, urine, stools, vomit, bruises). If urine discolored, determine cause, i.e., from drug therapy or hematuria. Indanedione-type anticoagulants turn alkaline urine a red-orange color; acidify urine or test for occult blood.

4. Sudden lumbar pain may indicate retroperitoneal hemorrhage.

5. GI dysfunction may indicate intestinal hemorrhage. Test for blood in urine and feces; check H&H to assess for abnormal bleeding.

6. Observe for "purple toes" syndrome related to inhibition of protein C and S.

CLIENT/FAMILY TEACHING

1. Take oral warfarin as prescribed and at the same time each day; must be compliant with therapy. Do not change brands of drug; may alter response.

2. This drug does not dissolve clots but decreases the clotting ability of the blood and helps to prevent the formation of harmful blood clots in the blood vessels and heart valves.

3. Avoid activities and contact sports that may cause injury or cuts and

W

bruises. Use a soft toothbrush, electric razor to shave, wear shoes and use a night light to avoid falls at night.

4. Report immediately any unusual bruising or bleeding, dark brown or blood-tinged body secretions, injury or trauma, dizziness, abdominal pain or swelling, back pain, severe headaches, and joint swelling and pain.

5. May carry vitamin K for emergency use. (The usual dosage is 5–25 mg parenterelly, to be used in the event of excessive bleeding.)

6. Avoid foods high in vitamin K: Asparagus, broccoli, cabbage, brussel sprouts, spinach, turnips, milk, and cheese, or consume in limited quantities as these may alter INR.

7. Use reliable birth control. Menstruation may be prolonged and flow slightly increased. Report if excessive and unusual.

8. Skin eruptions may develop as an allergic reaction; report.

9. Avoid OTC drugs. Check prior to taking any OTC drugs that have anticoagulant-type effects such as salicylates, NSAIDS, steroids, vitamin K, mineral preparations from health food stores, vitamins, or alcohol.

10. Wear identification and alert all providers of anticoagulant therapy.

11. Avoid smoking as this increases dose requirements.

12. Identify social/economic situations that may alter compliance; identify reliable resources.

13. Report as scheduled for labs to evaluate effectiveness of therapy and need for dosage changes.

14. Unusual hair loss and itching are common with the elderly; advise to report if intolerable or skin break down occurs.

15. The elderly are more prone to developing bleeding complications. Many elderly use multiple pharmacies and shop for value; stress that they know what they are taking and why and to carry the name and dosage of ALL drugs prescribed. Remind not to skip a dose as the drug works for only 24 hr and must be readministered in order to be effective.

OUTCOMES/EVALUATE

• PT within desired range (1.5–2 times the control)

• INR within desired range (2.0–3.0 with standard therapy; 2.5–4.0 with high-dose therapy)

• ↓ Risk of thromboembolism with prosthetic heart valves

• Resolution/prophylaxis of DVT

W

chapter 2
Therapeutic Drug Classifications

Refer to the accompanying website for additional drugs. Note that some drugs have recently been withdrawn from the market. Consult www.fda.gov for more information.

ALPHA-1-ADRENERGIC BLOCKING AGENTS

SEE ALSO THE FOLLOWING INDIVIDUAL ENTRIES:

Alfuzosin hydrochloride
Doxazosin mesylate
Prazosin hydrochloride
Tamsulosin hydrochloride
Terazosin

ACTION/KINETICS

Selectively block postsynaptic alpha-1-adrenergic receptors. Results in dilation of both arterioles and veins leading to a decrease in supine and standing BP. Diastolic BP is affected the most. Prazosin and terazosin do not produce reflex tachycardia. Terazosin also relaxes smooth muscle in the bladder neck and prostate, making it useful to treat BPH. Have many undesirable effects which, although not toxic, limit their use. Always start treatment at low doses and increase gradually.

USES

(1) Hypertension, alone or in combination with diuretics or beta-adrenergic blocking agents. (2) Doxazocin, terazosin, and tamulosin are used to treat BPH. *Investigational:* Prazosin is used for refractory CHF, management of Raynaud's vasospasm, and to treat BPH. Doxazosin, along with digoxin and diuretics, is used to treat CHF.

CONTRAINDICATIONS

Hypersensitivity to these drugs (i.e., quinazolines).

SPECIAL CONCERNS

The first few doses may cause postural hypotension and syncope with sudden loss of consciousness. Use with caution in lactation, with impaired hepatic function, or if receiving drugs known to influence hepatic metabolism. Safety and efficacy have not been established in children.

SIDE EFFECTS

The following side effects are common to alpha-1-adrenergic blockers. See individual drugs as well. **CV:** Marked hypotension and/or syncope with sudden loss of consciousness (first-dose effect), palpitations, postural hypotension, hypotension, tachycardia, chest pain, arrhythmia. **GI:** N&V, dry mouth, diarrhea, constipation, abdominal discomfort or pain, flatulence. **CNS:** Dizziness, depression, decreased libido, sexual dysfunction, nervousness, paresthesia, somnolence, anxiety, insomnia, asthenia, drowsiness. **Musculoskeletal:** Pain in the shoulder, neck, or back; gout, arthritis, joint pain, arthralgia. **Respiratory:** Dyspnea, nasal congestion, sinusitis, bronchitis, *bronchospasm,* cold symptoms, epistaxis, increased cough, flu symptoms, pharyngitis, rhinitis. **Ophthalmic:** Blurred vision, abnormal vision, reddened sclera, conjunctivitis. **GU:** Impotence, urinary frequency, incontinence, priapism. **Miscellaneous:** Tinnitus, vertigo, pruritus, sweating, alopecia, lichen planus, headache, edema, weight gain, facial edema, fever.

OD OVERDOSE MANAGEMENT

Symptoms: Extension of the side effects, especially on BP. *Treatment:* Keep supine to restore BP and normalize heart rate. Shock may be treated with volume expanders or vasopressors; support renal function.

DRUG INTERACTIONS

Ethanol / ↑ Risk of hypotension; advise clients to avoid alcohol

Clonidine / ↓ Antihypertensive effect of clonidine

LABORATORY TEST CONSIDERATIONS

↑ Urinary VMA.

DOSAGE

See individual agents.

NURSING CONSIDERATIONS

ADMINISTRATION/STORAGE

Take the first dose of prazosin and terazosin at bedtime to prevent dizziness.

ASSESSMENT

1. Note indications for therapy and characteristics of S&S. If history of PUD, use drug cautiously.

2. Assess for heart or lung disease; note currently prescribed therapy. Some agents may cause vasospasm with Prinzmetal or vasospastic angina.

3. Monitor electrolytes, ECG, and VS. Base titration on standing BP due to postural effects.

4. Use cautiously in older clients; may cause orthostatic hypotension. They may tolerate a slower, more gradual increase in dosage (i.e., terazosin 1 mg/day for 5 days followed by 2 mg/day for 5 days, etc., until desired response).

CLIENT/FAMILY TEACHING

1. May take with milk/meals to minimize GI upset. Do not stop abruptly; will have to re-titrate up to effective dose if stopped.

2. Take first dose at bedtime to minimize fainting and low BP effects. Do not drive or undertake hazardous tasks for 12–24 hr after first dose, after increasing dose, or following an interruption of dosage. Avoid low BP symptoms by rising slowly from a sitting or lying position and waiting until symptoms subside.

3. Record BP and weight. Report any weight gain or ankle swelling; without a diuretic, may experience retention of salt/water due to vessel dilation.

4. Dizziness, fatigue, headache, and palpitations may occur as well as transient apprehension, fear/anxiety. Report if persistent so dosage may be adjusted.

5. Report for yearly DRE and PSA to ensure lesion free.

6. Avoid excess caffeine and OTC agents (especially cold remedies). Review life-style changes needed for BP control (i.e., dietary restrictions of fat and sodium, weight reduction, regular physical exercise, decreased use of alcohol, stress reduction, and smoking cessation). For BPH control: no fluid intake 4 hr before bedtime, empty bladder before going to sleep, avoid caffeine and alcohol in the evening. If no improvement report to provider.

OUTCOMES/EVALUATE

- ↓ BP
- ↓ Nocturia, urgency/frequency

ANGIOTENSIN II RECEPTOR ANTAGONISTS ■

SEE ALSO THE FOLLOWING INDIVDIUAL ENTRIES:

Candesartan cilexetil
Eprosartan mesylate
Irbesartan
Losartan potassium
Olmesartan medoxomil
Telmisartan
Valsartan

ACTION/KINETICS

Angiotensin II, a potent vasoconstrictor, is the primary vasoactive hormone of the renin-angiotensin system; it is involved in the pathophysiology of hypertension. Angiotensin II increases systemic vascular resistance, causes sodium and water retention, and leads to increased HR and vasoconstriction. The angiotensin II receptor antagonists competitively block the angiotensin AT_1 receptor located in vascular smooth muscle and the adrenal glands, thus blocking the vasoconstrictor and aldosterone-secreting effects of angiotensin II. Thus, BP is reduced. No significant effects on HR with minimal orthostatic hypotension and no significant effect on potassium levels. Does not inhibit angiotensin converting enzyme (ACE).

USES
(1) Hypertension, alone or in combination with other antihypertensive drugs. (2) Nephropathy in type 2 diabetes mellitus (irbesartan and losartan). (3) Heart failure (NYHA class II to IV) in those intolerant to ACE inhibitors (valsartan). (4) Reduce risk of storke in those with hypertension and left ventricular hypertrophy (losartan). *Investigational:* Congestive heart failure. Can be combined with ACE inhibitors to reduce morbidity and mortality in clients with moderate to severe CHF.

CONTRAINDICATIONS
Hypersensitivity to any component of the products. Lactation.

SPECIAL CONCERNS
■When used during the second and third trimesters of pregnancy, drugs that act directly on the renin-angiotensin system can cause injury and even death to the developing fetus. When pregnancy is detected, discontinue angiotensin II receptor antagonists as soon as possible.■ Symptomatic hypotension may occur in those who are intravascularly volume-depleted. Fetal and neonatal morbidity and death are possible if given to pregnant women. Safety and efficacy have not been determined in children less than 18 years of age.

DOSAGE
See individual drugs.

NURSING CONSIDERATIONS

ASSESSMENT
1. Document indications for therapy, characteristics of S&S, and other agents trialed.
2. Ensure adequate hydration to prevent severe hypotensive episode.
3. Not for use during pregnancy or lactation. Observe infants exposed in utero for hypotension, oliguria, fetal defects, and ↑ K.

4. Monitor VS, CBC, electrolytes and renal function.
5. Assess for allergic reactions, i.e., rash, fever, itching, angioedema.

CLIENT/FAMILY TEACHING
1. Take only as directed usually once daily. May take with or without food.
2. Tell surgeon that ARB is prescribed; blockage of renin-angiotensin system following surgery may be problematic.
3. Avoid activities that may lead to reduction in fluid volume, i.e., excessive perspiration, vomiting, diarrhea, dehydration; may cause low BP.
4. Dizziness may occur; avoid activities that require mental alertness until drug effects realized. Change positions slowly to prevent sudden drop in BP.
5. Continue regular exercise, weight loss, dietary restrictions, including low salt, stop tobacco/alcohol; life style changes needed to lower BP.
6. Practice reliable contraception. Stop drug and report if pregnancy suspected; do not nurse.
7. Record BP regularly at different times of day for provider review. Continue regular medical followup and lab studies as scheduled; report unusual side effects or lack of response.

OUTCOMES/EVALUATE
• Control of BP
• Stabilization of CHF

ANGIOTENSIN-CONVERTING ENZYME (ACE) INHIBITORS ■

SEE ALSO THE FOLLOWING INDIVIDUAL ENTRIES:

Benazepril hydrochloride
Captopril
Enalapril maleate
Fosinopril sodium
Lisinopril
Moexipril hydrochloride
Perindopril erbumine
Quinapril hydrochloride
Ramipril
Trandolapril

ACTION/KINETICS
Believed to act by suppressing the renin-angiotensin-aldosterone   system.

Renin, synthesized by the kidneys, produces angiotensin I, an inactive decapeptide derived from plasma globulin substrate. Angiotensin I is converted to angiotensin II by ACE. Angiotensin II is a potent vasoconstrictor that also stimulates secretion of aldosterone from the adrenal cortex, resulting in sodium and fluid retention. The ACE inhibitors prevent the conversion of angiotensin I to angiotensin II. This results in a decrease in plasma angiotensin II and subsequently a decrease in peripheral resistance and decreased aldosterone secretion (leading to fluid loss) and therefore a decrease in BP. There may be either no change or an increase in CO. Several weeks of therapy may be required to achieve the maximum effect to reduce BP. Standing and supine BPs are lowered to about the same extent. Are also antihypertensive in low renin hypertensive clients. ACE inhibitors are additive with thiazide diuretics in lowering blood pressure; however, β-blockers and captopril have less than additive effects when used with ACE inhibitors.

USES

See individual drugs. Uses include, but are not limited to: (1) Hypertension, alone or in combination with other antihypertensive agents (especially thiazide diuretics). Can be used as first-line therapy in hypertensive African Americans with or at risk for renal dysfunction. (2) CHF often in combination with diuretics and/or digitalis. (3) MI (Lisinopril). (4) Left ventricular dysfunction (Enalapril). (5) Diabetic nephropathy (Captopril). (6) Reduction of risk of MI, stroke, and death from CV causes (Ramipril).

NOTE: Reduces incidence of stroke in high-risk hypertensive and normotensive clients.

CONTRAINDICATIONS

Hypersensitivity to the products or a history of angioedema due to previous treatment with an ACE inhibitor. Use of enalapril, enalaprilat, or lisinopril in clients with hereditary or idiopathic angioedema. Use of most ACE inhibitors during lactation.

SPECIAL CONCERNS

■Use during the second and third trimesters of pregnancy can result in injury and even death to the developing fetus. When pregnancy is detected discontinue the ACE inhibitor as soon as possible.■ May cause a profound drop in BP following the first dose; initiate therapy under close medical supervision. Use with caution in renal disease (especially renal artery stenosis) as increases in BUN and serum creatinine have occurred. Use with caution in clients with aortic stenosis due to possible decreased coronary perfusion following vasodilator use. It is possible that clients taking an ACE inhibitor and high-dose aspirin (325 mg/day) will have a higher mortality rate than those taking an ACE inhibitor alone or an ACE inhibitor plus low-dose aspirin (less than 160 mg/day). Most are used with caution during lactation. Geriatric clients may show a greater sensitivity to the hypotensive effects of ACE inhibitors although these drugs may preserve or improve renal function and reverse LV hypertrophy. For most ACE inhibitors, safety and effectiveness have not been determined in children. Compliance in taking the medication and inadequate dosage is a problem with ACE inhibitors.

SIDE EFFECTS

See individual entries. Side effects common to most ACE inhibitors include the following. **GI:** Abdominal pain, N&V, diarrhea, constipation, dry mouth, dyspepsia, hepatitis, pancreatitis. **CNS:** Sleep disturbances, insomnia, headache, dizziness, nervousness, paresthesias, depression, somnolence, drowsiness, vertigo. **CV:** Hypotension (especially following the first dose or in those volume- or salt-depleted), palpitations, angina pectoris, *MI, CVA, cardiac arrest,* orthostatic hypotension, chest pain, tachycardia. **Dermatologic:** Diaphoresis, sweating, flushing, pemphigus/pemiphigoid, pruritus, rash, urticaria. **Hepatic:** Rarely, cholestatic jaundice progressing to *hepatic necrosis and death.* **Respiratory:** Chronic cough, dyspnea, URTI. **Body as a**

whole: Fatigue, malaise, asthenia, fever, photosensitivity. **Miscellaneous:** Impotence, syncope, asthenia, anemia, tinnitus. **Angioedema** of the face, lips, tongue, glottis, larynx, extremities, and mucous membranes. **Anaphylaxis.**

OD OVERDOSE MANAGEMENT
Symptoms: Hypotension is the most common. *Treatment:* Supportive measures. The treatment of choice to restore BP is volume expansion with an IV infusion of NSS. Certain of the ACE inhibitors (captopril, enalaprilat, lisinopril, trandolaprilat) may be removed by hemodialysis.

DRUG INTERACTIONS
Allopurinol / ↑ Risk of hypersensitivity reactions
Anesthetics / ↑ Risk of hypotension if used with anesthetics that also cause hypotension
Antacids / Possible ↓ bioavailability of ACE inhibitors
Capsaicin / May cause or worsen cough associated with ACE inhibitor use
Digoxin / ↑ or ↓ Plasma digoxin levels; monitor digoxin plasma levels
Diuretics / Possible excess ↓ BP especially in those with intravascular volume depletion
Hypoglycemic drugs / Possible ↑ hypoglycemia
Indomethacin / ↓ Hypotensive effects of ACE inhibitors, especially in low renin or volume-dependent hypertensive clients
Insulin / Possible ↑ hypoglycemia
Lithium / ↑ Serum lithium levels → ↑ risk of toxicity
Loop diuretics / ↓ Effect of loop diuretics; possible inhibition of angiotensin II production by the ACE inhibitor
NSAIDs / ↓ Hypotensive effect of ACE inhibitors
Phenothiazines / ↑ Effect of ACE inhibitors
Potassium-sparing diuretics / ↑ Serum potassium levels
Potassium supplements / ↑ Serum potassium levels
Thiazide diuretics / Additive effect to ↓ BP

LABORATORY TEST CONSIDERATIONS
↑ BUN and creatinine (both transient and reversible). ↑ Liver enzymes, serum bilirubin, uric acid, blood glucose. Small ↑ serum potassium.
DOSAGE
See individual drugs.

NURSING CONSIDERATIONS
ADMINISTRATION/STORAGE
Do not interrupt or discontinue ACE inhibitor therapy without consulting provider.

ASSESSMENT
1. Note any previous therapy with ACE inhibitors or antihypertensive agents and the outcome.
2. Monitor VS (BP—both arms while lying, standing, and sitting), electrolytes, CBC, and renal and LFTs; check urine for protein if negative on urinalysis; check for microalbuminuria esp. in diabetics.
3. Document hereditary angioedema (especially if caused by a deficiency of C1 esterase inhibitor). Report any evidence of angioedema (swelling of face, lips, extremities, tongue, mucous membranes, glottis, or larynx) esp. after first dose (but may also be delayed response). Relieve S&S with antihistamines. If involves laryngeal edema, observe for airway obstruction. *Stop* drug; use epinephrine (1:1000 SC).
4. Monitor VS, I&O, weight, serum potassium, and renal function studies. Those hypovolemic due to diuretics, GI fluid loss, or salt restriction may exhibit severe hypotension after initial doses; supervise ambulation until drug response evident.
5. Assess for neutropenia (esp. with captopril); precludes drug therapy.
6. If undergoing surgery or general anesthesia with drugs that cause hypotension, ACE inhibitors will block angiotensin II formation; correct hypotension by volume expansion.
7. Document weight, risk factors, and medical problems. Identify life-style changes needed to achieve and maintain lowered BP. Assess motivation and ensure that a trial of 'good behavior' with dietary modifications and regular

exercise for 3–6 months has been done unless BP stage >2.

CLIENT/FAMILY TEACHING

1. Take 1 hr before or 2 hr after meals and only as directed. Medication controls but does not cure hypertension; take as prescribed despite feeling better and do not stop abruptly.

2. Review prescribed dietary guidelines; do not use potassium or salt substitutes containing potassium.

3. Do not perform activities that require mental alertness until drug effects realized; initially may cause dizziness, fainting, or lightheadedness. Rise slowly from a lying position and dangle feet before standing; avoid sudden position changes to minimize low BP effects.

4. Take BP readings at various times during the day and record to prevent treating 'white collar' readings.

5. Practice birth control; report if pregnancy suspected. Do not nurse.

6. Report adverse side effects:

- Nonproductive, persistent, cough
- Sore throat, fever, swelling of hands/feet, irregular heartbeat, chest pains, difficulty breathing, or hoarseness
- Excessive perspiration, dehydration, vomiting, and diarrhea
- Itching, joint pain, fever, or skin rash
- Swelling or weight gain of more than 3 lb/day or 5 lb/week

7. With diabetes (with/without hypertension), ACE inhibitors have been shown to reduce proteinuria and slow progression of renal disease.

8. Avoid excessive amounts of caffeine (e.g., tea, coffee, cola) and OTC medications, especially cold remedies.

9. NSAIDs and aspirin may impair the BP lowering effects of ACE inhibitors; antacids may decrease bioavailability.

10. Tell surgeon that ACE is being taken.

11. Avoid activities that may lead to a reduction in fluid volume, i.e., excessive perspiration, vomiting, diarrhea, dehydration may all cause drop in BP.

12. Regular exercise, proper diet, weight loss, stress management, and adequate rest in conjunction with medications are needed in the overall management of high BP. Additional interventions such as stopping alcohol/tobacco products, and salt intake may assist in BP control.

OUTCOMES/EVALUATE

- ↓ BP; ↓ Morbidity post-AMI
- Improvement in S&S of CHF
- ↓ Proteinuria/renal damage

ANTIANGINAL DRUGS— NITRATES/NITRITES

SEE ALSO BETA-ADRENERGIC BLOCKING AGENTS, CALCIUM CHANNEL BLOCKING DRUGS, AND THE FOLLOWING INDIVIDUAL ENTRIES:

Isosorbide dinitrate
Isosorbide mononitrate
Nitroglycerin IV
Nitroglycerin sublingual
Nitroglycerin sustained release capsules and tablets
Nitroglycerin topical ointment
Nitroglycerin transdermal system
Nitroglycerin translingual spray

ACTION/KINETICS

Nitrates relax vascular smooth muscle by stimulating production of intracellular cyclic guanosine monophosphate. Dilation of postcapillary vessels decreases venous return to the heart due to pooling of blood; thus, LV end-diastolic pressure (preload) is reduced. Relaxation of arterioles results in a decreased systemic vascular resistance and arterial pressure (afterload). The oxygen requirements of the myocardium are reduced and there is more efficient redistribution of blood flow through collateral channels in myocardial tissue. Diastolic, systolic, and mean BP are decreased. Also, elevated central venous and pulmonary capillary wedge pressures, pulmonary vascular resistance, and systemic vascular resistance are reduced. Reflex tachycardia may occur due to the overall decrease in BP. Cardiac index may increase, decrease, or remain the same; those with elevated left ventricular filling pressure and systemic vascular resistance values with a depressed cardiac index are likely to see improvement of the cardiac index. The onset and duration depend on the product and route of administration (sublingual, topical, transdermal, parenteral, oral, and buccal). **Onset:** 1 to 3 min for IV, sublingual, translingual, and transmucosal nitroglycerin or sublingual isosorbide dinitrate; 20 to 60 min for sustained-release, topical, and transdermal nitroglycerin or oral isosorbide dinitrate or mononitrate; and up to 4 hr for sustained-release isosorbide dinitrate. **Duration of action:** 3 to 5 min for IV nitroglycerin; 30 to 60 min for sublingual or translingual nitroglycerin; several hours for transmucosal, sustained-release, or topical nitroglycerin and all isosorbide dinitrate products; and up to 24 hr for transdermal nitroglycerin.

USES
(1) Treatment and prophylaxis of acute angina pectoris (use sublingual, transmucosal, or translingual nitroglycerin). (2) First-line therapy for unstable angina. (3) Prophylaxis of chronic angina pectoris (topical, transdermal, translingual, transmucosal), or oral sustained-release nitroglycerin; isosorbide dinitrate and mononitrate. (4) IV nitroglycerin is used to decrease BP in surgical procedures resulting in hypertension, as well as an adjunct in treating hypertension or CHF associated with MI. *Investigational:* Nitroglycerin ointment has been used as an adjunct in treating Raynaud's disease. Also, isosorbide dinitrate with prostaglandin E₁ for peripheral vascular disease. Sublingual and topical nitroglycerin and oral nitrates have been used to decrease cardiac workload in clients with acute MI and in CHF.

CONTRAINDICATIONS
Sensitivity to nitrites, which may result in severe hypotensive reactions, MI, or tolerance to nitrites. Severe anemia, cerebral hemorrhage, recent head trauma, postural hypotension, closed angle glaucoma, impaired hepatic function, hypertrophic cardiomyopathy, hypotension, recent MI. PO dosage forms should not be used in clients with GI hypermotility or with malabsorption syndrome. IV nitroglycerin should not be used in clients with hypotension, uncorrected hypovolemia, inadequate cerebral circulation, constrictive pericarditis, increased ICP, or pericardial tamponade.

SPECIAL CONCERNS
Use with caution during lactation and in glaucoma. Tolerance to the antianginal and vascular effects may occur. Safety and efficacy have not been determined during lactation and in children.

SIDE EFFECTS
• **SYSTEMIC. CNS:** Headaches (most common) which may be severe and persistent, restlessness, dizziness, weakness, apprehension, vertigo, anxiety, insomnia, confusion, nightmares, hypoesthesia, hypokinesia, dyscoordination. **CV:** Postural hypotension (common) with or without paradoxical bradycardia and increased angina, tachycardia, palpitations, syncope, rebound hypertension, crescendo angina, retrosternal discomfort, *CV collapse,* atrial fibrillation, PVCs, *arrhythmias.* **GI:** N&V, dyspepsia, diarrhea, dry mouth, abdominal pain, involuntary passing of feces and urine, tenesmus, tooth disorder. **Dermatologic:** Crusty skin lesions, pruritus, rash, exfoliative dermatitis, cutaneous vasodilation with flushing. **GU:** Urinary frequency, impotence, dysuria. **Respiratory:** URTI, bronchitis, pneumonia. **Allergic:** Itching, wheezing, tracheobronchitis. **Miscellaneous:** Perspiration, muscle twitching, methemoglobinemia, cold sweating, blurred vision, diplopia, *hemolytic anemia,* arthralgia, edema, malaise, neck stiffness, increased appetite, rigors.
• **TOPICAL.** Peripheral edema, contact dermatitis: Tolerance can occur following chronic use. Nitrites convert hemoglobin to methemoglobin, which impairs the oxygen-carrying capacity of the blood, resulting in *anemic hypoxia.* This interaction is dangerous in clients with preexisting anemia.

OD OVERDOSE MANAGEMENT
Symptoms (Toxicity): Severe toxicity is rarely encountered with therapeutic use. Symptoms include hypotension, flushing, tachycardia, headache, palpitations, vertigo, perspiring skin followed by cold and cyanotic skin, visual disturbances, syncope, nausea, diz-

Classifications

ziness, diaphoresis, initial hyperpnea, dyspnea and slow breathing, slow pulse, **heart block,** vomiting with the possibility of bloody diarrhea and colic, anorexia, and increased ICP with symptoms of confusion, moderate fever, and paralysis. Tissue hypoxia (due to methemoglobinemia) may result in **cyanosis, metabolic acidosis, coma, seizures, and death due to CV collapse.**

Treatment (Toxicity):

• Induction of emesis or gastric lavage followed by activated charcoal (nitrates are usually rapidly absorbed from the stomach). Gastric lavage may be used if the drug has been recently ingested.

• Maintain in a recumbent shock position and keep warm. Give oxygen and artificial respiration if required.

• Monitor methemoglobin levels.

• Elevate legs and administer IV fluids to treat severe hypotension and reflex tachycardia. Phenylephrine or methoxamine may also be helpful.

• Do not use epinephrine and similar drugs as they are ineffective in reversing severe hypotension.

DRUG INTERACTIONS

Acetylcholine / Effects ↓ when used with nitrates

Alcohol, ethyl / Hypotension and CV collapse R/T vasodilator effect of both agents

Antihypertensive drugs / Additive hypotension

Aspirin / ↑ Serum levels and effects of nitrates

Beta-adrenergic blocking drugs / Additive hypotension

Calcium channel blocking drugs / Additive hypotension, including significant orthostatic hypotension

Dihydroergotamine / ↑ Effect R/T ↑ bioavailability or antagonism resulting in ↓ antianginal effects

Heparin / Possible ↓ effect

Narcotics / Additive hypotensive effect

Phenothiazines / Additive hypotension

Sympathomimetics / ↓ Effect of nitrates; also, nitrates may ↓ effect of sympathomimetics → hypotension

LABORATORY TEST CONSIDERATIONS

↑ Urinary catecholamines. False negative ↓ in serum cholesterol.

DOSAGE

See individual agents.

NURSING CONSIDERATIONS

ADMINISTRATION/STORAGE

Store tablets and capsules tightly closed in their original container. Avoid exposure to air, heat, and moisture.

ASSESSMENT

1. Document location, intensity, duration, extent, and any precipitating factors (i.e., activity, stress) surrounding anginal pain. Use a pain-rating scale to rate pain.

2. Note any sensitivity to nitrites.

3. If history of anemia, administer with extreme caution.

4. Nitrates are contraindicated with elevated intracranial pressure and use of certain drugs for E.D.

5. Note any changes in ECG or elevated cardiac markers, results of echocardiogram, stress test, and/or catheterization.

INTERVENTIONS

1. Determine experience with self-administered medications; note if SL tablets ordered for bedside.

2. While hospitalized, record when consumed so effectiveness can be determined and usage monitored:

• Frequency given

• Duration and intensity of pain (use a pain-rating scale; rate pain initially and 5 min after administration) and if relief is partial or complete

• Time it takes for relief to occur

• Any side effects

3. Monitor VS. Assess for sensitivity to hypotensive effects (N&V, pallor, restlessness, and CV collapse). Monitor for hypotension when on additional drugs; adjust as needed. Supervise activities/ambulation until drug effects realized.

4. Assess for signs of tolerance, which occur following chronic use but may begin several days after starting treatment; manifested by absence of response to the usual dose. (Nitrites may be discontinued temporarily until tolerance is lost, and then reinstituted. During interim, other vasodilators may be used.) Managed by 12 hr nitrate rest.

---

5. Observe for N&V, drowsiness, headache, or visual disturbances with long-term therapy (may require a change in drug). Note change in activity and response to drug therapy. Determine if less discomfort experienced when performing regular activity.

CLIENT/FAMILY TEACHING

1. Take oral nitrates on an empty stomach with a glass of water. Drug decreases myocardial oxygen demand and reduces workload of the heart.

2. To prevent sudden drop in BP, use inhalation products or take SL tabs while sitting or lying down. Make position changes slowly and rise only after dangling feet for several minutes. The elderly should sit or lie down when taking NTG; may become dizzy and fall.

3. Avoid changing from one brand to another due to differences in effectiveness between different companies.

4. Always carry SL tablets for use in aborting an attack. Check expiration date; replace when needed or every 6 months. A burning sensation under the tongue attests to drug potency. Carry SL tablets in a *glass* bottle, tightly capped. Keep in original container as heat, moisture, and air cause deterioration. Do not use plastic containers; drug deteriorates in plastic; avoid child-proof caps as must get to tablets quickly.

5. If pain is not relieved in 5 min by first SL tablet, take up to 2 more tablets at 5-min intervals. If pain has not subsided 5 min after third tablet, client should be taken to the emergency room; *do not* drive; call 911.

6. Take SL tabs 5–15 min prior to any situation likely to cause pain (e.g., climbing stairs, sexual intercourse, exposure to cold weather). Record attacks; report any increase in the frequency/intensity of attacks and loss of NTG effectiveness. Schedule frequent rest periods, pace activities, and avoid stressful situations. Use acetaminophen for headaches.

7. Follow instructions on how to apply topical nitroglycerin. Remove at bedtime and apply upon arising; a nitrate-free period of 8 hr may reduce/prevent nitrate tolerance.

8. Avoid alcohol; nitrite syncope, a severe shock-like state, may occur. Inhalation products are flammable; do not use under situations where they might ignite.

9. Do not smoke. Review risks and lifestyle changes necessary to prevent further CAD (i.e., weight control, dietary changes, ↓ salt intake, modified regular exercise program, no alcohol/tobacco, and stress reduction).

10. Have family or significant other learn CPR; survival rate is greatly increased when CPR is initiated immediately. Carry ID with prescribed drugs. Know what you are taking and why.

OUTCOMES/EVALUATE

- ↓ Myocardial oxygen requirements; ↑ activity tolerance
- Improved myocardial perfusion
- Relief of pain/coronary artery spasm

ANTIARRHYTHMIC DRUGS

SEE ALSO THE FOLLOWING INDIVIDUAL ENTRIES:

Adenosine
Amiodarone hydrochloride
Bretylium tosylate
Calcium Channel Blocking Agents
Digoxin
Diltiazem hydrochloride
Dofetilide
Flecainide acetate
Ibutilide fumarate
Lidocaine hydrochloride
Moricizine hydrochloride
Phenytoin
Phenytoin sodium
Procainamide hydrochloride
Propafenone hydrochloride
Propranolol hydrochloride
Quinidine gluconate
Quinidine sulfate
Tocainide hydrochloride
Verapamil

GENERAL STATEMENT

Examples of cardiac arrhythmias are *premature ventricular beats, ventricular tachycardia, atrial flutter, atrial fibrillation, ventricular fibrillation,* and *atrioventricular heart block.* The various antiarrhythmic drugs are classified according to both their mechanism of action and their effects on the action potential of cardiac cells. Importantly, one drug in a particular class may be more effective and safer in an individual client. The antiarrhythmic drugs are classified as follows:

1. Class I. Decrease the rate of entry of sodium during cardiac membrane depolarization, decrease the rate of rise of phase O of the cardiac membrane action potential, prolong the effective refractory period of fast-response fibers, and require that a more negative membrane potential be reached before the membrane becomes excitable (and thus can propagate to other membranes). Class I drugs are further listed in subgroups (according to their effects on action potential duration) as follows:

• Class IA: Depress phase O and prolong the duration of the action potential. Examples: Disopyramide, procainamide, and quinidine.

• Class IB: Slightly depress phase O and are thought to shorten the action potential. Examples: Lidocaine, mexiletine, phenytoin, and tocainide.

• Class IC: Slight effect on repolarization but marked depression of phase O of the action potential. Significant slowing of conduction. Examples: Flecainide, and propafenone.

NOTE: Moricizine is classified as a Class I agent but it has characteristics of agents in groups IA, B, and C.

2. Class II. Competitively block beta-adrenergic receptors and depress phase 4 depolarization. Examples: Acebutolol, esmolol, and propranolol.

3. Class III. Prolong the duration of the membrane action potential (relative refractory period) without changing the phase of depolarization or the resting membrane potential. Examples: Amiodarone, bretylium, dofetilide, ibutilide, and sotalol.

4. Class IV. Diltiazem and verapamil, calcium channel blockers that slow conduction velocity and increase the refractoriness of the AV node.

Adenosine and digoxin are also used to treat arrhythmias. Adenosine slows conduction time through the AV node

and can interrupt the reentry pathways through the AV node. Digoxin causes a decrease in maximal diastolic potential and duration of the action potential; it also increases the slope of phase 4 depolarization.

SPECIAL CONCERNS

Monitor serum levels of antiarrhythmic drugs since some drugs can cause toxic side effects that can be confused with the purpose for which the drug is used. For example, toxicity from quinidine can result in cardiac arrhythmias. Antiarrhythmic drugs may cause new or worsening of arrhythmias, ranging from an increase in frequency of PVCs to severe ventricular tachycardia, ventricular fibrillation, or tachycardia that is more sustained and rapid. Such situations (called proarrhythmic effect) may make it difficult to distinguish the proarrhythmic effect from the underlying rhythm disorder.

DRUG INTERACTIONS

H *Aloe* / Chronic aloe use → ↑ serum potassium loss causing ↑ effect of antiarrhythmics

H *Buckthorn bark/berry* / Chronic buckthorn use → ↑ serum potassium loss causing ↑ effect of antiarrhythmics

H *Cascara sagrada bark* / Chronic cascara use → ↑ serum potassium loss causing ↑ effect of antiarrhythmics

H *Rhubarb root* / Chronic rhubarb use → ↑ serum potassium loss causing ↑ effect of antiarrhythmics

H *Senna pod/leaf* / Chronic senna use → ↑ serum potassium loss causing ↑ effect of antiarrhythmics

NURSING CONSIDERATIONS
ASSESSMENT

1. Note drug sensitivity and any previous experiences with these drugs. Assess extent of palpitations, fluttering sensations, chest pains, fainting episodes, or missed beats; obtain ECG documenting arrhythmia.

2. Assess heart sounds, VS and EF. Use cardiac monitor if administering drugs by IV route; monitor for rhythm changes.

3. Monitor BP and pulse. A HR < 50 bpm or > 120 should be avoided. Ob-

tain written parameters for BP and pulse limits.

4. Monitor BS, electrolytes, drug levels, liver and renal function studies. Ensure that serum pH, electrolytes, pO_2 and/or O_2 saturations are WNL.

5. Assess life-style related to cigarettes and caffeine use, alcohol consumption, and lack of regular exercise. Certain foods, emotional stress, and other environmental factors may also trigger arrhythmias; identify and eliminate before instituting drugs.

CLIENT/FAMILY TEACHING

1. Drugs work by controlling the irregular heart beats so the heart can pump more efficiently. Take as ordered. If a dose is missed, do not double up.

2. Avoid activities that require mental alertness until drug effects realized.

3. Avoid OTC products. Eliminate caffeine, cigarettes, salt, and alcohol; alters drug absorption and may precipitate arrhythmias or cause fluid retention with certain agents.

4. Record BP and pulse for review; identify with provider specific levels to hold drug i.e., HR < 50. Keep F/U visits so that therapy can be adjusted and evaluated.

5. Report concerns/fears or problems R/T sexual activity and side effects of drug therapy. Always carry list of prescribed medications and condition being treated.

6. Family/significant other should learn CPR; survival rates are greatly increased when CPR is initiated immediately.

OUTCOMES/EVALUATE

• ECG evidence of arrhythmia control; restoration of stable cardiac rhythm
• Serum drug concentrations within therapeutic range.

list

ANTIHYPERLIPIDEMIC AGENTS—HMG-COA REDUCTASE INHIBITORS

SEE ALSO THE FOLLOWING INDIVIDUAL ENTRIES:

Atorvastatin calcium
Fluvastatin sodium
Lovastatin
Pravastatin sodium
Rosuvastatin calcium
Simvastatin

GENERAL STATEMENT

The National Cholesterol Education Program Expert Panel on Detection, Evaluation, and Treatment of High Blood Cholesterol in Adults has developed guidelines for the treatment of high cholesterol and LDL in adults. Cholesterol levels less than 200 mg/dL are desirable. Cholesterol levels between 200 and 239 mg/dL are considered borderline-high while levels greater than 240 mg/dL are considered high. With respect to LDL, the following goals have been established: All people should be at 160 mg/dL or below; levels of 130 mg/dL are considered desirable in individuals with two or more risk factors (cigarette smoking, hypertension, HDL below 40 mg/dL, or family history of premature CAD). HDL above 60 mg/dL is a negative risk factor, i.e., its presence removes one of the previous risk factors from the total count. The LDL goal for those clients with diabetes and/or existing CAD is 100 mg/dL or lower. Depending on the levels of cholesterol and LDL and the number of risk factors present for CAD, the provider will develop a treatment regimen.

ACTION/KINETICS

The HMG-CoA reductase inhibitors competitively inhibit HMG-CoA reductase; this enzyme catalyzes the early rate-limiting step in the synthesis of cholesterol. HMG-CoA reductase inhibitors increase HDL cholesterol and decrease LDL cholesterol, total cholesterol, apolipoprotein B, VLDL cholesterol, and plasma triglycerides. The mechanism to lower LDL cholesterol may be due to both a decrease in VLDL cholesterol levels and induction of the LDL receptor, leading to reduced production or increased catabolism of LDL cholesterol. The maximum therapeutic response is seen in 4–6 weeks. Statins may help prevent infections in clients with diabetes. Statins cause a significant reduction in CV events.

USES

See individual drugs. Uses include primary hypercholesterolemia, mixed dyslipidemia, hypertriglyceridemia, prevention of coronary events, and prevention of CV events. *Investigational:* Treatment of osteoporosis. Lower risk of developing Type 2 diabetes and stroke when taken to reduce cholesterol. Lower cholesterol in women.

CONTRAINDICATIONS

Active liver disease or unexplained persistent elevated liver function tests. Pregnancy, lactation. Use in children.

SPECIAL CONCERNS

Use with caution in those who ingest large quantities of alcohol or who have a history of liver disease. May cause photosensitivity. Safety and efficacy have not been established in children less than 18 years of age.

SIDE EFFECTS

The following side effects are common to most HMG-CoA reductase inhibitors. Also see individual drugs. **GI:** N&V, diarrhea, constipation, abdominal cramps or pain, flatulence, dyspepsia, heartburn. **CNS:** Headache, dizziness, dysfunction of certain cranial nerves (e.g., alteration of taste, facial paresis, impairment of extraocular movement), tremor, vertigo, memory loss, paresthesia, anxiety, insomnia, depression, mental decline, aggressive behavior, *suicide attempts*. **Musculoskeletal:** Localized pain, myalgia, muscle cramps or pain, myopathy, rhabdomyolysis, arthralgia. **Respiratory:** URI, rhinitis, cough. **Ophthalmic:** Progression of cataracts (lens opacities), ophthalmoplegia. **Hypersensitivity:** *Anaphylaxis, angioedema,* vasculitis, purpura, thrombocytopenia, leukopenia, *hemolytic anemia,* lupus erythematosus-like syndrome, polymyalgia rheumatica, positive ANA, ESR increase, arthritis, arthralgia, eosinophilia, urticaria, photosensitivity, fever, chills, flushing, malaise, dyspnea, *toxic dermal necrolysis, Stevens-Johnson syndrome.* **Miscellaneous:** Rash, pruritus, cardiac chest pain, fatigue, influenza, alopecia, edema, dryness of skin and mucous membranes, changes to hair and nails, skin discoloration.

DRUG INTERACTIONS

SEE ALSO INDIVIDUAL DRUGS.

Antifungals, Azole / ↑ Levels of HMG-CoA inhibitors R/T ↓ metabolism

Clarithromycin / ↑ Levels of HMG-CoA inhibitors R/T ↓ metabolism

Clopidogrel / ↓ Clopidogrel effects on platelet function with atorvastatin or simvastatin

Cyclosporine / ↑ Risk of severe myopathy or rhabdomyolysis

Digoxin / Slight ↑ in digoxin levels

Erythromycin / ↑ Risk of severe myopathy or rhabdomyolysis

Gemfibrozil / Possibility of severe myopathy or rhabdomyolysis

Grapefruit juice / Possible ↑ AUC, C_{max}, and elimination t $\frac{1}{2}$ of certain HMG-CoA reductase inhibitors

Itraconazole / ↑ Levels of HMG-CoA inhibitors

Niacin, Nicotinic acid / Possibility of myopathy or severe rhabdomyolysis

Propranolol / ↓ Antihyperlipidemic activity

Protease inhibitors / ↑ Levels of HMG-CoA inhibitors R/T ↓ metabolism

Warfarin / ↑ Anticoagulant effect of warfarin.

LABORATORY TEST CONSIDERATIONS

↑ AST, ALT, CPK, alkaline phosphatase, bilirubin. Abnormal thyroid function tests.

DOSAGE

See individual drugs.

NURSING CONSIDERATIONS

ADMINISTRATION/STORAGE

1. Lovastatin should be taken with meals; fluvastatin, pravastatin, and simavastatin may be taken without regard to meals.

2. Step-down therapy (e.g., pravastatin) may decrease medication effectiveness.

ASSESSMENT

1. Review lifestyle, risk factors, attempts to control with diet, exercise, and weight reduction. Also review PMH, ROS, and physical exam; document risk factors. List other drugs trialed and drugs prescribed to ensure no adverse effects.

2. Note any alcohol abuse or liver disease. Monitor LFTs as recommended.

Bold Italic = life threatening side effect   ■ = black box warning   ✦ = Available in Canada

Transaminase levels 3 times normal may precipitate severe hepatic toxicity. If CK elevated, assess renal function as rhabdomyolsis with myoglobinuria could cause renal shutdown. Stop drug therapy and clearly mark chart and advise client not to take.

3. Note nutritional analysis by dietitian; assess cholesterol profile (HDL, LDL, cholesterol, and triglycerides) after 3–6 months of exercise and diet therapy if risk factors do not require immediate drug therapy. With diabetes and coronary heart disease a more aggressive drug approach should be instituted in addition to diet therapy with goals of reducing LDL below 100.

CLIENT/FAMILY TEACHING

1. Take only as directed. Drug is used to lower cholesterol levels and stabilize plaques in order to prevent CAD and control coronary risk factors.

2. Report any pain in skeletal muscles or unexplained muscle pain, tenderness, or weakness promptly, especially with fever or malaise. Stop drug with any major trauma, surgery, or serious illness.

3. May cause photosensitivity; avoid prolonged sun or UV light exposure. Use sunscreens, sunglasses, and protective clothing when exposed.

4. Continue life-style modifications that include low-fat, low-cholesterol, and low-sodium diets, weight reduction with obese clients, smoking cessation, reduction of alcohol consumption, and regular aerobic exercise in the overall goal of cholesterol reduction.

5. Avoid OTC agents. May use niaspan (SR form of niacin) with careful monitoring. Use a fibrate cautiously; lower statin dose is used and LFTs monitored. Report regularly for labs to prevent liver toxicity and to assess drug response.

OUTCOMES/EVALUATE

• ↓ LDL, triglycerides, and total cholesterol levels; ↓ risk of placque rupture and death

ANTIHYPERTENSIVE AGENTS

SEE ALSO THE FOLLOWING DRUG CLASSES AND INDIVIDUAL DRUGS:

Agents Acting Directly on Vascular Smooth Muscle

Diazoxide IV
Nitroprusside sodium

Alpha-1-Adrenergic Blocking Agents

Doxazosin mesylate
Prazosin hydrochloride
Terazosin

Angiotensin-II Receptor Blockers

Candesartan cilexetil
Eprosartan mesylate
Irbesartan
Losartan potassium
Olmesartan medoxomil
Valsartan

Angiotensin-Converting Enzyme Inhibitors

Benazepril hydrochloride
Captopril
Enalapril maleate
Fosinopril sodium
Lisinopril
Perindopril erbumine
Quinapril hydrochloride
Ramipril
Trandolopril

Beta-Adrenergic Blocking Agents

Atenolol
Betaxolol hydrochloride
Bisoprolol fumarate
Metoprolol succinate
Nadolol
Penbutolol sulfate
Propranolol hydrochloride
Timolol maleate

Calcium Channel Blocking Agents

Amlodipine
Bepridil hydrochloride
Diltiazem hydrochloride
Felodipine
Isradipine

Classifications

Nicardipine hydrochloride
Nifedipine
Nimodipine
Nisoldipine
Verapamil

Centrally-Acting Agents

Clonidine hydrochloride
Guanfacine hydrochloride
Methyldopa
Methyldopate hydrochloride

Combination Drugs Used for Hypertension

See Table in Appendix 14

Miscellaneous Agents

Bosentan
Carvedilol
Epoprostenol sodium
Labetalol hydrochloride
Minoxidil, oral

GENERAL STATEMENT

The Seventh Report of the Joint National Committee on Prevention, Detection, Evaluation and Treatment of High Blood Pressure classifies BP for adults aged 18 and over as follows: **Normal** as <120/<80 mm Hg, **Prehypertension** as 120–139/80–89 mm Hg, **Stage 1 Hypertension** as 140–159/90–99 mm Hg, and **Stage 2 Hypertension** as > or equal to 160/ > or equal to 100 mm Hg. Drug therapy is recommended depending on the BP and whether certain risk factors (e.g., smoking, dyslipidemia, diabetes, age, gender, target organ damage, clinical CV disease) are present. Lifestyle modification is an important component of treating hypertension, including weight reduction, diet, reduction of sodium intake, aerobic physical exercise, cessation of smoking, and moderate alcohol intake.

The risk of cardiovascular disease begins to increase when either the SPB exceeds 115 mm Hg or the DBP is greater than 75 mm Hg. Beyond 115/75 the risk of CV disease doubles with each advance of 20/10 mm Hg. In clients over 50 years of age, SBPs greater than 140 mm Hg are more important determinants of CV disease than are elevated DBPs. Generally speaking, the primary agents for initial monotherapy of Stage 1 hypertension to treat uncomplicated hypertension are thiazide diuretics; one may also consider ACE inhibitors, angiotensin receptor blockers, calcium channel blockers, and beta-adrenergic blocking agents. It should be noted that diet, exercise, and other life modifications are often sufficient to prevent or reduce hypertension. To treat Stage 2 hypertension, two drug combinations should be considered, i.e., usually a thiazide diuretic and an ACE inhibitor, or angiotensin receptor blocker, or a beta blocker, or a calcium channel blocker.

DRUG INTERACTIONS

See individual drugs

H *Black cohosh* / May potentiate antihypertensive drugs

H *Garlic* / May potentiate antihypertensive drugs

H *Hawthorn* / Cardioactive, hypotensive, and coronary vasodilator action of hawthorn may affect antihypertensive effect; monitor.

NURSING CONSIDERATIONS

ASSESSMENT

1. Note indications for therapy, other agents trialed and any family history of hypertension, stroke, CVD, CHD, MI, dyslipidemia, and diabetes.

2. Determine baseline BP before starting antihypertensive therapy. To ensure accuracy of baseline readings, take BP in both (bared and supported) arms (lying, standing, and sitting) 2 min apart (30 min after last cigarette or caffeine consumption) at least three times during one visit and on two subsequent visits. Document BMI (body mass index), or height, weight and risk factors.

3. Ascertain life-style modifications (weight reduction, ↓ alcohol intake, regular exercise, reduced sodium/fat intake, stress reduction, and smoking cessation) needed to achieve lowered BP. Offer a trial following these modifications and reassess in 3–6 months before starting therapy unless BP in severe range or > 2 risk factors.

4. Monitor ECG, chem-7, CBC, uric acid, urinalysis, cholesterol panel, and LFTs; always check for proteinuria.

5. Note funduscopic and neurologic exam findings. Assess for thyroid enlargement and presence of target organ damage. If difficult to control, assess for renal artery stenosis or secondary causes of HTN and refer for 24-hr ambulatory BP monitoring.

CLIENT/FAMILY TEACHING

1. Drugs control but do not cure hypertension. Take medications despite feeling fine and do not stop abruptly; may cause rebound hypertension. Drugs only provide protection/control of BP for the day in which they are taken. They must be taken daily as prescribed to ensure control. If dose missed, do not double up or take two doses close together.

2. There are generally no S&S of high blood pressure. When S&S become evident is when organ damage has already occurred. Keep a record of BP readings; helps identify 'white coat syndrome.'

3. Adhere to a low-sodium, low-fat diet; see dietitian as needed for education, meal planning, and food selections. Avoid excessive amounts of caffeine (tea, coffee, chocolate, or colas).

4. Weakness, dizziness, and fainting may occur with rapid changes of position from lying to standing (postural hypotension). Rise slowly from a lying or sitting position and dangle legs for several minutes before standing to minimize low BP effects. Exercising in hot weather may enhance these effects.

5. Report any swelling in hands or feet, increased SOB, chest pain, or changes in urination, i.e., pain, frequency or reduced amounts. Have yearly eye exams to detect early retinal changes from ↑ BP.

6. Avoid agents that may lower BP (e.g., alcohol, barbiturates, CNS depressants) or that could elevate BP (e.g., OTC cold remedies, oral contraceptives, steroids, NSAIDs, appetite suppressants, tricyclic antidepressants, MAO inhibitors). Sympathomimetic amines in products used to treat asthma, colds, and allergies must be used with extreme caution

7. Report if sexual dysfunction occurs as medication can usually be changed to minimize symptoms or other options for sexual dysfunction explored.

8. Identify holistic interventions/lifestyle modifications necessary for BP control: dietary restrictions of fat and sodium (2–3 g/day), weight reduction, ↓ alcohol (i.e., less than 24 oz beer or less than 8 oz of wine or less than 2 oz of 100-proof whiskey per day), tobacco cessation, ↑ physical activity, regular exercise programs, proper rest, and methods to reduce and deal with stress.

OUTCOMES/EVALUATE

• Understanding of disease/compliance with prescribed therapy

• ↓ BP (SBP < 120 and DBP < 80 mm Hg)

• Control/prevent target organ damage, stroke, MI, and/or death

BETA-ADRENERGIC BLOCKING AGENTS

SEE ALSO ALPHA-1-ADRENERGIC BLOCKING AGENTS AND THE FOLLOWING INDIVIDUAL AGENTS:

> Atenolol
> Betaxolol hydrochloride
> Bisoprolol fumarate
> Esmolol hydrochloride
> Levobunolol hydrochloride
> Metipranolol hydrochloride
> Metoprolol succinate
> Metoprolol tartrate
> Nadolol
> Penbutolol sulfate
> Propranolol hydrochloride
> Sotalol hydrochloride
> Timolol maleate

ACTION/KINETICS

Combine reversibly with beta-adrenergic receptors to block the response to sympathetic nerve impulses, circulating catecholamines, or adrenergic drugs. Beta-adrenergic receptors are classified as beta-1 (predominantly in the cardiac muscle) and beta-2 (mainly in the bronchi and vascular musculature). Blockade of beta-1 receptors decreases HR, myo-

Classifications

cardial contractility, and CO; in addition, AV conduction is slowed. These effects lead to a decrease in BP, as well as a reversal of cardiac arrhythmias. Blockade of beta-2 receptors increases airway resistance in the bronchioles and inhibits the vasodilating effects of catecholamines on peripheral blood vessels. The various beta-blocking agents differ in their ability to block beta-1 and beta-2 receptors (see individual drugs); also, certain of these agents have intrinsic sympathomimetic action.

Certain of these drugs (betaxolol, carteolol, levobunolol, metipranolol, and timolol) are used for glaucoma; act by reducing production of aqueous humor; metipranolol and timolol may also increase outflow of aqueous humor. Drugs have little or no effect on the pupil size or on accommodation.

USES
See individual drugs. Depending on the drug uses include, but are not limited to (1) Hypertension. (2) Angina pectoris. (3) MI. Are important in clients who have survived a first MI. (4) Migraine. (5) Part of the standard therapy for CHF. (6) May increase survival if taken prior to coronary artery bypass surgery.

CONTRAINDICATIONS
Sinus bradycardia, second- and third-degree AV block, cardiogenic shock, CHF unless secondary to tachyarrhythmia treatable with beta blockers, overt cardiac failure. Most are contraindicated in chronic bronchitis, bronchial asthma or history thereof, bronchospasm, emphysema, severe COPD.

SPECIAL CONCERNS
Use with caution in diabetes, thyrotoxicosis, cerebrovascular insufficiency, and impaired hepatic and renal function. Withdrawing beta blockers before major surgery is controversial. Safe use during pregnancy and lactation and in children has not been established. May be absorbed systemically when used for glaucoma; thus, there is the potential for an additive effect with beta blockers used systemically. Certain of the products for use in glaucoma contain sulfites, which may result in an allergic reaction. Also, see individual agents.

SIDE EFFECTS
CV: Bradycardia, hypotension (especially following IV use), CHF, cold extremities, claudication, worsening of angina, strokes, edema, syncope, arrhythmias, chest pain, peripheral ischemia, flushing, SOB, sinoatrial block, pulmonary edema, vasodilation, increased HR, palpitations, conduction disturbances, *first-, second-, and third-degree heart block,* worsening of AV block, thrombosis of renal or mesenteric arteries, precipitation/worsening of Raynaud's phenomenon. Sudden withdrawal of large doses may cause angina, ventricular tachycardia, *fatal MI, sudden death,* or *circulatory collapse.* **GI:** N&V, diarrhea, flatulence, dry mouth, constipation, anorexia, cramps, bloating, gastric pain, dyspepsia, distortion of taste, weight gain/loss, retroperitoneal fibrosis, ischemic colitis. **Hepatic:** Hepatomegaly, acute pancreatitis, elevated liver enzymes, liver damage (especially with chronic use of phenobarbital). **Respiratory:** Asthma-like symptoms, *bronchospasms, bronchial obstruction, laryngospasm with respiratory distress,* wheezing, worsening of cold, dyspnea, cough, nasal stuffiness, rhinitis, pharyngitis, rales. **CNS:** Dizziness, fatigue, lethargy, vivid dreams, depression, hallucinations, delirium, psychoses, paresthesias, insomnia, nervousness, nightmares, headache, vertigo, disorientation of time and place, hypoesthesia or hyperesthesia, decreased concentration, short-term memory loss, change in behavior, emotional lability, slurred speech, lightheadedness. In the elderly, paranoia, disorientation, and combativeness have occurred. **Hematologic:** *Agranulocytosis,* thrombocytopenia. **Allergic:** Fever, sore throat, respiratory distress, rash, pharyngitis, *laryngospasm, anaphylaxis.* **Skin:** Pruritus, rashes, increased skin pigmentation, sweating, dry skin, alopecia, skin irritation, psoriasis (reversible). **Musculoskeletal:** Joint/back/muscle pain, arthritis, arthralgia, muscle cramps, muscle weakness when used in clients with myasthenic symptoms. **GU:** Impotence, decreased libido, dysuria, UTI, nocturia,

---

Bold Italic = life threatening side effect　　■ = black box warning　　✦ = Available in Canada

urinary retention or frequency, pollakiuria. **Ophthalmic:** Visual disturbances, eye irritation, dry or burning eyes, blurred vision, conjunctivitis. **When used ophthalmically:** Keratitis, blepharoptosis, diplopia, ptosis, and visual disturbances including refractive changes. **Other:** Hyper/hypoglycemia, lupus-like syndrome, Peyronie's disease, tinnitus, increase in symptoms of myasthenia gravis, facial swelling, decreased exercise tolerance, rigors, speech disorders. **Systemic effects due to ophthalmic beta-1 and beta-2 blockers:** Headache, depression, arrhythmia, heart block, CVA, syncope, CHF, palpitation, cerebral ischemia, nausea, localized and generalized rash, bronchospasm (especially in those with preexisting bronchospastic disease), respiratory failure, masked symptoms of hypoglycemia in IDDM, keratitis, visual disturbances (including refractive changes), blepharoptosis, ptosis, diplopia.

OD OVERDOSE MANAGEMENT

Symptoms: CV symptoms include bradycardia, hypotension, CHF, ***cardiogenic shock,*** intraventricular conduction disturbances, ***AV block, pulmonary edema, asystole,*** and tachycardia. Also, overdosage of pindolol may cause hypertension and overdosage of propranolol may result in systemic vascular resistance. CNS symptoms include respiratory depression, decreased consciousness, ***coma, and seizures.*** Miscellaneous symptoms include ***bronchospasm*** (especially in clients with COPD), hyperkalemia, and hypoglycemia.

Treatment:

• To improve blood supply to the brain, place client in a supine position and raise the legs.

• Measure blood glucose and serum potassium. Monitor BP and ECG continuously.

• Provide general supportive treatment such as inducing emesis or gastric lavage and artificial respiration.

• *Seizures:* Give IV diazepam or phenytoin.

• *Excessive bradycardia:* If hypotensive, give atropine, 0.6 mg; if no response,

give q 3 min for a total of 2–3 mg. Cautious administration of isoproterenol may be tried. Also, glucagon, 5–10 mg rapidly over 30 sec, followed by continuous IV infusion of 5 mg/hr may reverse bradycardia. Transvenous cardiac pacing may be needed for refractory cases.

• *Cardiac failure:* Digitalis, diuretic, and oxygen; if failure is refractory, IV aminophylline or glucagon may be helpful.

• *Hypotension:* Place client in Trendelenburg position. IV fluids unless pulmonary edema is present; also vasopressors such as norepinephrine (may be drug of choice), dobutamine, dopamine with monitoring of BP. If refractory, glucagon may be helpful. In intractable cardiogenic shock, intra-aortic balloon insertion may be required.

• *Premature ventricular contractions:* Lidocaine or phenytoin. Disopyramide, quinidine, and procainamide should be avoided as they depress myocardial function further.

• *Bronchospasms:* Give a beta-2-adrenergic agonist, epinephrine, or theophylline.

• *Heart block, second or third degree:* Isoproterenol or transvenous cardiac pacing.

DRUG INTERACTIONS

Aluminum salts / ↓ Bioavailability of certain beta-blockers → ↓ effect

Ampicillin / ↓ Bioavailability of certain beta-blockers → ↓ effect

Anesthetics, general / Additive depression of myocardium

Anticholinergic agents / Counteract bradycardia produced by beta-adrenergic blockers

Antihypertensives / Additive hypotensive effect

Barbiturates / ↓ Bioavailability of certain beta-blockers → ↓ effect

Benzodiazepines / ↑ Effect of certain benzodiazepines by lipophilic beta-blockers

Calcium channel blockers / ↑ Effect of certain beta-blockers

Calcium salts / ↓ Bioavailability of certain beta-blockers → ↓ effect

Chlorpromazine / Additive beta-adrenergic blocking action

Cholestyramine / ↓ Bioavailability of certain beta-blockers → ↓ effect

Cimetidine / ↑ Effect of beta blockers R/T ↓ liver breakdown

Clonidine / Paradoxical hypertension; also, ↑ severity of rebound hypertension

Colestipol / ↓ Bioavailability of certain beta-blockers → ↓ effect

Diphenhydramine / ↑ Plasma levels and CV effects of certain beta-blockers R/T ↓ metabolism

Disopyramide / ↑ Effect of both drugs

Epinephrine / Beta blockers prevent beta-adrenergic action of epinephrine but not alpha-adrenergic action → ↑ SBP/DBP and ↓ HR

Ergot alkaloids / ↑ Risk of peripheral ischemia R/T ergot alkaloid-mediated vasoconstriction and peripheral effects of beta-blockers

Flecainide / Possible ↑ bioavailability of either drug → ↑ effects

Furosemide / ↑ Beta-adrenergic blockade

Haloperidol / ↑ Risk of hypotensive episodes

Hydralazine / ↑ Effect of both beta-blockers and hydralazine

Hydroxychloroquine / ↑ Plasma levels and CV effects of certain beta-blockers R/T ↓ metabolism

Indomethacin / ↓ Effect of beta blockers possibly due to inhibition of prostaglandin synthesis

Insulin / Beta blockers ↑ hypoglycemic effect of insulin

Lidocaine / ↑ Drug effect R/T ↓ liver breakdown

Methyldopa / Possible ↑ BP to alpha-adrenergic effect

Muscle relaxants, nondepolarizing / Beta-blockers may potentiate, counteract, or have no effect on action of nondepolarizing muscle relaxants

NSAIDs / ↓ Effect of beta blockers, possibly R/T inhibition of prostaglandin synthesis

Ophthalmic beta blockers / Additive systemic beta-blocking effects if used with oral beta blockers

Oral contraceptives / ↑ Effect of beta blockers R/T ↓ liver breakdown

Phenformin / ↑ Hypoglycemia

Phenobarbital / ↓ Effect of beta blockers R/T ↑ liver breakdown

Phenothiazines / ↑ Effect of both drugs

Phenytoin / Additive depression of myocardium; also ↓ effect of beta blockers R/T ↑ liver breakdown

Prazosin / ↑ First-dose effect of prazosin (acute postural hypotension)

Propafenone / ↑ Plasma levels of certain beta-blockers R/T ↓ liver metabolism

Quinidine / ↑ Plasma levels of beta-blockers in extensive metabolizers → ↑ effects

Quinolone antibiotics / ↑ Bioavailability of beta-blockers metabolized by the cytochrome P450 system

Rifampin / ↓ Effect of beta blockers due to ↑ breakdown by liver

Ritodrine / Beta blockers ↓ effect of ritodrine

Salicylates / ↓ Effect of beta blockers, possibly R/T inhibition of prostaglandin synthesis

SSRIs / Possible excessive beta-blockade R/T ↓ metabolism

Succinylcholine / Beta blockers ↑ effects of succinylcholine

Sulfonylureas / ↓ Effect of sulfonylureas

Sympathomimetics / Reverse effects of beta blockers

Theophylline / Beta blockers reverse the effect of theophylline; also, beta blockers ↓ renal drug clearance

Thioamines / ↑ Effects of beta-blockers

Thyroid hormones / Effects of certain beta-blockers may be ↓ when hypothyroid client is converted to euthyroid state

Tubocurarine / Beta blockers ↑ effects of tubocurarine

Verapamil / Possible side effects since both drugs ↓ myocardial contractility or AV conduction; bradycardia and asystole when beta blockers are used ophthalmically

LABORATORY TEST CONSIDERATIONS
↓ Serum glucose.

DOSAGE
See individual drugs.

Bold Italic = life threatening side effect   ■ = black box warning   ✦ = Available in Canada

NURSING CONSIDERATIONS

ADMINISTRATION/STORAGE

1. Sudden cessation of beta blockers may precipitate or worsen angina.

2. Lowering of intraocular pressure (IOP) may take a few weeks to stabilize when using betaxolol or timolol.

3. Due to diurnal variations in IOP, the response to twice a day therapy is best assessed by measuring IOP at different times during the day.

4. If IOP is not controlled using beta blockers, add additional drugs to the regimen, including pilocarpine, dipivefrin, or systemic carbonic anhydrase inhibitors.

ASSESSMENT

1. Note indications for therapy, symptom characteristics, and other agents trialed. List any history of depression; assess mental status. Review drugs currently prescribed to ensure none interact.

2. Note any history of asthma, diabetes, or impaired renal function. With asthma, avoid nonselective beta antagonists due to beta-2 receptor blockade which may lead to increased airway resistance.

3. Determine pulse and BP in both arms lying, sitting, and standing. Monitor EKG, glucose, CBC, electrolytes, renal and LFTs. Note MUGA, echocardiogram, or stress test results.

INTERVENTIONS

1. Monitor HR and BP; obtain written parameters for holding (e.g., for SBP < 90 for HR < 45).

2. When assessing respirations note rate and quality; may cause dyspnea and bronchospasm.

3. Monitor I&O and daily weights. Observe for increasing dyspnea, coughing, difficulty breathing, fatigue, or edema—symptoms of CHF, may require digitalization, diuretics, and/or drug discontinuation.

4. Complaints of cold S&S, easy fatigue, or feeling lightheaded may require a drug change.

5. With diabetics watch for S&S of hypoglycemia, such as hypotension or tachycardia; signs may be masked.

6. During IV administration, monitor EKG (may slow AV conduction and increase PR interval) and activities closely until drug effects evident.

CLIENT/FAMILY TEACHING

1. When prescribed for BP control, drug helps control hypertension but does not cure it. Must continue to take despite feeling better. With MI, drug is prescribed to prevent remodeling and to decrease sudden death after heart attack.

2. Record BP and take pulse immediately prior to first dose each day so medication can be adjusted. Review instructions for when to call provider, i.e., if HR < 45 beats/min or SBP < 80 mm Hg.

3. Review lifestyle changes for BP control: regular exercise, weight loss, low-fat and reduced-calorie diet, decreased salt and alcohol intake, smoking cessation, and relaxation techniques.

4. Always consult provider before interrupting therapy; abrupt withdrawal may precipitate angina, MI, or rebound hypertension. A 2-week taper is useful.

5. May cause blurred vision, dizziness, or drowsiness; avoid activities that require mental alertness until drug effects realized.

6. Rise from a sitting or lying position slowly and dangle legs before standing to avoid S&S of sudden drop in BP. Elastic support hose may help decrease symptoms.

7. Dress warmly during cold weather. Diminished blood supply to extremities may cause cold sensitivity; check extremities for warmth.

8. Avoid excessive intake of alcohol, coffee, tea, or cola. Avoid OTC agents without approval.

9. If diabetic, monitor BS and report S&S of hypoglycemia. With heart failure, check weight daily and report unusual weight gain (>2 lbs per day or 5 lbs per week.)

10. Report any asthma-like symptoms, cough, or nasal stuffiness; may be symptoms of CHF. Report any bothersome side effects or changes, especially new-onset depression or marked fatigue. Keep all F/U appointments.

OUTCOMES/EVALUATE

- ↓ BP; ↓ IOP; ↓ Remodeling
- ↓ Frequency/severity of anginal attacks; improved exercise tolerance
- ↓ Anxiety levels; ↓ tremors
- Migraine prophylaxis
- Control of cardiac arrhythmias

CALCIUM CHANNEL BLOCKING AGENTS

SEE ALSO THE FOLLOWING INDIVIDUAL ENTRIES:

Amlodipine
Diltiazem hydrochloride
Felodipine
Isradipine
Nicardipine hydrochloride
Nifedipine
Nimodipine
Nisoldipine
Verapamil

ACTION/KINETICS

For contraction of cardiac and smooth muscle to occur, extracellular calcium must move into the cell through openings called *calcium channels*. The calcium channel blocking agents (also called *slow channel blockers* or *calcium antagonists*) inhibit the influx of calcium through the cell membrane, resulting in a depression of automaticity and conduction velocity in both smooth and cardiac muscle. This leads to a depression of contraction in these tissues. Drugs in this class have different degrees of selectivity on vascular smooth muscle, myocardium, and conduction and pacemaker tissues. In the myocardium, these drugs dilate coronary vessels in both normal and ischemic tissues and inhibit spasms of coronary arteries. They also decrease total peripheral resistance, thus reducing energy and oxygen requirements of the heart. Also effective against certain cardiac arrhythmias by slowing AV conduction and prolonging repolarization. In addition, they depress the amplitude, rate of depolarization, and conduction in atria.

USES

See individual drugs. Uses include, but are not limited to: (1) Vasospastic (Prinzmetal's or variant) angina. (2) Chronic stable (classic-associated) angina. (3) Unstable angina at rest. (4) Paroxysmal supraventricular tachycardias. (5) Essential hypertension. (6) Atrial fibrillation/flutter.

CONTRAINDICATIONS

Sick sinus syndrome, second- or third-degree AV block (except with a functioning pacemaker). Use of bepridil, diltiazem, or verapamil for hypotension (< 90 mm Hg systolic pressure). Lactation.

SPECIAL CONCERNS

Abrupt withdrawal may result in increased frequency and duration of chest pain. Hypertensive clients treated with calcium channel blockers have a higher risk of heart attack than clients treated with diuretics or beta-adrenergic blockers. May also be an increased risk of heart attacks in diabetics (only nisoldipine studied). Safety and effectiveness of bepridil, diltiazem, felodipine, and isradipine have not been established in children.

SIDE EFFECTS

Side effects vary from one calcium channel blocker to another; refer to individual drugs.

OD OVERDOSE MANAGEMENT

Symptoms: Nausea, weakness, drowsiness, dizziness, slurred speech, confusion, marked and prolonged hypotension, bradycardia, junctional rhythms, *second- or third-degree block.*
Treatment:

- Treatment is supportive. Monitor cardiac and respiratory function.
- If client is seen soon after ingestion, emetics or gastric lavage should be considered followed by cathartics.
- *Hypotension:* IV calcium, dopamine, isoproterenol, metaraminol, norepinephrine. Also, provide IV fluids. Place client in Trendelenburg position.
- *Ventricular tachycardia:* IV procainamide or lidocaine; also, cardioversion may be necessary. Also, provide slow-drip IV fluids.
- *Bradycardia, asystole, AV block:* IV atropine sulfate (0.6–1 mg), calcium gluconate (10% solution), isoproterenol, norepinephrine; also, cardiac pacing

may be indicated. Provide slow-drip IV fluids.

DRUG INTERACTIONS

Anesthetics / Potentiation of cardiac effects and vascular dilation associated with anesthetics; possible severe hypotension

Beta-adrenergic blocking agents / Beta blockers may cause depression of myocardial contractility and AV conduction

Cimetidine / ↑ Effect of CCBs R/T ↓ first-pass metabolism

H *Dong quai* / Possible additive effect

Fentanyl / Severe hypotension or ↑ fluid volume requirements

H *Ginger* / May alter CCBs effect R/T ↑ calcium uptake by heart muscle

Grapefruit juice / ↑ Serum levels of most calcium channel blockers

Itraconazole / Edema when used with amlodipine or nifedipine

Ranitidine / ↑ Effect of CCBs R/T ↓ first-pass metabolism

DOSAGE————————————

See individual drugs.

NURSING CONSIDERATIONS

ASSESSMENT

1. Document indications for therapy, onset, and characteristics of symptoms. List other agents used and outcome. Note any experience with these agents and the response. List drugs prescribed to ensure none interact.

2. Assess/document CV and mental status. These drugs cause peripheral vasodilation. Any excessive hypotensive response and increased HR may precipitate angina. Record VS, weight, ECG and BP in both arms while lying, sitting, and standing. Assess for CHF (weight gain, peripheral edema, dyspnea, crackles, jugular vein distention).

3. Monitor BS, electrolytes, I&O, liver and renal function studies.

CLIENT/FAMILY TEACHING

1. These agents work by decreasing myocardial contractile force, which in turn decreases the heart's oxygen requirements. Take with meals to ↓ GI upset. Do not stop therapy suddenly.

2. Review goals of therapy (e.g., ↓ DBP by 10 mm Hg, ↓ HR by 20 beats/min). Record pulse and BP at least twice a week as well as weights; review instructions regarding when to hold medications and contact provider.

3. Do not perform activities that require mental alertness until drug effects realized. Report adverse effects such as dizziness, vertigo, unusual flushing, facial warmth, edema, nausea, constipation. Toxic drug effects are swelling of the hands or feet, pronounced dizziness, chest pain accompanied by sweating, SOB, or severe headaches.

4. If dizziness occurs (drop in BP), change positions slowly, especially when standing from a lying position. Sit down immediately if lightheadedness occurs. Move slowly from a lying to a sitting or standing position.

5. Avoid long periods of standing, excessive heat, hot showers or baths, and ingestion of alcohol; may exacerbate drop in BP.

6. Review lifestyle changes for BP control, i.e., regular exercise, weight loss, low-fat, low-cholesterol, reduced-calorie diet, decreased salt and alcohol consumption, smoking cessation, and stress reduction.

OUTCOMES/EVALUATE

• Control of BP; ↓ HR
• ↓ Frequency/intensity of angina
• Stable cardiac rhythm

CALCIUM SALTS

SEE ALSO THE FOLLOWING INDIVIDUAL ENTRIES:

Calcium carbonate
Calcium chloride
Calcium gluconate

ACTION/KINETICS

Calcium is essential for maintaining normal function of nerves, muscles, the skeletal system, and permeability of cell membranes and capillaries. The normal serum calcium concentration is 9–10.4 mg/dL (4.5–5.2 mEq/L). Hypocalcemia is characterized by muscular fibrillation, twitching, skeletal muscle spasms, leg cramps, tetanic spasms, cardiac arrhythmias, smooth muscle hyperexcitability, mental depression, and anxiety states. Excessive, chronic hypocalcemia is characterized by brittle, defective nails, poor dentition, and brittle hair. Calcium is well absorbed from the upper GI tract; Vitamin D is required for calcium absorption and increases the capability of the absorptive mechanisms. Food increases calcium absorption. Severe low-calcium tetany is best treated by IV administration of calcium gluconate. The hormone of the parathyroid gland is necessary for the regulation of the calcium level. Calcium is excreted mainly through the feces (as much as 250–300 mg/day in healthy adults eating a regular diet).

Recommended daily allowances for men and women, age 19–24 years is 1,200 mg/day; and, for men and women, 25 years of age and older is 800 mg/day. Dietary reference intakes for men and women, 19–50 years of age is 1,000 mg/day; for men and women over 51 years of age is 1,200 mg/day; and, for pregnant and breastfeeding women is 1000 mg/day.

USES

IV: (1) Acute hypocalcemic tetany secondary to renal failure. (2) Hypoparathyroidism. (3) Premature delivery. (4) Maternal diabetes mellitus in infants. (5) Poisoning due to magnesium, oxalic acid, radiophosphorus, carbon tetrachloride, fluoride, phosphate, strontium, and radium. (6) Treat depletion of electrolytes. (7) During cardiac resuscitation when epinephrine or isoproterenol has not improved myocardial contraction (may also be given into the ventricular cavity for this purpose). (8) To reverse cardiotoxicity or hyperkalemia. **IM or IV:** (1) Reduce spasms in renal, biliary, intestinal, or lead colic. (2) Relieve muscle cramps due to insect bites. (3) Decrease capillary permeability in various sensitivity reactions. **PO:** (1) Osteoporosis, osteomalacia. (2) Chronic hypoparathyroidism. (3) Rickets. (4) Latent tetany. (5) Hypocalcemia secondary to use of anticonvulsant drugs. (6) Myasthenia gravis. (7) Eaton-Lambert syndrome. (8) Supplement for pregnant, postmenopausal, or nursing women. (9) Prophylactically for primary osteoporosis. *Investigational:* As an infu-

sion to diagnose Zollinger-Ellison syndrome and medullary thyroid carcinoma. To antagonize neuromuscular blockade due to aminoglycosides.

CONTRAINDICATIONS

Digitalized clients, sarcoidosis, renal or cardiac disease, ventricular fibrillation. Cancer clients with bone metastases. Renal calculi, hypophosphatemia, hypercalcemia.

SPECIAL CONCERNS

Calcium requirements decrease in geriatric clients; thus, dose may have to be adjusted. Also, low levels of active vitamin D metabolites may impair calcium absorption in older clients. Use with caution in cor pulmonale, sarcoidosis, cardiac or renal disease, or in those receiving cardiac glycosides. May be irritating to the GI tract when given PO and may cause constipation.

SIDE EFFECTS

Following PO use: GI irritation, constipation. **Following IV use:** Venous irritation, tingling sensation, feeling of oppression or heat, chalky taste. Rapid IV administration may result in vasodilation, decreased BP and HR, *cardiac arrhythmias,* syncope, or *cardiac arrest.* **Following IM use:** Burning feeling, necrosis, tissue sloughing, cellulitis, soft tissue calcification. *NOTE:* If calcium is injected into the myocardium rather than into the ventricle, *laceration of coronary arteries, cardiac tamponade, pneumothorax, and ventricular fibrillation* may occur. **Symptoms due to excess calcium (hypercalcemia):** Lassitude, fatigue, GI symptoms (anorexia, N&V, abdominal pain, dry mouth, thirst), polyuria, depression of nervous and neuromuscular function (emotional disturbances, confusion, skeletal muscle weakness, and constipation), confusion, delirium, stupor, *coma,* impairment of renal function (polyuria, polydipsia, and azotemia), renal calculi, arrhythmias, and bradycardia.

OD **OVERDOSE MANAGEMENT**

Symptoms: Systemic overloading from parenteral administration can result in an acute hypercalcemic syndrome with symptoms including markedly increased plasma calcium levels, lethargy, intractable N&V, weakness, **coma, and sudden death.** *Treatment:* Discontinue therapy and lower serum calcium levels by giving an IV infusion of sodium chloride plus a potent diuretic such as furosemide. Consider hemodialysis.

DRUG INTERACTIONS
Atenolol / ↓ Drug effect R/T ↓ bioavailability and plasma levels
Cephalocin / Incompatible with calcium salts
Corticosteroids / Interfere with absorption of calcium from GI tract
Digitalis / ↑ Digitalis arrhythmias and toxicity. Death has resulted from combination of digitalis and IV calcium salts
Iron salts / ↓ Absorption of iron from the GI tract
[H] *Lily-of-the-valley herb* / ↑ Effectiveness and side effects of calcium
Milk / Excess of either may cause hypercalcemia, renal insufficiency with azotemia, alkalosis, and ocular lesions
Norfloxacin / ↓ Drug bioavailability
[H] *Pheasant's eye herb* / ↑ Effectiveness and side effects of calcium
Sodium polystyrene sulfonate / Metabolic alkalosis and ↓ binding of resin to potassium with renal impairment
[H] *Squill* / ↑ Effectiveness and side effects of calcium
Tetracyclines / ↓ Tetracycline effect R/T ↓ GI tract absorption
Thiazide diuretics / Hypercalcemia R/T to thiazide-induced renal tubular reabsorption of calcium and bone release of calcium
Verapamil / Calcium antagonizes the effect of verapamil
Vitamin D / Enhances intestinal absorption of dietary calcium

DOSAGE————————
See individual agents.

NURSING CONSIDERATIONS
ASSESSMENT
1. Perform a thorough nursing history, noting clinical presentation, indications for therapy and any precipitating causes. List drugs prescribed, especially if receiving digitalis products; drug may be contraindicated.
2. Monitor calcium levels and renal function; assess for renal or parathyroid

disease. Vitamin D facilitates absorption.
3. Assess for S&S of hypercalcemia, i.e., fatigue and CNS depression. With hypocalcemic tetany, protect client from injury.
4. Note bone density findings.

CLIENT/FAMILY TEACHING
1. General calcium requirements are best met by dietary sources (including milk in the diet). Supplements need vitamin D to facilitate absorption. Consult dietitian to assist with proper food selection and meal planning and preparation.
2. Multivitamin and mineral preparations are expensive and do not contain sufficient calcium to meet daily requirements. Review prescribed replacement regimen. Need follow-ups for dosage adjustments to prevent hypercalcemia and hypercalciuria.
3. Report adverse side effects, lack of desired response, and keep all F/U appointments to evalute drug response.

OUTCOMES/EVALUATE
• Resolution of hypocalcemia
• Relief of muscle cramps
• Osteoporosis prophylaxis
• Serum calcium levels within desired range (8.8–10.4 mg/dL)

CHOLINERGIC BLOCKING AGENTS

SEE ALSO THE FOLLOWING INDIVIDUAL ENTRIES:

Atropine sulfate
Benztropine mesylate
Biperiden hydrochloride
Dicyclomine hydrochloride
Ipratropium bromide
Scopolamine hydrobromide
Scopolamine transdermal
    therapeutic system

ACTION/KINETICS
Cholinergic blocking agents prevent the neurotransmitter acetylcholine from combining with receptors on the postganglionic parasympathetic nerve terminal (muscarinic site). Effects include reduction of smooth muscle spasms, blockade of vagal impulses to the heart,

[H] = Herbal   [IV] = Intravenous   ⓡ = sound-alike drug

decreased secretions (e.g., gastric, salivation, bronchial mucus, sweat glands), production of mydriasis and cycloplegia, and various CNS effects. In therapeutic doses, these drugs have little effect on transmission of nerve impulses across ganglia (nicotinic sites) or at the neuromuscular junction. Several anticholinergic drugs abolish or reduce the S&S of Parkinson's disease, such as tremors and rigidity, and result in some improvement in mobility, muscular coordination, and motor performance. These effects may be due to blockade of the effects of acetylcholine in the CNS.

USES
See individual drugs.

CONTRAINDICATIONS
Glaucoma, adhesions between iris and lens of the eye, tachycardia, myocardial ischemia, unstable CV state in acute hemorrhage, partial obstruction of the GI and biliary tracts, prostatic hypertrophy, renal disease, myasthenia gravis, hepatic disease, paralytic ileus, pyloroduodenal stenosis, pyloric obstruction, intestinal atony, ulcerative colitis, obstructive uropathy. Cardiac clients, especially when there is danger of tachycardia; older persons suffering from atherosclerosis or mental impairment. Lactation.

SPECIAL CONCERNS
Use with caution in pregnancy. Infants and young children are more susceptible to the toxic side effects of anticholinergic drugs. Use in children when the ambient temperature is high may cause a rapid increase in body temperature due to suppression of sweat glands. Geriatric clients are particularly likely to manifest anticholinergic side effects and CNS effects, including agitation, confusion, drowsiness, excitement, glaucoma, and impaired memory. Use with caution in hyperthyroidism, CHF, cardiac arrhythmias, hypertension, Down syndrome, asthma, spastic paralysis, blonde individuals, allergies, and chronic lung disease.

SIDE EFFECTS
These are desirable in some conditions and undesirable in others. Thus, the anticholinergics have an antisalivary effect that is useful in parkinsonism. This same effect is unpleasant when the drug is used for spastic conditions of the GI tract. Most side effects are dose-related and decrease when dosage decreases. **GI:** N&V, dry mouth, dysphagia, constipation, heartburn, change in taste perception, bloated feeling, paralytic ileus, epigastric distress, acute suppurative parotiditis, dilation of the colon, development of duodenal ulcer. **CNS:** Dizziness, drowsiness, nervousness, disorientation, headache, weakness, insomnia, fever (especially in children). Large doses may produce CNS stimulation including tremor and restlessness. **Anticholinergic psychoses:** Ataxia, euphoria, confusion, disorientation, loss of short-term memory, decreased anxiety, fatigue, insomnia, hallucinations, dysarthria, agitation. **CV:** Palpitations, tachycardia, hypotension, postural hypotension. **GU:** Urinary retention or hesitancy, dysuria, impotence. **Ophthalmologic:** Blurred vision, dilated pupils, diplopia, increased intraocular tension, angle-closure glaucoma, photophobia, cycloplegia, precipitation of acute glaucoma. **Dermatologic:** Urticaria, skin rashes, other dermatoses. **Musculoskeletal:** Muscle weakness, muscle cramping. **Other:** *Anaphylaxis,* flushing, decreased sweating, nasal congestion, numbness of fingers, suppression of glandular secretions including lactation. Heat prostration (fever and heat stroke) in presence of high environmental temperatures due to decreased sweating.

OD OVERDOSE MANAGEMENT
Symptoms ('Belladonna Poisoning'): Infants and children are especially susceptible to the toxic effects of atropine and scopolamine. Poisoning (dose-dependent) is characterized by the following symptoms: Dry mouth, burning sensation of the mouth, difficulty in swallowing and speaking, blurred vision, photophobia, dilated and sluggish pupils, rash, tachycardia, *circulatory collapse, cardiac arrest,* increased respiration, *increased body temperature* (up to 109°F, 42.7°C), restlessness, irritabili-

ty, confusion, anxiety, ataxia, hyperactivity, combativeness, toxic psychosis, anhidrosis, muscle incoordination, dilated pupils, hot dry skin, dry mucous membranes, dysphagia, foul-smelling breath, decreased bowel sounds, *respiratory depression and paralysis,* tremors, *seizures,* hallucinations, and *death.*
Treatment ('Belladonna Poisoning'):
• Gastric lavage or induction of vomiting followed by activated charcoal. General supportive measures.
• Anticholinergic effects can be reversed by physostigmine (Eserine), 1–3 mg IV (effectiveness uncertain; thus use other agents if possible). Neostigmine methylsulfate, 0.5–2 mg IV, repeated as necessary.
• If there is excitation, diazepam, a short-acting barbiturate, IV sodium thiopental (2% solution), or chloral hydrate (100–200 mL of a 2% solution by rectal infusion) may be given.
• For fever, cool baths may be used. Keep client in a darkened room if photophobia is manifested.
• Artificial respiration should be instituted if there is paralysis of respiratory muscles.

DRUG INTERACTIONS
Amantadine / Additive anticholinergic side effects
Antacids / ↓ Absorption of anticholinergics from GI tract
Antidepressants, tricyclic / Additive anticholinergic side effects
Antihistamines / Additive anticholinergic side effects
Atenolol / Anticholinergics ↑ effects of atenolol
Benzodiazepines / Additive anticholinergic side effects
Corticosteroids / Additive ↑ intraocular pressure
Digoxin / ↑ Drug effect R/T ↑ GI tract absorption
Disopyramide / Potentiation of anticholinergic side effects
Guanethidine / Reversal of inhibition of gastric acid secretion caused by anticholinergics
Haloperidol / Possible worsening of schizophrenic symptoms, ↓ haloperidol serum levels, and development of tardive dyskinesia
Histamine / Reversal of inhibition of gastric acid secretion caused by anticholinergics
Levodopa / Possible ↓ drug effect R/T ↑ breakdown of levodopa in stomach (R/T delayed gastric emptying time)
MAO inhibitors / ↑ Effect of anticholinergics R/T ↓ liver breakdown
Meperidine / Additive anticholinergic side effects
Methylphenidate / Potentiation of anticholinergic side effects
Metoclopramide / Anticholinergics block action of metoclopramide
Nitrates, nitrites / Potentiation of anticholinergic side effects
Nitrofurantoin / ↑ Bioavailability of nitrofurantoin
Orphenadrine / Additive anticholinergic side effects
Phenothiazines / Additive anticholinergic side effects; also, ↓ phenothiazine effects
Primidone / Potentiation of anticholinergic side effects
Procainamide / Additive anticholinergic side effects
Quinidine / Additive anticholinergic side effects
Sympathomimetics / ↑ Bronchial relaxation
Thiazide diuretics / ↑ Bioavailability of thiazide diuretics
Thioxanthines / Potentiation of anticholinergic side effects

DOSAGE
See individual drugs.

NURSING CONSIDERATIONS
ADMINISTRATION/STORAGE
Dosage is often small. To prevent overdosage, check dose and measure exactly.
ASSESSMENT
1. Document indications for therapy and clinical presentation. Assess for asthma, glaucoma, or duodenal ulcer (contraindications for therapy). Note any renal disease, cardiac problems, or hepatic disease.
2. Determine age; elderly clients, especially those with mental impairment or

atherosclerosis, should not receive these drugs. Assess for constipation, urinary retention, and tolerance. Monitor EKG, VS, I&O and respirations.

INTERVENTIONS
1. For complaints of a dry mouth, provide frequent mouth care and cold drinks, especially postoperatively. Sugarless hard candies/gum may also be of some benefit.
2. Drugs such as atropine may suppress thermoregulatory sweating; counsel client concerning activity (especially in hot weather) and appropriate clothing. Also, children and infants may exhibit 'atropine fever.'

CLIENT/FAMILY TEACHING
1. Certain side effects are to be expected, such as dry mouth or blurred vision, and may have to be tolerated because of the overall beneficial effects of drug therapy. These should be reported so symptoms may be alleviated by reducing the dose or temporarily stopping drug.
2. With parkinsonism, do not withdraw abruptly. If the medication is changed, one drug should be withdrawn slowly and the other started in small doses.

ADDITIONAL NURSING CONSIDERATIONS RELATED TO PATHOLOGIC CONDITIONS FOR WHICH THE DRUG IS ADMINISTERED

CARDIOVASCULAR
ASSESSMENT
Monitor VS and ECG. Assess for any hemodynamic changes and intraventricular conduction blocks. Note palpitations.

NURSING CONSIDERATIONS
OCULAR
ASSESSMENT
Determine any experience with these drugs and eye exam results. Document IOP; assess accommodation and pupillary response.

CLIENT/FAMILY TEACHING
1. Review methods for instillation of drops or ointment and frequency. Wash hands and do not permit container to come in contact with eye tissue. Vision

will be affected by the medications; temporary stinging and blurred vision will occur. Assess response and plan activities for safety.
2. Night vision may be impaired. Photophobia, which may occur, can be relieved by wearing dark glasses.
3. Report any marked changes in vision, eye irritation, eye pain after instillation, or persistent headaches immediately.
4. With large doses, tears may diminish; may experience dry/sandy eyes.

NURSING CONSIDERATIONS
GASTROINTESTINAL
ASSESSMENT
Note indications for therapy, other agents trialed and outcome. Document UGI and/or endoscopy findings.

CLIENT/FAMILY TEACHING
1. Take early enough before a meal (at least 20 min) so that it will be effective when needed. Review printed information related to the prescribed diet; see dietitian for assistance in meal planning.
2. Gastric emptying times may be prolonged and intestinal transit time lengthened. Drug-induced intestinal paralysis is temporary and should resolve after 1–3 days of therapy.

NURSING CONSIDERATIONS
GENITOURINARY
ASSESSMENT
Document indications for therapy, subjective reports of symptoms, and clinical presentation. Note PVR, cystoscopy and prostate exam results.

CLIENT/FAMILY TEACHING
1. Report urinary retention; may be more pronounced in elderly men with BPH. Monitor I&O and report evidence of bladder distention and need for catheterization if no urine output > 8 hr.
2. Consult with the provider for medication adjustment if impotence occurs; may be drug-related.

NURSING CONSIDERATIONS
CENTRAL NERVOUS SYSTEM
ASSESSMENT
Document indications for therapy, S&S of characteristics, other agents trialed,

---

and outcome. Note neurologist reports/ findings.

CLIENT/FAMILY TEACHING
1. Take only as directed. Do not skip or double up on doses if missed.
2. Avoid activities that require mental alertness until drug effects realized; may cause drowsiness. Use caution in hot weather as drugs may make one more susceptible to heat stroke.
3. Avoid OTC cough and cold remedies with alcohol and antihistamines unless specifically directed by provider.

DIURETICS, LOOP ■

SEE ALSO DIURETICS, THIAZIDES, AND THE FOLLOWING INDIVIDUAL ENTRIES:

Bumetanide
Ethacrynate sodium
Ethacrynic acid
Furosemide
Torsemide

ACTION/KINETICS
Loop diuretics inhibit reabsorption of sodium and chloride in the proximal and distal tubules and the loop of Henle. Metabolized in the liver and excreted primarily through the urine. Significantly bound to plasma protein.

USES
See individual drugs.

CONTRAINDICATIONS
Hypersensitivity to loop diruetics or to sulfonylureas. In hepatic coma or severe electrolyte depletion (until condition improves or is corrected). Lactation.

SPECIAL CONCERNS
■Loop diuretics are potent drugs; excess amounts can lead to a profound diuresis with water and electrolyte depletion. Careful medical supervision is required and dosage must be individualized.■ Sudden alterations of electrolytes in hepatic cirrhosis and ascites may precipitate hepatic encephalopathy and coma. SLE may be activated or worsened. Ototoxicity is most common with rapid injection, in severe renal impairment, with doses several times the usual dose, and with concurrent use of other ototoxic drugs. The risk of hospitalization is doubled in geriatric clients

who take diuretics and NSAIDs. Safety and efficacy of most loop diuretics have not been determined in children or infants.

SIDE EFFECTS
See individual drugs. Excessive diuresis may cause dehydration with the possibility of *circulatory collapse and vascular thrombosis or embolism.* Ototoxicity including tinnitus, hearing impairment, deafness (usually reversible), and vertigo with a sense of fullness are possible. Electrolyte imbalance, especially in clients with restricted salt intake. Photosensitivity. Changes include hypokalemia, hypomagnesemia, and hypocalcemia.

OD OVERDOSE MANAGEMENT
Symptoms: Acute profound water loss, volume and electrolyte depletion, dehydration, decreased blood volume, and *circulatory collapse with possibility of fascicular thrombosis and embolism.* *Treatment:* Replace fluid and electrolyte loss. Carefully monitor urine and plasma electrolyte levels. Emesis and gastric lavage may be useful. Supportive measures may include oxygen or artificial respiration.

DRUG INTERACTIONS
Aminoglycosides / ↑ Ototoxicity with hearing loss
Anticoagulants / ↑ Drug activity
Chloral hydrate / Transient diaphoresis, hot flashes, hypertension, tachycardia, weakness and nausea
Cisplatin / Additive ototoxicity
Digitalis glycosides / ↑ Risk of arrhythmias R/T diuretic-induced electrolyte disturbances
Lithium / ↑ Plasma levels of lithium → toxicity
Muscle relaxants, nondepolarizing / Effect of muscle relaxants either ↑ or ↓, depending on diuretic dose
Nonsteroidal anti-inflammatory drugs / ↓ Effect of loop diuretics
Probenecid / ↓ Effect of loop diuretics
Salicylates / Diuretic effect may be ↓ with cirrhosis and ascites
Sulfonylureas/ Loop diuretics may ↓ glucose tolerance
Theophyllines / Action of theophyllines may be ↑ or ↓

Classifications

Thiamine / High doses of loop diuretics → thiamine deficiency

Thiazide diuretics / Additive effects with loop diuretics → profound diuresis and serious electrolyte abnormalities

DOSAGE
See individual drugs.

NURSING CONSIDERATIONS

ASSESSMENT
1. Document indications for therapy. List other agents trialed and outcome. Note any sensitivity to sulfonamides; may exhibit cross-reactivity with furosemide.
2. Monitor BP, CBC, electrolytes, Mg, Ca, BS, uric acid, renal and LFTs.
3. Determine presence of SLE; drug may worsen condition. Assess auditory function carefully when large doses are anticipated or when used concurrently with other ototoxic agents. Ototoxicity is dose related and generally reversible.

INTERVENTIONS
1. Record VS, weights, I&O; keep bedpan or urinal within reach. Report absence/decrease in diuresis and note changes in lung sounds. Diuretics potentiate the effects of antihypertensive agents; monitor BP.
2. When ambulatory, check for edema in the extremities; if on bed rest, check for edema in the sacral area.
3. Monitor for serum electrolyte levels, pH, and the following *signs of electrolyte imbalance:*

• *Hyponatremia* (low-salt syndrome)— characterized by muscle weakness, leg cramps, dryness of mouth, dizziness, and GI upset.

• *Hypernatremia* (excessive sodium retention)—characterized by CNS disturbances, i.e., confusion, loss of sensorium, stupor, and coma. ↓ Skin turgor and postural hypotension not as prominent as with combined sodium and water deficits.

• *Water intoxication* (caused by defective water diuresis)—characterized by lethargy, confusion, stupor, and coma. Neuromuscular hyperexcitability with ↑ reflexes, muscular twitching, and convulsions if acute.

• *Metabolic acidosis*—characterized by weakness, headache, malaise, abdominal pain, and N&V. Hyperpnea occurs in severe metabolic acidosis. S&S of volume depletion: poor skin turgor, soft eyeballs, and dry tongue may be observed.

• *Metabolic alkalosis*—characterized by irritability, neuromuscular hyperexcitability, tetany if severe.

• *Hypokalemia (potassium deficiency)*— characterized by muscular weakness, peristalsis failure, postural hypotension, respiratory embarrassment, and cardiac arrhythmias.

• *Hyperkalemia (excess potassium)*— characterized by early signs of irritability, nausea, intestinal colic, and diarrhea; and by later signs of weakness, flaccid paralysis, dyspnea, dysphagia, and arrhythmias.

4. Hyper- or hypokalemia associated with diuretic therapy may potentiate the toxic effects of digitalis and precipitate arrhythmias.
5. With high doses monitor for hyperlipidemia and hyperuricemia; precipitating a gout attack. Assess for sore throat, skin rash, and yellowing of the skin or sclera; may be blood dyscrasias.
6. With liver dysfunction, assess for electrolyte imbalances, which could cause stupor, coma, and death.
7. If receiving EC potassium tablets, assess for abdominal pain, distention, or GI bleeding; can cause small bowel ulceration. Check stool for intact tablets.
8. May precipitate symptoms of diabetes with latent or mild diabetes. Test urine or perform finger sticks and monitor chemisty studies.

CLIENT/FAMILY TEACHING
1. Take with food or milk to decrease GI upset. May cause frequent, copious voiding. Plan activities/travel; take in the a.m. to prevent sleep disruption.
2. Include foods high in potassium, such as citrus, grape, cranberry, apple, pear, and apricot juices; bananas; meat, fish, or fowl; cereals; and tea and cola beverages. This is preferable to taking potassium chloride supplements but potassium supplements are usually pre-

---

scribed with non-potassium-sparing diuretics. Unless conditions such as gastric ulcer or diabetes exist, drink a large glass of orange juice daily. Consult dietitian as needed for assistance in selecting and preparing foods.

3. Weakness and/or dizziness may occur. Rise slowly from bed and sit down or lie down if evident. Use caution in driving a car or operating other hazardous machinery until drug effects apparent. The use of alcohol, standing for prolonged periods, and exercise in hot weather may enhance/lower BP.

4. Ensure adequate fluids; monitor BP and weight. Report excessive weight loss, loss of skin turgor or if dizziness, nausea, muscle weakness, cramps, or tingling of the extremities occur.

5. Wear protective clothing, sunscreens, and sunglasses to prevent photosensitivity reactions.

6. Avoid all OTC preparations without approval.

OUTCOMES/EVALUATE

• Symptomatic relief (↓ weight, ↓ swelling/edema, ↑ diuresis)
• Clinical improvement in S&S associated with CHF and renal failure

DIURETICS, THIAZIDES

SEE ALSO THE FOLLOWING INDIVIDUAL ENTRIES:

Hydrochlorothiazide
Indapamide

ACTION/KINETICS

Thiazides promote diuresis by decreasing the rate at which sodium and chloride are reabsorbed by the distal renal tubules of the kidney. By increasing the excretion of sodium and chloride, they force excretion of additional water. They also increase the excretion of potassium and, to a lesser extent, bicarbonate, as well as decrease the excretion of calcium and uric acid. Sodium and chloride are excreted in approximately equal amounts. Thiazides do not affect the glomerular filtration rate. Thiazides also have an antihypertensive effect which is attributed to direct dilation of the arterioles, as well as to a reduction in the total fluid volume of the body and altered sodium balance. The thiazide diuretics are related chemically to the sulfonamides. Although devoid of anti-infective activity, the thiazides can cause the same hypersensitivity reactions as the sulfonamides. A large fraction is excreted unchanged in urine.

USES

(1) Edema due to CHF, nephrosis, nephritis, renal failure, PMS, hepatic cirrhosis, corticosteroid or estrogen therapy. (2) Hypertension. (3) Premenstrual tension. *Investigational:* Thiazides are used alone or in combination with allopurinol (or amiloride) for prophylaxis of calcium nephrolithiasis. Nephrogenic diabetes insipidus.

CONTRAINDICATIONS

Hypersensitivity to drug, anuria, renal decompensation. Impaired renal function and advanced hepatic cirrhosis. Do not use indiscriminately in clients with edema and toxemia of pregnancy, even though they may be therapeutically useful, because the thiazides may have adverse effects on the newborn (thrombocytopenia and jaundice).

SPECIAL CONCERNS

Geriatric clients may manifest an increased risk of hypotension and changes in electrolyte levels. The risk of hospitalization is doubled in geriatric clients who take diuretics and NSAIDs. Administer with caution to debilitated clients or to those with a history of hepatic coma or precoma, gout, diabetes mellitus, or during pregnancy and lactation. Particular care must be exercised when thiazides are administered concomitantly with drugs that also cause potassium loss, such as digitalis, corticosteroids, and some estrogens. Clients with advanced heart failure, renal disease, or hepatic cirrhosis are most likely to develop hypokalemia. May activate or worsen SLE.

SIDE EFFECTS

The following side effects may be observed with most thiazides. See also individual drugs. **Electrolyte imbalance:** Hypokalemia (most frequent) characterized by cardiac arrhythmias. Hyponatre-

Classifications

Classifications

mia characterized by weakness, lethargy, epigastric distress, N&V. Hypokalemic alkalosis. **GI:** Anorexia, epigastric distress or irritation, N&V, cramping, bloating, abdominal pain, diarrhea, constipation, jaundice, pancreatitis. **CNS:** Dizziness, lightheadedness, headache, vertigo, xanthopsia, paresthesias, weakness, insomnia, restlessness. **CV:** Orthostatic hypotension, MIs in elderly clients with advanced arteriosclerosis, especially if the client is also receiving therapy with other antihypertensive agents. **Hematologic: *Agranulocytosis, aplastic or hypoplastic anemia, hemolytic anemia,*** leukopenia, thrombocytopenia. **Dermatologic:** Purpura, photosensitivity, photosensitivity dermatitis, rash, urticaria, necrotizing angiitis, vasculitis, cutaneous vasculitis. **Metabolic:** Neutropenia, hemolytic anemia. **Endocrine:** Hyperglycemia, glycosuria, hyperuricemia. **Miscellaneous:** Blurred vision, impotence, reduced libido, fever, muscle cramps, muscle spasm, respiratory distress.

OD OVERDOSE MANAGEMENT

Symptoms: Symptoms of plasma volume depletion, including orthostatic hypotension, dizziness, drowsiness, syncope, electrolyte abnormalities, hemoconcentration, hemodynamic changes. Signs of potassium depletion, including confusion, dizziness, muscle weakness, and GI disturbances. Also, N&V, GI irritation, GI hypermotility, CNS effects, cardiac abnormalities, ***seizures, hypotension, decreased respiration, and coma.*** *Treatment:*

• Induce emesis or perform gastric lavage followed by activated charcoal. Undertake measures to prevent aspiration.

• Electrolyte balance, hydration, respiration, CV, and renal function must be maintained. Cathartics should be avoided, as use may enhance fluid loss.

• Although GI effects are usually of short duration, treatment may be required.

DRUG INTERACTIONS

Allopurinol / ↑ Risk of hypersensitivity reactions to allopurinol

H *Aloe /* Hypokalemia as both drugs could potentiate effects of digoxin

Amphotericin B / Enhanced loss of electrolytes, especially potassium

Anesthetics / Thiazides may ↑ effects of anesthetics

Anticholinergic agents / ↑ Effect of thiazides R/T ↑ amount absorbed from GI tract

Anticoagulants, oral / Anticoagulant effects may be decreased

Antidiabetic agents / Thiazides antagonize hypoglycemic drug effects

Antigout agents / Thiazides may ↑ uric acid levels; thus, ↑ dose of antigout drug may be necessary

Antihypertensive agents / Thiazides potentiate drug effects

Antineoplastic agents / Thiazides may prolong drug induced leukopenia

Calcium salts / Hypercalcemia R/T renal tubular reabsorption or bone release of calcium may be ↑ by exogenous calcium

Cholestyramine / ↓ Effect of thiazides R/T ↓ GI tract absorption

Colestipol / ↓ Effect of thiazides R/T ↓ GI tract absorption

Corticosteroids / Enhanced potassium loss R/T potassium-losing properties of both drugs

Diazoxide / Enhanced hypotensive effect. Also, ↑ hyperglycemic response

Digoxin / Thiazides produce ↑ K and Mg loss with ↑ chance of digitalis-induced arrhythmias

Ethanol / Additive orthostatic hypotension

Fenfluramine / ↑ Antihypertensive effect of thiazides

Furosemide / Profound diuresis and electrolyte loss

Guanethidine / Additive hypotensive effect

Indomethacin / ↓ Effect of thiazides, possibly by inhibition of prostaglandins

Insulin / ↓ Effect R/T thiazide-induced hyperglycemia

H *Licorice root /* Potassium loss R/T thiazides and licorice → ↑ sensitivity to digitalis glycosides

Lithium / ↑ Risk of lithium toxicity R/T ↓ renal excretion; may be used together but monitored carefully

---

Bold Italic = life threatening side effect   ■ = black box warning   ✚ = Available in Canada

Loop diuretics / Additive effect to cause profound diuresis and serious electrolyte losses

Methenamine / ↓ Effect of thiazides R/T alkalinization of urine by methenamine

Methyldopa / ↑ Risk of hemolytic anemia (rare)

Muscle relaxants, nondepolarizing / ↑ Effect of muscle relaxants R/T hypokalemia

Norepinephrine / Thiazides ↓ arterial response to norepinephrine

Quinidine / ↑ Effect of quinidine R/T ↑ renal tubular reabsorption

Sulfonamides / ↑ Effect of thiazides R/T ↓ plasma protein binding

Sulfonylureas / ↓ Effect R/T thiazide-induced hyperglycemia

Tetracyclines / ↑ Risk of azotemia

Tubocurarine / ↑ Muscle relaxation and ↑ hypokalemia

Vasopressors (sympathomimetics) / Thiazides ↓ responsiveness of arterioles to vasopressors

Vitamin D / ↑ Effect of vitamin D R/T thiazide-induced hypercalcemia

LABORATORY TEST CONSIDERATIONS
Hypokalemia, hypercalcemia, hyponatremia, hypomagnesemia, hypochloremia, hypophosphatemia, hyperuricemia. ↑ BUN, creatinine, glucose in blood and urine. ↓ Serum PBI levels (no signs of thyroid disturbance). Initial ↑ total cholesterol, LDL cholesterol, and triglycerides.

DOSAGE
See individual drugs.

NURSING CONSIDERATIONS

ADMINISTRATION/STORAGE
1. Clients resistant to one type of thiazide may respond to another.
2. Liquid potassium preparations are bitter. Administer with fruit juice or milk to enhance palatability.
3. To minimize electrolyte imbalance, thiazides may be taken every other day or on a 3–5-day basis for treatment of edema.
4. To prevent excess hypotension, reduce dose of other antihypertensive agents when beginning therapy.

ASSESSMENT
1. Note any drug hypersensitivity. Document indications for therapy and any previous use of these drugs.
2. Monitor BP, hydration, CBC, glucose, electrolytes, Ca, Mg, renal and LFTs. Determine extent of edema; assess skin turgor, mucous membranes, extremities, and lung fields.
3. Note any history of heart disease or gout; check uric acid levels. With cirrhosis, avoid K$^+$ depletion and hepatic encephalopathy.

INTERVENTIONS
1. Stop drug at least 48 hr before surgery. Thiazide inhibits pressor effects of epinephrine.
2. Potassium supplements should be given only when dietary measures are inadequate. If required, use liquid preparations to avoid ulcerations that may be produced by potassium salts in the solid dosage form. Exceptions include slow-K forms (potassium salt imbedded in a wax matrix) and micro-K forms (microencapsulated potassium salt).

CLIENT/FAMILY TEACHING
1. Take with food or milk if GI upset occurs. Consume in the morning so that major diuretic effect occurs before bedtime.
2. Eat a diet high in potassium. Include orange juice, bananas, citrus fruits, broccoli, spinach, tomato juice, cucumbers, beets, dried fruits, and apricots. Avoid large amounts of black licorice; may precipitate severe hypokalemia.
3. Rise slowly and dangle legs before standing to minimize low BP effects. Sit or lie down if feeling faint or dizzy.
4. With gout, avoid foods that precipitate attacks and continue antigout agents as prescribed. With diabetes, monitor finger sticks more frequently; may need adjustment of insulin or oral hypoglycemic agent.
5. Avoid alcohol; causes severe drop in BP. Do not take any other medication (including OTC drugs for asthma, cough and colds, hay fever, weight control) unless approved.
6. Report any severe weight loss, muscle weakness, cramps, dizziness, or fatigue. Skin rashes may occur but severe

symptoms R/T allergic reactions include acute SOB (pulmonary edema), abdominal pain (acute pancreatitis), easy bruising/bleeding (thrombocytopenia), yellowing of skin/eyes; itching (cholestatic jaundice); and pale, weak/dizzy (hemolytic anemia); report immediately.

OUTCOMES/EVALUATE

• Control of hypertension; ↓ BP
• ↑ Urine output; ↓ edema; ↓ weight
• Adequate tissue perfusion with warm dry skin and good pulses
• Normal electrolyte levels and fluid balance

HEPARINS, LOW MOLECULAR WEIGHT   ■

SEE ALSO THE FOLLOWING INDIVIDUAL ENTRIES:

Dalteparin sodium
Enoxaparin
Tinzaparin sodium

ACTION/KINETICS

Obtained by depolymerization of unfractionated porcine heparin. Are antithrombotic drugs. They enhance the inhibition of Factor Xa and thrombin by binding to and accelerating antithrombin II activity. They potentiate the inhibition of Factor Xa preferentially; slightly affect thrombin and clotting time or activated partial thromboplastin time. They are primarily metabolized in the liver to lower molecular weight compounds with significantly less activity.

USES

See individual drugs. Uses include, but not limited to: (1) Prophylaxis of DVT. (2) Prophylaxis of ischemic complications in unstable angina and non-Q-wave MI when given together with aspirin. (3) With warfarin for inpatient treatment of acute DVT with and without pulmonary embolism or for outpatient treatment of acute DVT without pulmonary embolism.

CONTRAINDICATIONS

Hypersensitivity to heparin, pork products, methylparaben, sulfites, or benzyl alcohol. Active major bleeding. Thrombocytopenia with positive in vitro tests for antiplatelet antibody in presence of a low molecular weight heparin. IM or IV use.

SPECIAL CONCERNS

■(1) When spinal/epidural anesthesia or spinal puncture is used, those anticoagulated or scheduled to be anticoagulated with low molecular weight heparins or heparinoids to prevent thromboembolic complications are at risk of developing a spinal or epidural hematoma that can result in long-term or permanent paralysis. Risk is increased using indwelling epidural catheters for giving analgesics or by the concurrent use of drugs affecting hemostasis, such as NSAIDs, platelet inhibitors, or other anticoagulants. Risk also appears to increase by traumatic or repeated spinal or epidural puncture. (2) Frequently monitor for signs and symptoms of neurologic impairment. If observed, immediate treatment is required. (3) The physician should consider potential benefits vs risk before neuraxial intervention in clients anticoagulated or to be anticoagulated for thromboprophylaxis.■ Cannot be used interchangeably (unit for unit) with other low molecular weight heparins or with unfractionated heparin. Use with extreme caution in those with a history of heparin-induced thrombocytopenia. Use with caution in clients with an increased risk of hemorrhage, including those with severe uncontrolled hypertension, bacterial endocarditis, congenital or acquired bleeding disorders, active ulceration and angiodysplastic GI disease, or hemorrhagic stroke or shortly after brain, spinal, or ophthalmologic surgery. Also, use with caution in clients with bleeding diathesis, severe liver or kidney disease, hypertensive or diabetic retinopathy, and recent GI bleeding. Use with caution during lactation. Safety and efficacy have not been determined in children.

SIDE EFFECTS

See individual drugs. **Hemorrhagic side effects:** *Clinically significant bleeeding,* hemorrhage, injection site hematoma, wound hematoma. **Hemorrhagic complications:** Paralysis, paresthesia, headache, pain (chest, abdomen, joint, muscle, or other), dizziness, shortness of breath, difficulty breathing or swallowing, swelling, weakness, hypotension, shock, coma.

OD OVERDOSE MANAGEMENT
Symptoms: Hemorrhagic complications. *Treatment:* Slow IV protamine sulfate (1%) at a dose of 1 mg for every 100 anti-Xa international units of dalteparin and ardeparin or 1 mg for every 1 mg of enoxaparin. A second infusion of protamine sulfate, 0.5 mg per 100 anti-Xa international units of dalteparin or ardeparin or per 1 mg of enoxaparin may be given if the aPTT measured 2–4 hr after the first infusion of protamine sulfate remains prolonged. Take care not to give an overdose of protamine.

DRUG INTERACTIONS
Aspirin / ↑ Risk of bleeding
H *Bromelain* / ↑ Risk of bleeding
Clopidogrel ↑ Risk of bleeding
Dextran / ↑ Risk of bleeding
Dipyridamole / ↑ Risk of bleeding
H *Feverfew* / Possible additive antiplatelet effect
H *Garlic* / Possible additive antiplatelet effect
H *Ginger* / Possible additive antiplatelet effect
Ketorolac tromethamine / ↑ Risk of bleeding
NSAIDs / ↑ Risk of bleeding
Sulfinpyrazone / ↑ Risk of bleeding
Thrombolytics / ↑ Risk of bleeding
Ticlopidine / ↑ Risk of bleeding

LABORATORY TEST CONSIDERATIONS
↑ AST, ALT.

DOSAGE
See individual drugs.

NURSING CONSIDERATIONS

ASSESSMENT
1. Document indications for therapy (prophylaxis/treatment), other agents trialed, and outcome. Assess for any sensitivity to heparin, sulfite, methylparaben, or pork products.
2. Review list of special concerns that may preclude client receiving drugs. Those who received spinal anesthesia or taps require special monitoring to assess for neurologic S&S and spinal/

epidural hematoma formation which may cause permanent paralysis.
3. Note any evidence of active bleeding, bleeding disorders, or thrombocytopenia. Assess carefully for masked bleeding. Drug does not usually affect PT/PTT values yet client may be hemorrhaging. Monitor VS, I&O, mental status, H&H, U/A, electrolytes, and renal and LFTs; routinely check all potential bleeding sites. Any unexplained fall in BP or HCT should lead to a search for a bleeding site.

CLIENT/FAMILY TEACHING
1. Many clients are treated with low molecular weight heparins at home. Review indications for therapy, self administration techniques, length/frequency of therapy, and site rotation. Educate about SC injection techniques and recognizing signs of complications. To minimize bruising do not rub site after administering.
2. Avoid aspirin, NSAIDs, and all OTC agents. Report any unusual effects, i.e., bruising, bleeding, chest pain, acute SOB, itching, rash, or swelling. Keep followup appointments as scheduled.

OUTCOMES/EVALUATE
DVT prophylaxis; inhibition of blood coagulation

SYMPATHOMIMETIC DRUGS

SEE ALSO THE FOLLOWING INDIVIDUAL ENTRIES:

Albuterol
Bitolterol mesylate
Brimonidine tartrate
Dobutamine hydrochloride
Dopamine hydrochloride
Ephedrine sulfate
Epinephrine
Epinephrine bitartrate
Epinephrine borate
Epinephrine hydrochloride
Isoproterenol hydrochloride
Isoproterenol sulfate
Metaproterenol sulfate
Phenylephrine hydrochloride
Pirbuterol acetate
Pseudoephedrine hydrochloride
Pseudoephedrine sulfate

H = Herbal   IV = Intravenous   ℂ = sound-alike drug

Salmeterol xinafoate
Terbutaline sulfate

ACTION/KINETICS

Adrenergic drugs act: (1) by mimicking the action of norepinephrine or epinephrine by combining with alpha and/or beta receptors (directly acting sympathomimetics) or (2) by causing or regulating the release of the natural neurohormones from their storage sites at the nerve terminals (indirectly acting sympathomimetics). Some drugs exhibit a combination of both effects.

Adrenergic stimulation of receptors will manifest the following general effects:

Alpha-1-adrenergic: / Vasoconstriction, decongestion, constriction of the pupil of the eye, contraction of splenic capsule, contraction of the trigone-sphincter muscle of the urinary bladder.

Alpha-2-adrenergic: / Presynaptic to regulate amount of transmitter released; decrease tone, motility, and secretory activity of the GI tract (possibly involved in hypersecretory response also); decrease insulin secretion.

Beta-1-adrenergic: / Myocardial contraction (inotropic), regulation of heartbeat (chronotropic), improved impulse conduction, ↑ lipolysis.

Beta-2-adrenergic: / Peripheral vasodilation, bronchial dilation; ↓ tone, motility, and secretory activity of the GI tract; ↑ renin secretion.

Beta adrenergic drugs stimulate adenyl cyclase which catalyzes the formation of cyclic AMP from ATP. The formed cyclic AMP inhibits release of mediators from mast cells and basophils that cause hypersensitivity reactions. The increase in cyclic AMP leads to activation of protein kinase A, which inhibits phosphorylation of myosin and lowers intracellular ionic calcium levels causing smooth muscle relaxation.

USES

See individual drugs.

CONTRAINDICATIONS

Tachycardia due to arrhythmias; tachycardia or heart block caused by digitalis toxicity. See individual drugs.

SPECIAL CONCERNS

Use with caution in hyperthyroidism, diabetes, prostatic hypertrophy, seizures, degenerative heart disease, especially in geriatric clients or those with asthma, emphysema, or psychoneuroses. Also, use with caution in clients with coronary insufficiency, CAD, ischemic heart disease, CHF, cardiac arrhythmias, hypertension, or history of stroke. Asthma clients who rely heavily on inhaled beta-2-agonist bronchodilators may increase their chances of death. Thus, use to "rescue" clients but do not prescribe for regular long-term use. Beta-2 agonists may inhibit uterine contractions.

SIDE EFFECTS

See individual drugs; side effects common to most sympathomimetics are listed. **CV:** Tachycardia, arrhythmias, palpitations, BP changes, anginal pain, precordial pain, pallor, skipped beats, chest tightness, hypertension. **GI:** N&V, heartburn, anorexia, altered taste or bad taste, GI distress, dry mouth, diarrhea. **CNS:** Restlessness, anxiety, tension, insomnia, hyperkinesis, drowsiness, weakness, vertigo, irritability, dizziness, headache, tremors, general CNS stimulation, nervousness, shakiness, hyperactivity. **Respiratory:** Cough, dyspnea, dry throat, pharyngitis, *paradoxical bronchospasm,* irritation. **Other:** Flushing, sweating, *allergic reactions.*

OD OVERDOSE MANAGEMENT

Symptoms: Following inhalation: Exaggeration of side effects resulting in anginal pain, hypertension, hypokalemia, *seizures.* Following systemic use: CV symptoms include bradycardia, tachycardia, palpitations, extrasystoles, *heart block,* elevated BP, chest pain, hypokalemia. CNS symptoms include anxiety, insomnia, tremor, delirium, *convulsions, collapse, and coma.* Also, fever, chills, cold perspiration, N&V, mydriasis, and blanching of the skin.

Treatment:
• For overdosage due to inhalation: General supportive measures with sedatives given for restlessness. Use metoprolol or atenolol cautiously as they may induce an asthmatic attack in clients with asthma.

Bold Italic = life threatening side effect ▮ = black box warning ♣ = Available in Canada

• For systemic overdosage: Discontinue or decrease dose. General supportive measures. For overdose due to PO agents, emesis, gastric lavage, or charcoal may be helpful. In severe cases, propranolol may be used but this may cause airway obstruction. Phentolamine may be given to block strong alpha-adrenergic effects.

DRUG INTERACTIONS

Ammonium chloride / ↓ Effect of sympathomimetics R/T ↑ kidney excretion

Anesthetics / Halogenated anesthetics sensitize heart to adrenergics—causes cardiac arrhythmias

Anticholinergics / Concomitant use aggravates glaucoma

Antidiabetics / Hyperglycemic effect of epinephrine may necessitate ↑ dosage of insulin or oral hypoglycemic agents

Beta-adrenergic blocking agents / Inhibit adrenergic stimulation of the heart and bronchial tree; cause bronchial constriction; hypertension, asthma, not relieved by adrenergic agents

Corticosteroids / Chronic use with sympathomimetics may result in or aggravate glaucoma; aerosols containing sympathomimetics and corticosteroids may be lethal in asthmatic children

Digitalis glycosides / Combination may cause cardiac arrhythmias

Furazolidone / ↑ Effects of mixed-acting sympathomimetics

Guanethidine / Direct-acting sympathomimetics ↑ drug effects, while indirect-acting sympathomimetics ↓ effects of guanethidine; also reversal of hypotensive drug effects

H *Indian snakeroot* / Initial significant ↑ BP

Lithium / ↓ Pressor effect of direct-acting sympathomimetics

MAO inhibitors / All effects of sympathomimetics are potentiated; symptoms include hypertensive crisis with possible intracranial hemorrhage, hyperthermia, convulsions, coma; death may occur

Methyldopa / ↑ Pressor response

Methylphenidate / Potentiates pressor effect of sympathomimetics; combination hazardous in glaucoma

Oxytocics / ↑ Chance of severe hypertension

Phenothiazines / ↑ Risk of cardiac arrhythmias

Sodium bicarbonate / ↑ Effect of sympathomimetics R/T ↓ kidney excretion

Theophylline / Enhanced toxicity (especially cardiotoxicity); also ↓ drug levels

Thyroxine / Potentiation of pressor response of sympathomimetics

Tricyclic antidepressants / ↑ Effect of direct-acting sympathomimetics and ↓ effect of indirect-acting sympathomimetics

DOSAGE ————
See individual drugs.

NURSING CONSIDERATIONS
ADMINISTRATION/STORAGE
Discard colored solutions.
ASSESSMENT
1. Note indications for therapy, contributing factors/triggers, clinical presentation, and anticipated response. Determine any sensitivity/previous experience to adrenergic drugs/drugs in this class and the outcome.
2. Document any history of CAD, tachycardia, endocrine disturbances, or respiratory tract problems.
3. Obtain baseline data regarding general physical condition, hemodynamic status including ECG, VS, labs, oxygen saturation, smoking history, work history with any exposure to chemicals/asbestos. Monitor PFTs and lab data.
CLIENT/FAMILY TEACHING
1. Take exactly as directed. Do not increase dosage or take more frequently than prescribed. Consult provider if symptoms progress. Take early in the day to prevent insomnia.
2. Review prescribed drug therapy and potential side effects. Feelings/symptoms of fear or anxiety may be evident; these drugs mimic body's stress response. Avoid all OTC preparations.
3. Stop smoking to preserve current lung function. Attend formal smoking cessation classes.

SPECIAL NURSING CONSIDERATIONS FOR ADRENERGIC BRONCHODILATORS
ASSESSMENT
1. Obtain history and PE prior to starting therapy. Note any experience with this class of drugs.

2. Monitor VS; assess CV response. Evaluate cardiac function and note ejection fraction.

3. Document lung assessment, ABGs (or O_2 saturation), and PFTs. Note characteristics of cough and sputum production.

INTERVENTIONS

1. Observe effects on CNS; if pronounced, adjust dosage/frequency of administration.

2. With status asthmaticus and abnormal ABGs, continue to provide oxygen and ventilating assistance even though the symptoms appear to be relieved by the bronchodilator. To prevent depression of respiratory effort, administer oxygen based on client's clinical symptoms and ABGs or O_2 saturations.

3. If three to five aerosol treatments of the same agent have been administered within the last 6–12 hr, with no relief, further evaluation is warranted. If dyspnea worsens after repeated excessive use of the inhaler, paradoxical airway resistance may occur. Be prepared to assist with alternative therapy and respiratory support.

CLIENT/FAMILY TEACHING

1. Review technique for use/care of inhalers and respiratory equipment. Rinsing of equipment and mouth after use is imperative to prevent oral fungal infections. Maintain record of peak flow readings and seek medical attention as directed.

2. To improve lung ventilation and reduce fatigue during eating, start inhalation therapy upon arising in the morning and before meals.

3. Regular, consistent use of the drug is essential for maximum benefit, but overuse can be life-threatening. If using inhalable medications and bronchodilators, use the bronchodilator first and wait 5 min before using the other medication.

4. A single aerosol treatment is usually enough to control an asthma attack. Overuse of adrenergic bronchodilators may result in reduced effectiveness, paradoxical reaction, and death from cardiac arrest. Consult provider if more than three (or prescribed number) aerosol treatments in a 24-hr period are required for relief.

5. With postural drainage, review how to cough productively and show family how to clap and vibrate the chest and position client to promote good respiratory hygiene.

6. Increased fluid intake will aid in liquefying secretions and removal. Consult provider if dizziness or chest pain occurs, or if there is no relief when the usual dose is used.

7. Avoid OTC preparations and any other unprescribed adrenergic medications.

8. **Stop smoking,** avoid crowds during 'flu seasons,' dress warmly in cold weather and cover mouth with scarf to filter cold air, receive the pneumonia vaccine and seasonal flu shot, and stay in air conditioning during hot, humid days to prevent exacerbations of illness. Identify triggers and practice avoidance. Have family/significant other learn CPR.

Index

Boldface = generic drug name   CAPITALS = combination drugs

Boldface = generic drug name   CAPITALS = combination drugs

INDICATIONS

Plavix® (clopidogrel bisulfate) is indicated for the reduction of atherothrombotic events as follows:

Recent MI, Recent Stroke, or Established Peripheral Arterial Disease
For patients with a history of recent myocardial infarction (MI), recent stroke, or established peripheral arterial disease, PLAVIX has been shown to reduce the rate of a combined end point of new ischemic stroke (fatal or not), new MI (fatal or not), and other vascular death.

Acute Coronary Syndrome
For patients with acute coronary syndrome (unstable angina/non–Q-wave MI), including patients who are to be managed medically and those who are to be managed with percutaneous coronary intervention (with or without stent) or CABG, PLAVIX has been shown to decrease the rate of a combined end point of cardiovascular death, MI, or stroke as well as the rate of a combined end point of cardiovascular death, MI, stroke, or refractory ischemia.

IMPORTANT RISK INFORMATION
PLAVIX is contraindicated in patients with active pathologic bleeding such as peptic ulcer or intracranial hemorrhage. PLAVIX should be used with caution in patients who may be at risk of increased bleeding from trauma, surgery, or coadministration with NSAIDs or warfarin. **(See CONTRAINDICATIONS and PRECAUTIONS.*)**

The rates of major and minor bleeding were higher in patients treated with PLAVIX plus aspirin compared with placebo plus aspirin in a clinical trial. **(See ADVERSE REACTIONS.*)**

As part of the worldwide post marketing experience with PLAVIX, there have been cases of reported thrombotic thrombocytopenic purpura (TTP), some with fatal outcome. TTP has been reported rarely following use of PLAVIX, sometimes after a short exposure (<2 weeks). TTP is a serious condition that can be fatal and requires urgent treatment including plasmapheresis (plasma exchange). **(See WARNINGS.*)**

In clinical trials, the most common clinically important side effects were pruritus, purpura, diarrhea, and rash; infrequent events included intracranial hemorrhage (0.4%) and severe neutropenia (0.05%). **(See ADVERSE REACTIONS.*)**

* PLEASE SEE FULL PRESCRIBING INFORMATION ON INSIDE BACK COVER.